Petty's

PRINCIPLES of MUSCULOSKELETAL TREATMENT and MANAGEMENT

A Handbook for Therapists

FOURTH EDITION

Petty's PRINCIPLES of MUSCULOSKELETAL TREATMENT and MANAGEMENT

A Handbook for Therapists

EDITED BY

Kieran Barnard MSc PG Cert BSc (Hons) MCSP MMACP
Advanced Practitioner Physiotherapist
Sussex MSK Partnership, Brighton, UK
Private Practitioner
Flex Physiotherapy, Burgess Hill, UK

Dionne Ryder MSc MCSP MMACP FHEA
Visiting Lecturer
School of Health and Social Work
University of Hertfordshire, Hatfield, UK
Private Practitioner
Move and Improve Physiotherapy, St Albans, UK

FOREWORD BY

Nicola J Petty DPT MSc GradDipPhys FMACP FHEA
Formerly Associate Professor
School of Health Sciences
University of Brighton, UK

ELSEVIER

First edition 2004
Second edition 2011
Third edition 2018
Fourth edition 2024

Notices

Practitioners and researchers must always rely on their own experience and knowledge in evaluating and using any information, methods, compounds or experiments described herein. Because of rapid advances in the medical sciences, in particular, independent verification of diagnoses and drug dosages should be made. To the fullest extent of the law, no responsibility is assumed by Elsevier, authors, editors or contributors for any injury and/or damage to persons or property as a matter of products liability, negligence or otherwise, or from any use or operation of any methods, products, instructions, or ideas contained in the material herein.

ISBN: 978-0-323-87228-7

Content Strategist: Andrae Akeh
Content Project Manager: Shravan Kumar
Design: Margaret M. Reid
Marketing Manager: Deborah Watkins

Printed in Scotland

Last digit is the print number: 9 8 7 6 5 4 3 2 1

CONTENTS

FOREWORD

I started to write the first edition of this textbook in 2001, and it was finally published three years later in 2004. I was at the time teaching musculoskeletal physiotherapy to undergraduate and postgraduate students at a university, and qualified clinicians on weekend courses. Textbooks on the market at that time tended to describe different treatment techniques, for example for a joint, muscle or nerve, and this was also reflected by the clinicians on weekend courses who often were more interested in the practical skill of applying a technique, than the theory and principles underpinning it. Just focusing on skill development can result in a therapist-centred one size fits-all-approach of techniques to patients, which is neither professional nor ethical. So my aim was to write a companion text to Musculoskeletal Examination and Assessment that focused entirely on the theory and principles underpinning musculoskeletal treatment and management to enable the reader to critically understand their practice and be able to individualise their approach to patients. The book was well received and further editions followed in 2011 and 2018.

For the second edition, published in 2011, I chose to move from author to editor, and bring the expertise of well-respected and well-known clinicians and academics to build on the work of the first edition, and they did a sterling job. Kieran Barnard contributed to two chapters and seemed to me to be a gifted writer who could also deliver on time — a key requisite for publishing houses! I first got to know Kieran in 2007 as his course leader when he started his MSc Musculoskeletal Physiotherapy at the University of Brighton. During his studies, I remember being impressed by his thoughtful and questioning approach to theoretical issues underpinning practice and his excellence in writing essays.

For the third edition, published in 2018, I asked Kieran to co-edit with me and I was delighted when he agreed. As an Advanced Practitioner and clinical mentor for MSc Musculoskeletal Physiotherapists, Kieran has both clinical and educational expertise which is a perfect mix for knowing what knowledge and skill the reader needs to know to enhance their practice and develop clinical expertise. He took the lead in developing and updating the third edition, and we invited respected clinicians and academics to contribute to chapters to broaden and deepen the scope of the text.

During the preparation for the third edition, I made the decision, with a tinge of sadness, to withdraw completely from any future edition of the book, as my retirement from academia was on the horizon. I asked Kieran and Dionne Ryder to co-edit the fourth edition of the book, as well as co-edit the sixth edition of the companion text Petty's Musculoskeletal Examination and Assessment, and I was delighted when they both agreed.

I first met Dionne over 20 years ago. We were both teaching Musculoskeletal Physiotherapy in Higher Education Institutions and we were both involved with the Musculoskeletal Association of Chartered Physiotherapists (MACP). Dionne was an ideal editor for the fourth edition of the book as she has extensive clinical and educational experience, and knows first-hand how to guide the reader in the principles of treatment and management of the musculoskeletal system.

I feel honoured and delighted to be invited to write the foreword to this edition. The process of writing has allowed me to finally let go of the baton and pass it completely over to Kieran and Dionne in a very tangible and public way. I do so with complete confidence in their stewardship of my work and with my blessing, gift it to them.

Like a bottle of wine, this textbook is getting better with age. While the overall structure of the book remains much the same, the text, tables and figures have been updated and refreshed and findings from recent research have been added. It is wonderful to see the same contributors from the last edition: Paul Comfort, Clair Hebron, Catherine Hennessy, Lee Herrington, Ioannis Paneris, Colette Ridehalgh, Simon Spencer and Hubert van Griensven come alongside quite a number of new well-respected contributors: Laura Finucane, Sue Greenhalgh, Giles Hazan, Nathan Hutting, Matthew

Low, Chris McCarthy, Chris Mercer, Tim Noblet, James Selfe, Alan Taylor and Jennifer Ward.

The most substantive change has been the addition of three brand new chapters related to the vascular system, serious pathology and advancing practice. A new chapter on the vascular system is an excellent addition to the book as people with problems with the vascular system can appear to have a musculoskeletal problem. It is written by two eminent therapists in the field, Alan Taylor and Nathan Hutting. A new chapter on serious pathology by four influential and well-known contributors, Laura Finucane, Sue Greenhalgh, Chris Mercer and James Selfe, is also an important addition to the book to help the reader recognise patients who have an underlying serious pathology and may need to be referred on. The third new chapter, Advancing Practice, highlights the attributes of a musculoskeletal advanced physiotherapy practitioner, and is written by well-respected practitioners working at advanced level, Tim Noblet and Matthew Low and a General Practitioner specialised in musculoskeletal, Giles Hazan. Case studies in the chapter enable the reader to grasp the knowledge and skills required to work at this level. A reader starting their undergraduate physiotherapy course may be inspired by this chapter to become an advanced practitioner.

If the reader is looking for a textbook that gives them a comprehensive and evidence-enhanced guide to the principles underpinning musculoskeletal treatment and management, they need look no further. Developing expertise in this area is quite a challenge with the requirement to learn hands-on practical skill as well as learning the theory and research that underpins it. The text while well written and presented, is no easy read, there is effort required of the reader to engage and make sense of the theory, but the reward is potentially great. Critically understanding the principles underpinning treatment and management enables the clinician to logically and rationally choose, with best effect, an approach for an individual patient.

May you, the reader, be blessed as you seek to develop expertise in the art and science of musculoskeletal treatment and management.

Dr Nicola Petty
Hexham, UK

PREFACE

In the brand-new edition of this popular textbook, we have sought to build upon the content conceived and developed by Dr Nicola J Petty over the course of three previous editions. This edition has been significantly updated and new chapters have been added to reflect the direction of travel in modern musculoskeletal practice. There are eleven new contributors to this edition, and the book has benefitted enormously from the richness of their experience and clinical expertise. There are three new chapters including one on vascular pathology (an area often overlooked in musculoskeletal practice), a chapter on serious pathology and one on advancing clinical practice. With career opportunities for clinicians to develop into advanced practice and first contact practitioner roles within primary care settings, it is more vital than ever for them to have an appreciation of the wider medical picture including screening for serious pathologies. This book has sought to provide some grounding for the aspiring clinician looking towards more advanced roles. We are grateful, not only for the valuable input each contributor has made to the text, but also for the energy and enthusiasm to complete their contribution under tight timescales.

Thanks must go to Elsevier and in particular, Poppy Garraway who was instrumental in launching this project and Shravan Kumar for his guidance and support throughout the publishing process.

The overall aim of the book is to provide a clear and accessible text for pre-registration students that provides theory and research evidence underpinning musculoskeletal treatment and management; it is not a manual of how to treat and manage, rather it provides the principles of how to do this. We hope this provides the reader with the underpinning theory to be able to work creatively to meet the needs of individual patients.

Kieran Barnard
Dionne Ryder
Brighton and St Albans 2022

CONTRIBUTORS

The editors would like to acknowledge and offer grateful thanks for the input of all previous editions' contributors, without whom this new edition would not have been possible.

Kieran Barnard, MSc PG Cert BSc (Hons) MCSP MMACP
Advanced Practitioner Physiotherapist
Sussex MSK Partnership, Brighton, UK
Private Practitioner
Flex Physiotherapy, Burgess Hill, UK

Paul Comfort, PhD ASCC CSCS*D
Professor of Strength and Conditioning
University of Salford, Salford, UK
Adjunct Professor of Strength and Conditioning
Edith Cowan University, Western Australia

Laura Finucane, MSc BSc(Hons) FMACP FCSP
Consultant Physiotherapist Clinical Director
Sussex MSK Partnership, Physiotherapy
NHS, Brighton, UK
Honorary Associate Professor
St George's University
London, UK

Sue Greenhalgh, OBE PhD MA GD Phys
Consultant Physiotherapist and Clinical Fellow
Orthopaedic Interface Service
Bolton NHS FT and Manchester Metropolitan University, Bolton, UK

Giles Hazan, MBBS BSc MRCGP Dip MSM PG Cert Med Ed
GP, Dolphins Practice
Dolphins Practice, Haywards Heath, UK
GP (with an extended role), Community Pain Service
Sussex Partnership Foundation Trust, Eastbourne
East Sussex, UK

Clair Hebron, BSc(Hons) PgCERT MSc PhD MMACP FHEA
Principal Lecturer
School of Health Sciences, University of Brighton
Eastbourne, UK

Catherine Hennessy, BSc(Hons) MSc PCAP FHEA PhD
Lecturer/Acting Deputy Head of Anatomy
Brighton Sussex Medical School, University of Sussex
Brighton, UK

Lee Herrington, PhD MSc BSc Hons
Senior Lecturer in Sports Rehabilitation
School of Health Sciences
University of Salford, Salford
Greater Manchester, UK
Technical Lead Physiotherapist
Physiotherapy
English Institute of Sport, Manchester
Greater Manchester, UK

Nathan Hutting, PhD
Associate Professor
Occupation & Health Research Group
HAN University of Applied Sciences, Nijmegen
Netherlands

Matthew Low, MSc BSc(Hons) MSCP MMACP
Consultant Physiotherapist
University Hospitals Dorset NHS Foundation Trust
Christchurch, UK
Visiting Fellow, Orthopaedic Research Institute
University of Bournemouth, UK

Christopher McCarthy, PhD FCSP FMACP
Clinical Lead
Manchester School of Physiotherapy
Manchester Metropolitan University
Manchester, UK

Chris Mercer, MSC PgCert FMACP FCSP Grad Dip Phys
Consultant Physiotherapist
Physiotherapy, University Hospitals Sussex Trust
Worthing, UK

Tim Noblet, PhD MSc BSc(Hons) Physiotherapy MMACP MCSP
Consultant Musculoskeletal & Spinal Pain Physiotherapist
St George's University Hospitals NHS Foundation Trust, London, UK
Adjunct Professor of Research, Western University, London, Ontario, Canada
Hon. Associate Professor, Macquarie University, Sydney, NSW, Australia
Hon. Associate Professor, St George's University of London, London, UK

Ioannis Paneris, BSc(Hons) MSc MCSP MMACP
Advanced Clinical Practitioner MSK
Community and Medicine
Central Manchester University Hospitals - NHS
Foundation Trust, Manchester, UK
Associate Lecturer
Health, Psychology & Social Care
Manchester Metropolitan University, Manchester, UK

Colette Ridehalgh, PhD MSc BSc(Hons) MCSP MMACP
Principal Lecturer
School of Sport and Health Sciences
University of Brighton, Eastbourne
East Sussex, UK
Senior Research Fellow
Department of Neuroscience
Brighton and Sussex Medical School
University of Sussex
Brighton, East Sussex, UK

Dionne Ryder, MSc MCSP MMACP FHEA
Visiting Lecturer
Department of Allied Health Professions
Midwifery and Social Work
School of Health and Social Work
University of Hertfordshire, Hatfield, UK
Private Practitioner, Move and Improve
Physiotherapy
St Albans, UK

James Selfe, DSc PhD MA GDPhys FCSP
Professor of Physiotherapy
Health Professions
Manchester Metropolitan University
Manchester, UK

Simon Spencer, MSc BSc(Hons) MCSP
Head of Physical Health
English Institute of Sport, UK

Alan Taylor, MSc MCSP
Assistant Professor
Academic Plan Lead for PG Physiotherapy
Physiotherapy & Rehabilitation Sciences/School of Health Sciences/Faculty of Medicine & Health Sciences
University of Nottingham, Medical School
Queens Medical Centre, Nottingham, UK

Hubert van Griensven, PhD MSc(Pain) MCSP DipAc FHEA
St George's, University of London
Institute of Medical and Biomedical Education
Cranmer Terrace, London, UK

Jennifer Ward, BSc(Hons) MSc MCSP MMACP
Advanced Practitioner MSK Physiotherapy and NIHR PCAF Candidate
HEE Training Program Lead for Advanced Practice in Primary Care
University Hospital Sussex, Worthing, West Sussex, UK

1

Introduction

Kieran Barnard and Dionne Ryder

The management of neuromusculoskeletal conditions continues to evolve, and care looks different now to even a few short years ago when the last edition of this book was published. Whilst the underlying principles of function and dysfunction remain fairly constant and resolute, approaches to tissue management continue to progress as evidence emerges to underpin practice. With the evolution of Advanced Practice and the introduction of First Contact Practitioner roles, clinicians are increasingly working in multidisciplinary environments, developing new skills and a range of competencies combined with advancing clinical reasoning. These skills and competencies are essential to appropriately manage musculoskeletal conditions, but also to detect non-musculoskeletal conditions and possibly serious pathologies that may present in clinic.

The aim of this book is therefore to take the reader on a journey: Firstly, we help the reader understand the underlying principles of function and dysfunction and the management of different tissue states. After discussing joint, muscle and nerve, we have added a new vascular chapter as the vascular system has often been overlooked in neuromusculoskeletal assessment and management. Secondly, the book seeks to instil an understanding of pain states and the overarching principles of exercised-based rehabilitation. Finally, two new chapters considering serious pathology and Advanced Practice are presented.

This book has been written as a companion text to the examination and assessment of the musculoskeletal system (Ryder & Barnard, 2024). This introductory chapter aims to help the reader understand how the information has been laid out, by giving a brief résumé of what is contained within each chapter.

Chapter 2 provides key information on the anatomy, biomechanics, physiology and movement of joint structures and, on the basis of this summary of joint function, classifies and discusses common clinical presentations of joint dysfunction. Using this classification of dysfunction, Chapter 3 provides the principles underpinning joint treatment.

Chapter 4 provides key information on the anatomy, biomechanics and physiology of muscle and tendon and, from this summary of function, classifies and discusses common clinical presentations of muscle and tendon dysfunction. Using this classification of dysfunction, Chapter 5 provides the principles underpinning muscle treatment.

Chapter 6 provides key information on the anatomy, biomechanics, physiology and movement of nerves and, from this summary of nerve function, classifies and discusses common clinical presentations of nerve dysfunction. Using this classification of dysfunction, Chapter 7 provides the principles underpinning nerve treatment.

Chapter 8 encourages the reader to consider the vascular system as a source of symptoms when examining the neuromusculoskeletal system. It offers a guide to how a range of vascular dysfunctions, often masquerading as musculoskeletal presentations, can be recognized and managed using different relevant vascular pathologies as examples.

Treatment is very often aimed to relieve pain as this is why most patients will seek help, and, for this reason, Chapter 9 provides information related to understanding and managing people with persistent pain. Treatment of an individual patient is not simply the physical treatment of joint, muscle and nerve to relieve pain and other symptoms. The patient is a person with a mind and spirit, as well as a body, and the person lives within a particular context, all of which need to be understood when managing people with musculoskeletal conditions. This potent combination creates a complex therapeutic relationship, which defies a simple cause-and-effect analysis of our therapeutic interaction. The reader is referred to the updated communication chapter that has been moved to the companion assessment text, as developing a therapeutic relationship must be fostered through careful communication from the outset (Ryder & Barnard, 2024).

Chapter 10 considers the principles of exercise rehabilitation, so critical for full recovery and reducing the likelihood of recurrence of musculoskeletal problems.

Finally, Chapters 11 and 12 deal with serious pathology and Advanced Practice. Chapter 11 builds the framework for recognition of serious pathology and helpfully consolidates learning with highly clinically relevant case studies. Chapter 12 goes on to explore Advanced Practice, reflecting developments in neuromusculoskeletal practice.

In contemporary practice it is important to understand that there is still much we do not know about the human body. Anatomy, biomechanics, physiology and pathology textbooks provide general information that is often articulated in a straightforward manner; textbooks often aim to enhance the broad understanding of the reader. In contrast, articles published in scientific journals often awaken the reader to a more complex and uncertain view of the subject. Anatomy journals, for example, describe variations in joint architecture, muscle attachments and nerve pathways, demonstrating the uniqueness of individuals. So, while anatomy textbooks describe what is generally true, they do not describe what is particularly true for any one individual—the content of this textbook is no different. This has important implications for clinical practice.

Our knowledge of the neuromusculoskeletal system is far from complete and when we add patient individuality into the mix, neuromusculoskeletal care will no doubt always be a rich and challenging clinical field. We encourage you as clinicians to never forget the patient in front of you as you wrestle with a given clinical conundrum. Each patient who enters the treatment room has their own thoughts, feelings, hopes and fears which will inevitably influence their experience and their recovery. Whilst an understanding of the theoretical underpinning of contemporary neuromusculoskeletal management is crucial, and our sincere hope is that this book will create a robust foundation in exploring these, we must not lose sight of patients themselves.

REFERENCE

Ryder, D., Barnard, K., 2024. Musculoskeletal examination and assessment: a handbook for therapists, sixth ed. Elsevier, Oxford.

2

Function and Dysfunction of Joints

Ioannis Paneris and Catherine M. Hennessy

LEARNING OUTCOMES

After studying this chapter, you should be able to:

- Explain the structure and function of joints in terms of anatomy, physiology and biomechanics.
- Identify impact of dysfunction on joint structures and function.
- Consider how this information can be utilized in clinical practice to inform examination findings and justify management decisions.

CHAPTER CONTENTS

In this text, the term 'joint' refers to both the intra-articular and periarticular structures. The function of the neuromusculoskeletal system is to produce movement. This is dependent on each component of the system (i.e. normal function of joint, nerve and muscle). This interrelationship is depicted in Fig. 2.1, which shows a theoretical model originally devised to describe stability of the spine (Panjabi, 1992a); however, it is applicable to the entire neuromusculoskeletal system. Similarly, the stability of the knee joint has been described as 'a synergistic function in which bones, joint capsules, ligaments, muscles, tendons, and sensory receptors and their spinal and cortical neural projects and connections function in harmony' (Solomonow & Krogsgaard, 2001).

For a joint to function optimally there must be normal functioning of the relevant muscles and nerves. Stability of a joint is a function of joint stiffness (Panjabi, 1992b), and this is provided not only by the joint capsule but also by skin, muscle and tendon. In the human lumbar spine, a number of the ligaments are considered too weak to contribute significantly to joint stiffness and are regarded as transducers serving a proprioceptive function (Panjabi, 1992a; Adams et al.,

2013), while muscle augments segmental stability during functional movement (McGill et al., 2003). There is substantial evidence throughout the body that stability of joints is enhanced by muscle (Hortobagyi & DeVita, 2000; Solomonow & Krogsgaard, 2001; Delahunt et al., 2006; Veeger & Van Der Helm, 2007).

The nervous system underpins this stabilising function of muscle. For example, stimulation of afferents of the dorsal scapholunate interosseous ligament in the wrist causes activation of muscles adjacent to it (flexor carpi radialis, flexor carpi ulnaris and extensor carpi radialis brevis). This is thought to be a protective reflex to avoid excessive ligamentous tension (Hagert et al., 2009).

JOINT FUNCTION

The previous section has highlighted the complex, interdependent nature of joint, muscle and nerve. This should be borne in mind when reading the next section on aspects of joint function. Aspects of joint function that will be discussed are:

- classification of joints
- anatomy, biomechanics and physiology of joints
- nerve supply of joints
- classification of synovial joints
- joint movement
- biomechanics of joint movement.

A joint is the junction between two or more bones, and the function of a joint is to permit limited movement and to transfer force from one bone to another (Nigg & Herzog, 2007).

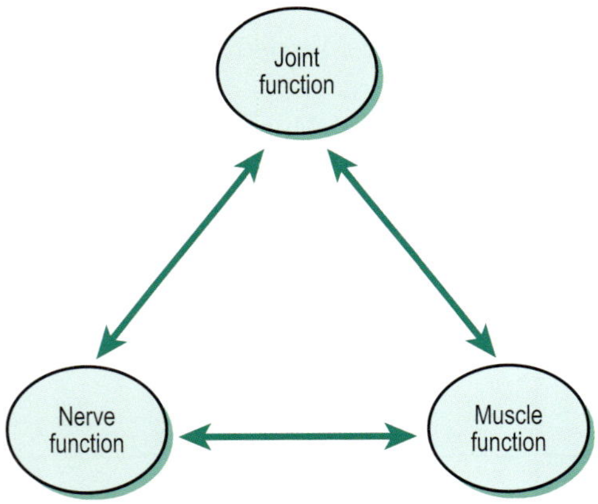

Fig. 2.1 Interdependence of the function of joint, nerve and muscle for normal movement. Normal function of the neuromusculoskeletal system requires normal function of joint, nerve and muscle. (*After Panjabi 1992a, with permission.*)

Classification of Joints

Joints can be classified as either synarthrosis (non synovial) or diarthrosis (synovial) (Levangie & Norkin, 2011). Synarthrosis joints are further divided into fibrous and cartilaginous joints (Fig. 2.2).

Fibrous joints can be further subdivided into suture joints, as in the joints of the skull, gomphosis joints, as in the joints between a tooth and the mandible or maxilla, and a syndesmosis joint between the shaft of the radius and ulna (Fig. 2.3A). As the name suggests, in each type of joint, fibrous tissue unites the joint surfaces and, as a result, only a small amount of movement is possible.

Cartilaginous joints can be further subdivided into symphysis, as in the symphysis pubis and the interbody joint (two vertebral bodies and the intervening disc) in the vertebral column (Fig. 2.3B), and synchondroses, as in the first chondrosternal joint. In this type of joint, fibrocartilage or hyaline cartilage directly unites the bone, and, again, only a small amount of movement is possible.

Diarthrosis or synovial joints are characterized by having no tissue uniting each end of the bones; rather, a joint space exists, thus allowing movement to occur.

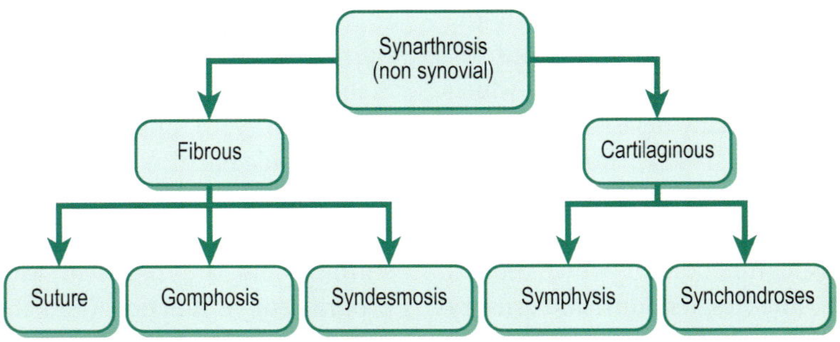

Fig. 2.2 Classification of synarthrosis joints. (*From Levangie & Norkin, 2011.*)

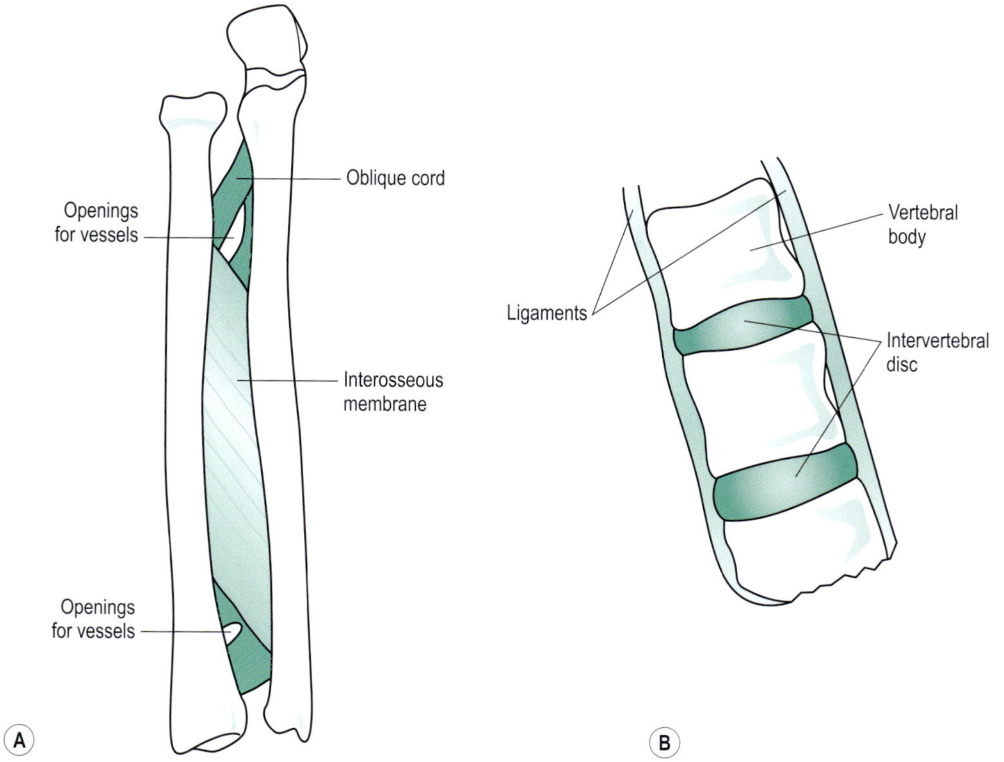

Fig. 2.3 (A) The syndesmosis joint between the shaft of the radius and ulna; the fibrous interosseous membrane unites the two bones. (B) The symphysis joint between the vertebral bodies in the spine. (*From Palastanga & Soames, 2012, with permission.*)

Synovial joints are characterized by a fibrous joint capsule lined with a synovial membrane; the bone end being covered by hyaline cartilage with a film of synovial fluid. Fat pads lie within the synovial membrane, filling the irregularities and potential spaces within the joint, and ligaments and tendons lie either within or adjacent to the joint. There may be a meniscus, for example in the knee joint, fibroadipose meniscoids in the zygapophyseal joints, a labrum in the glenohumeral or hip joints, an interarticular disc in the temporomandibular joint and in some cases bursae within the joint. Fig. 2.4 identifies the features of two synovial joints.

KNOWLEDGE CHECK

1. What type of joint is the symphysis pubis?
2. Can you name the types of the synarthroses?
3. What are the characteristics of the synovial joint?

Anatomy, Biomechanics and Physiology of Joint Tissues

Ligaments

Ligaments attach directly from one bone to another and may be:

- named parallel bundles of the outer fibrous capsule
- intraarticular, as in the cruciate ligaments of the knee
- periarticular, as in the lateral collateral ligament of the knee.

Ligaments consist of approximately two-thirds water and one-third solids, with the solids made up of 75% collagen with the balance being made up of elastin, proteoglycans and other proteins and glycoproteins (Frank, 2004). The aforementioned substances constitute the extracellular matrix. The principal cells responsible for the production and turnover of the extracellular matrix are fibroblastic-type cells called tenocytes if they are located in tendons and fibroblasts

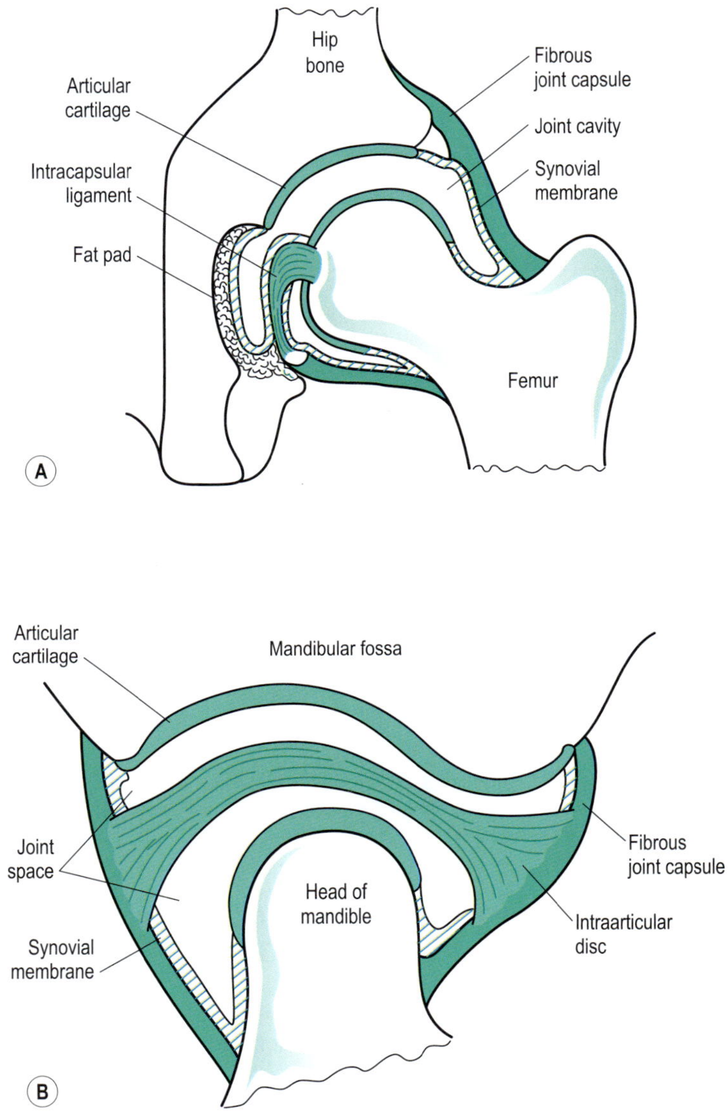

Fig. 2.4 Two synovial joints. (A) Hip joint. (B) Temporomandibular joint with an intraarticular disc. (*From Palastanga & Soames, 2012, with permission.*)

if located in ligaments (Asahara et al., 2017; Milz et al., 2009).

The collagen fibres in ligament are arranged in parallel bundles which have an undulated or 'crimping' appearance under the microscope (Frank & Shrive, 1999; Stanish, 2000) when they are relaxed. The ligament buckles under compression, so it is only the stretching of ligament with tensile loading that is functionally important (Panjabi & White, 2001). The crimping gives some slack to the ligament during minimal tensile loading (longitudinal stretching), and as it straightens out, it provides some resistance (Frank & Shrive, 1999). Fig. 2.5 demonstrates the change in fibre alignment during lengthening of a typical ligament.

The strength of connective tissue to tensile loading can be depicted on a force (or load)–displacement curve, shown in Fig. 2.6. The load or force is plotted against the stretch or deformation. In both load–displacement and stress–strain curves, the slope of the

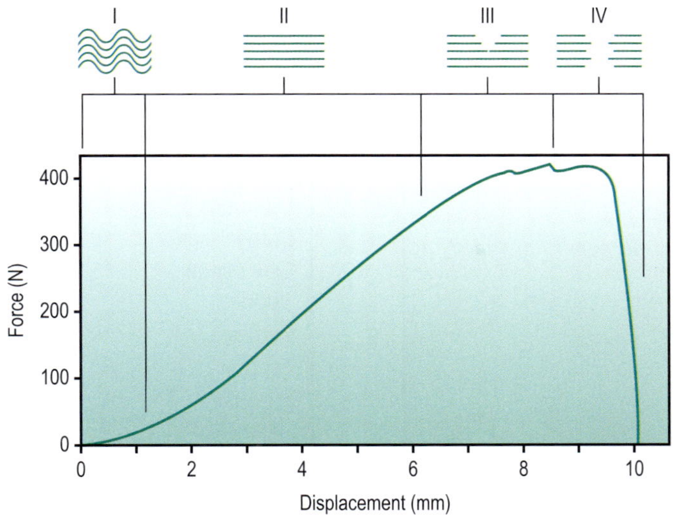

Fig. 2.5 A typical force–displacement curve for a ligament. I, Toe region where the collagen is crimped (schematic representation); II, linear region where the collagen is straightened out; III, microfailure; IV, failure region. (*After Frank & Shrive, 1999, with permission.*)

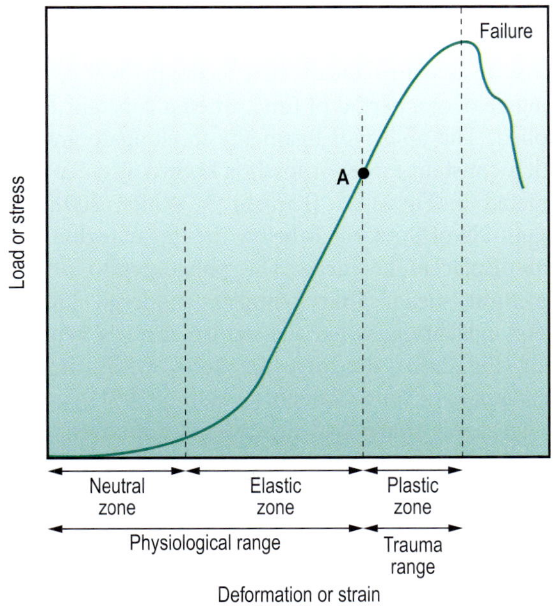

Fig. 2.6 Load (or force)–displacement curve or stress–strain curve of connective tissue. The physiological range is divided into an initial neutral zone followed by an elastic zone. Further force causes trauma and enters the plastic zone. Point A is the junction between the elastic and temporary displacement and the plastic and permanent displacement. This point is known as the yield stress and is the minimum stress necessary to cause a residual strain in the material. (*After Panjabi & White, 2001, with permission.*)

curve is the modulus of elasticity and is a measure of the 'stiffness' of the ligament (Panjabi & White, 2001). It can be seen in Fig. 2.6 that very little force is initially required to deform the ligament; a region referred to as the 'neutral zone' (Panjabi & White, 2001). Stiffness then increases, so that greater force is required to deform the ligament; this region is referred to as the elastic zone (Panjabi & White, 2001). Forces within the elastic zone will result in no permanent change in length; as soon as the force is released the tissue returns to its preload shape and size (Panjabi & White, 2001). The neutral zone and elastic zone fall within the normal physiological range of forces and deformation on ligament during everyday activities (Nordin & Frankel, 2012).

Towards the end of a joint's physiological range the force and deformation may be sufficient to cause microtrauma of individual ligament collagen fibres because microfailure of connective tissue begins at approximately 3% elongation and macrofailure at approximately 8% (Noyes et al., 1983; Lundon, 2007). The point at which there is permanent deformation is termed the 'yield stress', and the region beyond this point is known as the plastic zone (Panjabi & White, 2001; Lundon, 2007). A further increase in force will lead to trauma and eventually failure of the ligament (i.e. a strain injury).

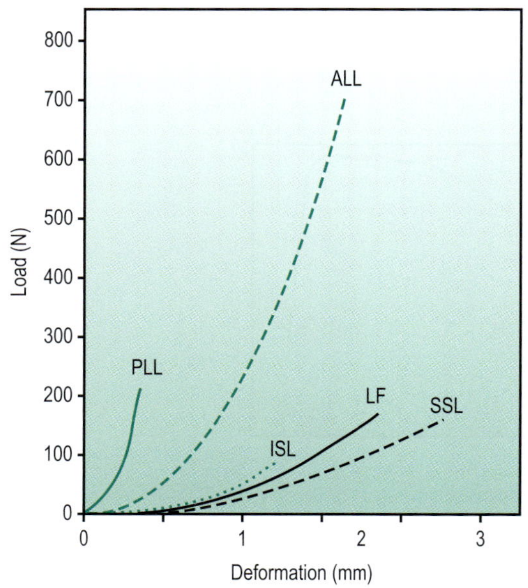

Fig. 2.7 Load–displacement curves for various spinal ligaments. The slope of the curve of the posterior longitudinal ligament *(PLL)* is greatest, demonstrating greatest stiffness. Stiffness values gradually lessen with the anterior longitudinal ligament *(ALL)*, interspinous ligament *(ISL)*, ligamentum flavum *(LF)* and finally supraspinous ligament *(SSL)*. (*From Panjabi & White, 2001, with permission.*)

Fig. 2.7 depicts various force–displacement curves for other ligaments in the body. It can be readily seen that there are quite large variations between ligaments, reflecting differences in function.

If the strength of a ligament is to be compared with another tissue, then a stress–strain curve can be drawn, where stress is the force per unit area (measured in Pa or N/m^2) and strain is the percentage change in length (from the resting length). The stress–strain tensile properties of ligament compared with bone, cartilage, muscle and nerve are shown in Table 2.1. The stress–strain curve of collagen, of which ligament is mostly composed, is shown in Fig. 2.6.

Ligaments are viscoelastic (i.e. they have time-dependent mechanical properties). These properties affect the behaviour of ligaments to movement and forces, hence important principles for clinicians. They can be summarized as:

- elastic nature
- viscous nature
- creep phenomena
- stress relaxation
- load dependent
- hysteresis.

TABLE 2.1 Tensile Properties of Ligament Compared With Bone, Cartilage, Muscle and Nerve

Tissue	Stress at Failure (MPa)	Strain at Failure (%)
Ligament	10–40	30–45
Cortical bone	100–200	1–3
Cancellous bone	10	5–7
Cartilage	10–15	80–120
Tendon	55	9–10
Muscle (passive)	0.17	60
Nerve roots	15	19

Panjabi and White (2001).

The elastic nature means that ligaments will stretch and return to their original shape like an elastic band. The viscous nature means that ligaments will gradually elongate over a period of time, when a constant force is applied. The ability of ligaments to elongate gradually with a constant force (or load) is known as creep and is depicted in Fig. 2.8A (Panjabi & White, 2001). The magnitude of the force is below the linear region of the load–displacement curve. The phenomenon of stress relaxation means that ligaments undergo load (or stress) relaxation; when the deformation is kept constant (Fig. 2.8B), the force (or stress) within ligament decreases over time (Panjabi & White, 2001).

Ligaments share load-dependent properties; that is, the stress–strain (or load–displacement) curve depends on the rate of loading. When the ligament is loaded quickly, it will be stiffer and will deform less than when it is loaded more slowly (Fig. 2.9). This is relevant when applying therapeutic force, as a slower rate will result in less resistance and more movement. The additional effect of having load-dependent properties is that the failure point of the ligament will be higher with a higher loading rate; in other words, the ligament will be stronger and less likely to rupture when the force is applied at a faster rate.

Ligaments demonstrate the phenomenon of hysteresis—energy loss during loading and unloading of the tissue, which results in elongation (Fig. 2.10)

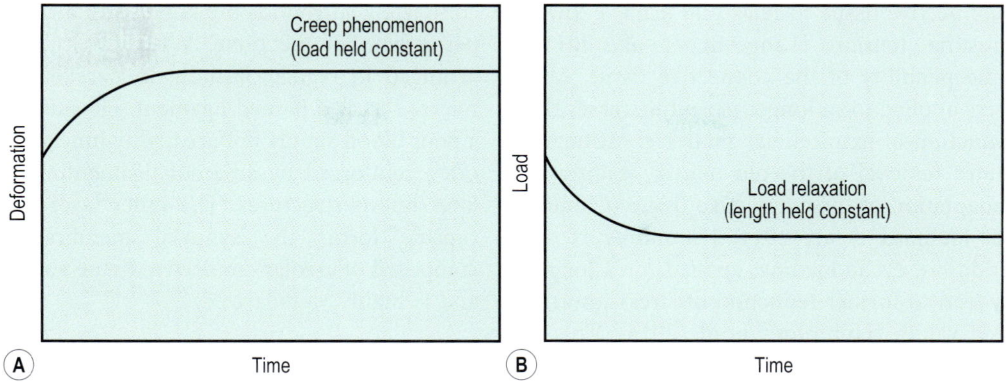

Fig. 2.8 Creep and load relaxation. (A) Creep is the increase in deformation that occurs when a constant load is applied over time. (B) Load relaxation is the decrease in stress within a ligament when a constant force is applied over a period of time. (*From Nordin & Frankel, 1989, with permission.*)

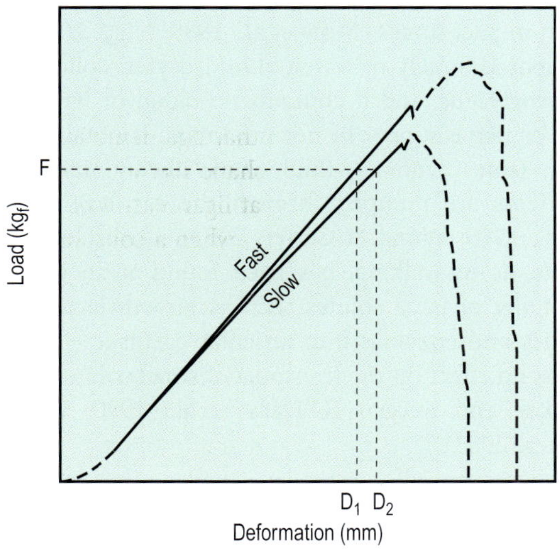

Fig. 2.9 Ligament is load dependent. It can be seen that a given force (F) applied quickly will produce a certain deformation (D_1) and if applied more slowly will produce a greater deformation (D_2). (*After Noyes et al., 1974, with permission.*)

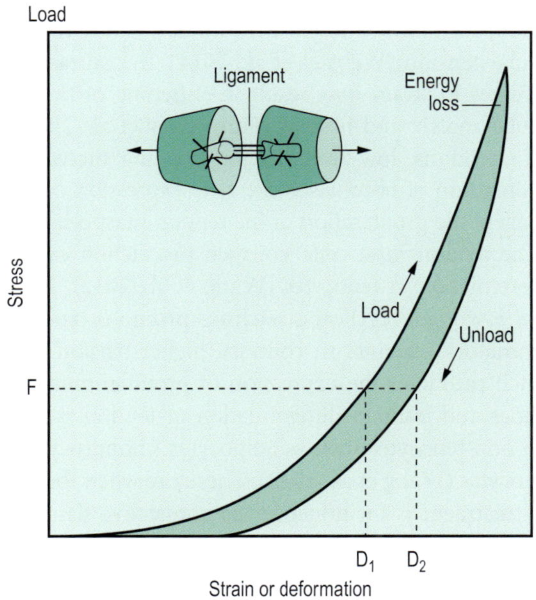

Fig. 2.10 Loading and unloading curves to indicate hysteresis. The shaded area depicts the loss of energy with deformation and is a measure of hysteresis. The unloading curve does not return to the same point on the strain or deformation axis; there is an increase in length as a result of the application of load. For a given force (F), there is a lengthening from the loading curve (D_1) to the unloading curve (D_2). (*After Panjabi & White, 2001, with permission.*)

(Panjabi & White, 2001). If the force applied is less than the yield stress, then the elongation will be temporary, and if it is the same as, or greater than, the yield stress, the elongation will be permanent.

On the microscopic level, the ligament fibroblasts are tethered to the extracellular matrix and thus are able to translate mechanical loads into biochemical processes that regulate cellular functions such as inflammation, cellular proliferation and migration, stem cell differentiation and maturation, and tissue remodelling and repair; this process is termed mechanotransduction (Chaitow, 2013; Dunn & Olmedo, 2016).

Sustained low-grade tension (for a few seconds to minutes) induces remodelling of the fibroblasts that allows the connective tissue to relax and achieve lower levels of resting tension (Langevin et al., 2011), increasing the pliability of the connective tissue. Mechanical stress applied for a longer period increases the cellular production of extracellular matrix constituents and accelerates removal of the old matrix, leading to long-term adaptation of the connective tissue (Chiquet et al., 2003; Jaumard et al., 2011; Humphrey et al., 2014). In addition, cyclic loading, applied for a longer period, may lead to further reduction of stress towards the preloaded values (Humphrey et al., 2014). This is clinically relevant as it provides another mechanism by which application of therapeutic force, by means of stretching and soft-tissue and joint mobilizations, may affect the connective tissue.

However, it is worth noting that fibroblasts respond optimally to slow rate stretch that allows cell reorganisation, accommodation to deformation and reduction in cellular tension (Webster et al., 2014). In contrast, acute increases in strain may result in stiffening of the extracellular matrix and fibrosis (Humphrey et al., 2014).

In tendons, low-grade cycling loading increases the proliferation of fibroblasts, the gene expression of type 1 collagen, the proliferation of the tendon mast cells as well as the tendon mast cells' collagen production and their differentiation in tenocytes (Wang et al., 2012). In addition, low-grade cyclical stretching promotes an antiinflammatory reaction. In contrast, higher-tension cyclical stretch promotes the expression of proinflammatory cytokines and leads to differentiation of tendon stem cells into non-tenocytes such as adipocytes, chondrocytes and osteocytes (Wang et al., 2012). Therefore when the aim of the treatment is to influence the connective tissue, slow rate loading and low-grade tension techniques may be more efficient.

The biomechanical properties of ligaments change with age; in younger subjects (16–26 years) ligaments fail after 44% elongation, whereas in older subjects (older than 60 years), failure occurs at 30% elongation (Noyes & Grood, 1976). Ageing causes changes in collagen and elastin, which result in reduced compliance of ligamentous structures, thus making them more susceptible to injury. This effect can be reduced or retarded, to an extent, by exercise (Menard, 2000).

Fibrous Joint Capsules and Synovial Membranes

The outer layer of a fibrous capsule is composed of dense irregular and regular fibrous tissue and completely surrounds the bone ends, attaching into the periosteum of the bone. Where the fibrous tissue is arranged in regular fashion, in parallel bundles, it is referred to as a named ligament. Fibrous capsules have a poor blood supply but are highly innervated. They are often reinforced by adjacent ligamentous and musculotendinous structures. The inner layer of the fibrous capsule forms the synovial membrane, which is composed of areolar connective tissue and elastic fibres, and is highly vascularized.

Articular Cartilage

Articular cartilage is white, dense connective tissue covering the bone ends of synovial joints and is between 1 and 5 mm in thickness. The function of articular cartilage is to distribute load, minimize friction of opposing joint surfaces and provide shock absorption from impact forces (Mow et al., 1989; Nigg, 2000). It is composed largely of water, chondrocytes, collagen and proteoglycans, and it contains no blood or lymph vessels or nerve supply in normal joints. It obtains nutrients from synovial fluid, and during movement, nutrients are pumped through the cartilage (O'Hara et al., 1990; Wong & Carter, 2003). Cyclic loading of joints, as in walking, has been found to increase the pumping of large solutes such as growth factors, hormones and enzymes into articular cartilage—although it has no effect on the transport of small solutes such as glucose and oxygen (O'Hara et al., 1990; Wong & Carter, 2003).

Microscopically, articular cartilage has a layered appearance. The most superficial layer is densely packed with collagen fibrils which are oriented parallel to the articular surface. This arrangement is thought to help resist shear forces at the joint (Shrive & Frank, 1999). The middle layer is characterized by the collagen fibrils being further apart, and the deepest layer has fibrils lying at right angles to the articular surface (Fig. 2.11). The collagen fibrils in this layer cross the interface between the articular cartilage and the underlying calcified cartilage beneath, a region known as the tidemark. This arrangement anchors the cartilage to the underlying bone.

This varying orientation of collagen fibre layers allows for tensile forces to be distributed across the articular surface (Nigg, 2000; Wong & Carter, 2003) because collagen fibrils are able to resist high tensile forces (Fig. 2.12). Meanwhile the water and

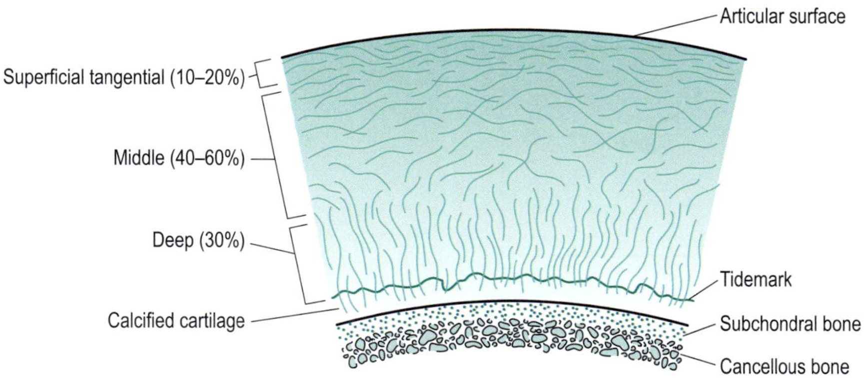

Fig. 2.11 Longitudinal section of articular cartilage demonstrating the varied orientation of collagen fibrils in the superficial, middle and deep layers. (*After Mow et al., 1989, with permission.*)

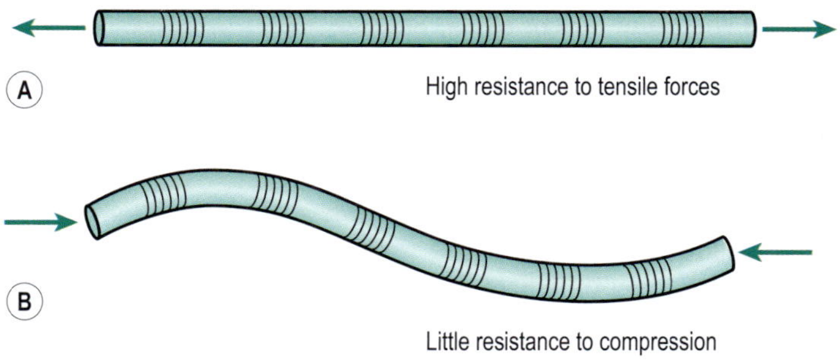

Fig. 2.12 Mechanical properties of collagen fibrils. (A) Resistance to tension. (B) Resistance to compression. (*From Mow et al., 1989, with permission.*)

proteoglycans surrounding the collagen fibrils create a fluid-filled matrix that has the mechanical characteristics of a solid object (Mow et al., 1989).

Articular cartilage is viscoelastic, therefore displaying creep, stress relaxation and hysteresis, and has a sensitivity to the rate of loading.

Compressive loading of articular cartilage. The compressive properties of articular cartilage depend on which layer is tested; the deepest layer is the stiffest because of its higher glycosaminoglycan and type II collagen content (Wong & Carter, 2003). The creep response of articular cartilage, when a constant compressive force is applied, is due to exudation of fluid (Fig. 2.13). The rate of fluid loss reduces over time until the compressive stress within the cartilage equals the applied compressive load so that equilibrium is reached. At this point, the compressive load is resisted by the matrix of collagen and proteoglycan.

The stress relaxation of articular cartilage is shown in Fig. 2.14. A compressive force is applied to the

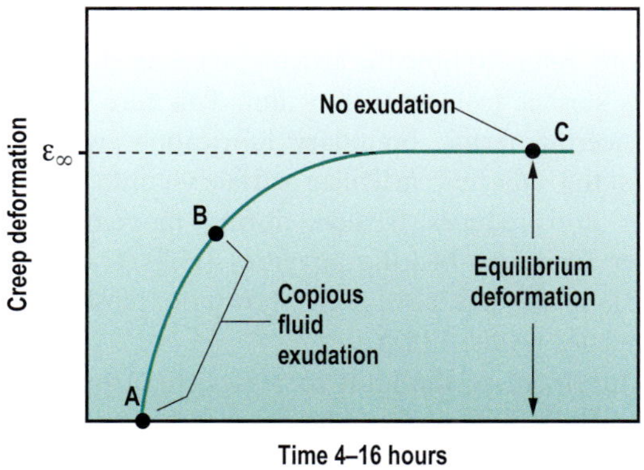

Fig. 2.13 Creep response of articular cartilage with a constant compressive load. (*After Mow et al., 1989, with permission.*)

cartilage until a specific amount of deformation is reached; the force is then held constant. During the initial compression phase the stress within the cartilage increases (to point B), but, once the force is held constant, there is a gradual reduction in stress (from point

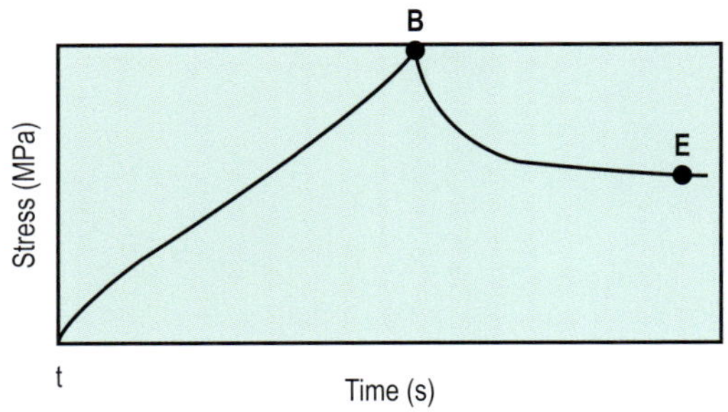

Fig. 2.14 Stress relaxation of articular cartilage with a constant rate of compression. Point B is the maximum stress within the tissue, followed by the gradual reduction in stress until equilibrium is reached at point E. (*After Mow et al., 1989, with permission.*)

B to point E). Point E indicates the point where equilibrium is reached.

The effect of hysteresis on articular cartilage is ultimately a reduction in cartilage thickness; however, this is dependent on the rate of loading: the faster the rate of loading, the stiffer the articular cartilage becomes and the less deformation occurs; with slower rates of loading the articular cartilage is more compliant, and there is greater deformation (Shrive & Frank, 1999).

Synovial Fluid

Synovial fluid contains surface-active phospholipid (SAPL), which is adsorbed as the outermost layer of articular cartilage (Hills & Crawford, 2003). The term 'adsorb' refers to how the articular cartilage holds SAPL to its surface to form a thin film. This film creates, in engineering terms, boundary lubrication, which prevents the adjacent articular surfaces contacting each other and reduces friction during movement, even under high-load-bearing activities (Hills & Crawford, 2003). SAPL has also been shown to have antiwear properties (Hills, 1995).

Movement of the joint increases the production of synovial fluid (Levick, 1983) and helps to distribute synovial fluid over the articular cartilage (Levick, 1984). The flow of synovial fluid into the joint cavity depends, to some extent, on the intraarticular fluid pressure and on the removal of fluid via the synovial lymphatic system (Levick, 1984). Intraarticular fluid pressure depends on a large number of factors, including the volume of fluid, rate of change of volume, joint angle, age of the person and muscle action (Levick, 1983). Joint movement is also required to remove fluid via the synovial lymphatic system. Lack of movement will reduce the removal of synovial fluid and so will result in an increase in intraarticular volume and pressure. Moderate amounts of movement will increase both the volume of synovial fluid and also the removal of fluid via the lymphatic system. Excessive movement causes a greater increase in the volume of synovial fluid than the removal of fluid, resulting in increased intraarticular volume and pressure (Levick, 1984).

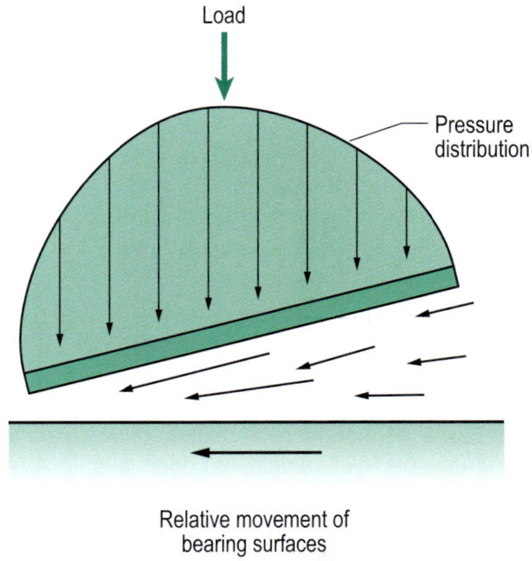

Fig. 2.15 Hydrodynamic lubrication. (*From Nordin & Frankel, 1989, with permission.*)

Synovial joint lubrication. Apart from boundary lubrication, a variety of other mechanisms are thought to ensure that synovial joints are able to maintain almost friction-free movement under a variety of functional activities. These mechanisms include the following.

Fluid lubrication. A thin film of lubricant separates the adjacent articular surfaces and is thought to operate under low loads and high speeds (Nordin & Frankel, 2012), using the following three mechanisms:

1. Hydrodynamic lubrication occurs when the articular surfaces do not lie parallel and then one articular surface slides on the other. A wedge of viscous fluid provides a lifting pressure to support the load (Fig. 2.15).
2. Squeeze film lubrication occurs when the two articular surfaces move towards each other—the fluid pressure between them increases and helps to support the load (Fig. 2.16).

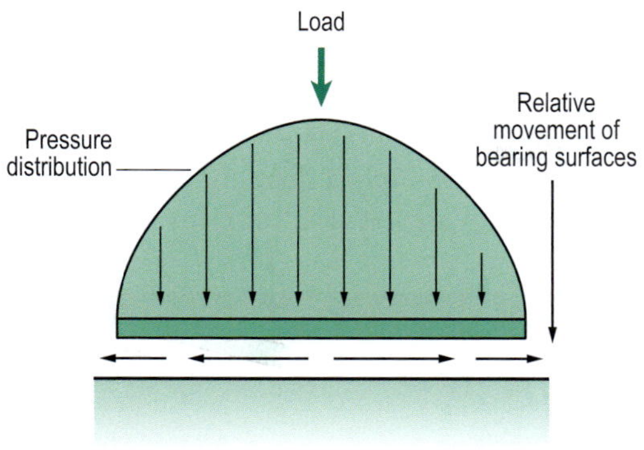

Fig. 2.16 Squeeze film lubrication. *(From Nordin & Frankel, 1989, with permission.)*

3. Elastohydrodynamic lubrication occurs due to the fact that articular cartilage is not rigid. This allows fluid pressures developed from the previous two mechanisms to cause deformation of the articular surface, which increases its surface area. This increases the time taken for the fluid to be squeezed out and therefore enhances the ability to withstand load.

Fat Pads

Fat pads are generally considered to act like cushions, occupying the potential spaces which often occur between the synovial membrane and capsule as synovial joints move. At the elbow, for example, there are a number of fat pads, including one in the olecranon, coronoid and radial fossae which accommodate the related bony prominences during elbow flexion and extension (Drake et al., 2015).

Menisci and Meniscoids

Fibrocartilage menisci are found in the temporomandibular, knee and sternoclavicular joints. The menisci in the knee joint increase the congruence between the articular surfaces of the femur and tibia, distribute weight-bearing forces, act as shock absorbers and reduce friction (Levangie & Norkin, 2011; Palastanga & Soames, 2012). Messner and Gao (1998) summarized that a further important function of knee menisci is to provide proprioceptive feedback, particularly at the extremes of joint range, due to the presence of mechanoreceptors and free nerve endings, with greatest density at the anterior and posterior horns (Albright et al., 1987). Fibroadipose meniscoids in the zygapophyseal joints are thought to protect the joint by preventing articular surface apposition during movement and by reducing friction (Bogduk, 2005).

Bursae

Bursae are sacs made of connective tissue lined by a synovial membrane and filled with fluid similar to synovial fluid. A bursa acts as a cushion to reduce friction. Bursae can be found between skin and bone, muscle and bone, tendon and bone, and ligament and bone. Some named bursae include the subacromial bursa, lying between the acromion and the glenohumeral joint capsule, and the prepatellar bursa, lying between the tendon skin and the patella (Drake et al., 2015).

Labra

Two joints in the human body contain a labrum: the glenohumeral joint and the hip joint. They form a fibrocartilaginous wedge-shaped rim around the glenoid and acetabular fossae, respectively. They deepen the articulating socket and may aid lubrication of the joints (Drake et al., 2015).

Intervertebral Disc

Intervertebral discs comprise an outer ring of thick fibrous cartilage, the annulus fibrosus, which contains the gelatinous inner core, the nucleus pulposus, with the superior and inferior cartilaginous end plates completing the structure.

KNOWLEDGE CHECK

1. What are the main constituents of ligaments?
2. What type of loading should be applied to promote lengthening of the ligaments and lower resting tension?
3. What is boundary lubrication, and how is it achieved?
4. What are bursae, and where can they be found?

Nerve Supply of Joints

Most of the components of joints, such as capsule, ligament, articular disc, meniscus, fat pad and articular blood vessels, are innervated; the only structure that is not innervated is the avascular articular cartilage (Messner, 1999).

The nerve endings in joints can be classified into four types:

1. Ruffini end organs
2. Pacinian corpuscles
3. Golgi endings
4. Free nerve endings.

For further information of these nerve endings, please see Table 2.2 and Chapter 6.

Classification of Synovial Joints

Although all synovial joints share the features described earlier, they vary a great deal in terms of the shape of

TABLE 2.2 Nerve Endings and Afferents Supplying Joints

Type of Nerve Ending	Descriptive Name for Nerve Ending	Function	Position	Afferent Nerve
Type I	Ruffini endings Golgi–Mazzoni endings Meissner corpuscles Spray-type endings Basket endings Ball-of-thread endings Bush-like endings	Low-threshold slowly adapting static and dynamic mechanoreceptors signal static joint position, changes in intraarticular pressure and direction, amplitude and velocity of joint movement	Joint capsule (superficial layer) Ligaments Meniscus Articular disc	Aβ fibre, myelinated, diameter 5–10 μm or group II afferent
Type II	Pacinian corpuscle Krause Endkörperchen Vater'schen Körper Vater–Pacinian corpuscle Modified Pacini(an) corpuscle Simple Pacinian corpuscle Paciniform corpuscle Golgi–Mazzoni body Meissner corpuscle Gelenknervenkörperchen Corpuscle of Krause Club-like ending Bulbous corpuscle Corpuscula nervosa articularia	Low-threshold rapidly adapting dynamic mechanoreceptors—signal beginning and end of movement, deceleration and acceleration, change in vibration or stress	Joint capsule (deeper layer) Ligaments Meniscus Articular disc Fat pads Synovium	Aβ fibre, myelinated diameter 8–12 μm or group II afferent
Type III	Golgi endings Golgi–Mazzoni corpuscles	High-threshold, very slowly adapting mechanoreceptors signal extreme ranges of movement or when there is considerable stress	Ligaments Meniscus Articular disc	Aβ fibre, myelinated diameter 13–17 μm Group II axons
Type IVa	Free nerve terminals	High-threshold, non-adapting pain receptors	Joint capsule (superficial and deep layers) Ligaments Meniscus Articular disc Fat pads	C fibre, unmyelinated, diameter 1–2 μm and thinly myelinated A fibre, diameter 2–4 μm Type III and IV axons

Continued

TABLE 2.2 **Nerve Endings and Afferents Supplying Joints—cont'd**

Type of Nerve Ending	Descriptive Name for Nerve Ending	Function	Position	Afferent Nerve
Type IVa	Free nerve endings	High-threshold, non-adapting pain receptors	Articular blood vessels	Aδ fibre, myelinated diameter 2–5 μm Group II/III axons
Type IVb	Free nerve endings	Vasomotor function	Articular blood vessels	C fibre, unmyelinated diameter <2 μm Group IV axons

Freeman and Wyke (1967), Wyke (1970), Kennedy et al. (1982), Albright et al. (1987), Zimny and St Onge (1987), Strasmann and Halata (1988), Zimny (1988), Messner (1999), Palastanga and Soames (2012).

the articular surfaces and subsequent movement that occurs.

Joint surfaces can be classified as:

- Flat: where the articular surfaces are flat, or plane, although no surface is completely flat.
- Ovoid: where the articular surfaces are wholly concave or wholly convex.
- Sellar: where the articular surfaces are concave in one plane and convex in another. (MacConaill, 1966, 1973).

Synovial joints are classified as:

- Gliding joints: The articular surfaces are more or less flat (MacConaill, 1953), gliding or translational movement occur (e.g. intercarpal and intertarsal joints, zygapophyseal joints in the cervical and thoracic spine, patellofemoral joints) (Fig. 2.17).
- Hinge joints: One articular surface is convex and the other concave, allowing rotational flexion and extension movement (e.g. tibiofemoral, humeroulnar, talocrural and interphalangeal joints in the hand and foot) (Fig 2.8B).
- Pivot joints: One articular surface is round and sits within a ring formed partly by bone and partly by ligament (e.g. include the atlantoaxial and the superior radioulnar joints) (MacConaill, 1973). Rotational movement is around the longitudinal axis (i.e. producing forearm, pronation and supination) (Fig 2.8C).
- Condyloid or ellipsoidal joints: One articular surface is oval and the other elliptical; movement can occur in two planes (e.g. at the radiocarpal joint, there is both flexion and extension and radial and ulnar deviation) (Fig 2.8D).
- Saddle joints: The articular surfaces are like the saddle on a horse: each articular surface is reciprocally concave in one plane and convex in another, sometimes referred to as sellar (MacConaill, 1953) (e.g. the first carpometacarpal joint, as in the condyloid joints, movement occurs in two planes, allowing flexion and extension and abduction and adduction).
- Ball-and-socket joints: One articular surface is shaped like a ball, and the other articular surface is shaped as a hand, which holds the ball. Movement occurs in three planes of movement, allowing flexion and extension, abduction and adduction, and medial and lateral rotation (e.g. the glenohumeral and hip joints).

KNOWLEDGE CHECK

1. How would you describe a hinge joint?
2. Where in the body might you find a pivot joint?
3. Why is the first carpometacarpal joint described as a saddle joint?

Joint Movement

The study of the movement of joint surfaces is termed arthrokinematics. The type of movement at a joint surface can be classified as slide, roll or spin:

- Slide or glide is a pure translation of one surface on another.
- Roll is when the bone rolls or rotates over the articular surface as a wheel rolls along the ground.
- Spin is pure rotation; it occurs at the radiocapitellar joint during pronation and supination of the forearm

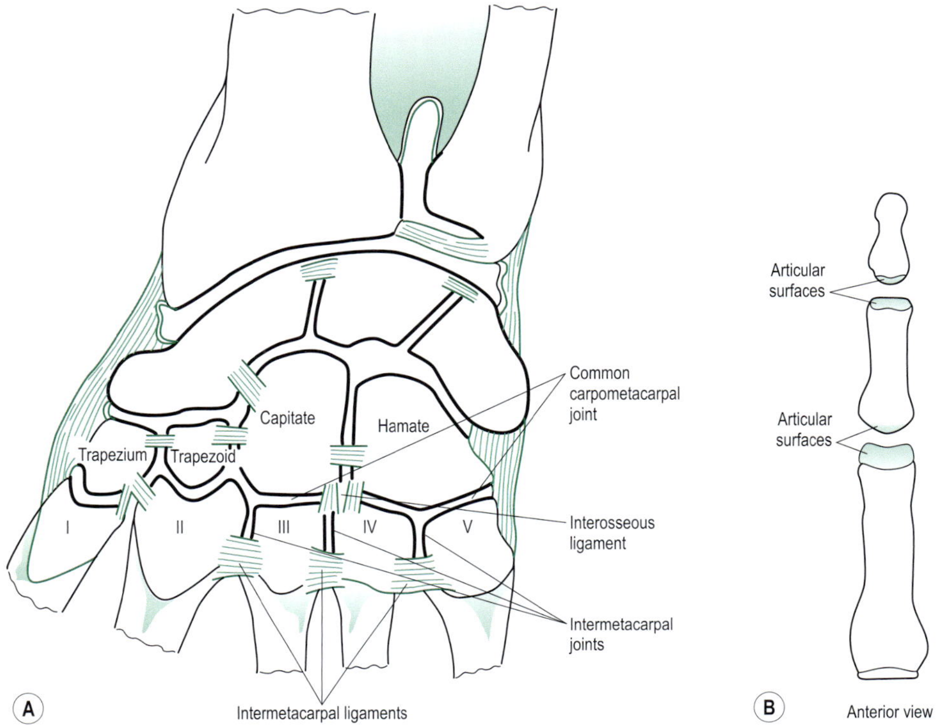

Fig. 2.17 Types of synovial joint. (A) Gliding joints of the intercarpal joints at the wrist. (B) Hinge: interphalangeal joints.

and at the hip and glenohumeral joint during flexion and extension (MacConaill, 1966).

The movement that occurs at a plane (or gliding) joint is slide or glide, but at all the other types of joint (hinge, pivot, condyloid, saddle, ball and socket) movement is a combination of slide with roll or spin.

Movement at a joint is further complicated by conjunct rotation, where a secondary rotation occurs during a rotational movement. For example, during flexion of the elbow and the knee joint, there is lateral rotation of the humerus and femur, respectively (MacConaill, 1966).

At any joint, there are potentially six degrees of freedom (Fig. 2.18), which can be described in terms of movement in a plane, or according to the axis of movement (Middleditch & Oliver, 2005). Movements according to the plane of movement are:

- rotation and translation in the sagittal plane
- rotation and translation in the coronal plane
- rotation and translation in the horizontal plane.

During lumbar spine flexion, for example, there is at each spinal level a combination of anterior sagittal rotation and anterior sagittal translation; during extension there is posterior sagittal rotation and posterior sagittal translation. More information and measurements of these movements can be obtained from Pearcy et al. (1984) and Pearcy and Tibrewal (1984).

Joint Glide During Physiological Movements

Movement at a joint is a combination of roll or spin with a glide or translation. The axis of movement constantly changes and is referred to as the instantaneous axis of rotation (e.g. during elbow flexion, the radial head rotates around the capitulum of the humerus and translates (i.e. slides) anteriorly). During knee flexion, non-weight bearing, the tibia rotates

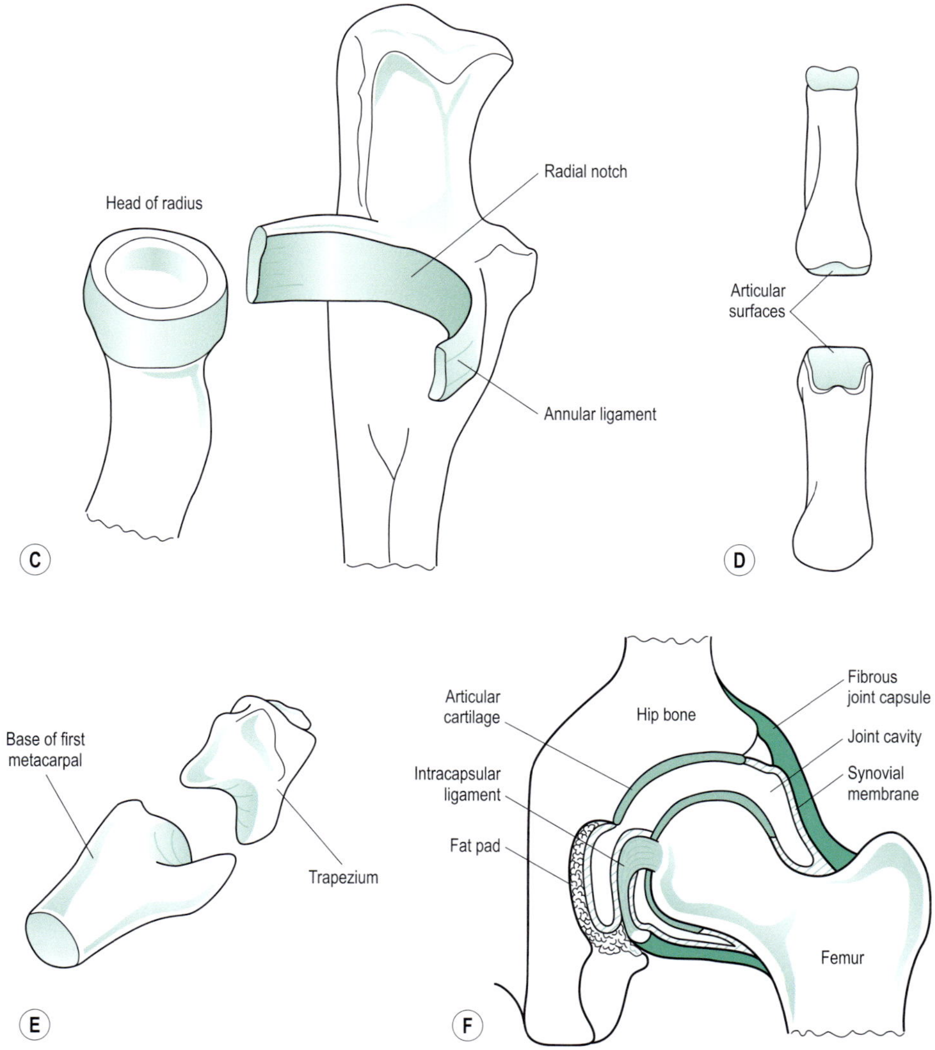

Fig. 2.17 cont'd (C) Pivot: superior radioulnar joint. (D) Condyloid: metacarpophalangeal joint of the thumb. (E) Saddle: carpometacarpal of the thumb. (F) Ball and socket: hip joint. (*After Palastanga & Soames, 2012, with permission.*)

posteriorly around the femur and slides posteriorly. Table 2.3 identifies, for each joint movement, the direction of the bone translation.

The direction in which the bone glides (or translates) depends upon the shape of the moving articular surface (Fig. 2.19) (MacConaill, 1973; Kaltenborn, 2014). When the joint surface of the moving bone is concave, the glide usually occurs in the same direction as the bone is moving so that, with flexion on the knee joint (in non-weight bearing), posterior glide of the tibial condyles occurs on the femoral condyles. When the joint surface is convex, the glide is usually in the opposite direction to the bone movement so that, with ankle dorsiflexion, there is a posterior glide of the talus on the inferior tibia and fibula.

Another consideration is the relative size of the articular surfaces; for example, in the glenohumeral joint the head of the humerus has a much larger surface area than the glenoid cavity. The effect of this is that the head of the humerus, as it rolls, would run out of articular surface on the glenoid. This is overcome by a glide and also by accompanying movement of the

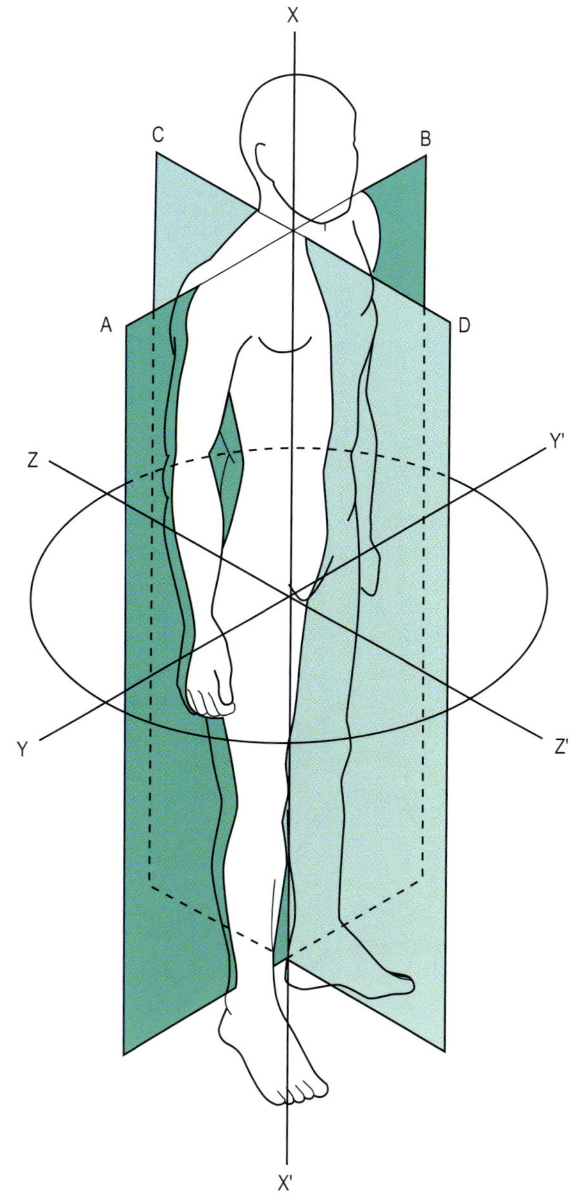

Fig. 2.18 Planes of the body and axes of movement. AB is the coronal plane, CD is the sagittal plane and the horizontal circle surrounding the person depicts the horizontal plane; XX′ is the vertical axis, YY′ is the frontal axis and ZZ′ is the sagittal axis. *(From Middleditch & Oliver, 2005, with permission.)*

scapula, during humeral movements (Levangie & Norkin, 2011).

The spinal joints follow the same principles as the peripheral joints but are worth describing separately here. Each spinal segmental level, between C2 and S1,

TABLE 2.3 Direction of Bone Translation During Active Physiological Movements

Movement	Translation
Glenohumeral	
Flexion	Anterior and superior
Extension	Posterior and inferior
Abduction	Inferior
Elbow: Humeroulnar	
Flexion	Anterior
Extension	Posterior
Elbow: Radiohumeral	
Flexion	Anterior
Extension	Posterior
Forearm: Superior Radioulnar	
Pronation	Posterior
Supination	Anterior
Forearm: Inferior Radioulnar	
Pronation	Anterior
Supination	Posterior
Wrist: Proximal Row of Carpus on Radius and Ulnar	
Flexion	Posterior
Extension	Anterior
Radial deviation	Medial
Ulnar deviation	Lateral
Thumb: Base of First Metacarpal on Trapezium	
Flexion	Anterior
Extension	Posterior
Abduction	Medial
Adduction	Lateral
Hip	
Flexion	Posterior
Extension	Anterior
Abduction	Medial
Adduction	Lateral
Knee, Non-Weight Bearing	
Flexion	Posterior
Extension	Anterior
Ankle, Non-Weight Bearing Talus on Tibia and Fibula	
Dorsiflexion	Posterior
Plantarflexion	Anterior

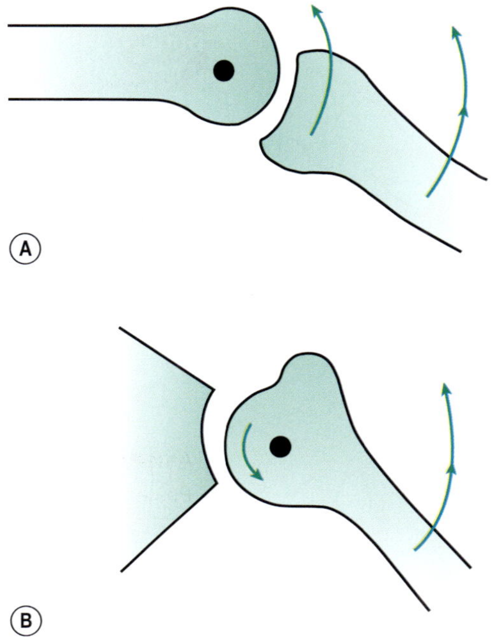

Fig. 2.19 Movement of articular surfaces during physiological movements. The single arrow depicts the direction of movement of the articular surface, and the double arrow depicts the physiological movement. (A) With knee extension (non–weight bearing), the concave articular surface of the tibia slides superiorly on the convex femoral condyles. (B) With shoulder elevation through abduction, the convex articular surface of the humerus slides inferiorly on the concave glenoid cavity. (*After Kaltenborn 2014, with permission.*)

consists of an interbody joint (two vertebral bodies and the intervening intervertebral disc) and two zygapophyseal joints (Middleditch & Oliver, 2005), functionally a triad joint. The shape and direction of the articular surfaces of the zygapophyseal joints vary throughout the spine (Table 2.4 and Fig. 2.20) and influence the gliding movement available at that segmental level (Table 2.5).

The upper cervical spine, C0–C1 (between the occiput and atlas) and C1–C2 (between the atlas and the axis) are, anatomically, different from the rest of the spine. The superior articular facets of C1 are concave and face upwards and medially; in addition, the lines of the two facets, when viewed superiorly, converge anteriorly (Fig. 2.21A). The occipital condyles are reciprocally shaped. The shape of the facets at C0–C1 facilitates flexion and extension movement. As the head rotates forwards on C1, the occipital condyles slide (or translate) in a posterior direction, following the aforementioned principle of a convex surface moving on a concave surface (Fig. 2.21B). With extension of the head on C1, the occipital condyles slide in an anterior direction. The flexion and extension at the C0–C1 articulation accounts for approximately one-third of the total sagittal plane movement of the cervical spine (Chancey et al., 2007).

The superior articular facets of C2 are large, oval and convex, and they lie in an anteroposterior direction. They face superiorly and laterally (Fig. 2.22A). The inferior articular facets of C1 are reciprocally shaped. The shape of the facets at C1–C2 facilitates rotation. With rotation to the right, the right inferior facet of C1 glides posteriorly and slightly caudal with the left inferior facet gliding anteriorly and slightly caudad (Fig. 2.22B). The ipsilateral posterior and contralateral anterior translations produce the rotation movement, and the caudal (inferior) movement usually produces a coupled left lateral flexion movement (Salem et al., 2013). Thus at this segmental level, rotation to the right

TABLE 2.4 Shape and Direction of the Superior Articular Surfaces of the Zygapophyseal Joints in the Spine

Spinal Level	Shape of Superior Facets	Direction of Superior Facets	Movement Facilitated by Direction of Facets
C1	Concave	Upwards and medial	Flexion and extension
C2	Large, oval, convex	Upwards and lateral	Rotation
C2–C7	Oval, flat	Upwards and backwards	All directions
T1–T12	Triangular, flat	Backwards, slightly upwards and lateral	Rotation Lateral flexion
L1–L5	Concave	Backwards and medial	Flexion, extension, lateral flexion

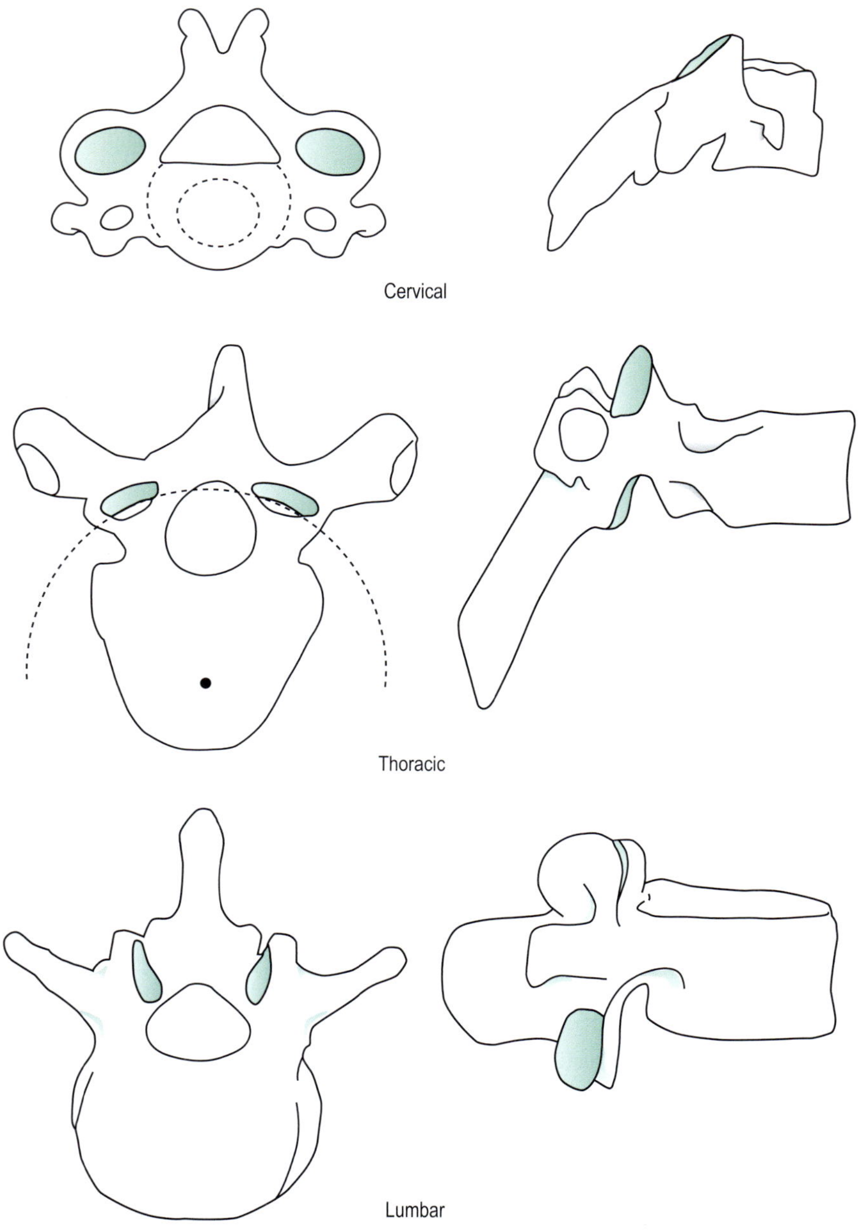

Fig. 2.20 Direction of articular surfaces in cervical, thoracic and lumbar spine. The superior articular facets of the cervical vertebrae face upwards and backwards, those of the thoracic vertebrae backwards and laterally and those of the lumbar vertebrae backwards and medially. (*From Palastanga & Soames, 2012, with permission.*)

is accompanied by contralateral (left) lateral flexion. During flexion, the inferior facets of C1 glide backwards on the superior facets of C2. During extension, the inferior facets of C1 glide forwards.

In the cervical spine (C3–C7 levels) the superior articular facets are oval and flat and face upwards and backwards (Fig. 2.20). During cervical spine flexion, the inferior articular facets of each cervical vertebra slide upwards and forwards on the superior articular facets of the vertebra below. For example, the inferior facets of C5 slide upwards and forwards on the superior facets of C6. On extension the reverse occurs throughout the cervical spine, so, for example, at C5–C6, the inferior facets of C5 slide downwards and backwards on the superior facets of C6.

TABLE 2.5 Glide of Inferior Articular Facets During Physiological Movements of the Spine

	Flexion	Extension	Left Lateral Flexion	Right Lateral Flexion	Left Rotation	Right Rotation
C3–C7						
Left inferior articular facet	Upwards	Downwards	Downwards	Upwards	Downwards	Upwards
	Forwards	Backwards	Backwards	Forwards	Backwards medial	Forwards lateral
Right inferior articular facet	Upwards	Downwards	Upwards	Downwards	Upwards	Downwards
	Forwards	Backwards	Forwards	Backwards	Forwards lateral	Backwards medial
T1–T12						
Left inferior articular facet	Upwards Forwards	Downwards Backwards	Downwards Backwards	Upwards Forwards	Medial	Lateral
Right inferior articular facet	Upwards Forwards	Downwards Backwards	Upwards Forwards	Downwards Backwards	Lateral	Medial
L1–S1						
Left inferior articular facet	Upwards Forwards	Downwards Backwards	Downwards Backwards	Upwards Forwards		
Right inferior articular facet	Upwards Forwards	Downwards Backwards	Upwards Forwards	Downwards Backwards		

On right lateral flexion, the left inferior articular facets of each cervical vertebra slide upwards but also forwards on the vertebra below, and on the right-hand side the inferior articular facets slide downwards but also backwards. Thus in the cervical spine, right lateral flexion is accompanied by right (ipsilateral) rotation (Fig. 2.23). It is the forward movement of the left inferior articular facet that produces the right rotation movement, and its upward movement produces a right lateral flexion movement (Bogduk & Mercer, 2000).

On cervical rotation to the right, the left inferior articular facets at each cervical level glide upwards, forwards and laterally on the superior facet of the vertebra below (Fig. 2.23), and on the right-hand side the inferior articular facets glide downwards, backwards and medially on the vertebra below, therefore producing right (ipsilateral) lateral flexion (Salem et al., 2013).

In summary, cervical lateral flexion is accompanied by ipsilateral rotation, and rotation is accompanied by ipsilateral lateral flexion (Bogduk & Mercer, 2000).

At the C2–C3 level, one can see a small deviation from the aforementioned rule. At this level and contrary to rest of the levels of the lower cervical spine, the superior articular surfaces in addition to facing upwards and backwards, they also face medially to approximately 40 degrees (Bogduk & Mercer, 2000). In addition, the superior articular facets of C3 lie slightly lower in relation to their vertebral body when compared with the rest of the lower cervical spine levels (Bogduk & Mercer, 2000). This morphological difference produces a change in kinematic behaviour of the C2–C3 segment, with rotation occasionally producing contralateral side flexion (Salem et al., 2013). Nevertheless, due to this anatomical variation at this level, the range of the coupled movement available is significantly less, compared with the rest of the levels (Salem et al., 2013), providing a more stable base for the atlantoaxial segment above.

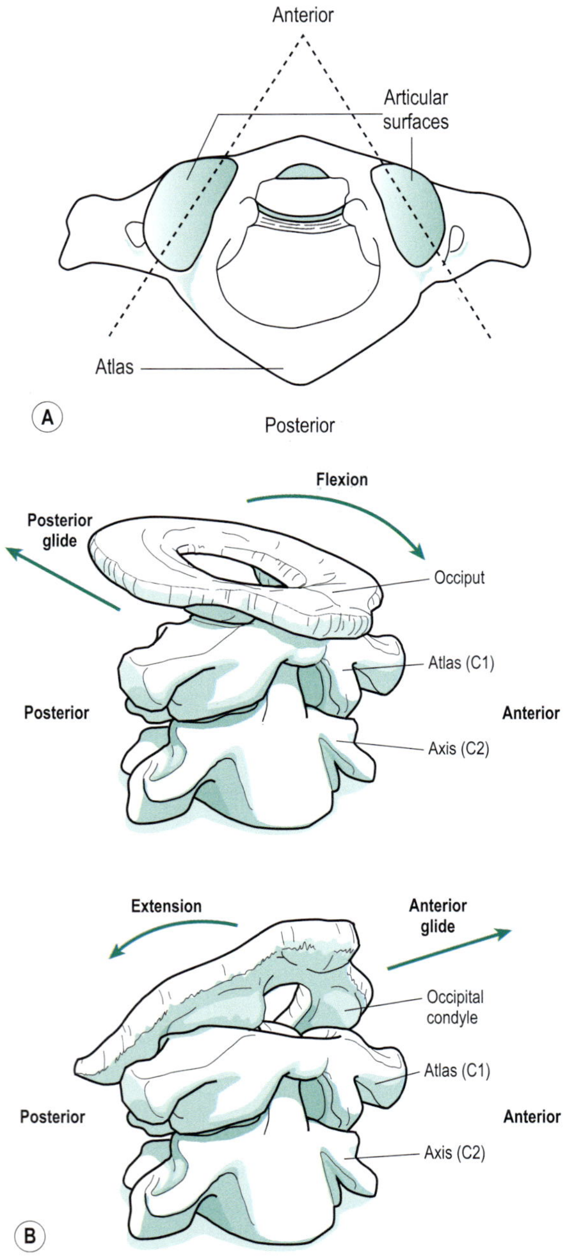

Fig. 2.21 (A) Superior surface of atlas. Superior articular facets of C1 are concave and face upwards and medial. The lines of the two facets, when viewed superiorly, converge anteriorly. *(From Palastanga & Soames, 2012, with permission.)* (B) Flexion and extension at the C0–C1 joint. During flexion the occipital condyles glide posteriorly, whereas during extension they glide anteriorly. (*After Edwards 1999, with permission.*)

In the thoracic spine, the flat, triangular superior articular facets face backwards and slightly upwards and lateral (Fig. 2.20). During thoracic flexion, the inferior articular facets at each level glide essentially upwards, with some forward translation (Fig. 2.24). On thoracic extension, the inferior articular facets glide downwards with some backward translation (Lee, 2003). The coupling of movements between rotation and side flexion at the thoracic spine varies significantly between studies and between subjects, showing both ipsilateral and contralateral rotation and side flexion coupling patterns at different levels. Variability may be due to differences between in vivo and cadaveric study protocols; the complexity posed by the presence and articulations of the rib cage with the thoracic spine; or the age of the subjects studied (McCarthy, 2010).

In the lumbar spine, the superior articular facets are concave, facing backwards and medially (Fig. 2.20). During lumbar flexion, the inferior articular facets glide upwards and forwards. On extension, the inferior articular facets glide downwards and backwards (Fig. 2.25). The movement of the articular facets during lateral flexion is less clear. With lateral flexion, there may be ipsilateral, contralateral rotation or no coupling (Cook, 2003). On lumbar rotation to the left (moving the trunk), the inferior articular facet on the right glides anteriorly and laterally to impact on to the superior articular facet of the vertebra below. The left inferior articular facet glides in a posterior and medial direction, so there is gapping of the joint space. Rotation of the lumbar spine from L1 to L4 is accompanied by contralateral lateral flexion, whereas rotation at L4–5 and L5–S1 is accompanied by ipsilateral lateral flexion (Fujii et al., 2007).

Normal function of any synovial joint requires the moving bone to rotate and translate. Normal rotational and translational movements would be full range and symptom free, with normal through-range and end-range resistance; normal muscle and nerve function is assumed. These movements can be examined in clinic during active and passive physiological movements assessment, and translation is examined during accessory movements assessment. The reader is directed to Hengeveld & Banks (2014a, 2014b) Ryder and Barnard (2024) chapter 4.

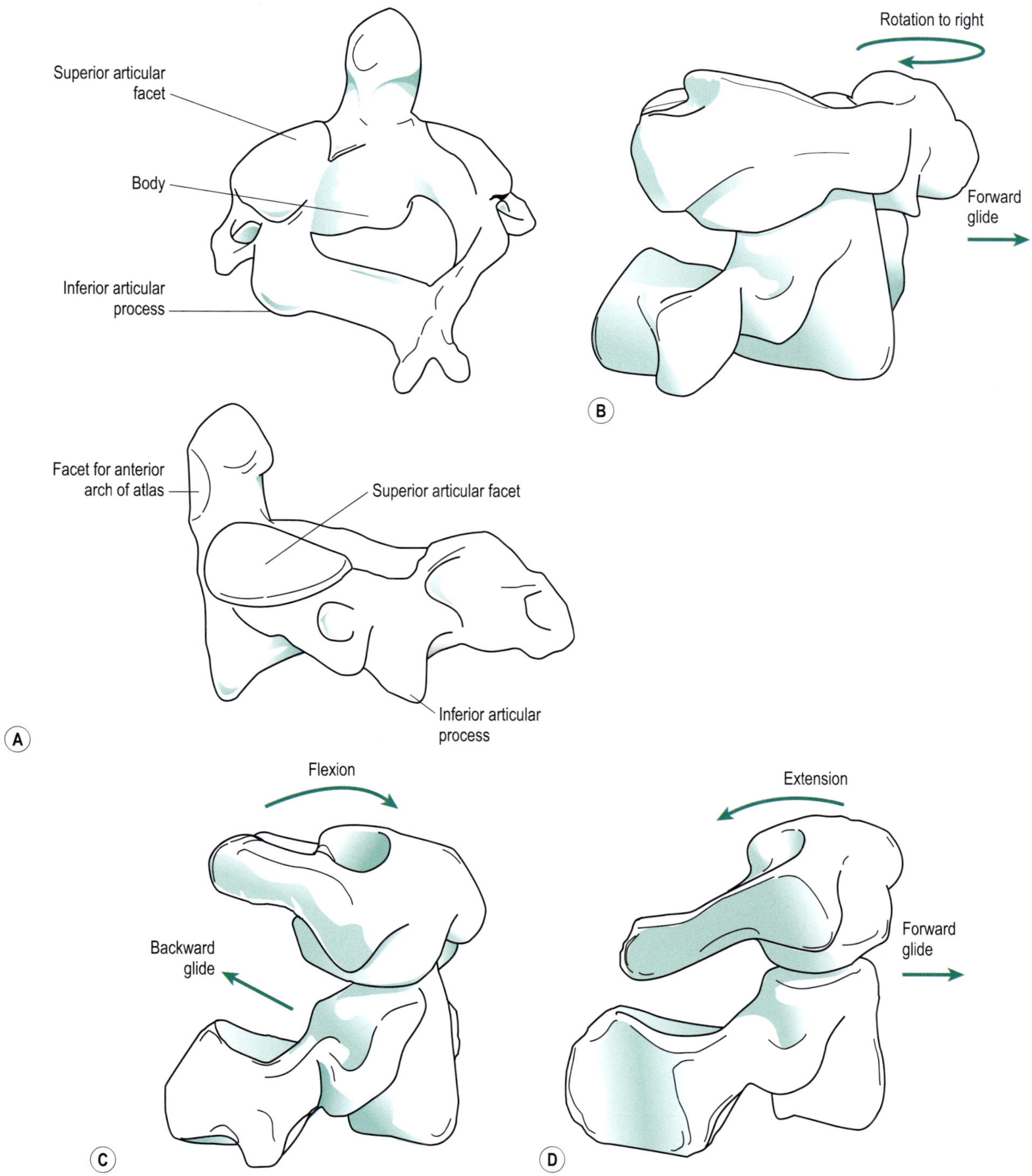

Fig. 2.22 (A) Superior surface of C2. The superior articular facets of C2 are large, oval and convex and face superiorly and laterally. *(After Middleditch & Oliver, 2005, with permission.)* (B) Rotation to the right at the C1–C2 joint. The right inferior facet of C1 glides posteriorly and slightly downwards, while the left inferior facet of C1 glides anteriorly and slightly upwards. *(After Edwards 1999, with permission).* (C) Flexion at the C1–C2 joint: the inferior facets of C1 glide backwards on the superior facets of C2. (D) Extension at the C1–C2 joint: the inferior facets of C1 glide forwards on the superior facets of C2.

Knowledge of the normal rotation and translation of bone during movement of a joint is important when attempting to restore normal joint function. For example, with the patient lying prone, to facilitate an increase in cervical flexion at the C4–C5 level, a central posteroanterior force with a cephalad inclination could be used on the C4 spinous process. This accessory movement will also enhance extension at the C3–C4 segmental level. Similar accessory movements can be applied to the thoracic and lumbar spine joints and to the peripheral joints (for further information, see Hengeveld & Banks, 2014a, 2014b).

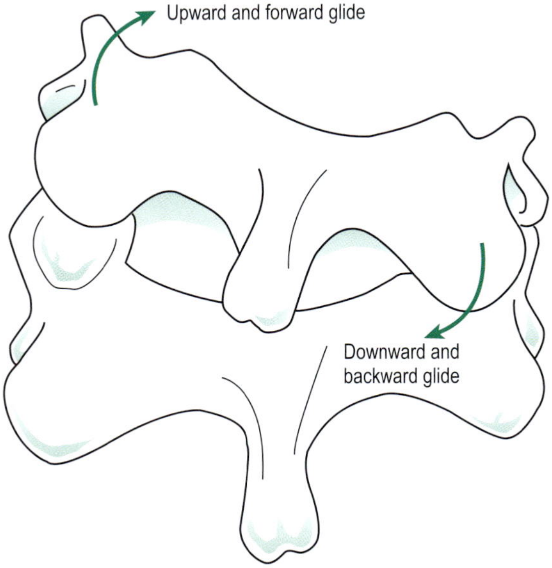

Fig. 2.23 Cervical rotation to the right is accompanied by lateral flexion to the right. The left inferior articular facet glides upwards and forwards, while the right inferior articular facet glides downwards and backwards. (*After Middleditch & Oliver, 2005, with permission*)

Another concept is that of close pack and loose pack position of a joint. Close pack usually found at the extremes of the range is where there is maximal congruency of joint surfaces, maximal tension in the joint capsule and ligaments and the least joint play (i.e. the amount of slack, or give, in the joint). Loose pack is any position other than close pack, where the joint capsule and ligaments are relatively slack and there is some joint play.

Joint position at the time of injury can ultimately predict the injury that occurs. For example, in a close-packed position, the application of force is likely to lead to a bony injury; due to the congruency of the adjoining bones the force is taken up through the bone rather than the supporting ligaments/capsular structures (e.g. a Colles fracture sustained by a fall on the outstretched hand and the wrist joint in extension). In the lower limb, for example, an anterior cruciate ligament tear may be sustained with the knee in a flexed and rotated position (Hertling & Kessler, 2006a).

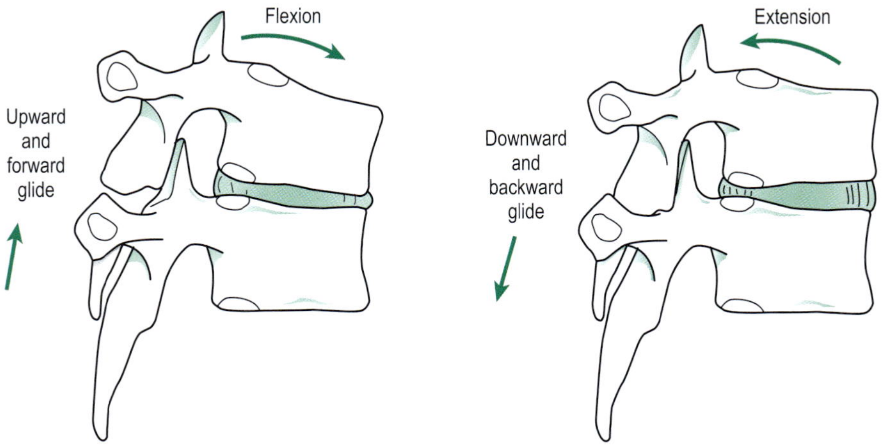

Fig. 2.24 Flexion and extension movements in the thoracic spine. During flexion the inferior articular facets glide upwards and slightly forwards, and on extension the inferior articular facets glide downwards and slightly backwards. (*After Palastanga & Soames, 2012, with permission.*)

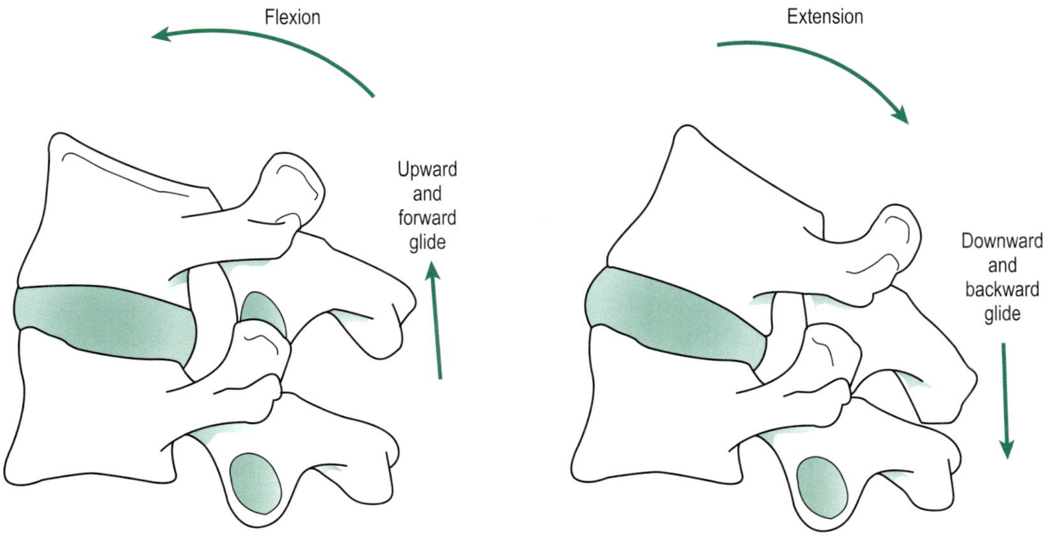

Fig. 2.25 Flexion and extension in the lumbar spine. During lumbar flexion the inferior articular facets glide upwards and forwards, while on extension they glide downwards and backwards. (*After Palastanga & Soames, 2012, with permission.*)

KNOWLEDGE CHECK

1. What is the close pack position of the ankle joint?
2. What term is used to describe the study of joint movement?
3. Can you describe how the articular surface shape influences the way the articular surface glides during movement?
4. How can this information help in clinical assessment and treatment?

Biomechanics of Normal Joint Movement

The normal function of most joints is to allow full-range movement of the adjacent bones. As the bones move towards the end range of joint movement, resistance to movement increases (Wright & Johns, 1961; Nigg & Herzog, 2007) as the surrounding joint capsule, ligaments and muscles become taut (Wright & Johns, 1961), eventually causing movement to stop. This is a protective mechanism so that the joint does not sub-luxate or dislocate.

End-feel. Different joints are limited by different structures at the end of a particular range of movement. For example, elbow extension is limited by bony opposition of the olecranon process of the ulna in the olecranon fossa, knee flexion is limited by soft-tissue opposition between the calf and the thigh, and wrist flexion is limited by the wrist dorsal ligaments as well as the bony configuration of the carpus. This resistance at the end of range of a joint movement and when felt by a clinician in clinical assessment of joint movement is referred to as end-feel. End-feel varies in different joints whether pathology is present or not.

Classification of end-feel as normal or pathological is based on the ability to interpret the movement occurring at the joint, in conjunction with anatomical knowledge and the point in the range at which the resistance is felt.

End-feel can be normal or indicative of pathology and therefore requires interpretation by an experienced clinician.

- **Capsular end-feel:** Normal—a firm, leathery feeling (Cyriax, 1982; Hertling & Kessler, 2006b; Atkins et al., 2010; Kaltenborn, 2014), when felt at the end of some ranges of movement (e.g. lateral rotation of the shoulder/hip). Abnormal—when felt early in the range and may be indicative of early degenerative changes in a joint.
- **Bony end-feel:** Normal—at end range when there is bony apposition of approximating surfaces (e.g. full-range elbow extension). Abnormal—when occurring before expected end range (e.g. degenerative change or malunion of an intraarticular fracture).
- **Soft-tissue end-feel:** Normal—a soft feeling at the end of range when muscular tissue is approximated

(e.g., knee flexion). Abnormal if joint range of motion is restricted due to muscle hypertrophy (Cyriax, 1982; Hertling & Kessler, 2006b; Kaltenborn, 2014).

- **Ligamentous end-feel:** Normal—firm end-feel with no appreciable give (e.g. when applying an abduction/adduction force to an extended knee). Abnormal—notable give may indicate ligamentous damage.

Abnormal end-feel may be categorized as follows:

- **Hard end-feel:** Seen in capsular and degenerative pathology. End-feel is harder than expected and/or occurs earlier in the range (Hertling & Kessler, 2006b; Atkins et al., 2010).
- **Springy end-feel:** (e.g. in the presence of a loose body); full range of joint movement is not achieved and an abnormal 'bouncy' feeling is felt by the clinician at the end of the available range (Atkins et al., 2010).
- **Muscle spasm end-feel:** often occurs with pain; end-feel—an abrupt stop to movement, often with visible muscle contraction present as a 'guarding' mechanism to prevent further movement.
- **Empty end-feel:** Rare but of high clinical significance. The sensation is described as 'empty' as the examiner experiences no resistance to continuation of movement, but the patient halts the movement due to severe pain. Interpretation of this response must be treated with caution but may be indicative of neoplasm, fracture, septic arthritis or acute bursitis.

Functional Movement

Functional activities often involve movement throughout the limb. For example, in standing, when a person bends at the knees this will be accompanied by hip flexion and ankle dorsiflexion. This predictable movement pattern can be referred to as a closed kinematic chain, a term used in engineering for linkages that make up a system. In contrast, the unpredictable movement patterns that can occur in the upper limb (and the lower limb when not weight bearing) can be termed an open kinematic chain. The concept of open and closed kinematic chains is useful in that it highlights that movement usually involves a number of joints. Furthermore, these patterns are used in clinical practice in varying stages of rehabilitation to mimic normal functional movement.

Proprioception

Joint stability occurs through the integration of dynamic and mechanical restraints (Myers et al., 2006; Munn et al., 2010). Mechanical restraints pertain to the joint capsule, ligaments, bony anatomy and intra-articular pressures, whereas dynamic restraints include muscle activation and the force produced from this muscle activity. These dynamic and mechanical restraints are mediated by the sensorimotor system, which includes sensory, motor, central integration and processing components. When functioning optimally, this provides a feedforward/feedback system, where mechanical restraints provide neural feedback via efferent motor pathways to the central nervous system. This in turn provides feedback to the dynamic restraints (Myers et al., 2006; Munn et al., 2010).

Proprioception is part of this sensorimotor system and forms the afferent feedback from joint and soft-tissue mechanoreceptors, present in muscle, ligaments, joint capsule and fascia, through mechanical and dynamic restraints. Proprioception, by definition, is a perception of position and movement (Boisgontier & Swinnen, 2014) gained from skin, joint and muscle receptors (Hewett et al., 2002). It has three main components: joint position sense, kinaesthesia and sensation of force. Damage to the joint, ligaments, muscle or skin can affect this feedback system and thus cause a loss of proprioception which may ultimately lead to muscle, joint and/or nerve dysfunction.

KNOWLEDGE CHECK

1. What are the main components of proprioception?
2. What do you understand by the terms open and close kinetic chain?
3. What might you find on examination of end-feel in a patient with significant ligamentous injury?

JOINT DYSFUNCTION

Just as the function of joints depends on the function of muscles and nerves, so dysfunction of joints can lead to dysfunction in muscles and nerves. They are dependent on each other in both normal and abnormal conditions, and this relationship is depicted in Fig. 2.26. The following examples explore how joint dysfunction is often accompanied by muscle and/or nerve dysfunction.

Joint Pathology and Muscle/Nerve Dysfunction

Joint pathology can lead to weakness of the overlying muscle and deficits in neuromuscular control (Myers & Lephart, 2000; Callaghan et al., 2014). This has been

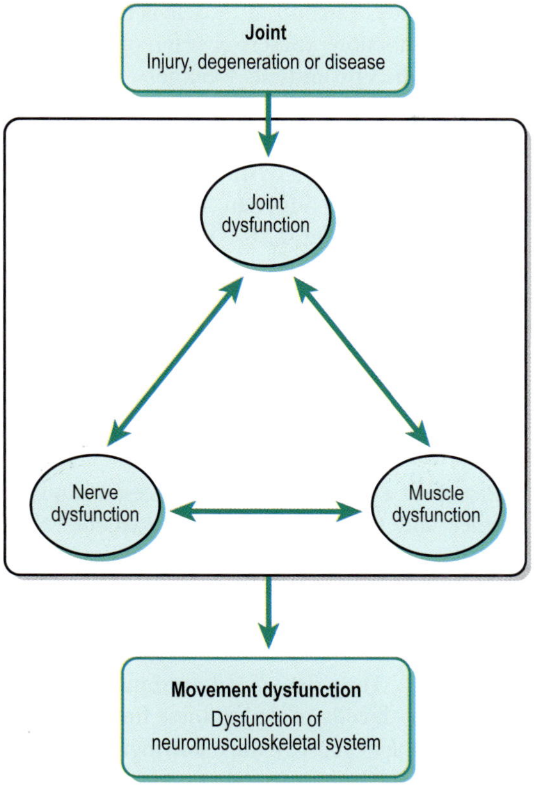

Fig. 2.26 Dysfunction of joint can produce muscle and/or nerve dysfunction.

demonstrated in the presence of a variety of pathologies: patellofemoral pain syndrome (Callaghan & Oldham, 2004); patellofemoral osteoarthritis (OA) (Callaghan et al., 2014); and ligamentous injuries (Urbach & Awiszus, 2002) following meniscectomy (Malliou et al., 2012). The presence of effusion has been shown to result in muscle inhibition in the knee (Palmieri-Smith et al., 2007) and in the hip joint (Freeman et al., 2013). However other research has failed to find a direct association between joint distension and muscle inhibition (Callaghan et al., 2014). The inhibition of muscle is thought to be due to inhibitory (Suter & Herzog, 2000; Torry et al., 2000) or abnormal (Rice et al., 2011) input from joint afferents. Thus joint pathology leads to altered nervous system activity, which leads to altered muscle activity.

Joint Immobilization and Muscle/Nerve Dysfunction

Joint immobilization can also have a negative effect on muscular and neural function. Joint immobilization for 3 weeks has been shown to cause a reduced maximal voluntary contraction of the muscle around the joint and a decrease in the maximal firing rate of motor neurons supplying muscle (Seki et al., 2001; Kazuhiko & Hiroshi, 2007). Thus immobilization of a joint leads to muscle weakness and altered nervous system activity.

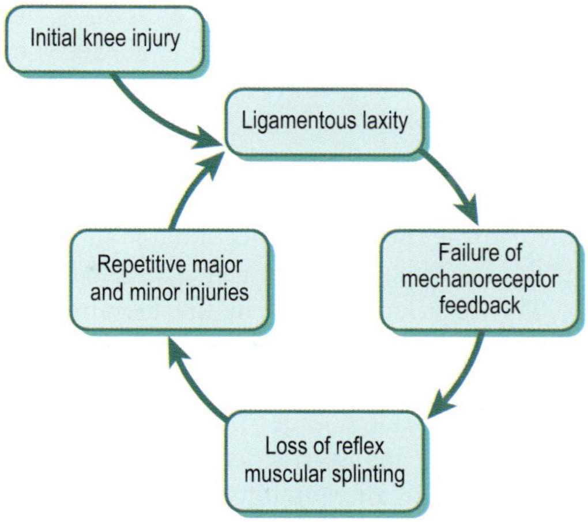

Fig. 2.27 A proposed cycle of progressive knee instability following an initial ligament injury. (*From Kennedy et al., 1982, with permission.*)

Joint Instability and Muscle/Nerve Dysfunction

Joint instability and ligament insufficiency have been shown to alter nervous system activity, which leads to altered muscle activity. In the ankle joint, arthrogenic muscle inhibition was found to be present post ankle sprain (McVey et al., 2005), and at the knee, anterior cruciate ligament deficiency has been found to alter activity of quadriceps and hamstring muscle groups during knee movement (Suarez et al., 2016), gait (Serrancoli et al., 2016) and negotiating stairs (Hall et al., 2015). A cycle of events leading to dysfunction in ligament, muscle and nerve is shown in Fig. 2.27 (Suter & Herzog, 2000).

Proprioceptive deficits have been identified in human arthritic conditions and are attributed to reduced activity of the joint, local muscle atrophy (Cuomo et al., 2005) and the presence of pain, where increased nociceptor activity causes a reduction in proprioception (Safran et al., 2001; Fortier & Basset, 2012) and joint swelling. Although it was previously thought that swelling had a negative influence on proprioception, it is now believed that the loss of proprioception in the presence of swelling is more likely to be due to the nature of the fluid contents or the length of time the effusion is present (e.g. in arthritic conditions (Palmieri et al., 2003) or the presence of pain (Callaghan et al., 2014)).

It has also been hypothesized that loss of proprioceptive mechanisms either due to age or due to decreased muscle mass may initiate or accelerate arthritic damage through its effect on a joint's dynamic and mechanical restraints (Ikeda et al., 2005; Kim et al., 2016). This is acknowledged in the literature, where ligamentous injury such as damage to the anterior cruciate ligament can affect postural control in both the injured and uninjured side (Ageberg, 2002). Joint damage, such as in arthritic conditions, may evoke abnormal articular afferent information, causing subsequent loss of muscle activation and altered neuromuscular control (Myers & Lephart, 2000). Problems with muscle activation are also reported following joint injury and proprioceptive loss and can contribute to recurrent instability problems, through suppressed reflexive activation and slow coactivation patterns from muscles with stabilizing roles (Myers et al., 2006).

Joint Nociception and Muscle Dysfunction

Joint nociceptor activity directly affects muscle activity. Joint pain is directly associated with muscle inhibition and weakness. Quadriceps muscle inhibition was found to be directly associated with the severity of pain from osteoarthritic patellofemoral joints (Callaghan et al., 2014), and more than 3 months' history of pain caused by lumbar disc herniation is linked to reduction in the cross-sectional area of multifidus (Kim et al., 2011).

Conversely, dysfunction in muscle is thought to lead to joint dysfunction (Suter & Herzog, 2000). For example, quadriceps muscle weakness is thought to alter knee joint loading which may, in the long term, lead to OA in the joint (Herzog & Longino, 2007; Hall et al., 2012). Thus joint dysfunction may occur as a result of a muscle dysfunction, and this sequence of events is outlined in Fig. 2.28.

KNOWLEDGE CHECK
1. Can you outline the impact of joint immobilization?
2. What is the impact of nociception on muscle activity?

Classification of Joint Dysfunction

The function of a joint is to transfer force from one bone to another and to permit limited movement (Nigg & Herzog, 2007). Some joints, such as the sacroiliac joint (SIJ), transmit very high forces and have hardly any movement, whereas other joints, such as the glenohumeral joint, transmit less force and have a large range of movement. The signs and symptoms of joint dysfunction are directly related to these functions; that is, there may be one or more of the following: reduced range of joint movement (hypomobility), increased range of joint movement (hypermobility) or altered quality of movement or production of symptoms. These signs and symptoms can occur in isolation or in any combination.

Hypomobility

Hypomobility can affect accessory or physiological movements. It seems reasonable to suggest that if there

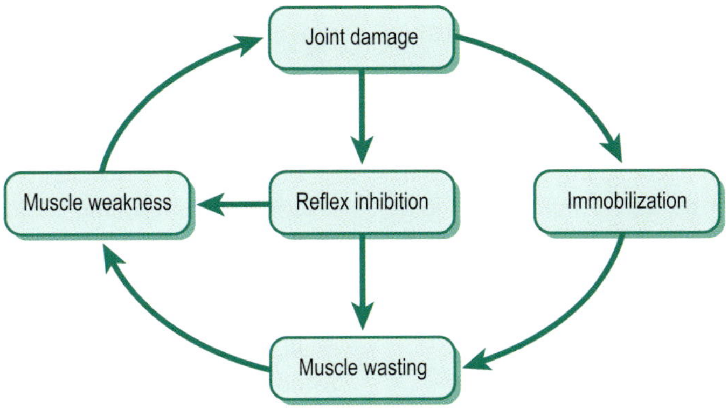

Fig. 2.28 Effect of joint damage and/or immobilization on muscle and nerve tissue. (*From Stokes, M., Young, A. 1984.* The contribution of reflex inhibition to arthrogenous muscle weakness. Clin. Sci. *67, 7–14. © The Biochemical Society and the Medical Research Society, with permission.*)

is a reduced range of translation this will affect, to some degree, the range of rotation of the bone. In the same way, if there is a reduced range of rotation movement, this will affect the range of translation movement.

Limited range of accessory or physiological movement is often associated with an altered quality of movement. This is most commonly increased resistance to movement or production of symptoms. These can be represented visually on a movement diagram Fig. 2.29. Details on how to draw a movement diagram can be found in Chapter 4 Ryder and Barnard (2024).

Traumatized or pathological tissues, which may produce alteration to the movement quality, include intraarticular structures, such as joint capsule, a torn meniscus or a loose body, and periarticular structures such as ligament, muscle or nerve overlying the joint. Each joint has its own unique range and resistance to movement, owing to its particular intraarticular and periarticular arrangement.

Limited range of accessory or physiological movements may be caused by the production of symptoms. Symptoms can be any sensation felt by the patient and can include pain, ache, pulling, pins and needles, numbness or a sense of something crawling along the skin, as well as apprehension by the patient to move further into range.

Hypomobility can be more fully appreciated by exploring the effects of immobilization on joint structures, as this produces the most profound joint hypomobility.

The Effects of Immobilization

Knowledge of the effects of immobilization on joint tissue has come about largely from research on animals.

The effects on of knee joint immobilization on the joint space, articular cartilage, joint capsule, synovial membrane and subchondral bone as wells as timescales involved in tissue changes are summarized in Table 2.6. All the knees investigated following immobilization had reduced range of movement and joint stiffness due to the connective tissue and adhesion formation in the joint space (Ando et al., 2010; Lee et al., 2010; Iqbal et al., 2012). The detailed changes of articular cartilage following immobilization are listed in Box 2.1.

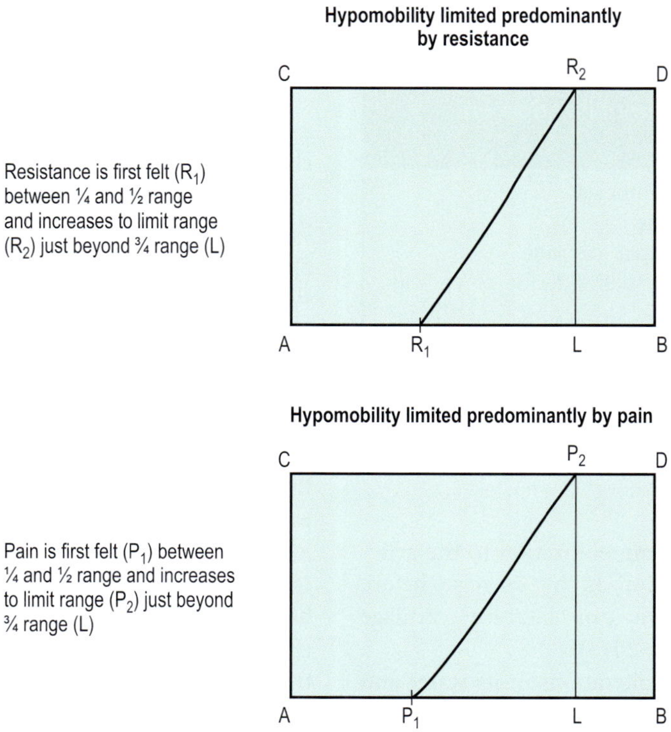

Fig. 2.29 Movement diagram of hypomobility due to resistance or production of symptoms, where L is the limit of range, R_1 is the first point of resistance felt by the examiner, R_2 is the maximum intensity of resistance which limits further movement, P_1 is the point in the range where pain is first felt and P_2 is the maximum intensity of pain which limits further movement.

TABLE 2.6 Effect of Immobilization on Joint

Tissue	Time	Effect	Study
Joint space	15 days; well established at 1 month	Fibrofatty connective tissue within the joint space	Evans et al. (1960)
Adhesions	2 weeks	Adhesions between synovial membrane and meniscus	Ando et al. (2010)
	4 weeks	Adhesions bridged the synovial membrane meniscus and articular cartilage	
	Between 8 and 16 weeks	Adhesions become hypocellular and fibrous	
Articular cartilage	1 month	Cartilage thinning with necrotic areas and erosion	Iqbal et al. (2012)
	2 months	Atrophy of unapposing cartilage and ulceration of the articular cartilage	Evans et al. (1960)
Subchondral bone	2 months	Proliferation of vascular connective tissue under areas of articular cartilage lesion and erosion of subchondral bone	Evans et al. (1960)
Synovial membrane	2–4 weeks	Shortening	Ando et al. (2010)
	16 weeks	Non-distinguishable synovial membrane	
Joint capsule	3 days	Cell proliferation hypoxia and inflammation	Yabe et al. (2013)
	8 and 16 weeks	Shortening	Ando et al. (2010)

BOX 2.1 Effect of Immobilization on Articular Cartilage

Decrease in proteoglycan synthesis
Softening of articular cartilage
Decreased thickness of articular cartilage
Adherence of fibrofatty connective tissue to cartilage surfaces
Pressure necrosis at points of cartilage–cartilage contact
Chondrocyte death

Vanwanseele et al. (2002).

However, the effects of immobilization to the articular cartilage can be minimized by exercise before immobilization, as exercise can increase cartilage thickness (Maldonado et al., 2013).

The ligament undergoes alterations in its water and glycosaminoglycan content, degradation in collagen synthesis, increase in collagen cross-links after 9 weeks, bone resorption at the bone–ligament junction, reduced stiffness and increased extensibility of the ligament and a reduction in load to failure (Box 2.2). The substantial change in the load–displacement curve of the rabbit femur–medial collateral ligament–tibia complex, after 9 weeks of immobilization, compared with a control group is depicted in Fig. 2.30 (Woo et al., 1988). The structural and mechanical effects of immobilization and remobilization of the bone–ligament–bone complex are depicted in Fig. 2.31 (Woo et al., 1987), showing that the ligament substance recovers quicker than the ligament insertion sites.

Hypermobility

Joint hypermobility is a condition in which synovial joints move excessively beyond normal limits, even after age, gender and race are taken into account (Grahame, 2003). Joint hypermobility may be inherited (Ferrell et al., 2004) or acquired through years of training or stretching (Grahame, 2003). In many cases it is asymptomatic and can be advantageous in areas such as the performing arts (Hakim & Grahame, 2003).

There may be hypermobility of one or more physiological movements and/or accessory movements in

BOX 2.2 Effect of Immobilization on Ligament

Effect on Ligament	Author
Decrease in water content and glycosaminoglycan level in collagen at 9 weeks	Akeson et al. (1973)
Initially an increase in collagen synthesis and degradation then a decrease in synthesis and degradation of collagen by 3 months	Amiel et al., (1983) Tipton et al., (1970)
Increase in collagen cross-links at 9 weeks	Akeson et al., (1977)
Decrease in cross-sectional area	Tipton et al. (1970)
Increase in osteoclastic activity at the bone–ligament junction, causing an increase in bone resorption in that area	Woo et al. (1987)
Reduced stiffness	Akeson et al. (1987)
Increased extensibility	Akeson et al. (1987)
Reduction in load to failure and reduction in energy-absorbing capabilities	Woo et al. (1987)

one or more joints. This increased range of motion may cause an increase in the range of translation of the joint surfaces and vice versa. This type of hypermobility may be due to injury/recurrent injury or inherited causing symptoms of increased joint range on active or passive testing.

It is important to note that in the presence of symptoms there are diagnostic criteria that would rule in hypermobility spectrum disorder (HSD) and hypermobile Ehlers–Danlos syndrome (hEDS) (Russek et al., 2019). Individuals with this inherited connective disorder tissue disorder may present with a range of signs and symptoms beyond the musculoskeletal system (e.g. cardiovascular, gastrointestinal) (Russek et al., 2019).

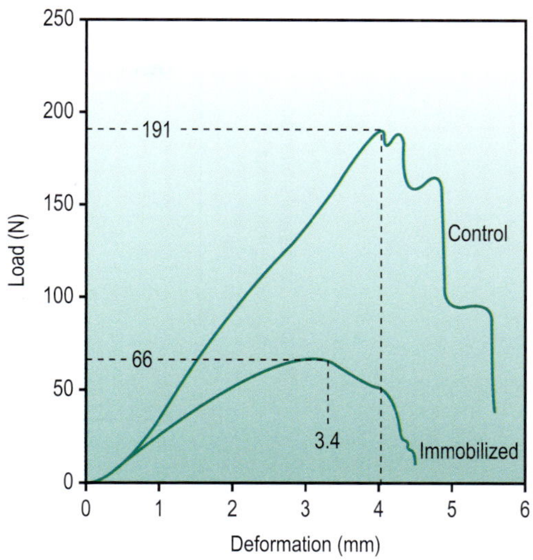

Fig. 2.30 The load–displacement curve of the rabbit femur–medial collateral ligament–tibia complex after 9 weeks of immobilization compared with a control group. *(From Woo, S., Buckwalter, J. 1988. Injury and Repair of the Musculoskeletal Soft Tissues. Rosemont, IL: American Academy of Orthopaedic Surgeons, with permission.)*

Joint Instability

Joint instability may be due to a deficit in the ligamentous, muscular and/or neural functioning around a joint. Instability may be described as mechanical or functional in nature. Mechanical instability refers to laxity of a joint due to injury of the ligamentous tissues which support the joint (Hertel & Kaminski, 2005). Functional instability refers to deficits in proprioceptive and neuromuscular control secondary to joint injury (Hertel & Kaminski, 2005). This is hypothesized to be due to the damage of the mechanoreceptors within the ligamentous structures following injury, which causes a reduction in perception of movement and particularly changes in direction (Hughes & Rochester, 2008). The relationship between the two is unclear, although mechanical instability can cause functional instability over time (Richie, 2001).

Altered Quality of Joint Movement

Alteration to the quality of movement encapsulates anything that is considered to be abnormal either by comparison with the other side or from the clinician's or the patient's experience of what is 'normal'. Abnormalities may include instability; increased or decreased

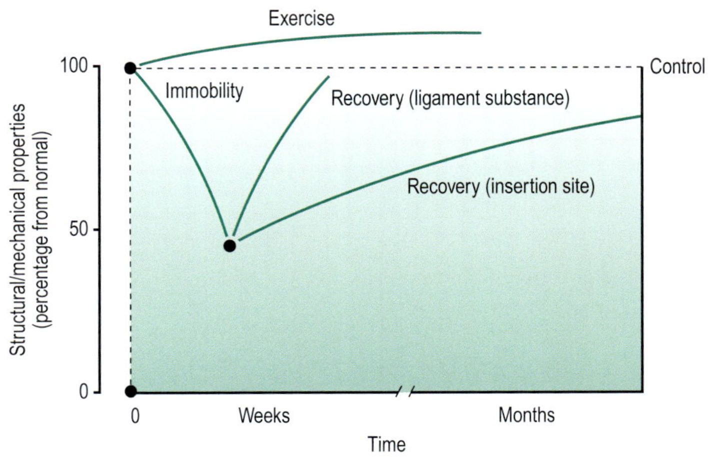

Fig. 2.31 The structural and mechanical properties of bone–ligament–bone complex following immobilization and recovery. (*From Woo et al., 1988, with permission of the American Academy of Orthopaedic Surgeons.*)

resistance to movement; poor control of movement; the presence of joint noise such as a clunk or crepitus; excessive effort or reluctance of the patient to move. Alterations in the quality of movement can directly or indirectly affect local or remote neuromuscular systems, leading to dysfunction, injury and musculoskeletal pathology. For example, weakness of hip abductors and external rotators can lead to increased hip internal rotation and adduction at the hip during dynamic activities and could lead to pathologies such as iliotibial band syndrome and patellofemoral joint dysfunction (Powers, 2010).

KNOWLEDGE CHECK

1. What is the impact of immobilization on articular cartilage?
2. Explain difference between functional and mechanical instability.

Joint Degeneration

OA is essentially the failure of the synovial joint that results from an increase in intraarticular stress. The increase in the articular stress may be due to a decrease in the load-bearing joint surface area or a quantitative increase of load (Brandt et al., 2009). Excessive loading of articular cartilage leads to depletion of proteoglycans, increase of water content of the cartilage and degradation of collagen fibres. The by-products of the breakdown of the cartilage and shards of cartilage that break off from the cartilage become incorporated into the synovial membrane causing inflammation and pain (Brandt et al., 2009). The subchondral bone also undergoes changes. In early-stage OA it becomes thinner and porous with an increased separation and thinning of the trabeculae. In later-stage OA the subchondral bone and trabeculae become thicker and sclerotic, increasing the damage to the overlying cartilage, in response to loading (Li et al., 2013). Bone marrow lesions (BMLs) develop in the subchondral bone under the areas of cartilage damage (Xu et al., 2012) that are associated with pain (Felson et al., 2001; Callaghan et al., 2015). Joint degeneration leads to loss of joint function due to pain and limitation of motion, frequently in a defined pattern, which is unique for every joint. This is termed a 'capsular pattern' (Atkins et al., 2010). The presence of a capsular pattern restriction, during clinical assessment, may be indicative of the presence of arthritis, but this association is not widely supported by research (Atkins et al., 2010). Thus capsular patterns should not be considered in isolation for the clinical diagnosis of arthritis Table 2.7.

There are a number of factors and aetiologies that are considered responsible for the onset of OA. Amongst them are, in no particular order of importance, genetic predisposition, gender, muscle power and

TABLE 2.7 Capsular Patterns

Joint	Pattern
Shoulder joint	Most lateral rotation, less than abduction, least medial rotation
Elbow	Flexion more than extension
Wrist	Flexion and extension equally limited
Trapeziometacarpal joint	Most limitation of extension
Cervical spine	Equal limitation in side flexions Equal limitation in rotations Some limitation in extension Usually, full flexion
Thoracic spine	Equal limitation in rotations Equal limitation in side flexions Some limitation in extension; usually full flexion
Lumbar spine	Limitation in extension Equal limitation in side flexions Usually, full flexion
Hip joint	Most limitation of medial rotation Less limitation of flexion and abduction Least limitation of extension
Knee joint	More limitation of flexion than extension
Ankle joint	More limitation of plantarflexion than dorsiflexion
First metatarsophalangeal joint	Marked limitation in extension. Some limitation in flexion

coordination, obesity, joint shape and malalignment, joint injury, instability and ageing.

Studies have shown 50% or more heritability for OA, with genes acting via different mechanisms such as injury avoidance and response to injury, body weight and obesity, muscle mass, bone structure and turnover and cartilage structure and turnover (Spector & MacGregor, 2004). Furthermore, genetic mutations that are responsible for the development and architecture of the joint may lead to malformations of the joint structure and thus alteration of the joint biomechanics which may lead to OA (Baker-LePain & Lane, 2010; Li et al., 2013). Typical examples of this, at the hip, are acetabular dysplasia, pistol grip deformity, wide femoral neck and altered femoral neck-shaft angle (Baker-LePain & Lane, 2010) At the knee, valgus and varus deformities are strongly associated with the development of OA. (Brouwer et al., 2007). Gender has also been shown to play a role in the development of OA. Men have a higher incidence of OA before the age of 50. Women have a higher prevalence of OA after the age of 50, with a high risk of hip and knee OA found amongst menopausal women on oestrogen replacement therapy (Li et al., 2013).

Joint trauma is strongly associated with the development of OA. The risk of developing OA is reported to be as high as 75% and with the risk to increase by more than 20-fold with articular fractures (Schenker et al., 2014). The exact mechanism for developing posttraumatic OA is not well understood. However, cartilage trauma has been shown to lead to chondrocyte death, matrix disruption and release of proinflammatory cytokines and reactive oxygen species that lead to further cell death and extracellular matrix disruption. In addition, the chronic joint overload secondary to posttraumatic instability, incongruity and malalignment may also play a role in the development of posttraumatic OA (Schenker et al., 2014).

Joint instability induced by resection of the anterior cruciate ligament, leading to OA, has been demonstrated in animal experimentation (Brandt et al., 2009). In humans, significant increase in the risk of developing knee OA has been demonstrated, after meniscal rupture and repair, partial or complete rupture of the anterior cruciate ligament (Gillquist & Messner, 1999). However, the development of OA may be as a result of altered muscle strength proprioception and joint kinematics secondary to instability. Hall et al. (2012) have shown a knee flexor strength reduction in subjects with anterior cruciate ligament reconstruction and alteration in the knee joint loading. This has been shown to increase the compressive loading of the articular cartilage. Reduced strength of the quadriceps muscle has been implicated in the onset of OA in animal studies (Herzog & Longino, 2007). Regarding the knee, the strength and seamless function of quadriceps, as well as the other muscles in the lower limb, are crucial for the protection of the joint. The muscles act as shock absorbers, absorbing significant loads when they work eccentrically during every day activity (Brandt et al., 2009). A reduction of the capacity of the muscle to adsorb these loads, leads to excessive loading of the articular cartilage and subchondral bone and eventual degeneration (Brandt et al., 2009). Furthermore, microincoordination of neuromuscular control of subjects with knee pain, termed 'microklutziness', seems to cause repetitive impulse loading in the joint which leads to OA (Radin et al., 1991).

Age-related changes promote the development of OA (Loeser et al., 2016). With ageing there is a decline in muscle mass, a reduction in strength and endurance, and deterioration of motor and locomotor skills (McCarthy et al., 2015). In addition, there is a reduction in the organization and number of cortical cells and fibres in the white matter of the brain. A reduction in peripheral proprioceptive fibres and loss of the efficacy of the afferent transmission to the muscles lead to deteriorating proprioception (McCarthy et al., 2015). These changes in muscle strength and coordination may be contributing to the high risk of developing OA with advanced age. However, changes at the joint, relating to ageing, such as increase matrix calcification and increase accumulation to advanced glycation end products, may directly contribute to cartilage degeneration (McCarthy et al., 2015).

KNOWLEDGE CHECK

1. Summarize articular cartilage changes in OA.
2. What is the impact of ageing as a contributor to OA?

Production of Symptoms

Symptoms from joint dysfunction are most commonly a pain or an ache. Other symptoms include soreness, pulling and apprehension by the patient to move further into range. Symptoms can come on at any point or increase through the joint range of movement and/or at the end of the range of joint movement. Sometimes a symptom is felt only during a part of the range through a particular arc of the movement and is referred to as an 'arc or catch of pain'. More commonly, symptoms are produced some time during the range and increase towards the limit of the range. The symptom may be sufficiently intense to be the cause of the limitation in range, depicted as P_2 on a movement diagram (Fig. 2.32), or may reach a particular intensity at the limit of range (P'). Symptoms may be produced in a joint with 'normal', hypomobile or hypermobile range of movement, with or without altered quality of movement. For further information on movement diagrams, see Ryder and Barnard 2024.

Nociception and Pain

Most of the tissues that make up a joint (capsule, ligament, articular disc, meniscus and fat pad) are innervated (McDougall, 2006); in fact, the only structure that is not innervated is the avascular articular cartilage (McDougall & Linton, 2012). All of these tissues are therefore capable of being a source of pain. The fibres that signal pain are type IV, an unmyelinated meshwork, usually associated with blood vessels, or myelinated, type III fibres with unmyelinated free nerve terminals lying between the collagen and elastic fibres of the connective tissue in which they lie (McDougall, 2006). These fibres are supplied by myelinated Aδ and unmyelinated C fibres.

Nociceptors in joint tissues can be activated by a noxious mechanical force or chemical stimulus (Jessell & Kelly, 1991). To produce the sensation of pain, this noxious stimulus must be transduced to a relevant neural neurophysiological signal (Giordano, 2005). The primary afferent fibres for pain are the Aδ and C fibres. The Aδ fibres are fast-conducting myelinated fibres that are modality specific (e.g. Aδ fibres respond to intense mechanical or thermal stimulus). The Aδ fibres have a small receptive field producing sharp, localized and well-defined pain (Giordano, 2005). In contrast, C fibres are thin, unmyelinated slow-conducting fibres, and they have a broad receptive field and thus produce a poorly localized, burning, throbbing, gnawing pain. C fibres are polymodal, responding to mechanical, thermal and chemical stimuli (Giordano, 2005).

Mechanical pain (Box 2.3) occurs when certain movements stress injured tissue or when a noxious

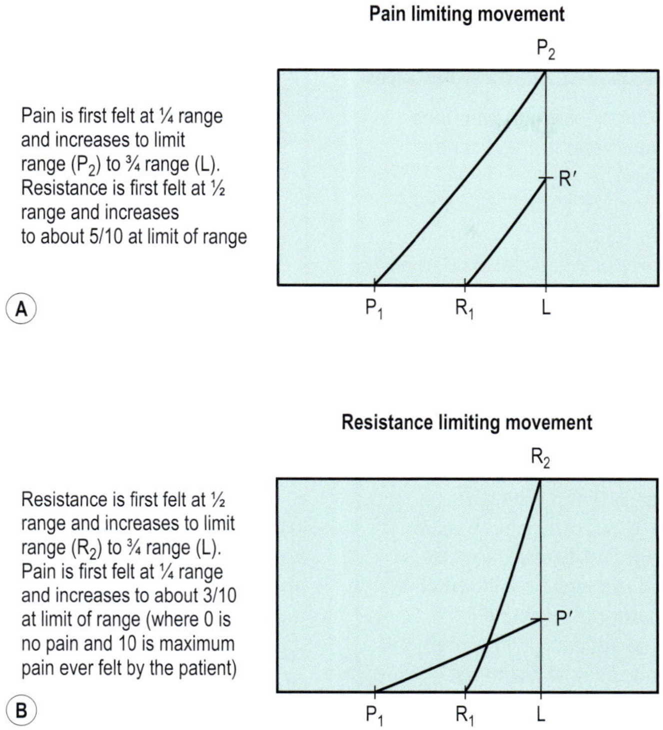

Fig. 2.32 Movement diagram depicting (A) P_2 with some resistance and normal range, and (B) P′ and resistance limiting movement.

movement or stress is applied to a joint, increasing the mechanical deformation and thus dramatically increasing the firing rate of nociceptors which the central nervous system interprets as pain (McDougall, 2006). This mechanical pain is present in the absence of inflammation and transmitted by the fast-conducting Aδ fibres. Thus with mechanical pain, there are particular movements which aggravate and ease the pain, sometimes referred to as 'on/off pain'. The magnitude of the mechanical deformation may be directly related to the magnitude of nociceptor activity (Garell et al., 1996).

Chemical nociceptive pain can be produced by the chemicals released as a result of inflammation, ischaemia or activity of the sympathetic nervous system (Gifford, 1998).

Tissue injury causes release of fatty acids and free ions from damaged cell membranes. This release activates a chain of reactions inducing an inflammatory cascade and production of chemicals that affect the sensitivity of the nociceptors and/or modify the configurational state of their ion channels, thus reducing the nociceptors' membrane thresholds (Giordano, 2005). This phenomenon is called peripheral sensitization (Cousing & Power, 2003).

This sensitization of nociceptors leads to phenomena of hyperalgesia (termed 'primary hyperalgesia'), where there is heightened pain intensity as a response to a noxious stimulus, and phenomena of 'allodynia', where innocuous stimuli, over the area of peripheral sensitization, are causing pain (McDougall, 2006).

Continuous stimulation of nociceptors causes an antidromic impulse causing the release of inflammatory mediators from the nerve fibre into the target tissues, causing in turn local inflammatory responses resulting in vasodilation and swelling in a process termed neurogenic inflammation (Butler, 2000; Giordano, 2005). Some joint afferents and some nociceptors have been found to contain proinflammatory chemicals (Levine et al., 1985a, 1985b; Salo & Theriault, 1997); this suggests that mechanoreceptors and nociceptors may contribute to the development of joint inflammation (Levine et al., 1985a; Holzer, 1988).

Normally, the nociceptors' high threshold causes some of them to become 'silent nociceptors'; that is, they may never fire (Butler, 2000; McDougall, 2006). However, joint injury and inflammation cause silent nociceptors to become active and hyperresponsive to

BOX 2.3 Clinical Features of Mechanical, Inflammatory and Ischaemic Pain

Mechanical	Specific movements/actions aggravating or easing the pain Intensity of stimulus and pain are related Usually pain is localized (small receptive field)
Inflammatory	May be associated with swelling redness and heat Pain may be present at rest Hyperalgesia/allodynia as a response to stimulus Diffuse pain areas/not localized (large receptive field) Close association with acute pain and tissue damage Good response to antiinflammatory medication
Ischaemic	Pain associated with prolonged and unusual postures Rapid reduction of symptoms with change of position Worsening of symptoms at the end of the day or after accumulation of activity Usually no evidence of acute tissue injury Poor response to antiinflammatory medication

Butler (2000).

normal and noxious stimulus by increasing their firing frequency. This increased sensitivity and firing frequency is interpreted by the central nervous system as pain, causing the phenomena of hyperalgesia and allodynia in acutely inflamed joints (McDougall, 2006). Activated silent nociceptors and sensory nerves may also continue to fire spontaneously in the absence of any mechanical stimulation. This accounts for the pain at rest experienced by patients with arthritis (McDougall, 2006).

In addition to the peripheral sensitization, prolonged nociceptive input drives changes in the dorsal horn that lead to the phenomenon of central sensitization. There is a reduction of the threshold so that stimulations arriving in the dorsal horn that are not normally noxious will activate neurons that transmit nociceptive information. Another change involves the increase in responsiveness of the neurons so that there is an increase in duration and magnitude of the stimuli. In addition, there is an expansion of the receptive field so that neurons will respond to nociceptive stimulation coming from areas outside the ones they normally serve (Butler, 2000; Cousing & Power, 2003). At the periphery, these changes result in an area of hyperalgesia and allodynia, with no change to thermal threshold, extending to uninjured tissues surrounding the site of injury or inflammation. This phenomenon is termed secondary hyperalgesia (Meyer, 1995; Cousing & Power, 2003).

TABLE 2.8 Degenerative Versus Inflammatory Arthropathy

Parameter	Degenerative	Inflammatory
Exercise	Worse	Better
Rest	Better (but stiffness may follow prolonged periods of rest)	Worse
Morning stiffness	<30 min	>30 min
Night pain	Not disturbing sleep	Disturbing sleep
Age of onset	Usually >40 years	<40 years

Clinical features of inflammatory pain are listed in Box 2.3 (Butler, 2000). More specifically, joint inflammatory arthropathy symptoms also include pain on waking in the morning which improves with activity but gets worse with rest and disturbs night sleep (Rudwaleit et al., 2006; Sieper et al., 2009; Walker & Williamson, 2009; Bailly et al., 2014). A comparison of the clinical features of degenerative (Gaskell, 2013) versus inflammatory arthropathy is displayed in Table 2.8.

Ischaemic nociceptive pain is caused by a lowered pH (acidosis) in tissues (Issberner et al., 1996), which stimulates nociceptor activity (Steen et al., 1995). Lowered pH level is frequently related to both painful ischaemic conditions and painful inflammatory conditions (Steen et al., 1995; Issberner et al., 1996). The clinical features of ischaemic pain are listed in Box 2.3 (Butler, 2000). In the presence of tissue injury or inflammation, sympathetic nervous system activity can maintain the perception of pain or enhance nociception in inflamed tissue. Sympathetically maintained pain can occur with complex regional pain syndromes and may play a part in chronic arthritis and soft-tissue trauma (Raja et al., 1999).

Clinicians must also be aware of the possibility of joint infection, referred to as septic arthritis, which can occur in both natural and artificial joints. A number of possible organisms (bacterial, fungal or viral) can be responsible, and possible associated factors are recent surgery or injection, human immunodeficiency virus (HIV) infection, immune deficiency, intravenous drug use or pre-existing systemic inflammatory arthritis. Local signs of inflammation will be present, as well as systemic signs such as fever and chills.

Although the commonest symptom from a joint is pain, it is essential to appreciate that the perception of pain occurs in the central nervous system and is multidimensional with sensory, physiological, affective, cognitive, behavioural and sociocultural factors (Ryder and Barnard 2024, Chapter 9).

KNOWLEDGE CHECK
1. How do C fibres and Aδ fibres differ in their structure, function and output?
2. How would you define the term allodynia?
3. What are the clinical features of inflammatory pain?

Pain Referral Areas

An understanding of pain referral from joint structures informs clinical reasoning. Cervical spine discs are capable of referring pain to distal axial and extremity regions (Slipman et al., 2005) (Fig. 2.33).

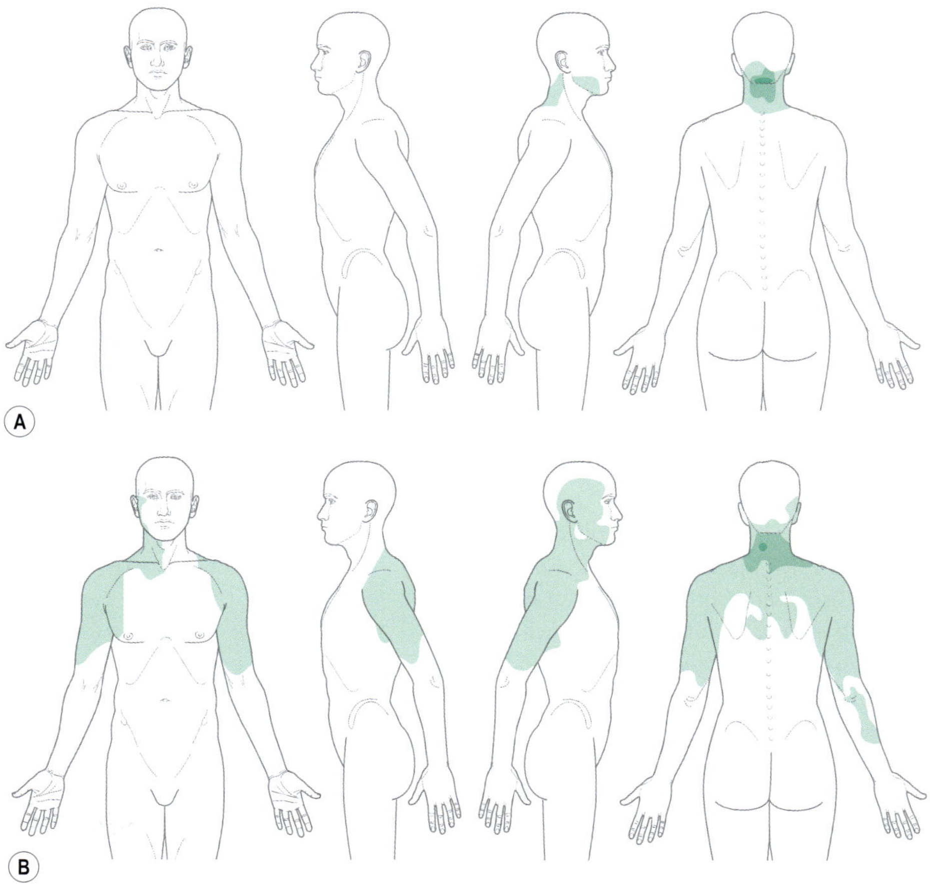

Fig. 2.33 Discography-produced pain referral map. (A) C2–C3 discogram pain referral map. (B) C4–C5 discogram pain referral map. (C) C6–C7 discogram pain referral map. (D) C7–T1 discogram pain referral map. (*From Slipman et al., 2005, with permission.*)

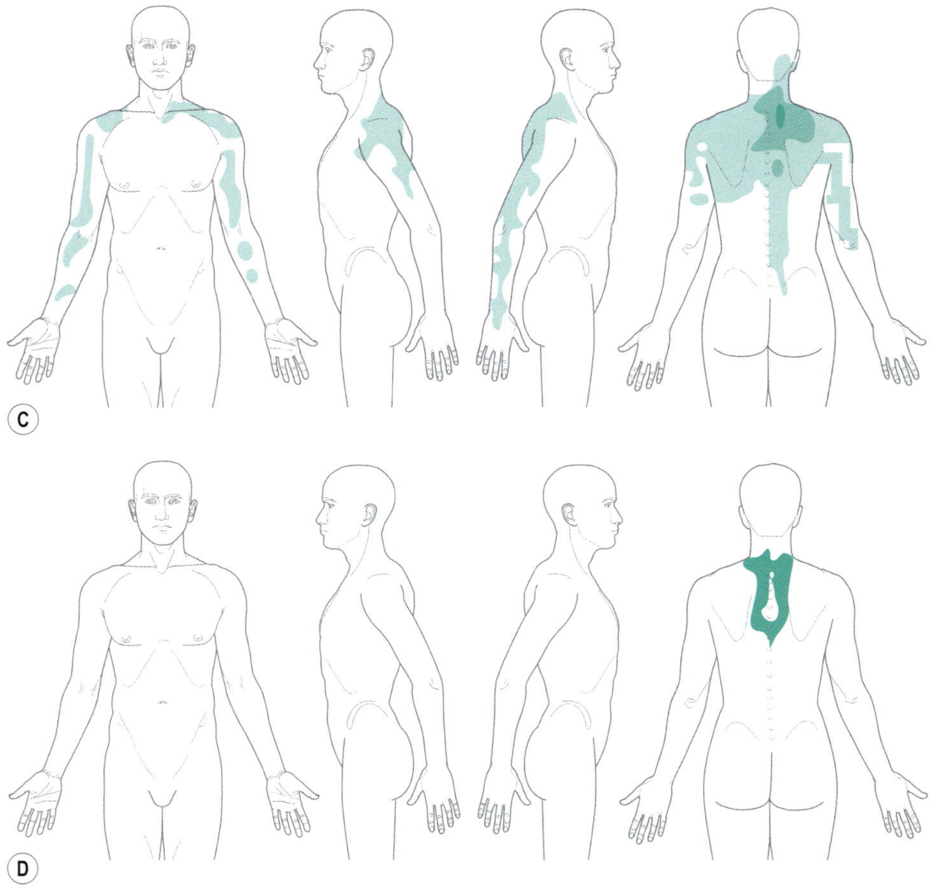

Fig. 2.33 cont'd (C) C6–C7 discogram pain referral map. (D) C7–T1 discogram pain referral map. (*From Slipman et al., 2005, with permission.*)

Cephalad cervical spine facets refer pain closer to the level as the painful joint. More caudal levels refer pain more distally and caudally (Dwyer et al., 1990; Fukui et al., 1996) (Fig. 2.34).

Common areas of lumbar facet joint pain referral are shown in Figs. 2.35 and 2.36 (Marks, 1989; Fukui et al., 1997; Jung et al., 2007). Absence of referred pain does not exclude facet joints as a cause of symptoms, whilst coccygeal pain is unlikely to be caused by facet joint pathology (Marks, 1989). In agreement with previous studies (McCall et al., 1979; Marks, 1989), Fukui et al. (1997) found significant overlap of pain referral regions from facet joints of different levels, which makes interpretation of this information in the clinical field difficult.

SIJ pain explored in 10 asymptomatic subjects using radiopaque injection into the joint (Fortin et al., 1994a)

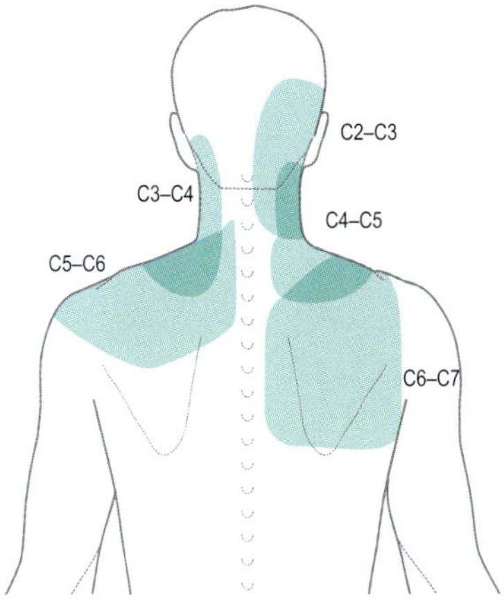

Fig. 2.34 Distribution of pain following contrast medium injections in the cervical spine zygapophyseal joints of normal volunteers. (*From Dwyer et al., 1990, with permission.*)

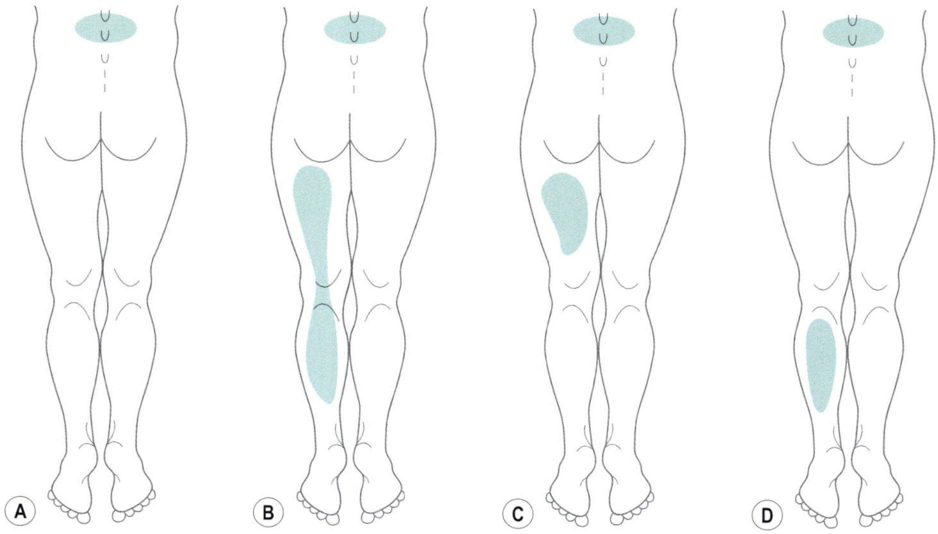

Fig. 2.35 (A–D) Types of pain distribution patterns in lumbar zygapophyseal joint arthropathy. (*From Jung et al., 2007, with permission.*)

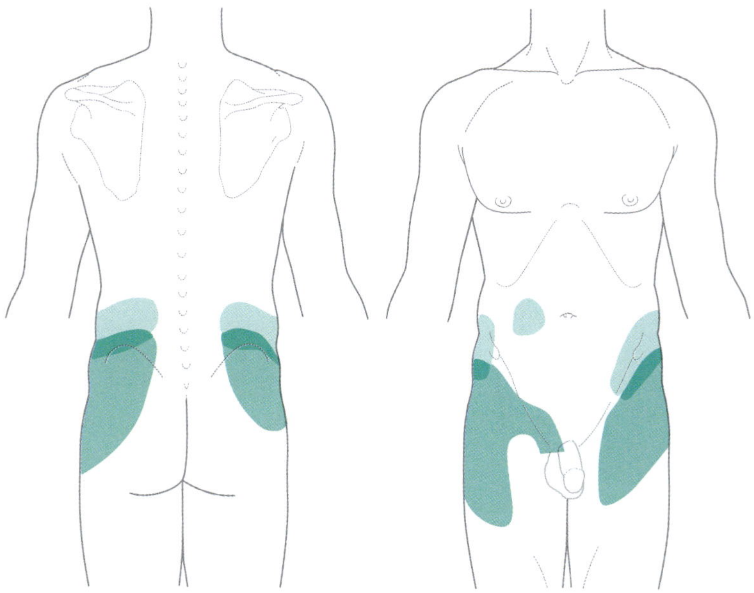

Fig. 2.36 Distribution of pain following injection of saline into the L1–L2 (lighter shading) and L4–L5 (darker shading) zygapophyseal joint. (*After McCall et al., 1979, with permission.*)

identified a fairly local distribution around the posterior superior iliac spine. However, this area of referral could not be used to identify accurately patients with SIJ pain (Fortin et al., 1994b). Indeed, in a study by Dreyfuss et al. (1996), the SIJ pain pattern was found to be widespread, covering wide areas of the pelvis and lower limbs. However, in contrast with the pain arising from the lumbar spine, SIJ pain was rarely referring above the level of L5. A more recent study of mapping of the pain from patients with confirmed SIJ pathology has found more concentrated but still wide pain referral areas (Jung et al., 2007) (Fig. 2.37).

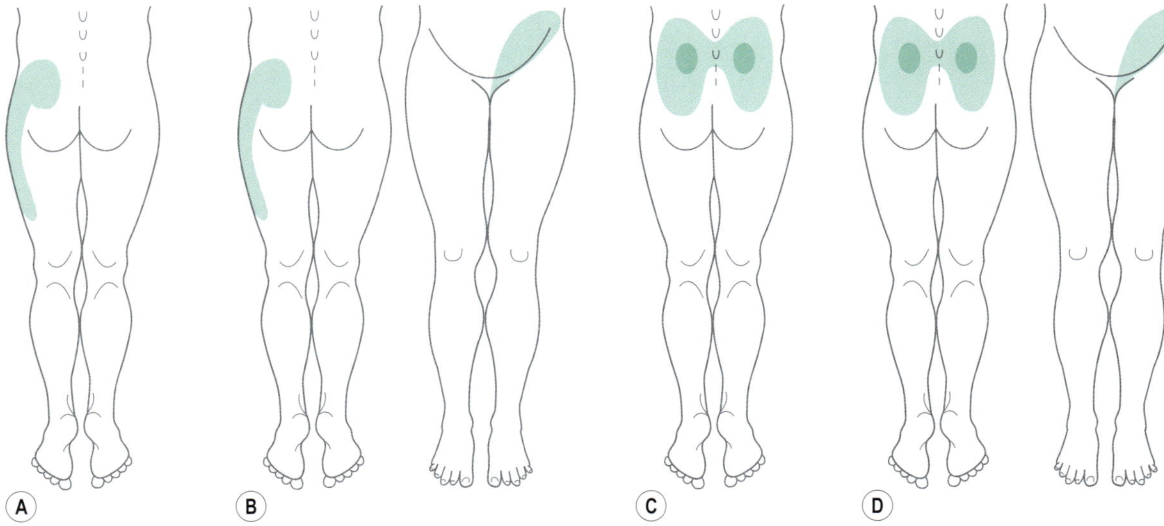

Fig. 2.37 (A–D) Types of pain distribution patterns in sacroiliac joint arthropathy. (*From Jung et al., 2007, with permission.*)

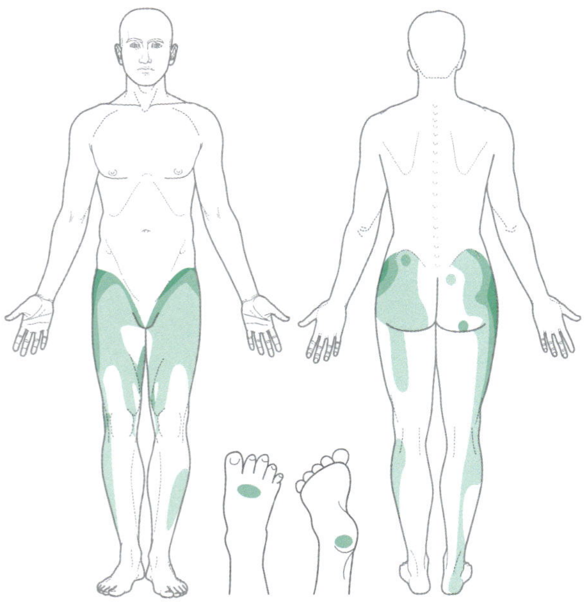

Fig. 2.38 Distribution of pain from the hip joint. (*From Lesher et al., 2008, with permission.*)

Hip joint pathology tends to produce pain that is mostly localized around the groin, anterior hip joint, lateral hip and buttock (Khan et al., 2004; Lesher et al., 2008; Arnold et al., 2011). However, hip OA can refer pain below the knee joint (Khan et al., 2004; Lesher et al., 2008) (Fig. 2.38), whilst there are clinical cases where hip pathology can cause knee pain without hip pain (Emms et al., 2002).

Pain arising from joints in the upper or lower limb tends to be localized around the joint. A study by Bayam et al. (2011) has shown a variety of quality and distribution of pain in the upper limb produced by different shoulder girdle joint pathologies (Fig. 2.39).

SUMMARY

This chapter outlined the principles of the joint function and dysfunction. The aim was to provide a background of the physiological function of the joints

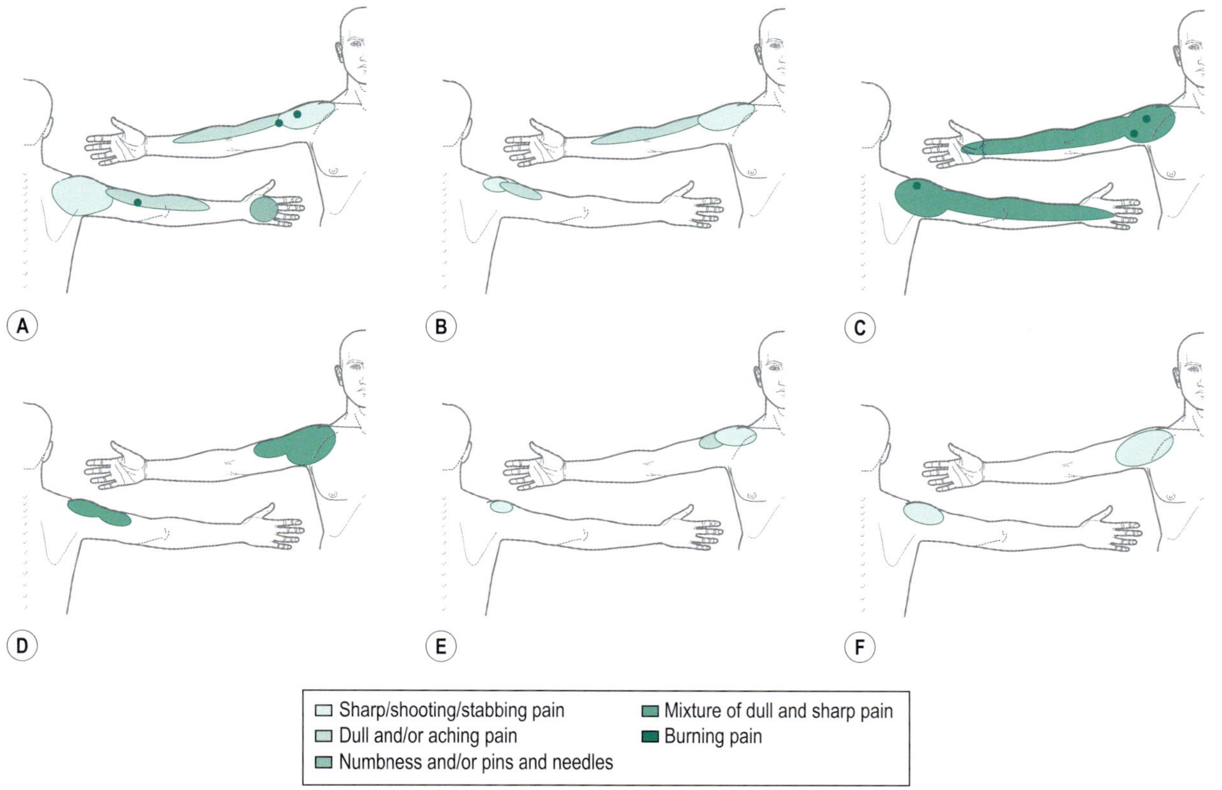

Fig. 2.39 Patterns of referred pain from different pathologies of the shoulder. (A) Impingement syndrome, (B) rotator cuff tear, (C) glenohumeral joint arthritis, (D) instability, (E) acromioclavicular joint pathology and (F) calcific tendonitis. *(From Bayam et al., 2011, with permission.)*

and the tissues that comprise them, pathological processes that the joint may be subject to and the symptoms that these processes may produce. It also aimed to provide rationale for the application of joint treatment, the principles of which are discussed on the following chapter.

REVIEW AND REVISE QUESTIONS

1. What type of joint is the knee? Explain why.
2. What type of loading should be used to achieve greater lengthening of a ligament?
3. Name two ball-and-socket joints.
4. When convex moves on concave, what direction is the gliding of the joint surface?
5. Describe a close kinetic and an open kinetic chain exercise for the hip.
6. Why would you be concerned if you ever find an empty end-feel on an assessment?
7. How does joint pain affect the muscle?
8. What is hypermobility, and what is instability?
9. What is a capsular pattern?
10. What are the differences between hyperalgesia and allodynia?
11. Which pain afferents can be sensitized by chemical stimulus.

REFERENCES

Adams, M.A., Bogduk, N., Burton, K., et al., 2013. The Biomechanics of Back Pain, third ed. Churchill Livingstone, Edinburgh.

Ageberg, E., 2002. Consequences of a ligament injury on neuromuscular function and relevance to rehabilitation – using the anterior cruciate ligament-injured knee as model. J. Electromyogr. Kinesiol. 12, 205–212.

Akeson, W.H., Amiel, D., Mechanic, G.L., et al., 1977. Collagen cross-linking alterations in joint contractures: changes in the reducible cross-links in periarticular connective tissue collagen after nine weeks of immobilization. Connect. Tissue Res. 5, 15–19.

Akeson, W.H., Amiel, D., Abel, M.F., et al., 1987. Effects of immobilization on joints. Clin. Orthop. Relat. Res. 219, 28–37.

Akeson, W.H., Woo, S.L.-Y., Amiel, D., et al., 1973. The connective tissue response to immobility: biochemical changes in periarticular connective tissue of the immobilized rabbit knee. Clin. Orthop. Relat. Res. 93, 356–362.

Albright, D.J., Zimny, M.L., Dabezies, E., 1987. Mechanoreceptors in the human medial meniscus. Anat. Record 218, 6A–7A.

Amiel, D., Akeson, W.H., Harwood, F.L., et al., 1983. Stress deprivation effect on metabolic turnover of the medial collateral ligament collagen. A comparison between nine- and 12-week immobilization. Clin. Orthop. Relat. Res. 172, 265–270.

Ando, A., Hagiwara, Y., Onoda, Y., et al., 2010. Distribution of type A and B synoviocytes in the adhesive and shortened synovial membrane during immobilization of the knee joint in rats. Tohoku J. Exp. Med. 221, 161–168.

Arnold, D.R., Keene, J.S., Blankenbaker, D.G., et al., 2011. Hip pain referral patterns in patients with labral tears: analysis based on intra-articular anesthetic injections, hip arthroscopy, and a new pain 'circle' diagram. Phys. Sportsmed. 39, 29–35.

Asahara, H., Inui, M., Lotz, M.K., 2017. Tendons and ligaments: connecting developmental biology to musculoskeletal disease pathogenesis. J. Bone Miner. Res. 32, 1773–1782.

Atkins, E., Kerr, J., Goodlad, E., 2010. A Practical Approach to Orthopaedic Medicine: Assessment, Diagnosis and Treatment, third ed. Churchill Livingstone Elsevier, Edinburgh.

Bailly, F., Maigne, J.-Y., Genevay, S., et al., 2014. Inflammatory pain pattern and pain with lumbar extension associated with Modic 1 changes on MRI: a prospective case-control study of 120 patients. Eur. Spine J. 23, 493–497.

Baker-Lepain, J.C., Lane, N.E., 2010. Relationship between joint shape and the development of osteoarthritis. Curr. Opin. Rheumatol. 22, 538–543.

Bayam, L., Ahmad, M.A., Naqui, S.Z., et al., 2011. Pain mapping for common shoulder disorders. Am. J. Orthop. (Belle Mead NJ) 40, 353–358.

Bogduk, N., Mercer, S., 2000. Biomechanics of the cervical spine. I: Normal kinematics. Clin. Biomech. (Bristol, Avon) 15, 633–648.

Bogduk, N., 2005. Clinical Anatomy of the Lumbar Spine and Sacrum, fourth ed. Elsevier Churchill Livingstone, Edinburgh.

Boisgontier, M.P., Swinnen, S.P., 2014. Proprioception in the cerebellum. Front. Hum. Neurosci. 8, 212.

Brandt, K.D., Dieppe, P., Radin, E., 2009. Etiopathogenesis of osteoarthritis. Med. Clin. North Am. 93 (1–24), xv.

Brouwer, G.M., van Tol, A.W., Bergink, A.P., et al., 2007. Association between valgus and varus alignment and the development and progression of radiographic osteoarthritis of the knee. Arthritis Rheum 56, 1204–1211.

Butler, D.S., 2000. The Sensitive Nervous System. Noigroup Publications, Adelaide, Australia.

Callaghan, M.J., Parkes, M.J., Hutchinson, C.E., et al., 2015. A randomised trial of a brace for patellofemoral osteoarthritis targeting knee pain and bone marrow lesions. Ann. Rheum. Dis. 74, 1164–1170.

Callaghan, M.J., Oldham, J.A., 2004. Quadriceps atrophy: to what extent does it exist in patellofemoral pain syndrome? Br. J. Sports Med. 38, 295–299.

Callaghan, M.J., Parkes, M.J., Hutchinson, C.E., et al., 2014. Factors associated with arthrogenous muscle inhibition in patellofemoral osteoarthritis. Osteoarthritis Cartilage 22, 742–746.

Chaitow, L., 2013. Understanding mechanotransduction and biotensegrity from an adaptation perspective. J. Bodyw. Mov. Ther. 17, 141–142.

Chancey, V.C., Ottaviano, D., Myers, B.S., et al., 2007. A kinematic and anthropometric study of the upper cervical spine and the occipital condyles. J. Biomech. 40, 1953–1959.

Chiquet, M., Renedo, A.S., Huber, F., et al., 2003. How do fibroblasts translate mechanical signals into changes in extracellular matrix production? Matrix Biol 22, 73–80.

Cook, C., 2003. Coupling behavior of the lumbar spine: a literature review. J. Man. Manip. Ther. 11, 137–145.

Cousing, M., Power, I., 2003. Acute and postoperative pain. In: Handbook of Pain Management: A Clinical Companion to Wall and Melzack's 'Textbook of Pain'. Churchill Livingstone, London.

Cuomo, F., Birdzell, M.G., Zuckerman, J.D., 2005. The effect of degenerative arthritis and prosthetic arthroplasty on shoulder proprioception. J. Shoulder Elbow Surg. 14, 345–348.

Cyriax, J., 1982. Textbook of Orthopaedic Medicine: Diagnosis of Soft Tissue Lesions, eighth ed. Baillière Tindall, London.

Delahunt, E., Monaghan, K., Caulfield, B., 2006. Altered neuromuscular control and ankle joint kinematics during walking in subjects with functional instability of the ankle joint. Am. J. Sports Med. 34, 1970–1976.

Drake, R., Vogl, A.W., Mitchell, A.W., 2015. Gray's Anatomy for Students, third ed. Elsevier Churchill Livingstone, Philadelphia.

Dreyfuss, P., Michaelsen, M., Pauza, K., et al., 1996. The value of medical history and physical examination in diagnosing sacroiliac joint pain. Spine 21, 2594–2602.

Dunn, S.L., Olmedo, M.L., 2016. Mechanotransduction: relevance to physical therapist practice – understanding our ability to affect genetic expression through mechanical forces. Phys. Ther. 96, 712–721.

Dwyer, A., Aprill, C., Bogduk, N., 1990. Cervical zygapophyseal joint pain patterns. I: a study in normal volunteers. Spine 15, 453–457.

Edwards, B.C., 1999. Manual of Combined Movements, second ed. Butterworth-Heinemann, Oxford.

Emms, N.W., O'Connor, M., Montgomery, S.C., 2002. Hip pathology can masquerade as knee pain in adults. Age Ageing 31, 67–69.

Evans, E.B., Eggers, G.W.N., Butler, J.K., et al., 1960. Experimental immobilization and remobilization of rat knee joints. J. Bone Joint Surg. Am. 42, 737–758.

Felson, D.T., Chaisson, C.E., Hill, C.L., et al., 2001. The association of bone marrow lesions with pain in knee osteoarthritis. Ann. Intern. Med. 134, 541–549.

Ferrell, W.R., Tennant, N., Sturrock, R.D., et al., 2004. Amelioration of symptoms by enhancement of proprioception in patients with joint hypermobility syndrome. Arthritis Rheumatol 50, 3323–3328.

Fortier, S., Basset, F.A., 2012. The effects of exercise on limb proprioceptive signals. J. Electromyogr. Kinesiol. 22, 795–802.

Fortin, J.D., Aprill, C.N., Ponthieux, B., et al., 1994b. Sacroiliac joint: pain referral maps upon applying a new injection/arthrography technique. Part II: clinical evaluation. Spine 19, 1483–1489.

Fortin, J.D., Dwyer, A.P., West, S., et al., 1994a. Sacroiliac joint: pain referral maps upon applying a new injection/arthrography technique. Part I: asymptomatic volunteers. Spine 19, 1475–1482.

Frank, C.B., 2004. Ligament structure, physiology and function. J. Musculoskelet. Neuronal Interact. 4, 199.

Frank, C.B., Shrive, N.G., 1999. Ligament. In: Nigg, B.M., Herzog, W. (Eds.), Biomechanics of the Musculo-Skeletal System, second ed. John Wiley, Chichester, pp. 107–126.

Freeman, M.A., Wyke, B., 1967. The innervation of the knee joint. An anatomical and histological study in the cat. J. Anat. 101, 505–532.

Freeman, S., Mascia, A., Mcgill, S., 2013. Arthrogenic neuromusculature inhibition: a foundational investigation of existence in the hip joint. Clin. Biomech. (Bristol, Avon) 28, 171–177.

Fujii, R., Sakaura, H., Mukai, Y., et al., 2007. Kinematics of the lumbar spine in trunk rotation: in vivo three-dimensional analysis using magnetic resonance imaging. Eur. Spine J. 16, 1867–1874.

Fukui, S., Ohseto, K., Shiotani, M., et al., 1996. Referred pain distribution of the cervical zygapophyseal joints and cervical dorsal rami. Pain 68, 79–83.

Fukui, S., Ohseto, K., Shiotani, M., et al., 1997. Distribution of referred pain from the lumbar zygapophyseal joints and dorsal rami. Clin. J. Pain 13, 303–307.

Garell, P.C., McGillis, S.L.B., Greenspan, J.D., 1996. Mechanical response properties of nociceptors innervating feline hairy skin. J. Neurophysiol. 75, 1177–1189.

Gaskell, L., 2013. Musculoskeletal assessment. In: Porter, S.B. (Ed.), Tidy's Physiotherapy, fifteenth ed. Churchill Livingstone, Elsevier, London.

Gifford, L., 1998. Pain. In: Pitt-Brooke, J., Reid, H., Lockwood, J., et al. (Eds.), Rehabilitation of Movement: Theoretical Basis of Clinical Practice. W.B. Saunders, London, pp. 196–232.

Gillquist, J., Messner, K., 1999. Anterior cruciate ligament reconstruction and the long term incidence of gonarthrosis. Sports Med 27, 143–156.

Giordano, J., 2005. The neuroscience of pain and analgesia. In: Boswell, M.V., Cole, B.E. (Eds.), Weiner's Pain Management: A Practical Guide for Clinicians, seventh ed. Informa, New York.

Grahame, R., 2003. Hypermobility and hypermobility syndrome. In: Keer, R., Grahame, R. (Eds.), Hypermobility Syndrome: Recognition and Management for Physiotherapists. Butterworth-Heinemann, London.

Hagert, E., Persson, J.K., Werner, M., et al., 2009. Evidence of wrist proprioceptive reflexes elicited after stimulation of the scapholunate interosseous ligament. J. Hand Surg. Am. 34, 642–651.

Hakim, A., Grahame, R., 2003. Joint hypermobility. Best Pract. Res. Clin. Rheumatol. 17, 989–1004.

Hall, M., Stevermer, C.A., Gillette, J.C., 2012. Gait analysis post anterior cruciate ligament reconstruction: knee osteoarthritis perspective. Gait Posture 36, 56–60.

Hall, M., Stevermer, C.A., Gillette, J.C., 2015. Muscle activity amplitudes and co-contraction during stair ambulation following anterior cruciate ligament reconstruction. J. Electromyogr. Kinesiol. 25, 298–304.

Hengeveld, E., Banks, K., 2014a. Maitland's Vertebral Manipulation: Management of Neuromuscular Disorders, eighth ed, vol. 1. Elsevier Churchill Livingstone, Edinburgh.

Hengeveld, E., Banks, K., 2014b. Maitland's Peripheral Manipulation: Management of Neuromusculoskeletal Disorders, eighth ed, vol. 2. Elsevier Churchill Livingstone, Edinburgh, p. 5.

Hertel, J., Kaminski, T.W., 2005. Second International Ankle Symposium, October 15–16, 2004, Newark, Delaware. J. Orthop. Sports Phys. Ther. 35, A1–A28.

Hertling, D., Kessler, R., 2006b. Assessment of musculoskeletal disorders and concepts of management. In: Hertling, D., Kessler, R.M. (Eds.), Management of Common Musculoskeletal Disorders: Physical Therapy, Principles and Methods. Lippincott, Williams and Wilkins, Philadelphia, pp. 61–107.

Hertling, D., Kessler, R.M., 2006a. Arthrology. In: Hertling, D., Kessler, R. (Eds.), Management of Common Musculoskeletal Disorders: Physical Therapy, Principles and Methods. Lippincott, Williams and Wilkins, Philadelphia, pp. 27–52.

Herzog, W., Longino, D., 2007. The role of muscles in joint degeneration and osteoarthritis. J. Biomech. 40 (Suppl 1), S54–63.

Herzog, W., Longino, D., 2007. The role of muscles in joint degeneration and osteoarthritis. J. Biomech. 40 (Suppl. 1), S54–S63.

Hewett, T.E., Paterno, M.V., Myer, G.D., 2002. Strategies for enhancing proprioception and neuromuscular control of the knee. Clin. Orthop. Relat. Res. 402, 76–94.

Hills, B.A., 1995. Remarkable anti-wear properties of joint surfactant. Ann. Biomed. Eng. 23, 112–115.

Hills, B.A., Crawford, R.W., 2003. Normal and prosthetic synovial joints are lubricated by surface-active phospholipid: a hypothesis. J. Arthroplasty 18, 499–505.

Hortobágyi, T., DeVita, P., 2000. Muscle pre- and coactivity during downward stepping are associated with leg stiffness in aging. J. Electromyogr. Kinesiol. 10, 117–126.

Hughes, T., Rochester, P., 2008. The effects of proprioceptive exercise and taping on proprioception in subjects with functional ankle instability: a review of the literature. Phys. Ther. Sport 9, 136–147.

Humphrey, J.D., Dufresne, E.R., Schwartz, M.A., 2014. Mechanotransduction and extracellular matrix homeostasis. Nat. Rev. Mol. Cell Biol. 15, 802.

Ikeda, S., Tsumura, H., Torisu, T., 2005. Age-related quadriceps-dominant muscle atrophy and incident radiographic knee osteoarthritis. J. Orthop. Sci. 10, 121–126.

Iqbal, K., Khan, M.Y., Minhas, L.A., 2012. Effects of immobilisation and re-mobilisation on superficial zone of articular cartilage of patella in rats. J. Pak. Med. Assoc. 62, 531-535.

Issberner, U., Reeh, P.W., Steen, K.H., 1996. Pain due to tissue acidosis: a mechanism for inflammatory and ischemic myalgia? Neurosci. Lett. 208, 191–194.

Jaumard, N.V., Welch, W.C., Winkelstein, B.A., 2011. Spinal facet joint biomechanics and mechanotransduction in normal, injury and degenerative conditions. J. Biomech. Eng. 133, 071010.

Jessell, T.M., Kelly, D.D., 1991. Pain and analgesia. In: Kandel, E.R., Schwartz, J.H., Jessell, T.M. (Eds.), Principles of Neural Science, third ed. Elsevier, New York, pp. 385–399.

Jung, J.H., Kim, H.I., Shin, D.A., et al., 2007. Usefulness of pain distribution pattern assessment in decision-making for the patients with lumbar zygapophyseal and sacroiliac joint arthropathy. J. Korean Med. Sci. 22, 1048–1054.

Kaltenborn, F.M., 2014. Manual Mobilization of the Joints: Joint Examination and Basic Treatment, eighth ed, vol. 1. The extremities. Olaf Norlis Bokhandel, Oslo.

Seki, K., Kizuka, T., Yamada, H., 2007. Reduction in maximal firing rate of motoneurons after 1-week immobilization of finger muscle in human subjects. J. Electromyogr. Kinesiol. 17, 113–120.

Kennedy, J.C., Alexander, I.J., Hayes, K.C., 1982. Nerve supply of the human knee and its functional importance. Am. J. Sports Med. 10, 329–335.

Khan, A.M., Mcloughlin, E., Giannakas, K., et al., 2004. Hip osteoarthritis: where is the pain? Ann. R. Coll. Surg. Engl. 86, 119–121.

Kim, H.-T., Kim, H.-J., Ahn, H.-Y., et al., 2016. An analysis of age-related loss of skeletal muscle mass and its significance on osteoarthritis in a Korean population. Korean J. Intern. Med. 31, 585–593.

Kim, W.H., Lee, S.-H., Lee, D.Y., 2011. Changes in the cross-sectional area of multifidus and psoas in unilateral sciatica caused by lumbar disc herniation. J. Korean Neurosurg. Soc. 50, 201–204.

Langevin, H.M., Bouffard, N.A., Fox, J.R., et al., 2011. Fibroblast cytoskeletal remodeling contributes to connective tissue tension. J. Cell Physiol. 226, 1166–1175.

Lee, D.G., 2003. The Thorax: An Integrated Approach. White Rock, BC, Canada, Orthopedic Physical Therapy.

Lee, S., Sakurai, T., Ohsako, M., et al., 2010. Tissue stiffness induced by prolonged immobilization of the rat knee joint and relevance of AGEs (pentosidine). Connect. Tissue Res. 51, 467–477.

Lesher, J.M., Dreyfuss, P., Hager, N., et al., 2008. Hip joint pain referral patterns: a descriptive study. Pain Med 9, 22–25.

Levangie, P.K., Norkin, C.C., 2011. Joint Structure and Function, a Comprehensive Analysis, fifth ed. F.A. Davis, Philadelphia.

Levick, J.R., 1983. Joint pressure-volume studies: their importance, design and interpretation. J. Rheumatol. 10, 353–357.

Levick, J.R., 1984. Blood flow and mass transport in synovial joints. In: Renkin, E.M., Michel, C.C. (Eds.), Handbook of

Physiology Section 2: The Cardiovascular System Volume IV: Microcirculation, Part 2. American Physiological Society, Bethesda, MD, pp. 917–947.
Levine, J.D., Dardick, S.J., Basbaum, A.I., et al., 1985a. Reflex neurogenic inflammation. I. Contribution of the peripheral nervous system to spatially remote inflammatory responses that follow injury. J. Neurosci. 5, 1380–1386.
Levine, J.D., Moskowitz, M.A., Basbaum, A.I., 1985b. The contribution of neurogenic inflammation in experimental arthritis. J. Immunol. 135, 843s–847s.
Li, G., Yin, J., Gao, J., et al., 2013. Subchondral bone in osteoarthritis: insight into risk factors and microstructural changes. Arthritis Res. Ther. 15, 223.
Loeser, R.F., Collins, J.A., Diekman, B.O., 2016. Ageing and the pathogenesis of osteoarthritis. Nat. Rev. Rheumatol. 12, 412–420.
Lundon, K., 2007. The effect of mechanical load on soft connective tissues. In: Hammer, W. (Ed.), Functional Soft-Tissue Examination and Treatment by Manual Methods, third ed. Jones and Bartlett, Boston, pp. 15–30.
MacConaill, M.A., 1953. The movements of bones and joints: 5. The significance of shape. J. Bone Joint Surg. Am. 35B, 290–297.
MacConaill, M.A., 1966. The geometry and algebra of articular kinematics. Biomed. Eng. 1, 205–211.
MacConaill, M.A., 1973. A structuro-functional classification of synovial articular units. Ir. J. Med. Sci. 142, 19–26.
Maldonado, D.C., Silva, M.C., Neto Sel, R., et al., 2013. The effects of joint immobilization on articular cartilage of the knee in previously exercised rats. J. Anat. 222, 518–525.
Malliou, P., Gioftsidou, A., Pafis, G., et al., 2012. Proprioception and functional deficits of partial meniscectomized knees. Eur. J. Phys. Rehabil. Med. 48, 231–236.
Marks, R., 1989. Distribution of pain provoked from lumbar facet joints and related structures during diagnostic spinal infiltration. Pain 39, 37–40.
McCall, I.W., Park, W.M., O'Brien, J.P., 1979. Induced pain referral from posterior lumbar elements in normal subjects. Spine 4, 441–446.
McCarthy, C., 2010. Combined Movement Theory: Rational Mobilization and Manipulation of the Vertebral Column. Churchill Livingstone, Edinburgh.
McCarthy, C., Money, A., Singer, K., 2015. Ageing and the musculoskeletal system. In: Jull, G., Moore, A., Falla, D., Lewis, J., Mccarthy, C., Sterling, M. (Eds.), Grieve's Modern Musculoskeletal Physiotherapy. Elsevier, London.
McDougall, J.J., 2006. Arthritis and pain. Neurogenic origin of joint pain. Arthritis Res. Ther. 8, 220.
McDougall, J.J., Linton, P., 2012. Neurophysiology of arthritis pain. Curr. Pain Headache Rep. 16, 485–491.
McGill, S.M., Grenier, S., Kavcic, N., et al., 2003. Coordination of muscle activity to assure stability of the lumbar spine. J. Electromyogr. Kinesiol. 13, 353–359.
McVey, E.D., Palmieri, R.M., Docherty, C.L., et al., 2005. Arthrogenic muscle inhibition in the leg muscles of subjects exhibiting functional ankle instability. Foot Ankle Int 26, 1055–1061.
Menard, D., 2000. The ageing athlete. In: Harries, M., Williams, C., Stanish, W. (Eds.), Oxford Textbook of Sports Medicine, second ed. Oxford University Press, Oxford, pp. 786–813.
Messner, K., 1999. The innervation of synovial joints. In: Archer, C.W., Caterson, B., Benjamin, M. (Eds.), Biology of the Synovial Joint. Harwood, Australia, pp. 405–421.
Messner, K., Gao, J., 1998. The menisci of the knee joint. Anatomical and functional characteristics, and a rationale for clinical treatment. J. Anat. 193, 161–178.
Meyer, R.A., 1995. Cutaneous hyperalgesia and primary afferent sensitization. Pulm. Pharmacol. 8, 187–193.
Middleditch, A., Oliver, J., 2005. Functional Anatomy of the Spine, second ed. Elsevier Butterworth-Heinemann, Edinburgh.
Milz, S., Ockert, B., Putz, R., 2009. Tenocytes and the extracellular matrix: a reciprocal relationship. Orthopade 38, 1071–1079.
Mow, V.C., Proctor, C.S., Kelly, M.A., 1989. Biomechanics of articular cartilage. In: Nordin, M., Frankel, V.H. (Eds.), Basic Biomechanics of the Musculoskeletal System, second ed. Lea & Febiger, Philadelphia, pp. 31–58.
Munn, J., Sullivan, S.J., Schneiders, A.G., 2010. Evidence of sensorimotor deficits in functional ankle instability: a systematic review with meta-analysis. J. Sci. Med. Sport 13, 2–12.
Myers, J.B., Lephart, S.M., 2000. The role of the sensorimotor system in the athletic shoulder. J. Athl. Train. 35, 351–363.
Myers, J.B., Wassinger, C.A., Lephart, S.M., 2006. Sensorimotor contribution to shoulder stability: effect of injury and rehabilitation. Man. Ther. 11, 197–201.
Nigg, B.M., 2000. Biomechanics as applied to sport. In: Harries, M., Williams, C., Stanish, W. (Eds.), Oxford Textbook of Sports Medicine, second ed. Oxford University Press, Oxford, pp. 153–171.
Nigg, B.M., Herzog, W., 2007. Biomechanics of the Musculo-Skeletal System, third ed. John Wiley, Chichester.
Nordin, M., Frankel, V.H., 1989. Basic Biomechanics of the Musculoskeletal System, second ed. Lea & Febiger, Philadelphia.
Nordin, M., Frankel, V.H., 2012. Basic Biomechanics of the Musculoskeletal System, fourth ed. Lippincott Williams & Wilkins, Baltimore.
Noyes, F.R., Butler, D.L., Paulos, L.E., et al., 1983. Intra-articular cruciate reconstruction. I: perspectives on graft strength, vascularization, and immediate motion after replacement. Clin. Orthop. Relat. Res. 172, 71–77.

Noyes, F.R., DeLucas, J.L., Torvik, P.J., 1974. Biomechanics of anterior cruciate ligament failure: an analysis of strain-rate sensitivity and mechanisms of failure in primates. J. Bone Joint Surg. Am. 56, 236–253.

Noyes, F.R., Grood, E.S., 1976. The strength of the anterior cruciate ligament in humans and rhesus monkeys, age-related and species-related changes. J. Bone Joint Surg. Am. 58, 1074–1082.

O'Hara, B.P., Urban, J.P.G., Maroudas, A., 1990. Influence of cyclic loading on the nutrition of articular cartilage. Ann. Rheum. Dis. 49, 536–539.

Palastanga, N., Soames, R., 2012. Anatomy and Human Movement: Structure and Function, sixth ed. Churchill Livingstone Elsevier, Edinburgh.

Palmieri, R.M., Ingersoll, C.D., Cordova, M.L., et al., 2003. The effect of simulated knee joint effusion on postural control in healthy subjects. Arch. Phys. Med. Rehabil. 84, 1076–1079.

Palmieri-Smith, R.M., Kreinbrink, J., Ashton-Miller, J.A., et al., 2007. Quadriceps inhibition induced by an experimental knee joint effusion affects knee joint mechanics during a single-legged drop landing. Am. J. Sports Med. 35, 1269–1275.

Panjabi, M.M., 1992a. The stabilizing system of the spine. Part 1. Function, dysfunction, adaptation, and enhancement. J. Spinal Disord. 5, 383–389.

Panjabi, M.M., 1992b. The stabilizing system of the spine. Part II. Neutral zone and instability hypothesis. J. Spinal Disord. 5, 390–396.

Panjabi, M.M., White, A.A., 2001. Biomechanics in the Musculoskeletal System. Churchill Livingstone, New York.

Pearcy, M., Portek, I., Shepherd, J., 1984. Three-dimensional X-ray analysis of normal movement in the lumbar spine. Spine 9, 294–297.

Pearcy, M.J., Tibrewal, S.B., 1984. Axial rotation and lateral bending in the normal lumbar spine measured by three-dimensional radiography. Spine 9, 582–587.

Powers, C.M., 2010. The influence of abnormal hip mechanics on knee injury: a biomechanical perspective. J. Orthop. Sports Phys. Ther. 40, 42–51.

Radin, E.L., Yang, K.H., Riegger, C., et al., 1991. Relationship between lower limb dynamics and knee joint pain. J. Orthop. Res. 9, 398–405.

Raja, S.N., Meyer, R.A., Ringkamp, M., et al., 1999. Peripheral neural mechanisms of nociception. In: Wall, P.D., Melzack, R. (Eds.), Textbook of Pain, fourth ed. Churchill Livingstone, Edinburgh.

Rice, D.A., McNair, P.J., Lewis, G.N., 2011. Mechanisms of quadriceps muscle weakness in knee joint osteoarthritis: the effects of prolonged vibration on torque and muscle activation in osteoarthritic and healthy control subjects. Arthritis Res. Ther. 13, R151.

Richie Jr., D.H., 2001. Functional instability of the ankle and the role of neuromuscular control: a comprehensive review. J. Foot Ankle Surg. 40, 240–251.

Rudwaleit, M., Metter, A., Listing, J., et al., 2006. Inflammatory back pain in ankylosing spondylitis: a reassessment of the clinical history for application as classification and diagnostic criteria. Arthritis Rheumatol 54, 569–578.

Russek, L.N., Stott, P., Simmonds, J., 2019. Recognizing and effectively managing hypermobility-related conditions. Phys. Ther. 99, 1189–1200.

Ryder, D., Barnard, K., 2024. Musculoskeletal Examination and Assessment: A Handbook for Therapists, sixth ed. Elsevier, Oxford.

Safran, M.R., Borsa, P.A., Lephart, S.M., et al., 2001. Shoulder proprioception in baseball pitchers. J. Shoulder Elbow Surg. 10, 438–444.

Salem, W., Lenders, C., Mathieu, J., et al., 2013. In vivo three-dimensional kinematics of the cervical spine during maximal axial rotation. Man. Ther. 18, 339–344.

Salo, P.T., Theriault, E., 1997. Number, distribution and neuropeptide content of rat knee joint afferents. J. Anat. 190, 515–522.

Schenker, M.L., Mauck, R.L., Ahn, J., et al., 2014. Pathogenesis and prevention of posttraumatic osteoarthritis after intra-articular fracture. J. Am. Acad. Orthop. Surg. 22, 20–28.

Seki, K., Taniguchi, Y., Narusawa, M., 2001. Effects of joint immobilization on firing rate modulation of human motor units. J. Physiol. 530, 507–519.

Serrancoli, G., Monllau, J.C., Font-Llagunes, J.M., 2016. Analysis of muscle synergies and activation-deactivation patterns in subjects with anterior cruciate ligament deficiency during walking. Clin. Biomech. (Bristol, Avon) 31, 65–73.

Shrive, N.G., Frank, C.B., 1999. Articular cartilage. In: Nigg, B.M., Herzog, W. (Eds.), Biomechanics of the Musculo-Skeletal System, second ed. John Wiley, Chichester, pp. 86–106.

Sieper, J., Van Der Heijde, D., Landewe, R., et al., 2009. New criteria for inflammatory back pain in patients with chronic back pain: a real patient exercise by experts from the Assessment of SpondyloArthritis international Society (ASAS). Ann. Rheum. Dis. 68, 784–788.

Slipman, C.W., Plastaras, C., Patel, R., et al., 2005. Provocative cervical discography symptom mapping. Spine J 5, 381–388.

Solomonow, M., Krogsgaard, M., 2001. Sensorimotor control of knee stability. A review. Scand. J. Med. Sci. Sports 11, 64–80.

Spector, T.D., Macgregor, A.J., 2004. Risk factors for osteoarthritis: genetics. Osteoarthritis Cartilage 12 (Suppl A), S39–44.

Stanish, W.D., 2000. Knee ligament sprains – acute and chronic. In: Harries, M., Williams, C., Stanish, W. (Eds.),

Oxford Textbook of Sports Medicine, second ed. Oxford University Press, Oxford, pp. 420–440.
Steen, K.H., Issberner, U., Reeh, P.W., 1995. Pain due to experimental acidosis in human skin: evidence for non-adapting nociceptor excitation. Neurosci. Lett. 199, 29–32.
Stokes, M., Young, A., 1984. The contribution of reflex inhibition to arthrogenous muscle weakness. Clin. Sci. 67, 7–14.
Strasmann, T., Halata, Z., 1988. Applications for 3-D image processing in functional anatomy: reconstruction of the cubital joint region and spatial distribution of mechanoreceptors surrounding this joint in *Mondelphius domestica*, a laboratory marsupial. Eur. J. Cell. Biol. 25, 107–110.
Suarez, T., Laudani, L., Giombini, A., et al., 2016. Comparison in joint-position sense and muscle coactivation between anterior cruciate ligament-deficient and healthy individuals. J. Sport Rehabil. 25, 64–69.
Suter, E., Herzog, W., 2000. Muscle inhibition and functional deficiencies associated with knee pathologies. In: Herzog, W. (Ed.), Skeletal Muscle Mechanics, From Mechanisms to Function. Wiley, Chichester, p. 365 (Chapter 21).
Tipton, C.M., James, S.L., Mergner, W., et al., 1970. Influence of exercise on strength of medial collateral knee ligaments of dogs. Am. J. Physiol. 218, 894–902.
Torry, M.R., Decker, M.J., Viola, R.W., et al., 2000. Intra-articular knee joint effusion induces quadriceps avoidance gait patterns. Clin. Biomech. (Bristol, Avon) 15, 147–159.
Urbach, D., Awiszus, F., 2002. Impaired ability of voluntary quadriceps activation bilaterally interferes with function testing after knee injuries. A twitch interpolation study. Int. J. Sports Med. 23, 231–236.
Vanwanseele, B., Lucchinetti, E., Stussi, E., 2002. The effects of immobilization on the characteristics of articular cartilage: current concepts and future directions. Osteoarthritis Cartilage 10, 408–419.
Veeger, H.E.J., Van Der Helm, F.C.T., 2007. Shoulder function: the perfect compromise between mobility and stability. J. Biomech. 40, 2119–2129.
Walker, B.F., Williamson, O.D., 2009. Mechanical or inflammatory low back pain. What are the potential signs and symptoms? Man. Ther. 14, 314–320.
Wang, J.H.-C., Guo, Q., Li, B., 2012. Tendon biomechanics and mechanobiology – a minireview of basic concepts and recent advancements. J. Hand Ther. 25, 133–140 quiz 141.
Webster, K.D., Ng, W.P., Fletcher, D.A., 2014. Tensional homeostasis in single fibroblasts. Biophys. J. 107, 146–155.
Wong, M., Carter, D.R., 2003. Articular cartilage functional histomorphology and mechanobiology: a research perspective. Bone 33, 1–13.
Woo, S.L., Maynard, J., Butler, D., et al., 1988. Ligament, tendon, and joint capsule insertions to bone. In: Woo, S.L., Buckwalter, J. (Eds.), Injury and Repair of the Musculoskeletal Soft Tissues. American Academy of Orthopaedic Surgeons, Park Ridge, IL, pp. 133–166.
Woo, S.L., Gomez, M.A., Sites, T.J., et al., 1987. The biomechanical and morphological changes in the medial collateral ligament of the rabbit after immobilization and remobilization. J. Bone Joint Surg. Am. 69, 1200–1211.
Wright, V., Johns, R.J., 1961. Quantitative and qualitative analysis of joint stiffness in normal subjects and in patients with connective tissue diseases. Ann. Rheum. Dis. 20, 36–46.
Wyke, B.D., 1970. The neurological basis of thoracic spinal pain. Rheumatol. Phys. Med. 10, 356–367.
Xu, L., Hayashi, D., Roemer, F.W., Felson, D.T., Guermazi, A., 2012. Magnetic resonance imaging of subchondral bone marrow lesions in association with osteoarthritis. Seminars in arthritis and rheumatism 42, 105–118.
Yabe, Y., Hagiwara, Y., Suda, H., et al., 2013. Joint immobilization induced hypoxic and inflammatory conditions in rat knee joints. Connect. Tissue Res. 54, 210–217.
Zimny, M.L., 1988. Mechanoreceptors in articular tissues. Am. J. Anat. 182, 16–32.
Zimny, M.L., St Onge, M., 1987. Mechanoreceptors in the temporomandibular articular disk. J. Dent. Res. 66, 237.

3

Principles of Joint Treatment

Clair Hebron and Chris McCarthy

LEARNING OUTCOMES

After studying this chapter, you should be able to:

- Understand the key principles of joint mobilization, manipulation treatment for joint dysfunction.
- Understand the key biomechanical and physiological mechanisms supporting joint treatments.
- Consider the principles of treatment selection, regression and progression.
- Understand the evidence for joint treatments.
- Critically reflect on if and when to include joint treatment within a person-centred framework of practice.

CHAPTER CONTENTS

This chapter will focus on the treatments which are directed at joints and associated structures; however, it is essential to emphasize that joints should not be treated in isolation but within a holistic approach to person-centred care. A person is embodied and is influenced by not just psychosocial factors, but by that person's being in the world, with its historical, contextual and situational influences (Heidegger, 1962). Thus treatment of people with musculoskeletal dysfunction should include consideration of the whole person and his or her embodied experience. The therapeutic value of communication in the therapeutic setting should not be underestimated and is considered further in Chapter 2, Ryder and Barnard (2024). Manual therapy can be considered to be a method of physical education and another physiotherapeutic modality facilitating communication about movement (McCarthy et al., 2020). Treatment of joints may comprise one aspect of management; however, health promotion is recognized as core to physiotherapy practice, and therefore treatment of joints should be complemented by recommendations regarding physical activity, smoking cessation, moderating alcohol consumption, basic nutrition, strategies in managing stress and sleep hygiene. Readers are recommended to refer to literature on behaviour change techniques, such as Michie et al. (2011) and Willett et al. (2019).

From a biomechanical perspective there is no pure treatment for joints; that is, treatment cannot be isolated to joints alone; it will always, to a greater or lesser extent, affect muscle, fascia and the nervous system. Some sort of classification system for treatment is needed in order to facilitate meaningful communication between clinicians, and this text follows the traditional classification of joint, muscle and nerve treatment. In this text, a 'joint treatment' is defined as a 'treatment to effect a change in a joint's function'; that is, the intention of the clinician is to produce a change in a joint's movement. Similarly, where a technique is used to effect a change in muscle function, it will be referred to as a 'muscle treatment', and where a technique is used to effect a change in nerve function, it will be referred to as a 'nerve treatment'. An example may help to illustrate the tissue non-specificity of a 'joint' mobilization technique. A posteroanterior (PA) glide on the head of the fibula will move the superior tibiofibular joint, the lateral collateral ligament of the tibiofemoral joint, the common peroneal nerve, local fascia and soleus / biceps femoris muscles. A PA glide to the head of the fibula can therefore be applied to affect any of these structures. It may be used to influence mechanoreceptors sited in the superior tibiofibular joint, in which case it could be described as a joint treatment, or it may be used to affect the sensitivity of the common peroneal nerve, in which case it might be referred to as a nerve treatment. Similarly, physiological joint movements will move local joint, fascia, nerve and muscle tissues.

The possible desired effects of joint mobilization on joint, nerve, fascia and muscle tissue are summarized in Box 3.1. For example, active shoulder flexion moves the glenohumeral and scapulothoracic joints, involves muscle contraction of numerous shoulder and scapular muscles, while also applying mechanical stress to the nerves of the brachial plexus. In this chapter it is assumed that joint mobilization or exercise treatment is being applied to affect joint tissues and their mechanoreceptors. The reader is reminded that there are a number of specific precautions and contraindications to joint mobilization treatment (Ryder & Barnard, 2024).

BOX 3.1 Desired Effects of Joint Mobilization

- Create an afferent barrage to initiate a neurophysiological response to reduce pain
- Glide joint surface parallel to plane of joint or rotate joint surfaces
- Move joint surface to lengthen periarticular tissues
- Move joint to affect nerve or muscle tissue
- Encourage normal patterns of movement
- Reduce fear of movement
- Improvement of somatosensory awareness of joint position and proprioception

Joint treatments are normally applied with the aim of decreasing pain or improving the range or quality of movement. The research evidence supporting the possible effects of treatment will be explored. However, it should be acknowledged that most clinical trials report on mean responses and do not necessarily represent individual patients. Therefore the physiotherapist should monitor the response to treatment on an individual basis and use joint treatment within an evidence-based framework of practice which considers evidence from the patient, therapist and research.

This chapter will examine joint mobilizations and manipulation and discuss the role of exercise in joint treatment. Readers are advised to refer to Chapter 10 for further details on exercise.

JOINT MOBILIZATIONS

Types of Joint Mobilizations

Joint mobilizations are passive joint movements performed in such a way that at all times they are within the control of the patient and within the physiological range of the joint. The direction of force applied is typically in parallel with the plane of the joint, thereby inducing no joint surface separation (McCarthy, 2010). This is in contrast to joint manipulation, which commonly involves a sudden movement, which is too sudden to be controlled by the patient's muscles. The direction of force applied is often approximately perpendicular to the plane of the joint and does induce joint surface separation (McCarthy, 2010).

Treatment aims to restore normal joint function, whether by reducing pain or by restoration of movement (the rotation movement, the translation movement or a combination of the two). This method of treating joints can therefore be broadly divided into physiological movements (which emphasize rotation of the bone) and accessory movements (which emphasize translation of the bone) or a combination of the two (Fig. 3.1). Combinations of accessory and physiological movements are also possible. Details of these accessory and physiological movements are provided in the companion text (Ryder & Barnard, 2024).

Accessory Movements

Every accessory movement (translational glide) available at a joint can be used as a treatment technique and

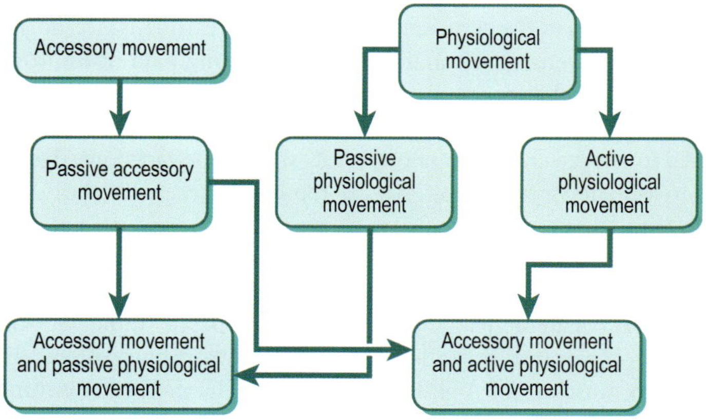

Fig. 3.1 Classification of joint mobilizations.

therefore can be induced at any point in range of movement. The starting position in which accessory movement is applied will influence the choice of treatment and the neuro-physiological impact the movement will have. Having examined and identified a dysfunction of an accessory movement, at a certain range of movement, the clinician could draw a movement diagram (see Chapter 4, Ryder & Barnard, 2024) and then choose a suitable treatment dose, described in the next section. The accessory movement can be carried out in any part of the physiological range of that joint; for example, an anteroposterior (AP) glide to the tibiofemoral joint can be applied with the knee in flexion, extension or tibial rotation. The chosen position depends on the desired effects of the treatment, discussed later in this chapter.

Physiological Movements

Every physiological movement available at a joint can be converted to a treatment technique and can be carried out actively by the patient or passively by the patient or clinician. Active repetitive movements of the spine have, for example, been advocated by McKenzie (1981, 1983, 1985), whilst others have advocated combining passive movements (McCarthy, 2010) and others a combination of active movement with passive movements combined (Hing, 2015). Having examined the physiological movement the clinician can then choose a suitable treatment dose, described in the next section.

The principles of applying passive physiological movement treatment are:

- The body part is adequately supported, to allow relaxation by the patient.
- The movement is fully controlled by the clinician or patient, in terms of where in the range the movement begins and ends, the amplitude, smoothness and speed of oscillations.
- The clinician constantly monitors symptoms during the application of the technique.
- In order to determine the immediate effects of the treatment the clinician reassesses the comparable signs.
- Changes in symptoms are discussed with the patient and explained in neurophysiological terms appropriate for the biopsychosocial profile of the patient.
- Treatment is converted to a home exercise/'stretching' manoeuvre which will be performed by the patient.

Passive Physiological Movement Combined With Accessory Movements

A physiological movement can be applied while also applying an accessory movement. Thus the physiological movement and the accessory movement can both be oscillated at the same time, the physiological movement can be oscillated while the accessory movement is sustained or the physiological movement can be sustained while the accessory movement is oscillated. For example, a longitudinal caudad glide and shoulder abduction can each be oscillated at the same time, the shoulder abduction can be oscillated while the longitudinal caudad glide is sustained or the shoulder abduction can be sustained while the longitudinal caudad glide is oscillated. These techniques can be applied in a variety of positions. For example, shoulder abduction with a longitudinal glide can be applied while sitting, lying or standing. Accessory mobilizations can also be applied during patients' functional aggravating movements. This may be limited by the ability of the therapist to apply force effectively, but explanations of sudden changes in symptoms can help to contextualize the treatment for the patient and may improve compliance with a home exercise programme (McCarthy et al., 2020).

Active Physiological Movement With Accessory Movement

As the patient performs an active physiological movement, the clinician can apply an accessory movement, often called a mobilization with movement (MWM) when applied to a peripheral joint or a sustained natural apophyseal glide (SNAG) when applied to the spine (Hing et al., 2015). For example, the clinician can apply an AP glide to the talus and ask the patient to dorsiflex the foot actively. For the cervical spine, the clinician can apply a transverse glide to a spinous process and then ask the patient to flex the head laterally. When the physiological movement is performed actively by the patient, as opposed to passively by the clinician, this can sometimes enable the technique to be carried out in a more functional position. For further information on accessory movement with active physiological movements, see Hing et al. (2015), or the review by Hing et al. (2008), which proposes an algorithm by which MWMs may be incorporated into patient management.

Clinicians might apply MWMs if they resulted in a reduction in symptoms or an increase in patients' confidence of movement. MWMs can often be applied by patients as a home exercise and can be performed during functional movements. Therefore they can be useful in empowering patients and helping them to gain control over their pain. Because they are encouraging movement in the painful direction they can also reduce fear avoidance, a factor that is associated with poor recovery (Wertli et al., 2014). Careful communication and use of language whilst the treatment technique is applied and during the whole patient encounter are essential in order to maximize the reduction of fear and empower patients (Chapter 2, Ryder and Barnard, 2024).

Manipulation

'Spinal Manipulation (SM) is the application of rapid movement to vertebral segments producing joint surface separation, transient sensory afferent input, and reduction in perception of pain. Joint surface separation will commonly result in intra-articular cavitation, which in turn, is commonly accompanied with an audible pop. Post manipulation reductions in pain perception are influenced by supra-spinal mechanisms including expectation of benefit' (McCarthy et al., 2015).

To minimize adverse events, manipulation should be applied using the same principles as for passive joint mobilization of the spine (Ryder & Barnard, 2024).

Further recommendations to promote the safe application of spinal manipulation are:

- Minimal force should be applied to any spinal structure. Low amplitude and short lever thrust techniques are preferable.
- Spinal manipulation techniques should at all times feel comfortable to the patient. In applying cervical spine manipulation, placing the patient's head on a pillow in supine lying is often more comfortable to the patient than alternative positions. This position also allows the practitioner to better monitor the patient's facial expression and for any nystagmus.
- Neck manipulation techniques should not be performed at the end of range of overall cervical spine physiological movement, especially for extension and rotation.
- When considering spinal manipulation, it is recommended that the clinician utilizes the International Federation of Orthopaedic Manipulative Physical Therapists (IFOMPT) International Cervical Framework (2020), which is designed to provide guidance for the assessment of the cervical spine region for potential vascular pathologies of the neck (www.ifompt.org).
- Repeated manipulation within the same session or over a number of consecutive sessions should be avoided, owing to potential dangers of frequent, repeated manipulations and a lack of longer-term benefit (McCarthy et al., 2015).

KNOWLEDGE CHECK

1. Which technique (either mobilization or manipulation) involves the induction of movement along the plane of joint surfaces, whilst the other technique involves the induction of movement in a plane perpendicular to the joint surface plane, thereby inducing joint surface separation?
2. What is the name of the technique which involves the application of a force, directed along a joint surface plane, whilst active movement is concurrently undertaken by the patient?
3. What is the difference between an accessory joint technique and a physiological joint technique?

Application of Joint Mobilizations

Dose

The term 'treatment dose' is often used by the medical profession when prescribing the quantity of a drug. The term is used here to describe the nature of the movement applied by the clinician or by the patient. The treatment dose incorporates quite a large number of factors, most of which have a number of variables outlined in Table 3.1.

An example of treatment dose, which might be used and documented in the patient's notes, is:

- IN: left side lying, with arm back and pelvis rotated.
- DID: right lumbar rotation grade II in line of femur, slowly and smoothly, for 30 seconds, to partial reproduction of patient's back pain.

This clinical note describes the patient in left side-lying, with the arm resting on the trunk and right hip and the knee flexed so that the knee rests on the couch, in front of the underlying leg. The clinician applied a slow and smooth passive physiological movement (grade II) to the pelvis, in the direction of the line of the femur, for 30 seconds, such that the patient felt only partial reproduction of the back pain.

Patient Position

This includes the general position of the patient, such as lying, sitting or standing, and the specific position of the body part; for example, the knee may be flexed or extended during the application of an AP glide on the tibia. For example, a patient with limitation of knee flexion due to resistance may be positioned in long sitting with the knee flexed to the end of the available range, while the clinician applies an AP glide to the tibia. The choice of general and specific positioning will depend on a number of factors, including:

- the comfort and support of the patient
- the comfort of the clinician applying the technique
- the desired effect of the treatment (e.g. decrease pain or increase range of movement)
- whether the joints are to be weight bearing or non-weight bearing
- to what extent the movement is to be functional
- to what extent symptoms are to be produced.

TABLE 3.1 Aspects of Treatment Dose for Joint Mobilization

Factors	Variables
Patient position	E.g. prone, side-lying, sitting, functional, aggravating
Starting position	Is it acceptable to induce movement in a position that reproduces pain or one in a starting position that allows pain free movement? (e.g. undertaking movement starting in flexion when extension positioning is painful)
Movement	This may be a physiological movement (e.g. flexion, lateral rotation, or an accessory movement or a mixture of the two)
Direction of force applied	E.g. anteroposterior, posteroanterior, medial, lateral, caudad, cephalad
Magnitude of force applied	Related to therapist's perception of resistance: grades I–V
Amplitude of oscillation	None: sustained (quasistatic) Small: grades I and IV Large: grades II and III
Speed	Slow or fast
Rhythm	Smooth or staccato
Time	Duration and number of repetitions
Symptom response	Short of symptom production Point of onset or increase in resting symptom Partial reproduction of symptom Full reproduction of symptom

Direction of Movement

Choice of treatment direction is generally based on the clinician's assessment of passive accessory and physiological motion and symptom response, including knowledge of the normal direction of bone translation. (See Chapter 4, Ryder & Barnard, 2024.) Where a physiological movement is used, a description of the physiological movement and naming the joint will describe this aspect of the treatment dose. For example, knee flexion, hip lateral rotation or lumbar rotation to the left each identifies the direction of the movement and the joint complex being influenced. Where an accessory movement is used, the direction of the force and the joint complex being influenced will describe the movement. Examples include an AP to the tibiofemoral joint, a lateral glide of the glenohumeral joint or an AP to the talocrural joint. Again, each identifies the direction of the force and the joint complex being influenced. The general convention would assume that the force was applied to the distal bone of the joint—in the above examples, to the tibia, humerus and talus, respectively. Techniques, of course, can be applied to the proximal bone; when this occurs the bone needs to be identified in the written description. For example, the description may read 'AP to tibiofemoral joint, on femur'.

In the spine, where each spinal level consists of a number of joints, an additional descriptor is added for accessory movements. The point of application of the force needs to be identified, for example, a central PA (angled caudad) on L3, a transverse glide to the left on T5, a unilateral PA on C5 (angled cephalad). In these examples, the word 'central' means that the force is applied over the spinous process, 'transverse' to the lateral aspect of the spinous process and 'unilateral' to the point on the back where the articular pillar or transverse process are sited (although not palpable). Where the severity, irritability and nature of the condition allow, treatment is normally directed at the most symptomatic level and in the most symptomatic direction as the movement will be influencing the most sensitized nociceptors and providing the central nervous system with 'new' and 'important' afferent information for processing (Ellingsen et al., 2016).

Magnitude of the Force/Grades of Movement

Whenever a clinician passively moves a joint, with either a physiological or accessory movement, the clinician is applying a force. Clearly, all movements have the features of amplitude, direction, acceleration, speed and force. The amplitude of a movement can be commonly described using a grade of movement (Magarey, 1985, 1986; Hengeveld & Banks, 2013). Grades of movement are defined according to where the movement occurs, in relation to the joint resistance typically felt as passive (and active muscle) structures begin to restrain movement. The resistance to movement, perceived by the operator inducing the movement, is depicted on a movement diagram (described in Chapter 4, Ryder & Barnard, 2024). Grades of movement (I–IV+) are then defined according to their relationship to the resistance profile, depicted in a movement diagram and an ascending sloped line and the amplitude of the movement. The grades of movement defined in this text (Table 3.2) are a modification of Magarey (1985, 1986). The modification allows every possible position in range to be described (Magarey, 1985, 1986) and each grade to be distinct from one another (Hengeveld & Banks, 2013). A grade V technique is a manipulative thrust described as a small amplitude movement applied at the very end of the range of movement and is no longer recommended in vertebral manipulation (McCarthy et al., 2015).

TABLE 3.2 Grades of Movement

Grade	Definition
I	Small-amplitude movement short of resistance
II	Large-amplitude movement short of resistance
III–	Large-amplitude movement in the first third of resistance
IV–	Small-amplitude movement in the first third of resistance
III	Large-amplitude movement in the middle third of resistance
IV	Small-amplitude movement in the middle third of resistance
III+	Large-amplitude movement in the last third of resistance
IV+	Small-amplitude movement in the last third of resistance
V	Quick, small-amplitude movement at the end of range

With most joint movements there is minimal resistance within the early range of movement. For example, elbow flexion or knee extension will have little resistance in the early part of the range, and the clinician may mark the onset of resistance (R_1) somewhere towards the end of the movement (Fig. 3.2A).

Grades of movement available for physiological movements include (I, II) small and large amplitude movement in a range where no resistance to movement is felt. Additionally, large amplitude movements at the beginning III−, middle III and end of movement III+ in resistance, or small amplitude movements at the beginning IV−, middle IV, or end of range IV+ (see Fig. 3.2A). The grade of movement is defined according to where the maximum force is applied in resistance and whether the clinician considers the movement to be large or small (see Fig. 3.2B).

Studies investigating force of shoulder and elbow mobilizations suggest that higher treatment force may result in better outcomes (Vicenzino et al., 2001; McLean et al., 2002; Vermeulen et al., 2006), and in participants with persistent low-back pain higher lumbar mobilization treatment forces were associated with a greater increase in pressure pain thresholds (reductions in perception of nociceptive afferent input) and concomitant reduction in verbal rating of pain (Hebron, 2014). Collectively these studies suggest that where pain allows using higher grades of treatment may be considered. One paradigm, useful in selecting grades of passive movement, is the combined movement approach (McCarthy, 2010). This approach advocates the exclusive use of grades of movement within the range where resistance is perceived deliberately to utilize this 'higher-dose' afferent input into the central nervous system (CNS) of patients. In order to allow this approach, the starting position in which the joint is placed, in order to undertake the passive movement, is critically important. If a joint complex has become directionally sensitized, pain perception is provoked in a certain range (for example lumbar extension); in order to allow comfortable movement in a range where resistance is felt (grades III & IV), the joint may need to be placed in a starting position that avoids that directional sensitivity (i.e. lumbar flexion) (McCarthy, 2010; McCarthy & Rivett, 2019).

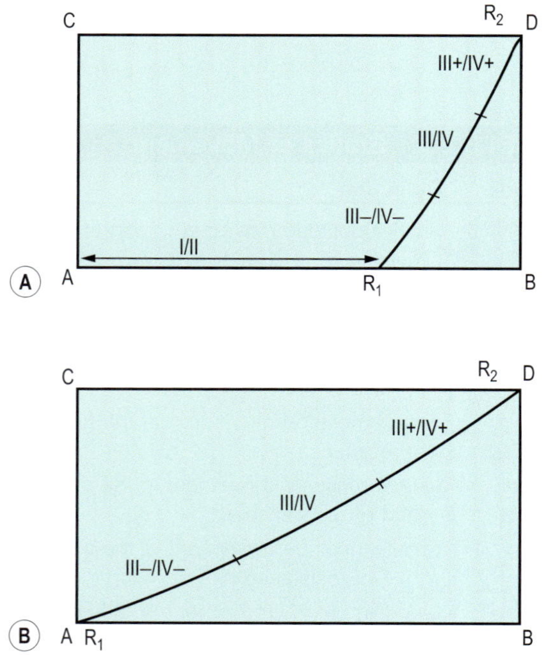

Fig. 3.2 Movement diagram with grades of movement for (A) a typical asymptomatic physiological movement and (B) a typical asymptomatic accessory movement. The resistance is divided into thirds, so that a large-amplitude movement within the middle third will be a grade III.

Amplitude of Oscillation

A movement can be a sustained or an oscillatory motion. If the force is deliberately oscillated it is described as having a small or large amplitude. The amplitude is relative to the available range of any particular movement, so it will vary quite dramatically between physiological and accessory movements. For example, small-amplitude accessory movements may be a few millimetres of movement compared with a 40-degree arc of movement for a physiological movement. The amplitude of oscillatory movement is described within the definition of grades of movement: grades I and IV are small-amplitude movements, and grades II and III are large-amplitude movements. The choice of grade of movement is determined by the relationship of pain (or other symptom) and resistance through the range of movement; this is depicted on a movement diagram (Hengeveld & Banks, 2013). Where resistance limits the range of movement (Fig. 3.3A), a grade III+ or IV+, provoking some pain, may be appropriate (pain would be 4 out of 10 or more in this example). The extent of pain reproduction can be altered according to what is acceptable to the patient, and thus with some patients a

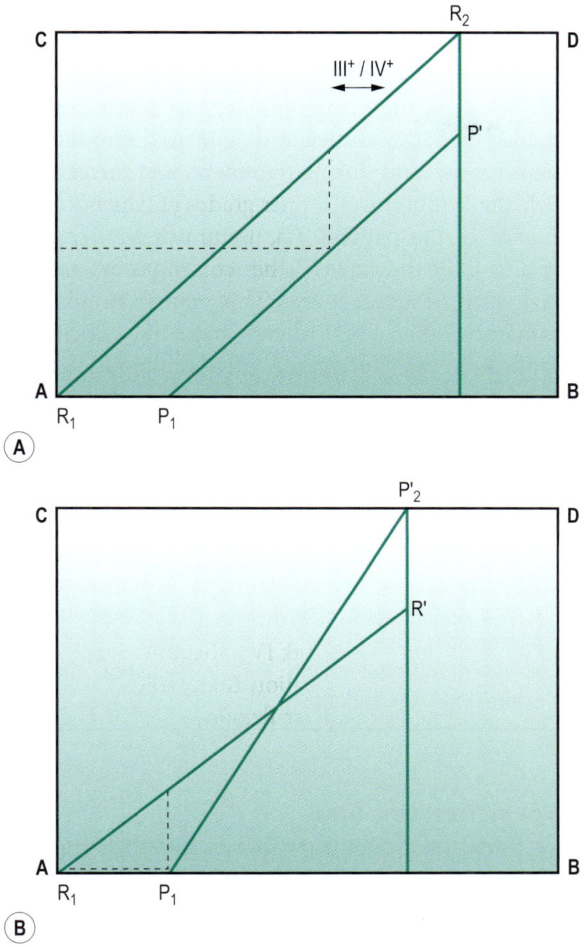

Fig. 3.3 Grades of movement are determined by the relationship of pain and resistance through the range of movement; this is depicted on a movement diagram. (A) Resistance limiting movement. (B) Pain limiting movement.

grade III or IV might be used in this example. Where pain limits the range of movement (see Fig. 3.3B), a grade III− or IV− that does not produce any pain may be appropriate.

There is little evidence to inform clinicians when deciding on the amplitude of mobilizations; theoretically increasing the amplitude will stimulate more mechanoreceptors and thus increase pain relief mediated via the pain gate mechanism (van Griensven, 2005; McCarthy, 2013). However, a study including asymptomatic participants did not find a difference in the hypoalgesic effect of different amplitudes of lumbar mobilization (Grades III or IV) oscillations (Krouwel et al., 2010). This methodology was recently replicated, with persistent low back pain and again demonstrated no difference between grade III or IV movements. The study did report hypoalgesic effects when compared with a no touch control (Khanmohammadi et al., 2021).

Speed and Rhythm of Movement

The speed of the movement can be described as slow or fast and the rhythm as smooth or staccato (jerky). Speed and rhythm go hand in hand; movements will tend to be slow and smooth, fast and smooth or fast and staccato. A manipulative thrust is often described as a high velocity low amplitude (HVLA) thrust and can be performed at any point in range. If it is performed at the beginning of resistance it is called a 'grade IV-thrust technique' (as recommended in spinal manipulation) (McCarthy, 2010; McCarthy et al., 2015). If an HVLA is undertaken at the very end of movement it would be called grade V and is not recommended in spinal manipulation (McCarthy, 2010; McCarthy et al., 2015). The tissues around a joint are viscoelastic and, as such, are sensitive to the speed of the applied force. A force applied quickly will produce less movement, provoking a greater stiffness in the tissues; a force applied more slowly, on the other hand, will cause more movement as the stiffness is relatively less (Noyes et al., 1974). Thus it is generally more comfortable to evoke movement slowly and smoothly rather than with short staccato motions. There is a paucity of evidence regarding the influence of different speeds of mobilizations. Chiu and Wright (1996) reported greater changes in skin conductance (indicating sympatho-excitation) following mobilization at 2 Hz than those at 0.5 Hz, but no difference in the hypoalgesic effect of different speeds of mobilization was reported in asymptomatic participants (Willett et al., 2010).

Time

In terms of treatment dose, this relates to the duration for which a movement is carried out in a treatment session, the number of times this is repeated within a treatment session and the frequency of appointments. When applying MWMs or SNAGs the movement and associated pressure are normally applied five to seven times (Hing et al., 2015). When using mobilizations clinical practice typically involves up to three repetitions (sets) of a treatment technique, each lasting between 30 seconds and 1 minute—most research exploring the effects of joint mobilizations has used this time range. However, there is some evidence that longer treatment duration may have a greater treatment effect: in asymptomatic participants a greater increase in ankle range of movement was found with 2 minutes than with 30 seconds or 1 minute of mobilization treatment (Holland et al., 2015), and more treatment sets of lumbar mobilizations were found to have a greater hypoalgesic effect (Pentelka et al., 2012). An association between lumbar mobilization treatment duration and change in pressure pain threshold has been found in participants with persistent low-back pain, with significantly more participants responding to 6 minutes than to 1 minute of treatment (Hebron, 2014).

The frequency of appointments is decided by the clinician and the patient and will depend on a number of factors, including the nature of the patient's condition, the severity and irritability of symptoms, the area of the symptoms, the functional limitations of the patient, the stage of the patient's condition, the prognosis and the available time the patient has to attend for treatment.

Symptom Response

The clinician decides which symptom and to what extent each symptom is to be provoked during assessment and treatment. Choices include:

- no provocation
- provocation to the point of onset, or increase, in resting symptoms
- partial reproduction
- total reproduction.

The decision as to what extent each symptom is provoked during treatment depends on the severity and irritability of the symptom(s) and the nature of the condition. If the symptoms are severe, that is, the patient is unable to tolerate the symptom being reproduced, the clinician would choose to apply treatment that did not provoke the symptoms. This may involve using lower grades of movement (I, II) or changing the starting position to allow use of high-grade movements (III, IV), in a position away from the patient's directional sensitivity (McCarthy, 2010). Clinicians will typically choose not to provoke symptoms if the patient is deemed to be 'irritable'; that is, symptoms that are quickly provoked and take some time to even begin to ease. Irritability is a feature of over-reactivity of pain responses to afferent inputs associated with nociplastic (central sensitivity) and neurogenic (neural source) pain (McCarthy, 2010) (see Chapter 3, Ryder & Barnard, 2024).

If, however, the symptoms are not severe and not irritable, then the clinician is able to reproduce the patient's symptoms during treatment, and the extent to which the symptoms are provoked will depend on the tolerance of the patient. The nature of the condition may also limit the extent to which symptoms are produced, such as a recent traumatic injury, an acute inflammatory state or where there is nociplastic amplification of nociceptor afferent input (central sensitization).

> **KNOWLEDGE CHECK**
> 1. What is the minimum time required to evoke a change in pain, when undertaking mobilization treatment?
> 2. What grades of movement occur in the range of movement where resistance to movement is perceived?
> 3. Is there a frequency of joint mobilization that is optimal for pain reduction?

Choice of Treatment Dose

An optimal treatment approach is one that improves the patient's signs and symptoms in the shortest period of time. Manual therapy aims to empower patients to get better quicker. Thus any physical test, undertaken during the patient's examination, that reproduces and eases the patient's symptoms can be converted to a treatment technique. Converting positive (symptom modifying) physical testing procedures to treatment techniques would seem the most logical approach to choosing treatment, as the clinician can be confident that the treatment is affecting the patient's sensitivity to pain and ability to function. The careful (non-threatening) reproduction of the patient's symptoms can be vital data to aid in the selection of treatments (Wertli et al., 2014). This may require some careful and time-consuming examination procedures, taking an attitude of an explorer, a researcher or a detective who can explore all components of the patient's movement impairment and pain. For example, testing elbow flexion is fully explored if variations of forearm pronation and supination and variations in direction of flexion medially and laterally are carried out. Similarly, when applying accessory movements, a wide variation in the directions of the force applied may be necessary.

The decision on the treatment of choice will be based on a number of factors, including:

- the desired therapeutic effect (e.g. to decrease pain or increase range of movement)
- the severity and irritability of the symptoms
- most symptomatic findings on physical examination: these are normally converted to treatment
- the results of reassessment of the comparable signs within the assessment; for example, if reassessment of active range of movement improves most after passive physiological intervertebral movement assessment, then passive physiological treatment might be the treatment of choice
- patients' aggravating factors: the treatment position, rate and rhythm may be designed to replicate elements of aggravating movements or positions.
- the starting position chosen for the application of a passive movement will be influenced by the patient's biopsychosocial profile; severity of directional sensitivity to a particular movement, the nature of the pain (predominant pain mechanism), psychological influences on movement such as fear avoidance, hypervigilance and guarding behaviours (McCarthy, 2013).
- the nature of the condition: for example, the stage in the healing process postinjury or the predominant pain mechanism; for example, in patients with nociplastic pain (central sensitization), where possible, treatment would be pain-free (or at least of a level that is considered non-threatening to the patient) to avoid triggering more nociceptive barrage (Nijs & Van Houdenhove, 2009; Wertli et al., 2014).
- the aim of treatment, in terms of the patient's functional goals
- patient's treatment preferences and expectations: there is evidence to suggest that patients have better outcomes when they receive their preferred treatment (Kalauokalani et al., 2001; Palmlöf et al., 2016)
- patients' beliefs: where patients display fear-avoidant behaviour, treatment may centre on encouraging normal joint movement and reducing fear. Desensitization to a particular directional sensitivity (for example lumbar flexion) can be induced with a gradual upgrading of exposure to the sensitized movement, reducing pain due to habituation within the nervous system (George & Zeppieri, 2009; May et al., 2012).
- what is feasible for patients to perform at home: in order to aid the transition to home exercise and help empower patients.

When choosing between manipulations and mobilizations, the particular treatment may be unimportant as studies have reported no difference in the effects of mobilization and manipulation (Gross et al., 2010, 2015; Leaver et al., 2010; Cook et al., 2013; Salom-Moreno et al., 2014; Young et al., 2014) or mobilizations and SNAGS (Ganesh et al., 2015). Furthermore, manual therapy treatment directed at an adjacent region may be equally effective, with studies reporting decreased neck pain following thoracic mobilizations (Cleland et al., 2005; Gross et al., 2015) and a similar pain-relieving effect of manipulation when applied to the painful lumbar levels or upper thoracic spine in patients with low-back pain (Fernando de Oliveira et al., 2013). Mobilization techniques applied according to clinician clinical reasoning and mobilizations applied in a set manner only at L4 and L5 have been equally effective in low back pain, suggesting the specific level for mobilization is less important than treating generally in a painful region (Donaldson et al., 2016). This is a finding also found in manipulation where a general thrust to the lumbar spine has been shown to be equally effective as a manipulation targeted at the clinically 'important' level (Sutlive et al., 2009; McCarthy et al., 2019).

Modification, Progression and Regression

The choice of treatment dose on second and subsequent treatment occasions needs to be informed by patients' response to the previous treatment (same, better, worse) as well as the level of presenting symptoms and irritability at the time. The decision may be to continue the initial treatment, to modify it in some way, to progress the treatment or to regress the treatment. For instance, if a quick improvement was expected but only some improvement occurred, the clinician may progress treatment. If the patient is worse after treatment the dose may be regressed, and if the treatment made no difference at all then a more substantial modification may be made.

A treatment is progressed or regressed by altering appropriate aspects of the treatment dose in such a way that more or less input is applied to the tissues/nervous system. The aspects of treatment dose that can be altered are outlined in Table 3.3. It may be important to

TABLE 3.3 Progression and Regression of Treatment Dose

Treatment Dose	Progression	Regression
Position	Joint towards end of available range/more pain provoking	Joint towards beginning of available range/less pain provoking
Direction of force	More provocative	Less provocative
Magnitude of force	Increased	Decreased
Amplitude of oscillation	Decreased	Increased
Rhythm	Staccato	Smoother
Time	Longer	Shorter
Speed	Slower or faster	Slower
Symptom response	Allowing more symptoms to be provoked	Allowing fewer symptoms to be provoked

TABLE 3.4 Examples of How a Treatment Dose Can Be Progressed and Regressed

Regression	Dose	Progression	Explanation
In cervical extension did central PA C4 IV ×3 (1 minute) slowly and smoothly to partial reproduction of patient's neck pain	In cervical neutral did central PA C4 IV ×3 (1 minute) slowly and smoothly to partial reproduction of patient's neck pain	In cervical flexion did central PA C4 IV ×3 (1 minute) slowly and smoothly to partial reproduction of patient's neck pain	The starting position has been altered. It might be assumed that extension is a position of ease and flexion a more provocative position.
In 90 degrees knee flexion did medial glide tibiofemoral joint III– ×3 (1 minute) slowly and smoothly short of P1	In 90 degrees knee flexion did medial glide tibiofemoral joint III slowly and smoothly ×3 (1 minute) short of P1	In 90 degrees knee flexion did medial glide tibiofemoral joint IIII+ ×3 (1 minute) slowly and smoothly short of P1	The grade of movement has been altered.
Physiological plantarflexion II ×3 (1 minute) slowly and smoothly to full reproduction of ankle pain	Physiological plantarflexion III– ×3 (1 minute) slowly and smoothly to full reproduction of ankle pain	Physiological plantarflexion III+ ×3 (1 minute) fast and staccato to full reproduction of ankle pain	Grade has been altered as a regression. Grade, speed and rhythm have been altered as a progression.

PA, Posteroanterior.

modify only one or two components of the treatment technique at any one time to avoid excessively irritating symptoms and to be able to identify the treatment components that are having an effect. Treatment should continue until the desired treatment goal is reached, or it is no longer having an effect and ceased if it is having any adverse effect.

Specific examples of how a treatment dose may be progressed and regressed are provided in Table 3.4.

Assessment of Outcome

The measurement of outcome is an important part of ensuring that the desired treatment effect is being achieved. In terms of joint mobilization, the typical outcome is likely to be a change in pain, and/or range of motion, which will be evaluated by reassessment of the subjective and physical asterisks. Measuring these variables before, during and after treatment is an appropriate way to assess the ongoing treatment effect. The clinician may choose a relevant joint movement (single plane, or a more functional combination, as relevant) and in a collaborative process, ask the patient to help evaluate whether there has been any effect by rating the pain while performing the movement by asking for their perception on whether there has been any change in the movement and pain (and possibly by using an 11-point numerical rating scale, an instrument found to be responsive in musculoskeletal pain) (Bolton & Wilkinson, 1998; Hefford et al., 2012). This same movement, and questioning regarding pain intensity, may be used between sets of joint mobilization to see if the pain level is changing. Equally the range of motion for a relevant movement may be measured using standard goniometry (Soames, 2003) or a more functional measure, and this can be repeated at intervals before and after treatment. The importance of person-based measures such as quality-of-life scales, return to work or sport, or satisfaction measures is an important component of measurement of the long-term effect of treatment.

Effect of Mobilizations

The underlying mechanisms by which joint mobilizations and manipulations can increase the range of movement and reduce pain can be broadly divided into mechanical effects and neurophysiological effects.

Mechanical Effects

It is recognized that mobilizations have a widespread mechanical effect, influencing other joints, subcutaneous tissues, muscles and local nerves. This is particularly evident in the spine where, for example, during the application of a central PA mobilization to the lumbar spine, movement occurs throughout the whole thoracolumbar region (Lee et al., 1996). This is made up of rotation of the pelvis and thoracic cage (Chansirinukor et al., 2001, 2003), compression of the skin and soft tissue (Lee et al., 1996; Lee & Evans, 2000) and movement at local and distant spinal joints (Lee & Evans, 1997; Powers et al., 2003; Kulig et al., 2004).

There is a mechanical effect on soft tissue; however, if the aim of treatment is to elongate periarticular tissues permanently then this will require application of force of sufficient magnitude to produce microtrauma (Threlkeld, 1992). The force needs to lie within the plastic zone of the force–displacement curve. A force of lesser magnitude, within the elastic zone, will result in only a temporary increase in length owing to creep and hysteresis (Panjabi & White, 2001). A rough guide to the amount of force needed to cause a permanent change in length has been estimated to be between 224 and 1136 N (Threlkeld, 1992). Forces used by clinicians during mobilization have been measured up to about 350 N in the lumbar spine (Harms & Bader, 1997) and 70 N in the cervical spine (Snodgrass et al., 2009). It is as yet unknown whether clinically applied forces are able to cause a permanent increase in length. There has been some suggestion that manual forces applied are insufficient to produce microtrauma and that the clinically applied forces lie within the elastic range of the tissues (McQuade et al., 1999). There is some initial evidence suggesting that movement can induce growth hormones and either provoke inflammatory mediators with excessive loading or reduce inflammatory mediators with gentle motion (Langevin et al., 2005). Thus fascial and ligament biomechanical and intracellular health can be adapted in response to the provision of motion stimulus to the tissues. The amount of movement required to evoke these changes appears to require at least a few minutes of motion and is likely to be dose respondent (Langevin et al., 2005; Leong et al., 2011; Parravicini & Bergna, 2017).

High intraarticular pressure can be caused by high levels of intraarticular fluid or increased muscle tension on the joint capsule (Levick, 1979) and is considered to be partly responsible for the pain and limitation of movement in injured or arthritic joints (Ferrell et al., 1986). Repetitive active joint movements (Giovanelli-Blacker et al., 1985) and passive joint movements (Nade & Newbold, 1983; Giovanelli-Blacker et al., 1985) have been found to cause a reduction in intraarticular pressure. Movement (such as long periods (>1 hour daily) of cyclical motion such as walking or cycling) has been shown to provide an important mechanical stimulus for both joint capsule and cartilage nutrition, growth and apoptosis (cell death—promoting new cell synthesis) (Leong et al., 2011).

A mechanical treatment effect, specific to manipulation, is cavitation, which commonly causes an audible ‘crack/pop’. Cavitation is caused by the separation of the joint space creating a vacuum effect and a resulting collapse of microbubbles within the joint (Cascioli et al., 2003). An increase in joint space has been reported following manipulation of a metacarpophalangeal joint (Unsworth et al., 1971; Kawchuk et al., 2015). There is debate as to whether cavitation is important in creating a treatment effect. A number of studies have shown that the hypoalgesic effect of manipulation is independent of cavitation, suggesting that it is not therapeutically important (Flynn et al., 2006; Cleland et al., 2007; Bialosky et al., 2010; Sillevis & Cleland, 2011). However, in another study, the stretch reflex following manipulation was attenuated only when cavitation was heard (Clark et al., 2011). One difficulty in assessing the clinical relevance of the audible pop, commonly observed during manipulative techniques, is that the noise can be originating from a joint two levels away and/or bilaterally at the same level (Dunning et al., 2017; Mourad et al., 2019). Thus whilst an audible pop may be observed it does not necessarily indicate that it originated from the region targeted with the technique. Thus it is sensible to not consider the presence of an audible pop to be the marker of a 'successful' technique and rather reassess motion which should be immediately improved due to the immediate reduction in local muscle activity and increase in local joint compliance (Pfluegler et al., 2020).

MWM of peripheral joints has been shown to increase range of movement of the ankle joint (Nisha et al., 2014; Holland et al., 2015), shoulder (Teys et al., 2008; Delgado et al., 2015) and hip (Beselga et al., 2016). However, evidence of increased range of movement following mobilizations to the spine is inconclusive; a systematic review reported mobilization treatment had no effect on range of movement in the lumbar spine and sacroiliac joint and a small effect on cervical range of movement (Millan et al., 2012b). Most evidence demonstrates that mobilizations do not reduce spinal stiffness (Goodsell et al., 2000; Allison et al., 2001). Current thinking suggests that there is an interaction between the biomechanical and neurophysiological effects, whereby a mechanical stimulus initiates a neurophysiological response (Bialosky et al., 2009a; Pickar & Bolton, 2012; Pfluegler et al., 2020).

KNOWLEDGE CHECK

1. How much time is required for movement to provide an important mechanical stimulus for both joint capsule and cartilage nutrition and growth?
2. What is cavitation phenomenon and is it important for patients to hear it for pain relief?

Neurophysiological Effects

Mobilization and manipulation techniques cause activation of afferents in skin, joints, muscles and nerves, and this biomechanical stimulus initiates a neurophysiological response, causing alteration of input to the central nervous system. An analgesic response is thought to occur through local effects (Teodorczyk-Injeyan et al., 2006; Molina-Ortega et al., 2014), through mechanisms at the level of the spinal cord (Boal & Gillette, 2004; George et al., 2006; Bialosky et al., 2009a) and via supraspinal mechanisms (Wright, 1995). It is likely that more than one of these mechanisms and the interaction between them results in analgesia induced by joint treatments (Pfluegler et al., 2020).

Local Immune Response Mechanisms

Mobilizations and manipulation are thought to have an anti-inflammatory effect as they have been found to result in an increase in the inflammatory mediator substance P (Brennan et al., 1991; Molina-Ortega et al., 2014) and reduction in local proinflammatory cytokines (Teodorczyk-Injeyan et al., 2006). However, the available evidence supporting the capacity of manual therapy to trigger a significant, systemic immune–endocrine response is mixed, and its clinical relevance remains to be established (Colombi & Testa, 2019).

Spinal Cord–Mediated Mechanisms

Manual therapy stimulates mechanosensitive receptors, which transmit afferent information via large-diameter nerve fibres, to the dorsal horn of the spinal cord. At this location this afferent input will influence the proportion of concomitant nociceptive input that is transmitted onto the ascending spinothalamic tracks via an interneural gating mechanism within the nociceptive and wide dynamic range cells in the dorsal horn (Wyke & Polacek, 1975; Pickar & Bolton, 2012) in accordance with the pain gate theory (Melzack & Wall, 1965). Afferent signals from type I mechanoreceptors, in joints, have been found to have an inhibitory effect, at the spinal cord, on type IV nociceptor afferent transmission (Wyke & Polacek, 1975). Nociplastic pain (central sensitization) is a factor in determining levels of ongoing pain and dysfunction, and it has been shown that the afferent stimulus provided by light touch and gentle movement in resistance reduces central sensitization through an inhibition of the dorsal horn 'wind up' (amplification) that occurs in nociplastic pain (Boal & Gillette, 2004). This is supported by studies that have measured temporal sensory summation, a phenomenon which occurs in nociplastic pain states. An immediate reduction in temporal summation has been reported following spinal manipulation in healthy participants (George et al., 2006; Bishop et al., 2011) and participants with low-back pain (Bialosky et al., 2009b). This was found to occur in the lumbar but not in the cervical innervated regions, leading the authors to conclude pain was modulated at the dorsal horn of the spinal cord (George et al., 2006; Bialosky et al., 2009b).

Supraspinal Mechanisms

Mobilizations and manipulations may reduce pain through the stimulation of supraspinal analgesic mechanisms. Wright (1995) proposed that mobilizations modulate pain-descending inhibition via the periaqueductal grey (PAG) area of the midbrain, an area important in the mediation of pain in both animals (Reynolds, 1969) and humans (Hosobuchi et al., 1977). The PAG projects to the dorsal horn and has a descending control on nociception (Fig. 3.4). It also projects upwards to the medial thalamus and orbital frontal cortex and so may have an ascending control of nociception (Fields & Basbaum, 1999). The PAG has two distinct regions: the dorsolateral PAG (dPAG) and the ventrolateral PAG (vPAG). In the rat, stimulation of the dPAG causes mechanical analgesia and sympatho-excitation, whereas stimulation of the vPAG causes analgesia associated with thermal analgesia and sympathetic inhibition (Lovick, 1991). The neurotransmitters used are noradrenaline (norepinephrine) from the dPAG and serotonin from the vPAG. The response to stimulation of the PAG in rats has been likened to the behaviour of animals under threat, which initially act with a defensive flight-or-fight response, followed by recuperation (Fanselow, 1991; Lovick, 1991); this is summarized in Fig. 3.5.

A number of research studies support the proposal of modulation of pain via the PAG, as they have reported concurrent sympatho-excitation and mechanical analgesia that mirror the effects of stimulation of the PAG in rats (Vicenzino, 1995; Vicenzino et al., 1996, 1998; Sterling et al., 2001). Furthermore, systematic reviews support the sympatho-excitatory effects of mobilizations (Kingston et al., 2014) and an increase in pressure pain threshold at local and remote sites (Coronado et al., 2012; Lascurain-Aguirrebena et al., 2016), although other reviews have reported local increases in pressure pain threshold following intervention but inconsistent effects at more remote locations (Millan et al., 2012a; Voogt et al., 2015).

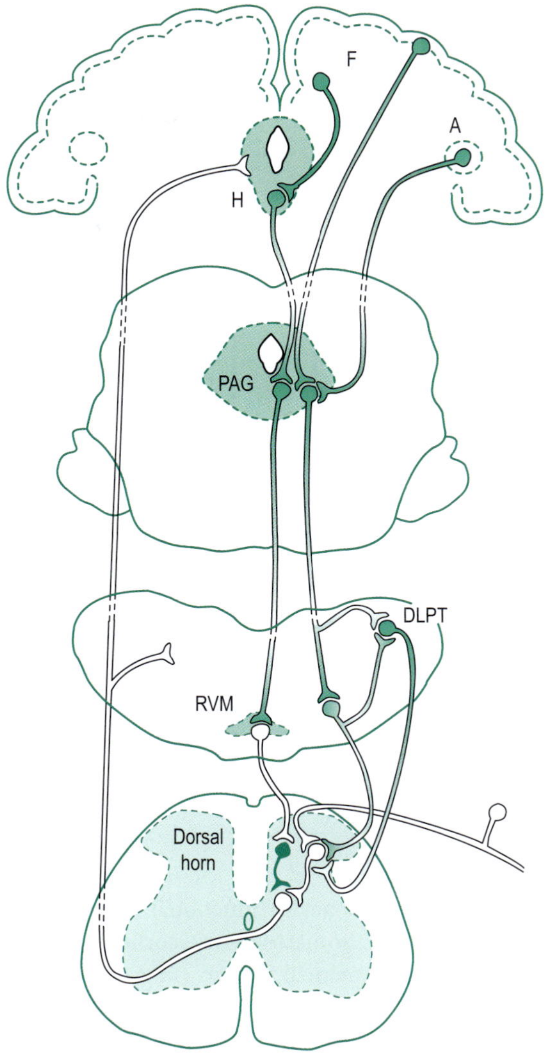

Fig. 3.4 Pain-modulating pathway. Periaqueductal grey (*PAG*) receives input from the frontal lobe (*F*), the amygdala (*A*) and the hypothalamus (*H*). Afferents from PAG travel to the rostral ventromedial medulla (*RVM*) and the dorsolateral pontomesencephalic tegmentum (*DLPT*) and on to the dorsal horn. The RVM has bidirectional control of nociceptive transmission. There are inhibitory (filled) and excitatory (unfilled) interneurones. (*From Fields & Basbaum, 1999, with permission.*)

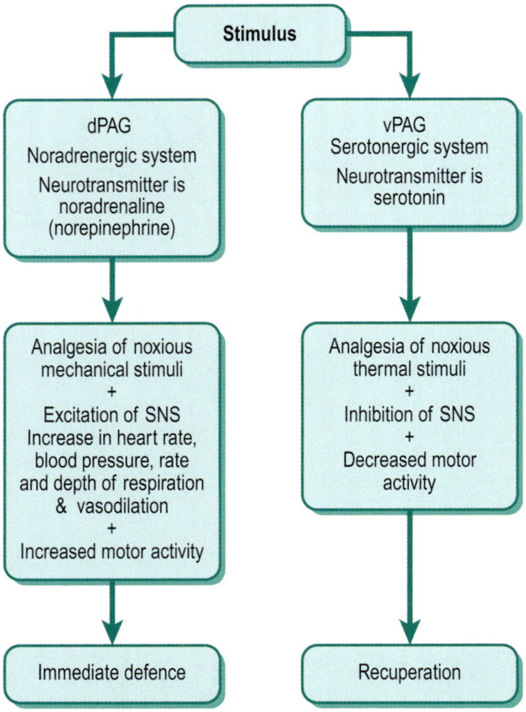

Fig. 3.5 Descending inhibition of mechanical nociception from the dorsolateral periaqueductal grey (*dPAG*: noradrenergic system), and thermal nociception from the ventrolateral periaqueductal grey (*vPAG*: serotonergic system). *SNS*, Sympathetic nervous system.

Furthermore, changes in functional connectivity in the insular cortex, somatosensory cortices and PAG were observed post manual therapy (in groups receiving mobilization, manipulation and therapeutic touch) in human participants with exercise-induced back pain (Gay et al., 2014). However, this was not compared with a control intervention and thus changes could result from natural history. A recent review of the effect of manipulative techniques on improving 'brain function' concluded that the evidence base is inconsistent across and—sometimes—within studies and that the clinical relevance of the observed responses in the brain is unknown (Meyer et al., 2019).

> **KNOWLEDGE CHECK**
> 1. What are the influences of manual therapy on the immune system?
> 2. What are the effects of manual therapy on inhibition of pain in the central nervous system?

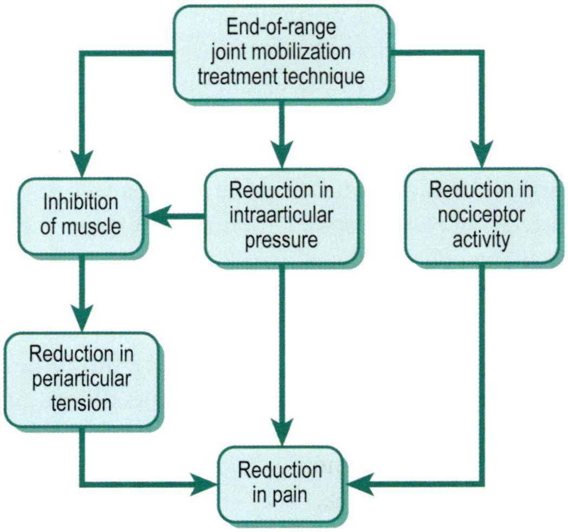

Fig. 3.6 Proposed mechanism for pain relief following end-of-range joint mobilization treatment. (*From Zusman, 1986.*)

Effect of Manual Therapy on Motor Activity

There is some evidence to suggest that joint treatment influences motor control and proprioception, thought to be factors in ongoing pain and dysfunction. Manual therapy may also reduce pain through interruption of the pain–muscle spasm–pain cycle. Zusman (1986) proposed a theory for the relief of pain with passive end-range joint movement through inhibiting reflex muscle contraction and reducing the level of joint afferent activity (Fig. 3.6). A number of studies investigating articular neurology have demonstrated that end-of-range passive joint movements cause a reduction in local and distant reflex muscle contraction (Freeman & Wyke, 1967; Baxendale & Ferrell, 1981; Taylor et al., 1994) and reduction in muscle tension at the limits of joint movement (Lundberg et al., 1978). This reduction in muscle contraction is thought to reduce ischaemic muscle pain (Freeman & Wyke, 1967) and to reduce muscle tension on periarticular and aponeurotic structures, with a subsequent reduction in the peripheral afferent activity (Millar, 1973; Grigg, 1976). Greater inhibition of muscle has been shown to occur with mechanical stimulation of joint afferents than with cutaneous or muscle stimulation, albeit in decerebrate cats (Baxendale & Ferrell, 1981).

The majority of studies directly investigating the effects of manual therapy on motor activity have focused on manipulation and have reported contradictory findings. Those using electromyography (EMG) to determine muscle response to manipulation provide some evidence that motor activity may be facilitated in response to manipulation (Herzog, 1999; Colloca & Keller, 2001; Colloca et al., 2003); however, the lack of control groups and low participant numbers in these studies cast doubt over the strength of this evidence. A stronger randomized controlled trial using patients with low-back pain reported similar results of an increase in EMG output during trunk extension in prone after manipulation; this was not observed in the control or sham manipulation groups (Keller & Colloca, 2000). In agreement with EMG studies, a study using transcranial magnetic stimulation reported postsynaptic facilitation of alpha and cortical motoneurons following manipulation (Dishman et al., 2002). In contrast, studies measuring the H-reflex have found that manipulation results in a transient suppression of motor neurone excitability (Dishman & Bulbulian, 2000; Dishman & Burke, 2003). Dishman and Burke (2003) proposed that this may be due to presynaptic inhibition of Ia fibres in the dorsal horn or changes in segmental and descending pathways mediating postsynaptic inhibition of motor neurons.

Pain can result in altered sensorimotor input, the process that coordinates afferent information and resultant control of the motor system. The afferent input from manipulation has been shown to alter somato-motor information by changing the way in which the somatosensory cortex responds to subsequent input (Haavik-Taylor & Murphy, 2007, 2008, 2009). For example, manipulation of the cervical spine in people with subclinical neck pain has been shown to improve suppression of somatosensory evoked potential indicating changes in cortical excitability (Haavik-Taylor & Murphy, 2007, 2008). In a later study the same research group found that manipulation in participants with subclinical neck pain resulted in cerebellar modulation which normalized sensorimotor integration and motor output in a subsequent motor task (Daligadu et al., 2013).

Studies investigating the effects of mobilizations on motor activity consistently report a reduction in motor activity following treatment, both at rest and during active movements. Gross et al. (2012) reported side-to-side differences in short-latency stretch reflexes of erector spinae in patients with persistent low-back pain which were normalized following mobilizations. This was proposed to be due to downregulation of the stretch reflex response in muscle spindles. A significant reduction in EMG activity has been reported in the superficial neck muscles following cervical spine mobilizations in patients with neck pain (Sterling et al., 2001), the erector spinae following lumbar mobilizations in an asymptomatic population (Krekoukias et al., 2009) and the masseter muscle following temporomandibular joint mobilization (Taylor et al., 1994). The effect in masseter muscle remained evident for 15 minutes post treatment and was apparent both at rest and during active movement (Taylor et al., 1994). Similarly reduced EMG activity during trunk extension has been found following mobilization of the thoracic spine (Pecos-Martin et al., 2017). The most recent review on this area (Pfluegler et al., 2020) concluded that 'the evidence suggests that passive joint mobilisations have the ability to immediately alter muscle function'. There is a moderate level of evidence that joint mobilization immediately decreases the activation of superficial muscles during low load conditions in symptomatic individuals, suggesting an increase in deep muscle recruitment, hence an improved motor pattern. There are contradictory findings regarding the ability to alter maximum muscle strength; a low level of evidence for asymptomatic individuals indicates that joint mobilization can improve maximum muscle strength, opposed to a very low level of evidence suggesting no such improvement in symptomatic individuals (Pfluegler et al., 2020). The effects of manual therapy treatments are short-term, and this should be acknowledged when making shared decisions related to treatment choice with the patient. Clinicians should help the patient to consider how a similar technique might be applied by them at home to stimulate these effects, if and when it is useful for them.

Evidence Base for Joint Mobilizations

As discussed earlier, there is a large amount of basic science research to support the therapeutic effects of joint mobilizations. However, it is also important to know that these effects translate to an improvement in clinical outcomes for patients. There are numerous systematic reviews and meta-analyses examining the effectiveness of joint mobilizations.

In spinal joint dysfunction, there is evidence from systematic reviews of moderate benefit for spinal manual therapy in neck disorders (Bronfort et al., 2004; Gross et al., 2004, 2015; Sarigiovannis & Hollins, 2005) although the effect size is no better than just exercise (Fredin & Lorås, 2017), cervicogenic headache (Bronfort et al., 2001) and acute low-back pain (Hettinga et al., 2008). The outcomes in persistent low-back pain have been variable, with some trials finding that manual therapy is an effective treatment (UK BEAM Trial, 2004) while others have found it not superior to other advocated treatments (Assendelft et al., 2004; Goldby et al., 2006; Goertz et al., 2012).

In the case of peripheral disorders, there is also a moderate level of evidence from systematic reviews for the use of joint mobilizations in lower-limb joint dysfunction (Brantingham et al., 2009), upper-limb joint injury (Michlovitz et al., 2004), adhesive capsulitis of the shoulder (Noten et al., 2016), lateral epicondylalgia (Herd & Meserve, 2008; Heiser et al., 2013) and ankle sprain (van der Wees et al., 2006; Loudon et al., 2014) and for the use of MWMs in a variety of peripheral disorders (Hing et al., 2008). A recent study has also shown the long-term clinical and cost effectiveness benefits of incorporating manual therapy within a programme of exercise for patients with knee osteoarthritis (Bove et al., 2018). In contrast, there have been trials that suggest that adding joint mobilizations to a standard physiotherapy programme of exercise and advice does not improve outcomes in peripheral disorders such as radial fractures (Kay et al., 2000), shoulder pain (Chen et al., 2009) and ankle fractures (Lin et al., 2008).

EXERCISE FOR JOINT DYSFUNCTION

Physical activity and exercise play an essential and distinct role in the maintenance of health. Physiotherapists have prolonged contact with patients and therefore have an important role in health education. With the roots of physiotherapy in exercise, physiotherapists are well placed to employ behavioural change techniques and empower patients to become more physically active and take more exercise. A holistic, person-centred approach recognizes the embodied experience of people in pain and the importance of exercise in health should not be underestimated; for example, a recent meta-analysis found strong evidence that exercise was effective in the treatment of depression (Schuch et al., 2016), and a reciprocal relationship between increased physical activity and improved sleep has been reported in patients with persistent pain (Tang & Sanborn, 2014). Furthermore, exercise is important in primary and secondary disease prevention. However, as with all treatment interventions persons should be involved in making decisions related to their care, and it should be acknowledged and respected that not all persons want to or can exercise. Physiotherapists should reflect on their own exercise identity and bias and be sensitive to how discussing exercise may stigmatize some persons, particularly non-white persons and persons living in larger bodies (Setchell & Abaraogu, 2018) or with disabilities.

From a biomechanical perspective, therapeutic exercise has been widely reported to reduce and prevent the incidence of spinal and peripheral pathology as well as influence the rate of healing (Hertling & Kessler, 2006a). The beneficial effects of exercise on pain and function in patients with osteoarthritis are proposed to result from increased leg muscle strength, and improvement in proprioception (Runhaar et al., 2015). Research supports the theory that exercise can help in improving the strength, integrity and organization of collagen, an important substance in the healing process (Taunton et al., 1998; Hertling & Kessler, 2006a). Furthermore, physical activity can help increase tensile strength in injured tendons and ligaments and has been shown to be superior to rest in relation to time taken to return to activity (Hertling & Kessler, 2006a). It is believed that early movement is crucial from the proliferative stage of ligament injury, owing to the profound effect it has on healing tissue (Taunton et al., 1998). Mobilizing exercises, whether passive, active or a combination of both, in these early stages post ligamentous or muscular injury, influence the alignment and orientation of collagen, increase the tensile strength of repair and enhance the proliferative stage of healing as well as the next stage of remodelling (Taunton et al., 1998; Hassenkamp, 2005). This emphasizes the necessity for early mobilization of periarticular structures postinjury (Jarvinen & Kaariainen, 2007), but mobilization is also vital for maintenance of healthy intraarticular structures.

Several types of exercise are utilized in rehabilitation, including strengthening, agility, power training, stabilization, proprioception and balance exercises, flexibility drills, aerobic exercise and endurance training. With regard to joint dysfunction, the aim of exercise is to restore previous function, while remaining cognizant of adequate tissue healing and pain control in the acute stages of healing. In patients with central pain mechanisms exercise can exacerbate pain (Lima et al., 2017), and it is pivotal that clinicians acknowledge and validate this experience and explore with the person whether graded exposure and pacing techniques may be useful for them.

The benefits of exercise include:

- reduction in pain (Frank et al., 1984; Hertling & Kessler, 2006b)
- reduced need for analgesia
- promotion of healing through circulatory effects and effects on collagen
- maintenance of muscle length and strength
- improved balance
- enhanced healing process due to increased protein synthesis
- improved psychological well-being
- improved sleep
- primary and secondary disease prevention.

KEY POINTS AND SUMMARY

Management of people with joint dysfunction should, where possible, restore and encourage normal movement while addressing people's beliefs and expectations, and listening to and acknowledging their lived experience.

- Treatments aimed at joints can be incorporated within a holistic approach to management of people with musculoskeletal pain and dysfunction.
- The physiotherapist should treat joints alongside addressing unhelpful pain beliefs and behaviours.
- Joint treatment should be complemented with promotion of healthy lifestyle choices.
- Joint mobilizations and exercise both form components of evidence-based treatment of joint dysfunction.
- The choice and application of joint mobilizations are dependent on thorough and ongoing assessment of the patient's symptoms and signs, with the need for appropriate modification as required.
- Treatment in functional positions should be considered, with a recognition of the importance of the choice of starting position for treatment.
- The effect of joint mobilizations is both mechanical and neurophysiological, occurring at local, spinal and supraspinal levels. These effects are short-term, and this should be acknowledged when making shared decisions related to treatment choice with the person. Clinicians should help the person to consider how a similar technique might be applied by them at home to stimulate these effects, if and when it is useful for them.
- In joint dysfunction, exercise aims to restore function in terms of range and quality of motion and proprioceptive control, while helping to manage pain and enhance tissue healing.

REVIEW AND REVISE QUESTIONS

1. Please review the effects of joint mobilizations, both mechanical and neurophysiological, occurring at local, spinal and supraspinal levels.
2. Consider how to prescribe similar techniques (stretches/exercises) that a patient could undertake at home to stimulate these effects.
3. Review your understanding of the difference between joint mobilization, mobilization with movement and manipulation to clarify the similarities and differences in the techniques.

REFERENCES

Allison, G., Edmonston, S., Kiviniemi, K., et al., 2001. Influence of standardized mobilization on the posteroanterior stiffness of the lumbar spine in asymptomatic subjects. Physiother. Res. Int. 6, 145–156.

Assendelft, W.J., Morton, S.C., Yu, E.I., et al., 2004. Spinal manipulative therapy for low back pain. Cochrane Database Syst. Rev. 1, CD000447.

Baxendale, R.H., Ferrell, W.R., 1981. The effect of knee joint afferent discharge on transmission in flexion reflex pathways in decerebrate cats. J. Physiol. 315, 231–242.

Beselga, C., Neto, F., Alburquerque-Sendin, F., et al., 2016. Immediate effects of hip mobilisation with movement in patients with hip osteoarthritis: a randomized controlled trial. Man. Ther. 22, 80–85.

Bialosky, J., Bishop, M., Price, D., et al., 2009a. The mechanism of manual therapy in the treatment of musculoskeletal pain: a comprehensive model. Man. Ther. 14, 531–538.

Bialosky, J., Bishop, M., Robinson, M., et al., 2009b. Spinal manipulative therapy has an immediate effect on thermal pain sensitivity in people with low back pain: a randomized controlled trial. Phys. Ther. 89, 1292–1303.

Bialosky, J., Bishop, M., Robinson, M., et al., 2010. The relationship of the audible pop to hypoalgesia associated with high-velocity, low-amplitude thrust manipulation: a secondary analysis of an experimental study in pain-free participants. J. Manipulative Physiol. Ther. 33, 117–124.

Bishop, M., Beneciuk, J., George, S., 2011. Immediate reduction in temporal sensory summation after thoracic spinal manipulation. Spine J. 11, 440–446.

Boal, R., Gillette, R., 2004. Central neuronal plasticity, low back pain and spinal manipulative therapy. J. Manipulative Physiol. Ther. 27, 314–326.

Bolton, J.E., Wilkinson, R.C., 1998. Responsiveness of pain scales: a comparison of three pain intensity measures in chiropractic patients. J. Manipulative Physiol. Ther. 21, 1–7.

Bove, A.M., Smith, K.J., Bise, C.G., et al., 2018. Exercise, manual therapy, and booster sessions in knee osteoarthritis: cost-effectiveness analysis from a multicenter randomized controlled trial. Phys. Ther. 98 (1), 16–27.

Brantingham, J.W., Globe, G., Pollard, H., et al., 2009. Manipulative therapy for lower extremity conditions: expansion of literature review. J. Manipulative Physiol. Ther. 32, 53–71.

Brennan, P., Kokjohn, K., Kaltinger, C., et al., 1991. Enhanced phagocytic cell respiratory burst induced by spinal manipulation: potential role of substance P. J. Manipulative Physiol. Ther. 14, 399–408.

Bronfort, G., Assendelft, W.J., Evans, R., et al., 2001. Efficacy of spinal manipulation for chronic headache: a systematic review. J. Manipulative Physiol. Ther. 24, 457–466.

Bronfort, G., Haas, M., Evans, R.L., et al., 2004. Efficacy of spinal manipulation and mobilization for low back pain and neck pain: a systematic review and best evidence synthesis. Spine J. 4 (3), 335–356.

Cascioli, V., Corr, P., Till, T., 2003. An investigation into the production of intra-articular gas bubbles and increase in joint space in the zygapophyseal joints of the cervical spine in asymptomatic subjects after spinal manipulation. J. Manipulative Physiol. Ther. 26, 356–364.

Chansirinukor, W., Lee, M., Latimer, J., 2001. Contribution of pelvic rotation to lumbar posteroanterior movement. Man. Ther. 6, 242–249.

Chansirinukor, W., Lee, M., Latimer, J., 2003. Contribution of ribcage movement to thoracolumbar posteroanterior stiffness. J. Manipulative Physiol. Ther. 26, 176–183.

Chen, J.F., Ginn, K.A., Herbert, R.D., 2009. Passive mobilisation of shoulder region joints plus advice and exercise does not reduce pain and disability more than advice and exercise alone: a randomised trial. Aust. J. Physiother. 55, 17–23.

Chiu, T.W., Wright, A., 1996. To compare the effects of different rates of application of a cervical mobilisation technique on sympathetic outflow to the upper limb in normal subjects. Man. Ther. 1, 198–203.

Clark, B., Gross, D., Walkoski, S., et al., 2011. Neurophysiologic effects of spinal manipulation in patients with chronic low back pain. BMC Musculoskelet. Disord. 12, 170.

Cleland, J.A., Childs, J.D., McRae, M., et al., 2005. Immediate effects of thoracic manipulation in patients with neck pain: a randomized clinical trial. Man. Ther. 10, 127–135.

Cleland, J.A., Flynn, T., Childs, J.D., et al., 2007. The audible pop from thoracic spine thrust manipulation and its relation to short-term outcomes in patients with neck pain. J. Manipulative Physiol. Ther. 15, 143–154.

Colloca, C., Keller, T., 2001. Stiffness and neuromuscular reflex response of the human spine to posteroanterior manipulative thrusts in patients with low back pain. J. Manipulative Physiol. Ther. 24, 489–500.

Colloca, C., Keller, T., Gunzburg, R., 2003. Neuromechanical characterization of in vivo lumbar spinal manipulation. Part II. Neurophysiological response. J. Manipulative Physiol. Ther. 26, 579–591.

Colombi, A., Testa, M., 2019. The effects induced by spinal manipulative therapy on the immune and endocrine systems. Medicina (Kaunas). 55 (8), 448.

Cook, C., Learman, K., Showalter, C., et al., 2013. Early use of thrust manipulation versus non-thrust manipulation: a randomized clinical trial. Man. Ther. 18 (3), 191–198.

Coronado, R., Gay, C., Bialosky, J., et al., 2012. Changes in pain sensitivity following manipulation: a systematic review and meta-analysis. J. Electromyogr. Kinesiol. 22, 752–756.

Daligadu, J., Haavik-Taylor, H., Yielder, P., et al., 2013. Alteration in cortical and cerebellar motor processing in subclinical neck pain patients following spinal manipulation. J. Manipulative Physiol. Ther. 36, 527–537.

Delgado, J., Prado-Robles, E., Rodrigues-de-Souza, D., et al., 2015. Effects of mobilisation with movement on pain and range of motion in patients with unilateral shoulder impingement syndrome: a randomized controlled trial. J. Manipulative Physiol. Ther. 38, 245–252.

Dishman, J., Bulbulian, R., 2000. Spinal reflex attenuation associated with spinal manipulation. Spine 25, 2519–2525.

Dishman, J., Burke, J., 2003. Spinal reflex excitability changes after cervical and lumbar spinal manipulation: a comparative study. Spine J. 3, 204–212.

Dishman, J.D., Ball, K.A., Burke, J., 2002. Central motor excitability changes after spinal manipulation: a transcranial magnetic stimulation study. J. Manipulative Physiol. Ther. 25, 1–9.

Donaldson, M., Petersen, S., Cook, C., Learman, K., 2016. A prescriptively selected nonthrust manipulation versus a therapist-selected nonthrust manipulation for treatment of individuals with low back pain: a randomized clinical trial. J. Orthop. Sports Phys. Ther. 46, 243–250.

Dunning, J., Mourad, F., Zingoni, A., et al., 2017. Cavitation sounds during cervicothoracic spinal manipulation. Int. J. Sports Phys. Ther. 12 (4), 642–654.

Ellingsen, D.M., Leknes, S., Løseth, G., et al., 2016. The neurobiology shaping affective touch: expectation, motivation, and meaning in the multisensory context. Front. Psychol. 6, 1986.

Fanselow, M.S., 1991. The midbrain periaqueductal gray as a coordinator of action in response to fear and anxiety. In: Depaulis, A., Bandler, R. (Eds.), The Midbrain Periaqueductal Gray Matter. Plenum Press, New York, pp. 151–173.

Fernando de Oliveira, R., Eloin Liebano, R., de Cunha Menezes Costa, L., et al., 2013. Immediate effects of region-specific and non-region specific spinal manipulative therapy on patients with chronic low back pain: a randomized controlled trial. Phys. Ther. 93, 748–756.

Ferrell, W.R., Nade, S., Newbold, P.J., 1986. The interrelation of neural discharge, intra-articular pressure, and joint angle in the knee of the dog. J. Physiol. 373, 353–365.

Fields, H.L., Basbaum, A.I., 1999. Central nervous system mechanisms of pain modulation. In: Wall, P.D., Melzack, R. (Eds.), Textbook of Pain, fourth ed. Churchill Livingstone, Edinburgh, pp. 309–329.

Flynn, T., Childs, J., Fritz, J., 2006. The audible pop from high-velocity thrust manipulation and outcome in individuals with low back pain. J. Manipulative Physiol. Ther. 29, 40–45.

Frank, C., Akesan, W., Woo, S.L.Y., et al., 1984. Physiology and therapeutic value of passive joint motion. Clin. Orthop. Relat. Res. 185, 113–125.

Fredin, K., Lorås, H., 2017. Manual therapy, exercise therapy or combined treatment in the management of adult neck pain – a systematic review and meta-analysis. Musculoskelet. Sci. Pract. 62–71.

Freeman, M.A.R., Wyke, B.D., 1967. Articular reflexes at the ankle joint: an electromyographic study of normal and abnormal influences of ankle-joint mechanoreceptors upon reflex activity in the leg muscles. Br. J. Surg. 54, 990–1001.

Ganesh, S., Mohanty, P., Pattnaik, M., et al., 2015. Effectiveness of mobilization therapy and exercise in mechanical neck pain. Physiother. Theory Pract. 31, 99–106.

Gay, C., Robinson, M., George, S., et al., 2014. Immediate changes after manual therapy in resting-state functional connectivity as measured by functional magnetic resonance imaging in participants with induced low back pain. J. Manipulative Physiol. Ther. 37, 615–627.

George, S., Bishop, M., Bialosky, J., et al., 2006. Immediate effects of spinal manipulation on thermal pain sensitivity: an experimental study. BMC Musculoskelet. Disord. 7, 1–10.

George, S.Z., Zeppieri, G., 2009. Physical therapy utilization of graded exposure for patients with low back pain. J. Orthop Sports Phys. Ther. 39 (7), 496–505.

Giovanelli-Blacker, B., Elvey, R., Thompson, E., 1985. The clinical significance of measured lumbar zygapophyseal intracapsular pressure variation. In: Proceedings of the Manipulative Therapists Association of Australia 4th Biennial Conference, Brisbane, Queensland, pp. 122–139.

Goertz, C., Pohlman, K., Vining, R., et al., 2012. Patient-centered outcomes of high velocity, low amplitude spinal manipulation for low back pain: a systematic review. J. Electromyogr. Kinesiol. 22, 670–691.

Goldby, L.J., Moore, A.P., Doust, J., et al., 2006. A randomized control trial investigating the efficiency of musculoskeletal physiotherapy on chronic back pain disorder. Spine 31, 1083–1093.

Goodsell, M., Lee, M., Latimer, J., 2000. Short-term effects of lumbar posteroanterior mobilization in individuals with low-back pain. J. Manipulative Physiol. Ther. 23, 332–342.

Grigg, P., 1976. Response of joint afferent neurons in cat medial articular nerve to active and passive movements of the knee. Brain Res. 118, 482–485.

Gross, A., Hoving, J.L., Haines, T., et al., 2004. Manipulation and mobilisation for mechanical neck disorders. Cochrane Database Syst. Rev. 1, CD004249.

Gross, A., Langevin, P., Burnie, S., et al., 2015. Manipulation and mobilisation for neck pain contrasted against inactive control or another active treatment. Cochrane Database Syst. Rev. (9), CD004249.

Gross, A., Miller, J., D'Sylva, J., et al., 2010. Manipulation and mobilisation for neck pain. Man. Ther. 15, 315–333.

Gross, D., Thomas, J., Walkowski, S., et al., 2012. Non-thrust manual therapy reduces erector spinae short-latency stretch reflex asymmetries I patients with chronic low back pain. J. Electryomyogr. Kinesiol. 22, 663–669.

Haavik-Taylor, H., Murphy, B., 2007. Cervical spine manipulation alters somatosensory integration: a somatosensory evoked potential study. Clin. Neurophysiol. 118, 391–402.

Haavik-Taylor, H., Murphy, B., 2008. Altered central integration of dual somatosensory input after cervical spine manipulation. J. Manipulative Physiol. Ther. 33, 178–188.

Haavik-Taylor, H., Murphy, B., 2009. The effects of spinal manipulation on central integration of dual somatosensory input observed after motor training: a crossover study. J. Manipulative Physiol. Ther. 33, 261–272.

Harms, M.C., Bader, D.L., 1997. Variability of forces applied by experienced therapists during spinal mobilization. Clin. Biomech. (Bristol, Avon) 12, 393–399.

Hassenkamp, A., 2005. Soft tissue injuries. In: Atkinson, K., Coutts, F., Hassenkamp, A. (Eds.), Physiotherapy in Orthopaedics, second ed. Elsevier Churchill Livingstone, London.

Hebron, C., 2014. The biomechanical and analgesic effects of lumbar mobilisations. Doctoral thesis, University of Brighton.

Hefford, C., Haxby-Abbott, J., Arnold, R., et al., 2012. The patient-specific functional scale: validity, reliability, and responsiveness in patients with upper extremity musculoskeletal problems. J. Orthop. Sports Phys. Ther. 42, 56–65.

Heidegger, M., 1962. Being and Time (J. Maquarrie and E. Robinson, Trans.). Blackwell, Oxford.

Heiser, R., O'Brien, V., Schwartz, D., 2013. The use of joint mobilization to improve clinical outcomes in hand therapy: a systematic review of the literature. J. Hand Ther. 26, 297–311.

Hengeveld, E., Banks, K., 2013. Maitland's Vertebral Manipulation, eighth ed. Churchill Livingstone, Edinburgh.

Herd, C.R., Meserve, B.B., 2008. Systematic review of the effectiveness of manipulative therapy in treating lateral epicondylalgia. J. Man. Manip. Ther. 16, 225–237.

Hertling, D., Kessler, R., 2006a. Introduction to manual therapy. In: Hertling, D., Kessler, R. (Eds.), Management of Common Musculoskeletal Disorders: Physical Therapy Principles and Methods. Lippincott, Williams and Wilkins, Philadelphia.

Hertling, D., Kessler, R.M., 2006b. Shoulder and shoulder girdle. In: Hertling, D., Kessler, R.M. (Eds.), Management of Common Musculoskeletal Disorders: Physical Therapy Principles and Methods. Lippincott, Williams and Wilkins, Philadelphia.

Herzog, W., 1999. Electromyographic responses of back and limb muscles associated with spinal manipulative therapy. Spine 24, 146–153.

Hettinga, D.M., Hurley, D.A., Jackson, A., et al., 2008. Assessing the effect of sample size, methodological quality and statistical rigour on outcomes of randomised controlled trials on mobilisation, manipulation and massage for low back pain of at least 6 weeks duration. Physiotherapy 94, 97–104.

Hing, W., Bigelow, R., Bremner, T., 2008. Mulligan's mobilisation with movement: a review of the tenets and prescription of MWMs. N. Z. J. Physiother. 36, 144–164.

Hing, W., Hallam, T., Rivett, D., et al., 2015. The Mulligan Concept of Manual Therapy. Churchill Livingstone, Edinburgh.

Holland, C., Campbell, K., Hunt, K., 2015. Increased treatment duration lead to greater improvements in non-weight bearing dorsiflexion range of motion for asymptomatic individuals immediately following an anteroposterior grade IV mobilisation of the talus. Man. Ther. 20, 598–602.

Hosobuchi, Y., Adams, J., Linchitz, R., 1977. Pain relief by electrical stimulation of the central gray matter in humans and its reversal by naloxone. Science 197, 183–186.

Jarvinen, T., Kaariainen, M., 2007. Muscle injuries: optimising recovery. Best Pract. Res. Clin. Rheumatol. 21, 317–331.

Kalauokalani, D., Cherkin, D., Sherman, K., et al., 2001. Lessons from a trial of acupuncture and massage for low back pain. Spine 26, 1418–1424.

Kawchuk, G.N., Fryer, J., Jaremko, J.L., et al., 2015. Real-time visualization of joint cavitation. PLoS One 10 (4), e0119470. https://doi.org/10.1371/ journal. pone. 0119470.

Kay, S., Haensel, N., Stiller, K., 2000. The effect of passive mobilisation following fractures involving the distal radius: a randomised study. J. Physiother. 46, 93–101.

Keller, T., Colloca, C., 2000. Mechanical force spinal manipulation increases trunk muscle strength assessed by electromyography: a comparative clinical trial. J. Manipulative Physiol. Ther. 23, 585–595.

Khanmohammadi, M.R., Rostami, M.R.A., Khazaeipour, M.S.Z., et al., 2021. Larger amplitude spinal mobilization is more effective to decrease pain systematically: q clinical trial using pressure pain thresholds in chronic low back pain participants. J. Bodyw. Mov. Ther. 25, 16–23.

Kingston, L., Claydon, L., Tumilty, S., 2014. The effects of spinal mobilization on the sympathetic nervous system: a systematic review. Man. Ther. 19, 281–287.

Krekoukias, G., Petty, N., Cheek, L., 2009. Comparison of surface electromyographic activity of erector spinae before and after the application of central posteroanterior mobilisation on the lumbar spine. J. Electromyogr. Kinesiol. 19, 39–45.

Krouwel, O., Hebron, C., Willett, E., 2010. An investigation into the potential hypoalgesic effects of different amplitudes of PA mobilisations on the lumbar spine as measured by pressure pain thresholds (PPT). Man. Ther. 15, 7–12.

Kulig, K., Landel, R., Powers, C., 2004. Assessment of lumbar spine kinematics using dynamic MRI: a proposed mechanism of sagittal plane motion induced by manual posterior-to-anterior mobilisation. J. Orthop. Sports Phys. Ther. 34, 57–64.

Langevin, H.M., Bouffard, N.A., Badger, G.J., et al., 2005. Dynamic fibroblast cytoskeletal response to subcutaneous tissue stretch ex vivo and in vivo. Am. J. Physiol. Cell. Physiol. 288 (3), C747–C756.

Lascurain-Aguirrebena, I., Newham, D., Critchley, D., 2016. Mechanism of action of spinal mobilizations: a systematic review. Spine 41, 159–172.

Leaver, A., Maher, C., Herbert, R., et al., 2010. A randomized controlled trial comparing manipulation with mobilisation for recent onset neck pain. Arch. Phys. Med. Rehabil. 91, 1313–1318.

Lee, M., Steven, G., Crosbie, R., 1996. Towards a theory of lumbar mobilisations – the relationship between applied manual force and movements of the spine. Man. Ther. 2, 67–75.

Lee, R., Evans, J., 1997. An in vivo study of the intervertebral movements produced by posteroanterior mobilization. Clin. Biomech. (Bristol, Avon) 12, 400–408.

Lee, R., Evans, J., 2000. The role of spinal tissues in resisting posteroanterior forces applied to the lumbar spine. J. Manipulative Physiol. Ther. 23, 551–555.

Leong, D.J., Hardin, J.A., Cobelli, N.J., et al., 2011. Mechanotransduction and cartilage integrity. Ann NY Acad. Sci. 1240, 32–37.

Levick, J.R., 1979. An investigation into the validity of subatmospheric pressure recordings from synovial fluid and their dependence on joint angle. J. Physiol. 289, 55–67.

Lima, L.V., Abner, T.S.S., Sluka, K.A., 2017. Does exercise increase or decrease pain? Central mechanisms underlying these two phenomena. J. Physiol. 595 (13), 4141–4150.

Lin, C.W., Moseley, A.M., Haas, M., et al., 2008. Manual therapy in addition to physiotherapy does not improve clinical or economic outcomes after ankle fracture. J. Rehabil. Med. 40, 433–439.

Loudon, J., Reiman, M., Sylvain, J., 2014. The efficacy of manual joint mobilisation / manipulation in treatment of lateral ankle sprains: a systematic review. Br. J. Sports Med. 48, 365–379.

Lovick, T.A., 1991. Interactions between descending pathways from the dorsal and ventrolateral periaqueductal gray matter in the rat. In: Depaulis, A., Bandler, R. (Eds.), The midbrain periaqueductal gray matter. Plenum Press, New York, pp. 101–120.

Lundberg, A., Malmgren, K., Schomburg, E.D., 1978. Role of joint afferents in motor control exemplified by effects on reflex pathways from 1b afferents. J. Physiol. 284, 327–343.

Magarey, M.E., 1985. Selection of passive treatment techniques. Proceedings of the Manipulative Therapists Association of Australia 4th Biennial Conference, Brisbane, pp. 298–320.

Magarey, M.E., 1986. Examination and assessment in spinal joint dysfunction. In: Grieve, G.P. (Ed.), Modern Manual Therapy of the Vertebral Column. Churchill Livingstone, Edinburgh, pp. 481–497.

May, A., Rodriguez-Raecke, R., Schulte, A., et al., 2012. Within-session sensitization and between-session habituation: a robust physiological response to repetitive painful heat stimulation. Eur. J. Pain 16, 401–409.

McCarthy, C., Rivett, D., 2019. Thoracic Spine Pain in a Soccer Player: A Combined Movement Theory Approach. Chapter 24 in Clinical Reasoning in Musculoskeletal Practice, second ed. Elsevier, Oxford, UK.

McCarthy, C., Lonnemann, E., Hindle, J., et al., 2020. The physiology of manual therapy. In: A Comprehensive Guide to Sports Physiology and Injury Management E-Book: An Interdisciplinary Approach. Elsevier, Oxford, UK.

McCarthy, C.J., 2010. Combined Movement Theory: Rational Mobilization and Manipulation of the Vertebral Column. Elsevier Science, Oxford UK, ISBN 978-0-443-06857-7.

McCarthy, C.J., 2013. Manual therapy and pain perception. In: Pain a Textbook for Therapists, second ed. Van Grievesen, Elsevier Healthscience, Oxford, UK.

McCarthy, C.J., Bialosky, J., Rivett, D., 2015. Manipulative Therapy. In: Jull, G., Moore, A., Falla, D., et al. (Eds.), Grieve's Modern Musculoskeletal Therapy, fourth ed. Elsevier Healthscience, Oxford, UK.

McCarthy, C.J., Potter, L., Oldham, J.A., 2019. Comparing targeted thrust manipulation with general thrust manipulation in patients with low back pain. A general approach is as effective as a specific one. A randomised controlled trial. BMJ Open Sport Exerc. Med. 5 (1), e000514. https://doi.org/10.1136/bmjsem-2019-000514.

McKenzie, R., 1981. The Lumbar Spine, Mechanical Diagnosis and Therapy. Spinal Publications, New Zealand.

McKenzie, R., 1983. Treat Your Own Neck. Spinal Publications, New Zealand.

McKenzie, R., 1985. Treat Your Own Back. Spinal Publications, New Zealand.

McLean, S., Naish, R., Reed, L., et al., 2002. A pilot study of the manual force levels required to produce manipulation induced hypoalgesia. Clin. Biomech. (Bristol, Avon) 17, 304–308.

McQuade, K.J., Shelley, I., Cvitkovic, J., 1999. Patterns of stiffness during clinical examination of the glenohumeral joint. Clin. Biomech. (Bristol, Avon) 14, 620–627.

Melzack, R., Wall, P.D., 1965. Pain mechanisms: a new theory. Science 150, 971–979.

Meyer, A.L., Amorim, M.A., Schubert, M., Schweinhardt, P., Leboeuf-Yde, C., 2019. Unravelling functional neurology: does spinal manipulation have an effect on the brain? – a systematic literature review. Chiropr. Man. Therap. 2 (27), 60.

Michie, S., van Stralen, M., West, R., 2011. The behavioural change wheel: a new method for characterizing and designing behavior change interventions. Implement. Sci. 6, 42.

Michlovitz, S., Harris, B.A., Watkins, M.P., 2004. Therapy interventions for improving joint range of motion: a systematic review. J. Hand Ther. 17, 118–131.

Millan, M., Leboeuf-Yde, C., Budgell, B., et al., 2012a. The effects of spinal manipulative therapy on experimentally induced pain: a systematic literature review. Chiropr. Man. Therap. 20, 1–22.

Millan, M., Leboeuf-Yde, C., Budgell, B., et al., 2012b. The effects of spinal manipulative therapy on spinal range of movement: a systematic literature review. Chiropr. Man. Therap. 20, 1–18.

Millar, J., 1973. Joint afferent fibres responding to muscle stretch, vibration and contraction. Brain Res. 63, 380–383.

Molina-Ortega, F., Lomas-Vega, R., Hita-Contreras, F., et al., 2014. Immediate effects of spinal manipulation on nitric oxide, substance P and pain perception. Man. Ther. 19, 411–417.

Mourad, F., Dunning, J., Zingoni, A., et al., 2019. Unilateral and Multiple Cavitation Sounds During Lumbosacral Spinal Manipulation. J. Manipulative Physiol. Ther. 42 (1), 12–22.

Nade, J.S., Newbold, P.J., 1983. Factors determining the level and changes in intra-articular pressure in the knee joint of the dog. J. Physiol. 338, 21–36.

Nijs, J., Van Houdenhove, B., 2009. From acute musculoskeletal pain to chronic widespread pain and fibromyalgia: application of pain neurophysiology in manual therapy practice. Man. Ther. 14, 3–12.

Nisha, K., Megha, N., Paresh, P., 2014. Efficacy of weight bearing distal tibiofibular joint mobilisation with movement (MWM) in improving pain, dorsiflexion range and function in patients with postacute lateral ankle sprain. Int. J. Physiother. 2, 542–548.

Noten, S., Meeus, M., Stassijns, G., et al., 2016. Efficacy of different types of mobilization techniques in patients with primary adhesive capsulitis of the shoulder: a systematic review. Arch. Phys. Med. Rehabil. 97, 815–825.

Noyes, F.R., DeLucas, J.L., Torvik, P.J., 1974. Biomechanics of anterior cruciate ligament failure: an analysis of strain-rate sensitivity and mechanisms of failure in primates. J. Bone Joint Surg. Am. 56A, 236–253.

Palmlöf, L., Holm, L.W., Alfredsson, L., Skillgate, E., 2016. Expectations of recovery: a prognostic factor in patients with neck pain undergoing manual therapy treatment. Eur. J. Pain 20 (9), 1384–1391.

Panjabi, M.M., White, A.A., 2001. Biomechanics in the Musculoskeletal System. Churchill Livingstone, New York.

Parravicini, G., Bergna, A., 2017. Biological effects of direct and indirect manipulation of the fascial system. Narrative review. J. Bodyw Mov. Ther. 21 (2), 435–445.

Pecos-Martín, D., de Melo Aroeira, A.E., Verás Silva, R.L., et al., 2017. Immediate effects of thoracic spinal mobilisation on erector spinae muscle activity and pain in patients with thoracic spine pain: a preliminary randomised controlled trial. Physiotherapy 103 (1), 90–97.

Pentelka, L., Hebron, C., Shapleski, R., et al., 2012. The effect of increasing sets (within one treatment session) and different set durations (between treatment sessions) of lumbar spine posteroanterior mobilisations on pressure pain thresholds. Man. Ther. 17, 526–530.

Pfluegler, G., Kasper, J., Luedtke, K., 2020. The immediate effects of passive joint mobilisation on local muscle function. A systematic review of the literature. Musculoskelet. Sci. Pract. 45, 102106.

Pickar, J.G., Bolton, P., 2012. Spinal manipulative therapy and somatosensory activation. J. Electromyogr. Kinesiol. 22, 785–794.

Powers, C., Kulig, K., Harrison, J., et al., 2003. Segmental mobility of the lumbar spine during a posterior to anterior mobilization: assessment using dynamic MRI. Clin. Biomech. 18, 80–83.

Reynolds, D., 1969. Surgery in the rat during electrical analgesia induced by focal brain stimulation. Science 164, 444–445.

Runhaar, J., Luijsterburg, P., Dekker, J., et al., 2015. Identifying potential mechanisms behind the positive effects of exercise therapy on pain and function in osteoarthritis; a systematic review. Osteoarthritis Cartilage 23, 1071–1082.

Ryder, D., Barnard, K., 2024. Petty's Musculoskeletal Examination and Assessment: A Handbook for Therapists, sixth ed. Elsevier, Oxford.

Salom-Moreno, R., Ortega-Santiago, R., Cleland, J., et al., 2014. Immediate changes in neck pain intensity and widespread pressure pain sensitivity in patients with bilateral chronic mechanical neck pain: a randomized controlled trial of thoracic thrust manipulation vs non-thrust mobilization. J. Manipulative Physiol. Ther. 37, 312–319.

Sarigiovannis, P., Hollins, B., 2005. Effectiveness of manual therapy in the treatment of non-specific neck pain: a review. Phys. Ther. Rev. 10, 35–50.

Schuch, F., Vancampfort, D., Richards, J., et al., 2016. Exercise as a treatment for depression: a meta-analysis adjusting for publication bias. J. Psychiatr. Res. 77, 42–51.

Setchell, J., Abaraogu, U., 2018. A critical perspective on stigma in physiotherapy: the example of weight stigma. In: Manipulating Practices: A Critical Physiotherapy Reader. Cappelen Damm, Norway.

Sillevis, R., Cleland, J., 2011. Immediate effects of the audible pop from a thoracic spine thrust manipulation on the autonomic nervous system and pain: a secondary analysis of a randomized controlled trial. J. Manipulative Physiol. Ther. 34, 37–45.

Snodgrass, S., Rivett, D., Robertson, V., et al., 2009. Cervical spine mobilisation forces applied by physiotherapy students. Physiotherapy 96, 120–129.

Soames, R., 2003. Joint Motion: Clinical Measurement and Evaluation. Churchill Livingstone, Edinburgh.

Sterling, M., Jull, G., Wright, A., 2001. Cervical mobilisation: concurrent effects on pain, sympathetic nervous system activity and motor activity. Man. Ther. 6, 72–81.

Sutlive, T.G., Mabry, L.M., Easterling, E.J., et al., 2009. Comparison of short-term response to two spinal manipulation techniques for patients with low back pain in a military beneficiary population. Mil. Med. 174 (7), 750–756.

Tang, N., Sanborn, A., 2014. Better quality sleep promotes daytime physical activity in patients with chronic pain? A multilevel analysis of the within-person relationship. PLoS One 9, e92158.

Taunton, J., Robertson Lloyd-Smith, D., Fricker, P., 1998. The ankle. In: Harries, M., Williams, C., Stanish, W. (Eds.), Oxford Textbook of Sports Medicine, second ed. Oxford University Press, Oxford.

Taylor, M., Suvinen, T., Reade, P., 1994. The effect of grade IV distraction mobilisation on patients with temporomandibular pain-dysfunction disorder. Physiother. Theory Pract. 10, 129–136.

Teodorczyk-Injeyan, J., Injeyan, S., Ruegg, R., 2006. Spinal manipulative therapy reduces inflammatory cytokines but not substance P production in normal subjects. J. Manipulative Physiol. Ther. 29, 14–21.

Teys, P., Bisset, L., Vicenzino, B., 2008. The initial effects of a Mulligan's mobilisation with movement technique on range of movement and pressure pain threshold in pain-limited shoulders. Man. Ther. 13, 37–42.

Threlkeld, A.J., 1992. The effects of manual therapy on connective tissue. Phys. Ther. 72, 893–902.

UK BEAM Trial, 2004. United Kingdom Back Pain Exercise and Manipulation (UK BEAM) randomised trial: effectiveness of physical treatments for back pain in primary care. Br. Med. J. https://doi.org/10.1136/bmj.38282.669225.AE.

Unsworth, A., Dowson, D., Wright, V., 1971. Cracking joints: a bioengineering study of cavitation in the metacarpophalangeal joint. Ann. Rheum. Dis. 30, 348–358.

van der Wees, P.J., Lenssen, A.F., Hendriks, E.J.M., et al., 2006. Effectiveness of exercise therapy and manual mobilisation in acute ankle sprain and functional instability: a systematic review. Aust. J. Physiother. 52, 27–37.

van Griensven, H., 2005. Pain in practice: theory and treatment strategies for manual therapists. Butterworth Heinemann, Elsevier, London.

Vermeulen, H., Rozing, P.M., Obermann, W.R., et al., 2006. Comparison of high-grade and low-grade mobilization techniques in the management of adhesive capsulitis of the shoulder: randomized controlled trial. Phys. Ther. 86, 355–368.

Vicenzino, B., 1995. An investigation of the effects of spinal manual therapy on forequater pressure and thermal pain thresholds and sympathetic nervous system activity in asymptomatic subjects: a preliminary report. In: Shacklock, M.O. (Ed.), Moving in on pain. Butterworth-Heinemann, Australia, pp. 185–193.

Vicenzino, B., Collins, D., Benson, H., et al., 1998. An investigation of the interrelationship between manipulative therapy-induced hypoalgesia and sympathoexcitation. J. Manipulative Physiol. Ther. 21, 448–453.

Vicenzino, B., Collins, D., Wright, A., 1996. The initial effects of a cervical spine manipulative physiotherapy treatment on the pain and dysfunction of lateral epicondylalgia. Pain 68, 69–74.

Vicenzino, B., McLean, S., Naish, R., 2001. Preliminary evidence of a force threshold required to produce manipulation inducted hypoalgesia. In: Procceedings of the 12th Biennial Conference Musculoskeletal Physiotherapy Australia, November.

Voogt, L., de Vries, J., Meeus, M., et al., 2015. Analgesic effects of manual therapy in patients with musculoskeletal pain: a systematic review. Man. Ther. 20, 250–256.

Wertli, M., Rasmussen-Barr, E., Held, U., 2014. Fear-avoidance beliefs – a moderator of treatment efficacy in patients with low back pain: a systematic review. Spine J. 14, 2658–2678.

Willett, E., Hebron, C., Krouwel, O., 2010. The initial effects of different rates of lumbar mobilisations on pressure pain thresholds in asymptomatic subjects. Man. Ther. 15, 173–178.

Willett, M., Duda, J., Fenton, S., et al., 2019. Effectiveness of behaviour change techniques in physiotherapy interventions to promote physical activity adherence in lower limb osteoarthritis patients: a systematic review. PLoS One 14 (7), e0219482. https://doi.org/10.1371/journal.pone.0219482.

Wright, A., 1995. Hypoalgesia post-manipulative therapy: a review of a potential neurophysiological mechanism. Man. Ther. 1, 11–16.

Wyke, B.D., Polacek, P., 1975. Articular neurology: the present position. J. Joint Bone Surg. 57B, 401.

Young, J.L., Walker, D., Snyder, S., et al., 2014. Thoracic manipulation versus mobilization in patients with mechanical neck pain: a systematic review. J. Man. Manip. Ther. 22, 141–153.

Zusman, M., 1986. Spinal manipulative therapy: review of some proposed mechanisms, and a new hypothesis. Am. J. Physiother. 32, 89–99.

4

Function and Dysfunction of Muscle and Tendon

Paul Comfort and Lee Herrington

LEARNING OUTCOMES

After studying this chapter, you should be able to:

- Understand the constituent parts of a muscle.
- Understand the physiology and biomechanics of muscle actions.
- Explain specific muscle characteristics, such as strength, power and muscular endurance.
- Explain the effects of ageing, injury and immobilization on muscle and tendon function.

CHAPTER CONTENTS

The function of the neuromusculoskeletal system is to produce efficient movement which is dependent on optimal functioning of each component: nerves, muscles, tendons, and joints (Fig. 4.1). This interrelationship has been described in relation to the knee, for instance, as 'a complex systematic sensory–motor synergy, which includes the ligaments, antagonistic muscle pairs (flexors and extensors), bones, and sensory mechanoreceptors in the ligaments, joint capsule, and associated muscles' (Solomonow et al., 1987). This description could equally be applied to the entire neuromusculoskeletal system. Therefore, although this chapter is concerned with the function of muscle, it is important to stress that muscles do not function in isolation but in a highly interdependent way with joints and nerves, the latter determining the level and rate of activation of the muscle.

SKELETAL MUSCLE FUNCTION

The following aspects of muscle function will be considered:

- anatomy, biomechanics and physiology of muscle
- nerve supply of muscle
- muscle action

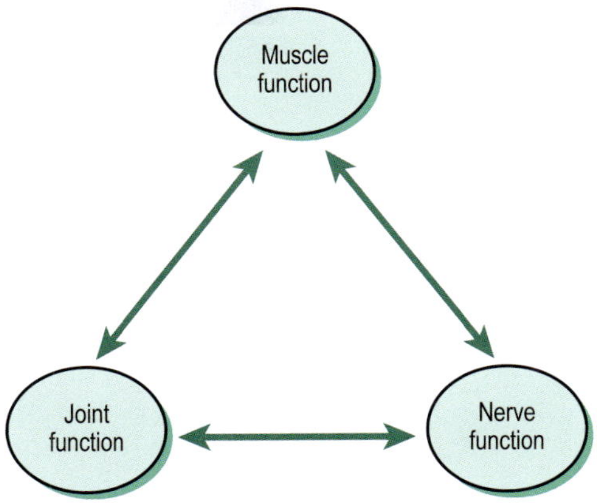

Fig. 4.1 Interdependence of the function of muscle, joint and nerve for normal movement (after Panjabi, 1992, with permission). Normal function of the neuromusculoskeletal system requires normal function of muscle, joint and nerve.

- muscle strength, power, endurance, motor control and muscle length
- simple classification of muscle

Anatomy, Biomechanics and Physiology of Muscle

Muscle constitutes approximately 40% of the total body weight, depending on the level of muscular development of the individual. A muscle (i.e. muscle and its tendons) can be divided grossly into contractile tissue and noncontractile tissue.

Contractile Tissue of Muscle

The smallest unit of muscle is the myofibril, made up of thin actin and thick myosin filaments, giving a striated appearance under the microscope (Fig. 4.2). The myosin filaments produce the dark A band, and the actin filaments produce the light I band. In addition, elastic titin filaments lie between the myosin filaments. The titin filaments act like a spring, with increased tension when the sarcomere is lengthened, thus enabling it to return to its resting length when the tension is removed; this is also thought to keep the myosin in the centre of the sarcomere when there is an asymmetrical pull (Horowits et al., 1989). The Z line demarcates the sarcomere, which is the basic contractile unit of muscle.

Individual muscle fibres (or cells) are covered in a membrane, called the sarcolemma, and by a connective tissue sheath called the endomysium (Fig. 4.3).

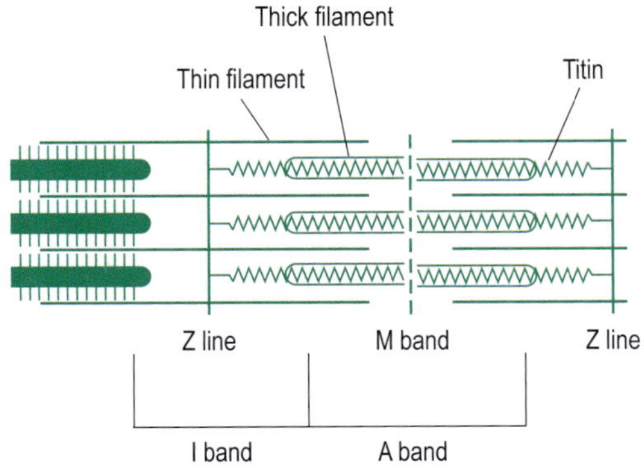

Fig. 4.2 The basic contractile unit of muscle, the sarcomere, formed by the thin actin and thick myosin filaments. (From Herzog, 1999, with permission.)

Individual muscle fibres are collected into bundles (or fascicles) by a connective tissue sheath called the perimysium. Numbers of muscle bundles constitute the muscle and are surrounded by a connective tissue sheath called the epimysium and by an outer layer of fascia. These muscle fibres are known as extrafusal fibres, compared with intrafusal fibres, which lie within the muscle spindle (discussed later under nerve supply).

Noncontractile Tissue of Muscle

The noncontractile tissue includes the connective tissue layers within muscle and the tendons. Connective tissue is found in layers within the muscle and tendons and consists of collagen fibres and some elastin fibres. The elastin fibres enable muscle to regain its shape, following both shortening and lengthening. Connective tissue makes up approximately 30% of muscle mass and is vital for normal muscle function.

Connective tissue forms a sheath around each muscle fibre (endomysium), around bundles of muscle fibres (perimysium) and around the whole muscle (epimysium), as shown in Fig. 4.3. The connective tissue, along with the nerves and blood vessels, form the noncontractile element of the muscle belly. The outer layer of connective tissue enables identification of particular muscles (e.g. the semitendinosus muscle in the thigh) and allows sliding of muscle on adjacent tissues (e.g. movement of semitendinosus on the biceps femoris and the sciatic nerve). The perimysium around a bundle of muscle fibres provides a channel for blood vessels and nerves. The endomysium, perimysium and epimysium join to form the tendon or aponeurosis that attaches the muscle to bone.

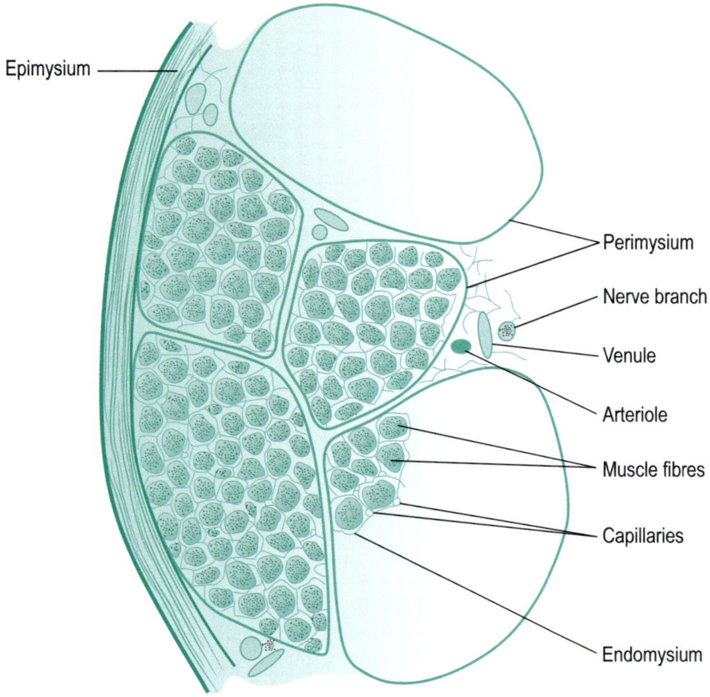

Fig. 4.3 Schematic illustration of the cross-sectional structure of muscle. (From McComas, 1996, with permission.)

Connective tissue is also the major constituent of fascia, which is divided into superficial and deep. Superficial fascia lies just below the skin and allows skin movement; it is thick on the plantar aspect of the hands and thin on the dorsum of the hands and feet. Deep fascia acts as retinacula, intermuscular septa, intermuscular aponeurosis and attachment for muscle. In the thoracic and abdominal cavities deep fascia covers and supports the viscera (e.g. the pleura, pericardium, and peritoneum). The flexor and extensor retinacula of the wrist and foot are deep fascia arranged as a transverse thickening to retain tendons deep to it. The intermuscular septa pass between groups of muscles and attach to bone. Muscles can take attachment from the intermuscular septa, which may then be better named intermuscular aponeurosis (e.g. the rectal sheath). The deep fascia can be a point of attachment for muscle to bone and from muscle to muscle. For example, the tensor fascia lata and gluteus maximus attach to the iliotibial tract (fascia), which then passes down the leg and attaches to the tibia. Deep fascia in the lower leg connects the peroneus longus to the biceps femoris and, in the upper arm, pectoralis minor to the short head of biceps.

Musculotendinous (Or Myotendinous) Junction

The musculotendinous junction is the junction between the muscle and the tendon. The contact area is characterized by the muscle cells forming finger-like projections in which the collagen fibres of the tendon insert (Fig. 4.4). This arrangement increases the surface area of the contact region and so reduces the tensile force applied to the tissue (Kvist et al., 1991). Interestingly, this is reflected in differences in surface area between type I and type II muscle fibres. The area is greater for type II fibres, which are involved in more forceful voluntary movements, than for type I fibres, which generate lower forces and are largely involved in postural control (Kvist et al., 1991) and prolonged lower intensity, aerobic activities. Despite this arrangement, the region is the weakest part of the tendon–muscle unit and is susceptible to strain injuries (Garrett, 1990; Tidball, 1991).

Osteotendinous Junctions

This is where tendon attaches to bone. Tendons usually attach directly to bone, where there is an abrupt well-defined area of attachment with a clear demarcation of tendon and bone; examples include supraspinatus,

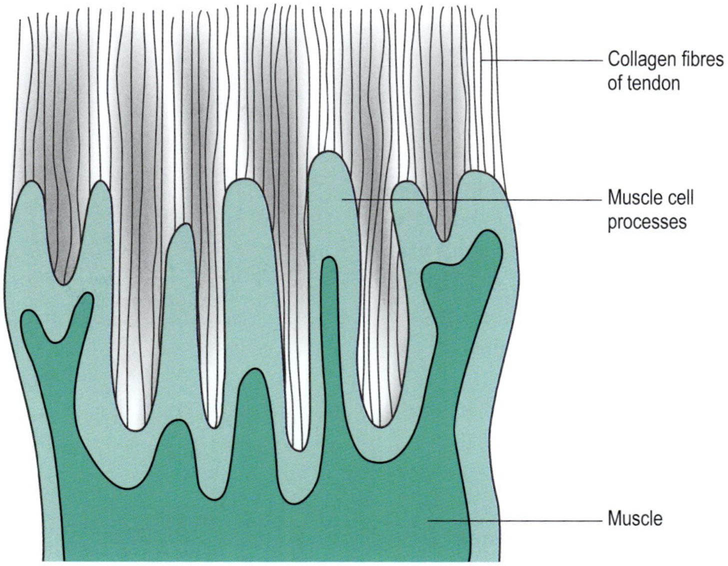

Fig. 4.4 Schematic figure of musculotendinous junction. (After Jozsa & Kannus, 1997, with permission.)

where it attaches to the superior facet on the greater tuberosity of the humerus, and the medial collateral ligament to the medial condyle of the femur (Woo et al., 1988). Tendons with direct attachments have a superficial layer which blends with periosteum and a larger deep layer which inserts directly into bone via a thin layer of fibrocartilage (Woo et al., 1988). Sometimes tendons attach indirectly, such that there is a more gradual and less distinct area of attachment; the superficial layer in this case provides the predominant attachment, blending with the periosteum and bone via Sharpey fibres, while the deep layer attaches directly to the bone (Woo et al., 1988).

Tendons

Tendons are designed to transmit high tensile force from muscle to bone. They are made up of approximately 70% longitudinally arranged collagen tissue, with some elastin tissue (Hess et al., 1989) and are relatively inextensible and able to withstand large tensile forces (Jozsa & Kannus, 1997). They have a sparse blood supply, with this avascular nature decreasing the rate of adaptation and increasing the time scales for rehabilitation.

Tendons sometimes contain a sesamoid bone which increases the mechanical advantage of the muscle and decreases friction between adjacent tissues. These are covered with hyaline cartilage. Examples include the pisiform bone within the flexor carpi ulnaris tendon and the patella within the quadriceps tendon. The existence and shape of sesamoid bones vary between individuals (McBryde & Anderson, 1988).

During a muscle action, tendon moves on adjacent tissue; the frictional resistance to this movement is minimized by bursae and sheaths, which can be classified as fibrous, synovial and paratenon sheaths.

1. A bursa may lie adjacent to tendon to aid gliding movement of the tendon on adjacent tissue
2. A fibrous sheath may surround a tendon, as in the tendons around the ankle. Bony grooves and notches contain a layer of fibrocartilage, and superficially the tendon is held in place by retinaculum.
3. A synovial sheath may surround a tendon where ease of movement with adjacent tissue is of paramount importance, as in the tendons of the hands and feet. Synovial sheaths are composed of an outer fibrotic sheath and an inner synovial sheath. A thin film of synovial fluid, rich in hyaluronic acid, fills the space between the sheaths and acts as a lubricant reducing frictional resistance (Jozsa & Kannus, 1997).
4. A paratenon sheath (or peritendinous sheet) may surround a tendon (e.g. the tendocalcaneus tendon). The paratenon is made up of collagen fibres, elastic

fibrils and synovial cells and acts as an elastic sleeve, facilitating movement between the tendon and its surrounding tissues (Hess et al., 1989; Jozsa & Kannus, 1997). The paratenon and epitenon are sometimes referred to as the peritendon.

Tendon tissue is plastic and will alter its composition and construction according to the physical demands placed upon it (Pearson & Hussain, 2014). For example, with exercise, there is an increase in tendon thickness and tensile strength (Brumitt & Cuddeford, 2015). The stimulus for tendon growth is the tension that is applied and is therefore correlated with the strength of the muscle (Muraoka et al., 2005).

Tendons have viscoelastic properties; the load–displacement curve for a tendon is shown in Fig. 4.5. The toe region is concave and is considered to reflect the straightening of the wavy collagen fibres shown in Fig. 4.6 (Hirsch, 1974). Little force is required to lengthen the tendon in this region. This region is responsible for the ability of tendon to absorb shock (Wood et al., 1988). With continued lengthening, the wave pattern straightens, and the tendon behaves like a stiff spring; this occurs after about 3% elongation (Herzog & Gal, 2007). As the force increases, stiffness increases in the tendon, producing the linear part of the curve; this occurs at about 4% elongation (Wainwright et al., 1982). Both toe and linear regions are temporary, and on removal of the force, the tendon will return to its resting length. During normal everyday activities, tensile forces on tendon are thought to lie within the toe and linear region and are thought to be less than 4% strain (Fung, 1993). If the force continues to elongate beyond this, a permanent deformation in the yield region of the curve occurs, up to a maximum of approximately 8% to 15% elongation, when failure occurs (Fung, 1993). During the yield region, a relatively small increase in force will produce a relatively large increase in displacement. The stiffness of tendon is not the same throughout its length (Kolz et al., 2015). Tendon is stiffest in the middle of its length and least stiff at its insertion, so when a tendon is lengthened there is greatest displacement at the insertion region (Woo et al., 1988, Kolz et al., 2015).

Blood supply of tendon. Tendons receive their blood supply at the osteotendinous junction, from vessels within bone and periosteum. At the musculotendinous junction, it receives blood from vessels within muscle and from the surrounding vessels within the paratenon, mesotenon and synovial sheath. The blood supply at the osteotendinous junction is sparse and is limited to where the tendon attaches to bone (Jozsa & Kannus, 1997).

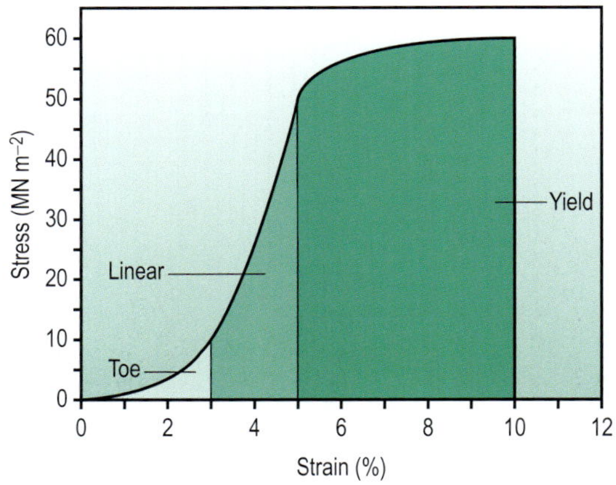

Fig. 4.5 Load–displacement (stress–strain) curve for tendon. (From Herzog & Gal, 2007, with permission.)

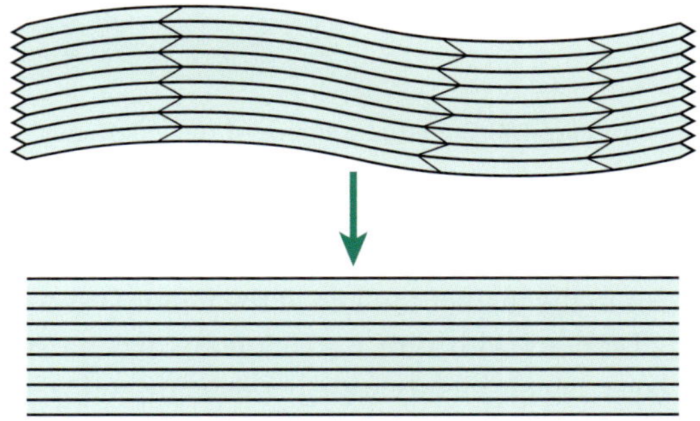

Fig. 4.6 The wavy pattern of a tendon in a relaxed state straightens out when it is stretched. (From Jozsa & Kannus, 1997, with permission.)

Biomechanics of the Muscle–Tendon Unit

It is useful to consider the biomechanical behaviour of the muscle–tendon unit as a single unit. The strength of the muscle–tendon unit with respect to tensile loading can be depicted on a force–displacement curve (Fig. 4.7); this curve was obtained from the whole tibialis anterior muscle–tendon unit of a rabbit (Taylor et al., 1990). Force is plotted against the stretch or deformation. The slope of the curve is the modulus of elasticity, measured in Pa or N/m^2 and is a measure of the 'stiffness' of the muscle–tendon unit (Panjabi & White, 2001). Only a low force is initially required to

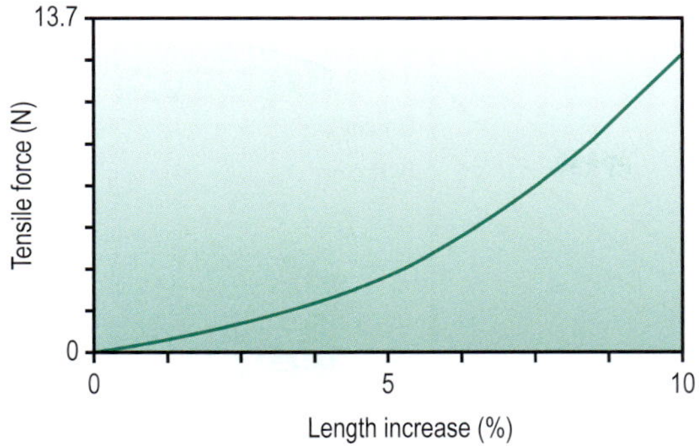

Fig. 4.7 Force–displacement curve of the muscle–tendon unit. (After Taylor et al., 1990, with permission.)

TABLE 4.1 Tensile Properties of Muscle and Tendon Compared With Bone, Cartilage, Ligament and Nerve

Tissue	Stress at Failure (MPa)	Strain at Failure (%)
Muscle (passive)	0.17	60
Tendon	55	9–10
Cortical bone	100–200	1–3
Cancellous bone	10	5–7
Cartilage	10–15	80–120
Ligament	10–40	30–45
Nerve roots	15	19

Panjabi and White (2001).

deform the muscle–tendon unit, a region referred to as the 'toe' region (Threlkeld, 1992) or 'neutral zone' (Panjabi & White, 2001). Stiffness then increases, so that greater force is required to deform the muscle–tendon unit; this region is referred to as the elastic zone. Forces within the elastic zone will result in no permanent change in length as soon as the force is released the muscle–tendon unit will return to its preload size (Panjabi & White, 2001). The neutral zone and elastic zone fall within the normal physiological range of forces and deformation on the muscle–tendon unit during everyday activities (Nordin & Frankel, 1989). The stress–strain properties of muscle and tendon are compared with those of bone, cartilage, ligament and nerve in Table 4.1. The ability of muscle to resist lengthening reduces with age (Panjabi & White, 2001), likely as a product of reductions in activity and therefore force production.

The muscle–tendon unit will elongate on loading; this is dependent on the rate of loading. When the muscle–tendon unit of tibialis anterior is loaded quickly, it will be stiffer and deform less than when it is loaded more slowly (Fig. 4.8). This is relevant when applying therapeutic force, as a slower rate will result in less resistance and more movement-elongation. An additional effect is that the failure point of the muscle–tendon unit will be higher with a higher loading rate; in other words, it will be stronger and less likely to rupture when the force is applied at a faster rate.

The muscle–tendon unit demonstrates the phenomenon of hysteresis, which is the energy loss during loading and unloading (Fig. 4.9) (Taylor et al., 1990). The unloading curve lies below the loading curve and reflects a greater energy expenditure on loading than the energy regained during unloading. The muscle belly is less stiff than the tendon, so when a muscle is passively lengthened most of the length change occurs in the muscle belly and the tendon is minimally affected (Jami, 1992). The primary outcome of stretching will be to lengthen/elongate the muscle to increase range of motion around the joint and not to lengthen the tendons.

Differences in muscle and tendon contribution can be observed in different jumping tasks; for example, there are distinct differences if we compare a drop jump and a depth jump:

- The drop jump is a fast stretch shortening cycle (SSC) task, characterized by a short ground contact time (<250 ms) requiring limited angular displacement of the hips, knees, and ankles on ground contact. Such a 'stiff' strategy results in minimal lengthening and shortening of the muscles but notable lengthening of the Achilles and gastrocnemius tendons. As such the tendons contribute to the propulsion phase of the jump to a greater extent than the muscles, and minimal, if any energy is lost via hysteresis
- The depth jump is a slow SSC task, characterized by a longer ground contact (usually ~500 ms) with a greater angular displacement of the hips, knees and ankles, resulting in notable lengthening and shortening of the associated musculature, increasing the

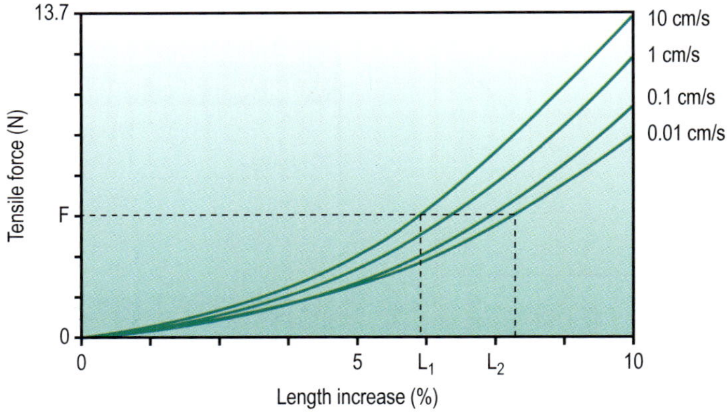

Fig. 4.8 The muscle–tendon unit and rate of loading. When it is loaded quickly, it will be stiffer and will sustain a higher force before breaking than when it is loaded more slowly. For example, a given force, if applied at 10 cm/s, will cause a displacement L_1, but if applied more slowly, at 0.01 cm/s, it will cause a greater displacement to L_2. These data are from the tibialis anterior muscle–tendon unit from New Zealand white rabbits. (After Taylor et al., 1990, with permission.)

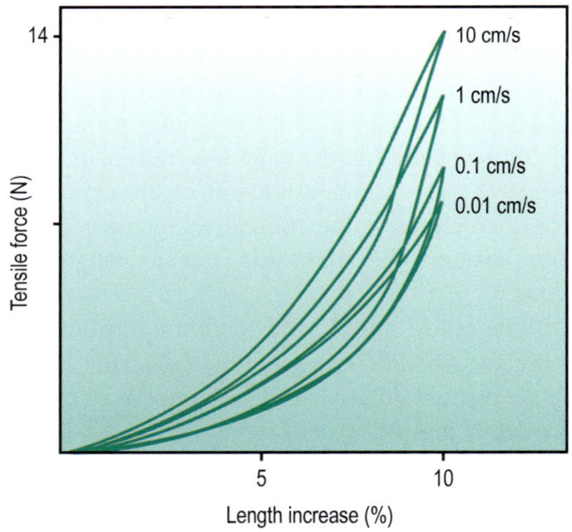

Fig. 4.9 The muscle–tendon unit demonstrates the phenomenon of hysteresis (From Taylor et al., 1990, with permission). The graph was produced from the tibialis anterior muscle–tendon unit of New Zealand white rabbits. The loading rate used was 0.01, 0.1, 1 and 10 cm/s.

contribution of the muscles, and decreasing the contribution of the tendons

Types of Muscle Fibre

Muscle fibres can be classified in various ways (Table 4.2). Initially, muscle fibres were described according to the speed of shortening and were identified by staining for myoglobin concentration (myoglobin binds oxygen). Muscles were divided into (1) slow muscles (type I), which stained red owing to a high concentration of myoglobin enabling aerobic energy metabolism, and (2) fast muscles (type II), which stained white owing to a low concentration of myoglobin enabling anaerobic energy metabolism (Pette & Staron, 1990). Fast-twitch fibres (type II) contract more quickly, generate higher forces but fatigue more quickly than slow-twitch (type I) fibres (Table 4.3).

An alternative classification system identified type I and type II myofibrillar actomyosin adenosine triphosphate (ATP) which related to different contractile properties (Pette & Staron, 1990). When this classification was combined with the myoglobin classification, a metabolic enzyme-based classification was developed (see Table 4.2). This classification includes three types of muscle fibre: slow-twitch oxidative (SO), fast-twitch oxidative (FOG) and fast-twitch glycolytic (FG) (Pette & Staron, 1990; McComas, 1996). Fibres that fall between slow-twitch (type I) and fast-twitch (type IIb) are termed intermediate (type IIa) (Pette et al., 1999) but adapt due to activity to become more like either the FG or SO fibres, dependent on the nature (usually the magnitude and rate of force production) of the activity. The characteristics of these types of muscle fibre are summarized in Table 4.3.

Although it is convenient to classify muscle fibres into three types, the reality is more of a continuum between fast-twitch and slow-twitch muscles; a third

TABLE 4.2 Classification of Muscle Fibre Types

Myosin ATPase	Myosin ATPase Hydrolysis Rate	Myosin Heavy Chain (MHC)	Biochemical Identification of Metabolic Enzymes
I	I	MHCI	Slow-twitch oxidative
	IC	MHCI and MHCIIa	
	IIC	MHCI and MHCIIa	
	IIAC	MHCI and MHCIIa	
IIA	IIA	MHCIIa	? Fast-twitch oxidative[a]
	IIAB	MHCIIa and MHCIIb	
IIB	IIB	MHCIIb	? Fast-twitch glycolytic[a]

[a]The question mark beside fast-twitch oxidative and fast-twitch glycolytic indicates that muscle fibre types IIA and IIB do not always rely on aerobic/oxidative and anaerobic/glycolytic metabolism (McComas 1996).
ATPase, Adenosine triphosphatase.
Staron (1997) and Scott et al. (2001).

TABLE 4.3 Characteristics of Skeletal Muscle and Motor Neurones

Characteristic	Type I	Type IIa	Type IIb
Muscle fibre type	Slow oxidative (SO)	Fast oxidative glycolytic (FOG)	Fast glycolytic (FG)
Motor unit type	Slow	Fast fatigue-resistant	Fast fatigable
Motor unit size	Small	Medium	Large
Conduction rate of motor neurone	Slow	Fast	Fast
Twitch tension	Low	Moderate	High
Speed of contraction	Slow	Fast	Fast
Resistance to fatigue	High	High	Low
Mitochondrial enzyme activity	High	Medium	Low
Myoglobin content	High	Medium	Low
Capillary density	High	Medium	Low

Newham and Ainscough-Potts (2001).

type of fast fibre has since been identified and is known as IIX (Pette et al., 1999). Prolonged aerobic exercise primarily recruits the SO fibres, whereas near-maximal efforts (e.g., strength/power training/short sprints) primarily recruits the FG fibres, resulting in specific adaptations in these specific fibres. In contrast, regular aerobic or anaerobic training can result in adaptation of the FOG fibres to adapt to resemble either the SO or FG fibres, respectively.

For any one motor unit, the characteristic of the muscle fibre type is mirrored by the motor nerve supply (Box 4.1). All muscle fibres that are innervated by the same motor neurone are of the same type; that is, the conduction rate of a motor neurone innervating fast-twitch fibres is faster than that for slow-twitch fibres. The motor neurone determines the characteristic of a muscle fibre and is described as a phasic or tonic motor neurone. Large, phasic high-threshold motor neurones discharge at the high frequency of 30–60 Hz compared with small, tonic low-threshold motor neurones with a lower frequency of 10–20 Hz. The nerve is so influential on muscle fibre type that, if the motor neurones to fast- and slow-twitch fibres are experimentally switched, the muscle fibre types will also switch characteristics (Lomo et al., 1980).

Smaller motor units tend to be composed of slow-twitch muscle fibres and larger motor units composed of fast-twitch fibres. The motor neurone of a slow-twitch motor unit innervates 12–180 muscle fibres compared with 300–800 muscle fibres of a fast-twitch

BOX 4.1 Characteristics of Motor Neurone and Muscle Fibre Type

Nerve	**Nerve**
Large motor neurone	Small motor neurone
Phasic	Tonic
High threshold	Low threshold
High frequency	Low frequency
Muscle Fibres	**Muscle Fibres**
Fast-twitch	Slow-twitch
Type Ia—fast oxidative glycolytic	Type I—slow-twitch oxidative
Type IIb—fast glycolytic	Small motor unit supplies 12–180 muscle fibres
Large motor unit supplies 300–800 muscle fibres	

Newham and Ainscough-Potts (2001).

motor unit. The fewer number of slow-twitch muscle fibres supplied by a motor neurone enables greater control of muscular action. The fact that any one muscle contains both small and large motor units providing fine control of muscle actions, as well as greater velocity and force of muscle actions, attests to the multiplicity of muscle functions, and it is an over-simplification to define individual muscles as specifically FG or SO twitch, as they will adapt to the environmental-training stresses applied to them.

Nerve Supply of Muscles

Sensory nerve endings in the muscle–tendon units include muscle spindles, Golgi tendon organs and free nerve endings. Large-diameter myelinated group Ia and II fibres supply the muscle spindles, slightly smaller myelinated IIb fibres supply Golgi tendon organs and fine myelinated Aδ (or group III fibres) and unmyelinated C (or group IV) fibres supply the free nerve endings.

Muscle Spindles

Muscle spindles are stretch receptors monitoring the length (or tension) and rate of change in length of muscle. The greater the rate of change in length or the greater the magnitude of change in length the greater the resultant stimulus via the stretch reflex.

Muscle spindles lie within the muscle belly, parallel to extrafusal fibres, and near the musculotendinous junction (Boyd, 1976). The muscle spindle consists of intrafusal fibres to distinguish it from the rest of muscle which, in turn, consists of a noncontractile central portion within a capsule with contractile ends. When a muscle is progressively stretched at a constant velocity, the primary endings initially have a burst of activity with the rate of activity depending on the velocity of the stretch; increased velocity results in an increased rate of activity (Hunt, 1990). Therefore maintaining a low lengthening velocity while progressively increasing range of motion during a stretch results in lower stimulation of the muscle spindle and therefore less muscle activation resulting in a greater range of motion, because of a reduction in the reflex resistance to elongation created by the muscle spindle. If the lengthened muscle is then maintained at its new length, there is a reduction in the rate of discharge and the perceived tension in the muscle will reduce. While the lengthened muscle is maintained at its new length, the fibres within the muscle spindle exhibit creep (i.e. they lengthen) (Boyd, 1976). The discharge rate from the secondary group II fibres increases with a maintained position and so appear to act as position detectors (Hunt, 1990). Because the intrafusal fibres lie parallel to the extrafusal fibres, the discharge from the sensory fibres in the muscle spindle diminishes or ceases when the muscle shortens and increases when the muscle is lengthened (Hunt, 1990).

Stimulation of the muscle spindle causes excitation of the α motor neurones leading to contraction of the extrafusal muscle fibres in which the spindle is situated and inhibition of the antagonistic muscles. This phenomenon is known as the stretch reflex (Fig. 4.10). Muscle spindles protect and limit the muscle from excessive lengthening. Clearly, this is a useful protective mechanism to regulate movement and maintain posture (Hunt, 1990).

Golgi Tendon Organs

Golgi tendon organs lie in the musculotendinous junctions, between the fascicles and the collagen strands coming from the tendons and aponeurosis; they are rarely found in the tendon itself (Jami, 1992). They are encapsulated corpuscles containing collagen fibres, lying in series with 15–20 muscle fibres and stimulated only by the tension in these muscle fibres in series (Shumway-Cook & Woollacott, 1995) (Fig. 4.11). They are sensitive to changes in tension within the

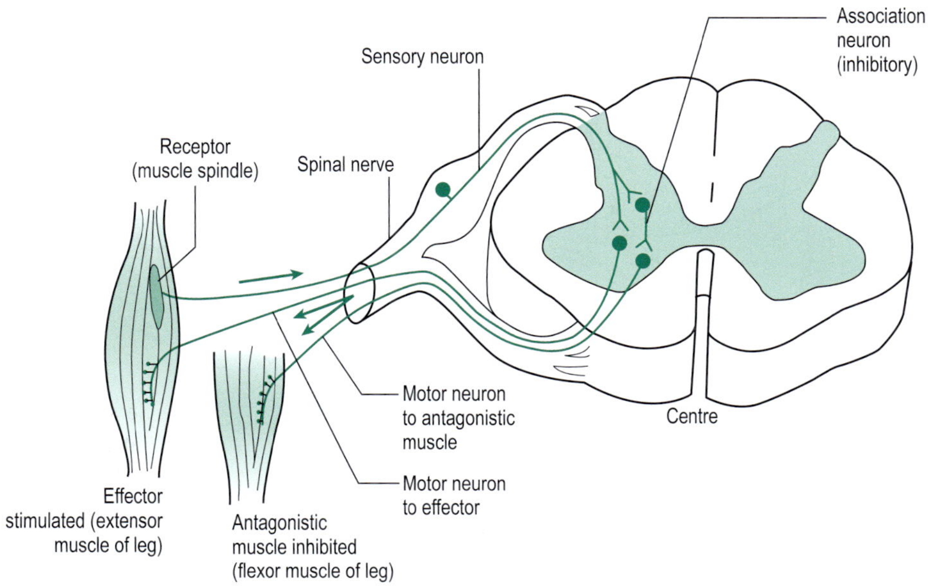

Fig. 4.10 Spindle stretch reflex. Excitation of the muscle spindle causes a reflex contraction of the muscle in which the spindle lies and inhibition of the antagonistic muscle. (From Crow & Haas, 2001, with permission.)

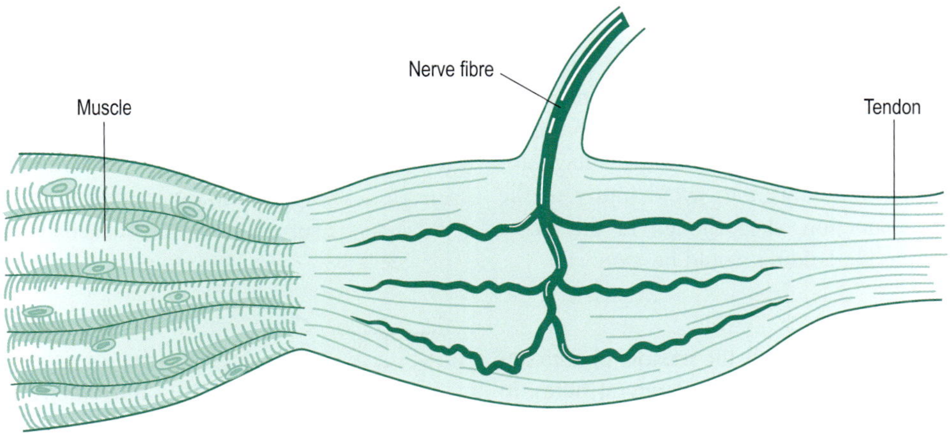

Fig. 4.11 Golgi tendon organ in series with 15–20 muscle fibres. (From Shumway-Cook & Woollacott, 1995, with permission.)

musculotendinous junction and to the rate of change in tension (Houk & Henneman, 1967). Golgi tendon organs can be stimulated by passive lengthening of the muscle–tendon unit; however, the threshold for discharge is very high and rarely persists with a maintained muscle stretch (Jami, 1992). Each is innervated by a large fast-conducting Ib afferent fibre, with the rate of firing from the Golgi tendon organ proportional to the muscle tension (Crow & Haas, 2001). When the muscle fibres contract, there is a lengthening of the musculotendinous junction and collagen fibres within the Golgi tendon organ; this compresses the nerve terminals and causes firing of the Ib afferent fibre.

Stimulation of Golgi tendon organs leads to inhibition of the muscle in which they are situated (inhibition of both α and γ motor neurones), a mechanism known as autogenic inhibition, and excitation of the antagonist muscles (Fig. 4.12) (Chalmers, 2002, 2004). So, for

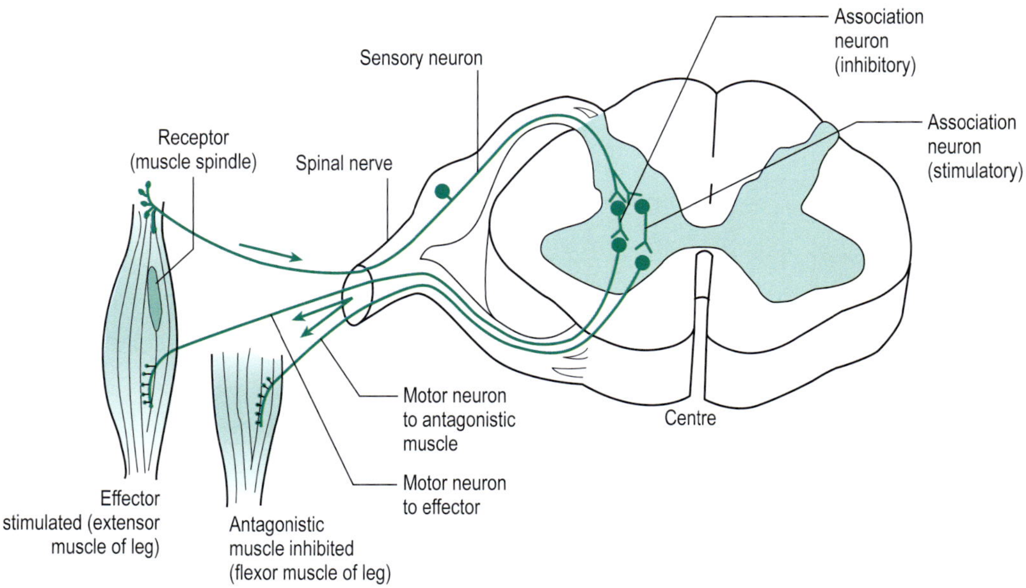

Fig. 4.12 The tendon reflex: stimulation of the Golgi tendon organ causes inhibition of the muscle in which it lies and excitation of the antagonistic muscle. (From Crow & Haas, 2001, with permission.)

example, when jumping off an object and landing, the muscles of the lower limbs perform an eccentric action to decelerate the individual; however, if the object was too high and the resultant impact causes excessive force that may damage the musculotendinous junction, the Golgi tendon organs will be stimulated, producing inhibition of the agonist muscles and stimulation of the antagonist. This is a protective mechanism to avoid injury to the musculotendinous junction, even though in the aforementioned example the landing would be 'poor'.

Free Nerve Endings

Free nerve endings lie throughout the muscle, in the connective tissue, between intrafusal and extrafusal fibres, in arterioles and venules, in the capsule of muscle spindles and tendon organs, in tendon tissue at the musculotendinous junction and in fat cells (Reinert & Mense, 1992). This is summarized in Box 4.2. Free nerve endings are supplied by myelinated Aδ (group III) and unmyelinated C (group IV) fibres. Type III afferents act as low-threshold mechanical pressure receptors, contraction-sensitive receptors and nociceptors (Mense & Meyer, 1985). Most type IV afferents are mainly nociceptors (to both noxious mechanical and chemical stimulation), with a smaller proportion being low-threshold mechanical pressure receptors, contraction-sensitive receptors and thermoreceptors (Mense & Meyer, 1985).

BOX 4.2 Position of Free Nerve Endings in Muscle and Predominant Function of Type III and IV Afferent Fibres

Connective tissue between:
Intrafusal and extrafusal fibres
Arterioles and venules
Capsule of muscle spindles
Capsule of tendon organs
Tendon tissue at the musculotendinous junction in fat cells

TYPE III	**TYPE IV**
Most are mechanical pressure contraction-sensitive	Most are nociceptors: mechanical and chemical

Mechanoreceptors

Mechanoreceptors respond to pressure, active muscle shortening (concentric action) and muscle lengthening (eccentric action). Most group III fibres respond to local pressure stimulation (Kaufman et al., 1984), whereas very few of the group IV fibres respond to low-threshold innocuous pressure (Franz & Mense, 1975). Group III and IV fibres are activated in a linear fashion to the force of a muscle contraction or the force of a stretch on a muscle (Mense & Stahnke, 1983; Mense & Meyer, 1985)—the greater the force, the greater the response. Approximately half of the afferents respond to both contraction and lengthening, and half are specific to one or other stimulus (Mense & Meyer, 1985). Afferents responsive to active contraction are often also chemical receptors responsive to bradykinin (Mense & Meyer, 1985), a chemical released with inflammation. Group III afferents appear to be stimulated by the mechanical effects of the contraction, whereas group IV receptors seem to be stimulated by the metabolic products produced by muscle actions (Kaufman et al., 1982, 1983).

Chemical Receptors

Some free nerve endings are sensitive to muscle pH, concentrations of extracellular potassium and sodium chloride and changes in oxygen and carbon dioxide. They help to regulate the cardiopulmonary system during exercise or activity (Laughlin & Korthuis, 1987). Group IV afferents in muscle are thought to be primarily responsible for producing the reflex changes in cardiorespiratory function with exercise (Kaufman et al., 1982, 1983). Inflammatory or chemically induced muscle pain in humans is thought to be due to activation of these free nerve endings (Mense, 1996).

Thermal Receptors

Some group IV receptors respond to small changes of temperature in muscle (Mense, 1996). Others have been identified to have a high threshold for thermal stimulation and are thus thermal nociceptors (Mense & Meyer, 1985). A high proportion of thermoreceptors have also been found to be sensitive to noxious mechanical pressure (Mense & Meyer, 1985).

Nociceptors

Muscle nociceptors have a high mechanical threshold, and some also have a high thermal threshold. It is also thought that group III muscle afferents may be capable of acting as nociceptors and thus mediating pain. Bradykinin, a chemical released with inflammation, has been found to sensitize muscle and tendon nociceptors (Mense & Meyer, 1985). This sensitization lowers the firing threshold such that an innocuous mechanical stimulus (e.g. movement or a light touch) causes excitation, a phenomenon known as allodynia (Raja et al., 1999).

Efferent Nerve Fibres

In general, the efferent fibres to muscle consist of the large myelinated α motor neurones that supply the extrafusal fibres, and the small, myelinated γ (or fusimotor) fibres that supply the intrafusal fibres within the muscle spindle. Type I muscle fibres are innervated by small, low-threshold, slowly conducting motor nerves, whereas type IIb fibres are innervated by large, higher-threshold, fast-conducting motor nerves.

The efferent fibres enter the muscle around the centre of the muscle belly, a region known as the motor point. Motor nerves divide into small branches to supply each muscle fibre; the presynaptic terminal synapses at the neuromuscular junction, with the motor end plate (Fig. 4.13). When an action potential arrives

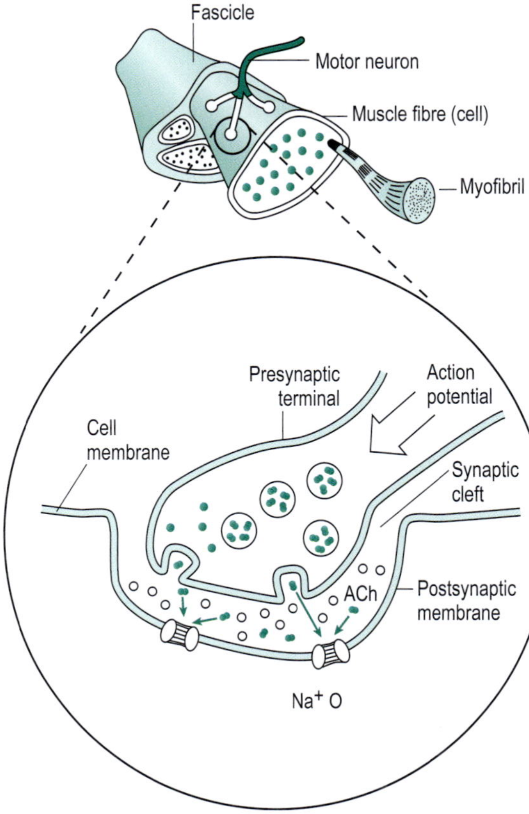

Fig. 4.13 Neuromuscular junction formed by the motor nerve and the motor end plate (After Herzog, 1999, with permission). *ACh,* Acetylcholine.

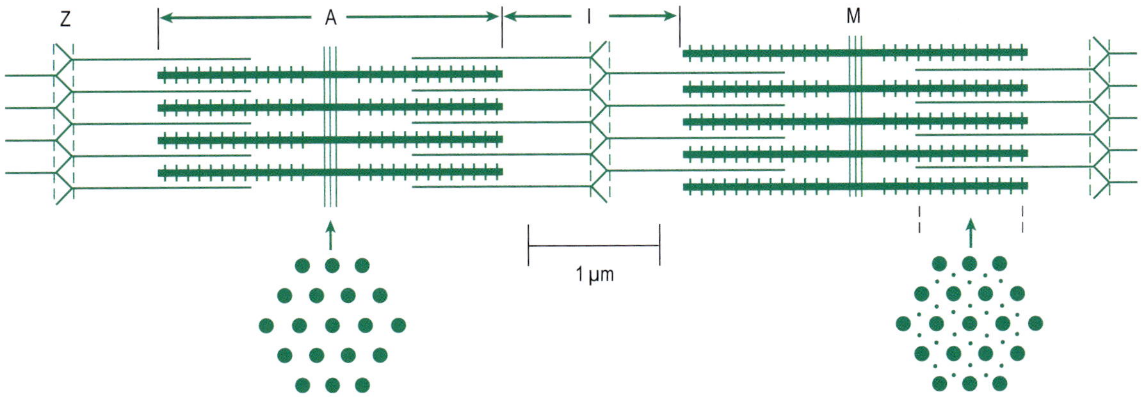

Fig. 4.14 The sliding filament model. (From Huxley, 2000, with permission.)

at the presynaptic terminal, a chain of chemical reactions is initiated which causes diffusion of acetylcholine across the synaptic cleft to the postsynaptic membrane. This chemical causes an increase in the permeability of sodium ions which, if sufficient, will initiate an action potential along the muscle fibre.

Each muscle fibre is supplied by a motor neurone. The motor neurone, and the muscle fibres it innervates, is termed a motor unit and is the functional unit of a muscle. Stimulation of the motor neurone initiates and maintains a series of complex events leading to either shortening (concentric contraction) or active lengthening (eccentric contraction) of muscle, and the development of muscle tension. Muscle contraction ceases when the stimulation of the motor nerve stops.

Muscle actions occur via the sliding of myosin and actin filaments so that the length of the sarcomere is shortened (during a concentric muscle action); this is termed the sliding filament theory (Fig. 4.14). Myosin contains proteins that extend towards the actin filaments, in the form of a tail and a head. The head contains a binding site for actin (Fig. 4.15) and forms the cross-bridge between myosin and actin. The reader is directed to a physiology textbook for a more detailed description of the sliding filament theory.

Muscle Strength

The force of a muscle action depends on the following factors.

1. The type and number of motor units recruited. The recruitment of muscle fibres is directly related to the size of the motor neurone (Milner-Brown et al., 1973), with an initial recruitment of small motor neurones and then recruitment of large motor neurones as more force is required (Henneman & Olson, 1965; Henneman et al., 1965), referred to as the Henneman size principle. Small motor units (type I) are recruited first and then large motor units (type II) if initial force is not sufficient.
2. The initial length of the muscle affects its force generating capacity. The optimal length is where there is maximum overlap between actin and myosin filaments. Where a muscle fibre is less or more than the optimal length, fewer cross-bridges between actin and myosin are formed and the tension is lessened. This phenomenon produces a length–tension relationship in muscle which can be depicted on a graph (Fig. 4.16). When a single muscle fibre is lengthened, there is an uneven lengthening such that the central portion of the muscle fibre lengthens more than the ends of the muscle; while there is a reduction in the cross-bridges in the central portion there are still cross-bridges at the ends (Huxley, 2000).
3. The nature of the neural stimulation of the motor unit. The frequency of the neural stimulation affects the force of the muscular action. A single neural stimulus will result in a muscle twitch. A muscle twitch consists of a brief latent period, then a muscle contraction and then a relaxation period. The total time this takes varies between 10 and 100 ms (Ghez, 1991). The force of the action and the total time will depend on the type of muscle fibre, with fast-twitch fibres contracting more quickly, and with more force, than slow-twitch fibres. If a series of neural stimuli are used (1–3 ms apart) (Ghez,

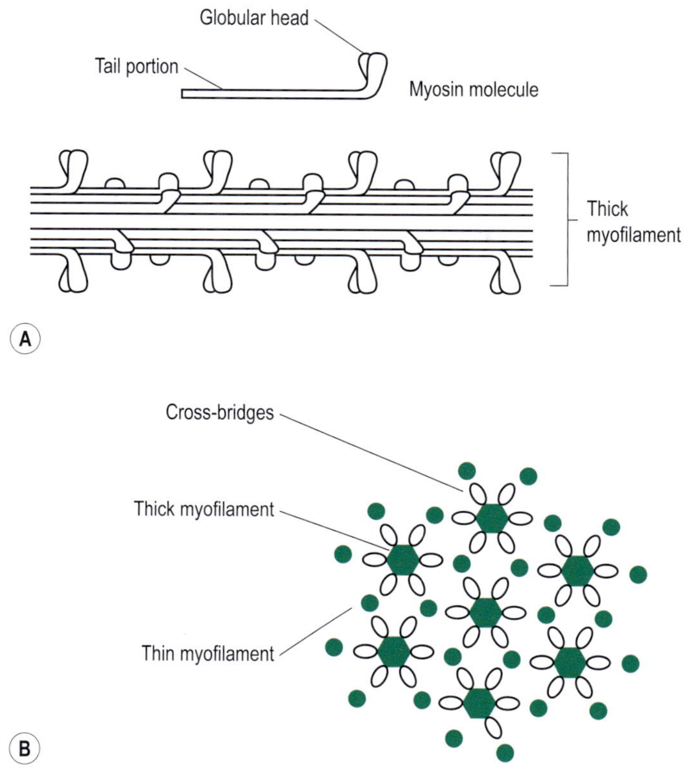

Fig. 4.15 (A) Myosin with tail and head projecting towards the actin filaments (From Herzog, 1999, with permission). (B) Cross-sectional arrangement of actin and myosin. (After Herzog, 1999, with permission.)

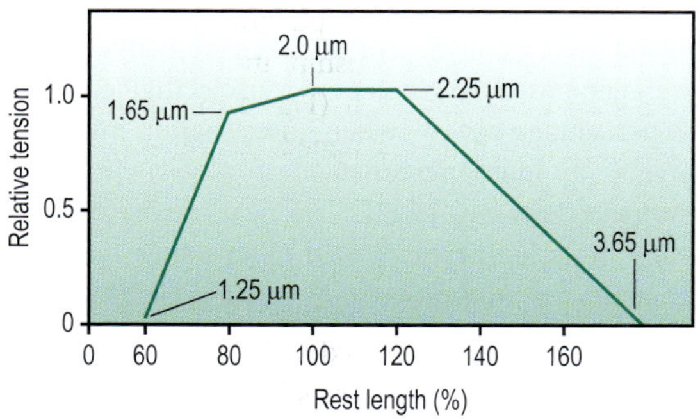

Fig. 4.16 Length–tension relationship in skeletal muscle (From Powers & Howley, 1997, with permission.)

1991), the muscle has not had time to relax and so an increase in muscle tension is produced due to the summation of each twitch. If the frequency of the neural stimuli is increased further, individual contractions are combined in a single sustained contraction known as fused tetanus (Ghez, 1991), which will continue until the neural stimulus is stopped or the muscle fatigues.

4. Muscle architecture. Muscle strength is proportional to the physiological cross-sectional area of the muscle, reflecting the number of sarcomeres in parallel (Aagaard et al., 2001; Seitz et al., 2016). However, architectural properties of skeletal muscle have been shown to affect both force and velocity of muscle actions. A decrease in pennation angle or an increase in fascicle length results in an increased potential for fascicle lengthening and shortening velocity, due to an increased length of the contractile component (Blazevich, 2006; Earp et al., 2010). In contrast, an increase in pennation angle results in an increase in the number of fibres for a given cross-sectional area, which increases force generation capacity (Blazevich, 2006; Manal et al., 2006, Earp et al., 2010)
5. The age of the patient. The cross-sectional area of muscle has been found to reduce with age, although

this is generally associated with reduced activity (reduced loading) and is somewhat reversible with appropriate activity (Mayer et al., 2011; Bouchonville & Villareal, 2013). A reduction in isokinetic (Gajdosik et al., 1996) and isometric strength with an increase in age (Grimby, 1995; Heyley et al., 1998) has been reported and is associated with a decreased level of activity and an associated muscle atrophy (Pedrero-Chamizo et al., 2015). Between the fourth and seventh decade a progressive decline in isokinetic quadriceps strength of approximately 14% per decade appears to be the 'normal' rate of decline (Hughes et al., 2001, Piasecki et al., 2016). However, this decline in force production, which is generally associated with a decrease in cross-sectional area of the muscle, can easily be reduced with increased activity levels, especially activities requiring high forces to be produced (Mayer et al., 2011; Bouchonville & Villareal, 2013), hence the importance of resistance training in the maintenance of independence in older adults.

Muscle Power

Internal muscle power is calculated from the force of contraction and the shortening velocity (force multiplied by velocity), with external power calculated as the force applied to the mass being accelerated, multiplied by the resultant velocity of the object at each specific time point (also calculated as work done divided by time) (Turner et al., 2020). Muscle power is influenced by the number of sarcomeres in series (muscle length), and the angle of pennation of the muscle fibres (the more parallel to the direction of force, the greater the fascicle shortening velocity during a concentric muscle action) (de Brito Fontana et al., 2014; Hauraix et al., 2015). For a given muscular force, the fascicle shortening velocity and therefore the external movement velocity is greater in muscles that contain a higher percentage of fast-twitch fibres (Fig. 4.17). For both fast- and slow-twitch muscle fibres, the greatest force occurs at the lowest fascicle shortening velocities, with a progressive decline in force production as fascicle shortening velocity increases (Kojima, 1991; Blazevich, 2006). Fast-twitch fibres can produce greater force at higher velocities than slow-twitch fibres; hence muscles with predominantly fast-twitch fibres can generate higher forces and greater power than muscles with predominantly slow-twitch fibres. It is worth noting that movement velocity is also related to neuromuscular coordination (Kerr,

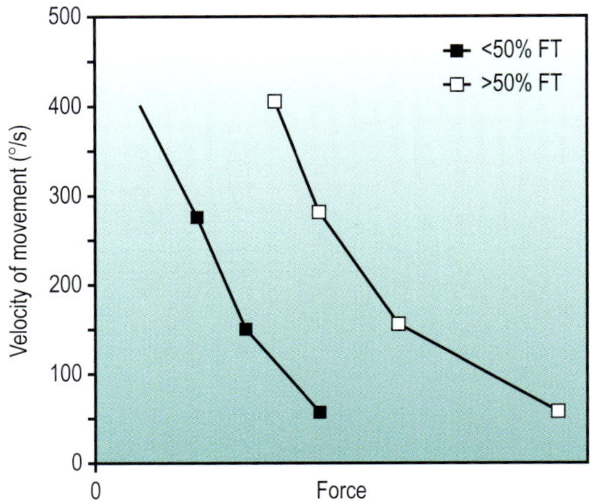

Fig. 4.17 Difference in muscular force and speed of movement between muscles predominantly with fast-twitch *(FT)* and with slow-twitch muscle fibres. (From Powers & Howley, 1997, with permission.)

1998), including the coordination of the relaxation of antagonists. Muscle power reduces with age as a product of muscle atrophy and the associated decline in force production capability (Gajdosik et al., 1996), although this can easily be reduced with increased activity levels and more specifically resistance training, especially at high intensities (Mayer et al., 2011; Bouchonville & Villareal, 2013).

The relationship of muscle power and velocity is depicted in Fig. 4.18. For a given velocity the peak power generated is greater in muscle that contains a high percentage of fast-twitch fibres than in muscle that contains a high percentage of slow-twitch fibres (Powers & Howley, 1997). The peak power generated by any muscle increases with increasing velocity of movement, up to a movement velocity of 200–400 degrees/s, when assessing single joint activities. During multi-joint activities, peak power occurs at different loads depending on the type of exercise and the nature of the exercise; for example, peak power during squats occurs at 56% one-repetition maximum (1RM), whereas during a jump squat peak power occurs at 0% 1RM back squat (Cormie et al., 2007). This is likely due to the nature of the movement, where the final stages of the squat (last 45% of the range of motion) result in a deceleration phase, whereas acceleration occurs almost until take off during jumping activities. More important than the relationship between power and velocity is the relationship between force and power, as force

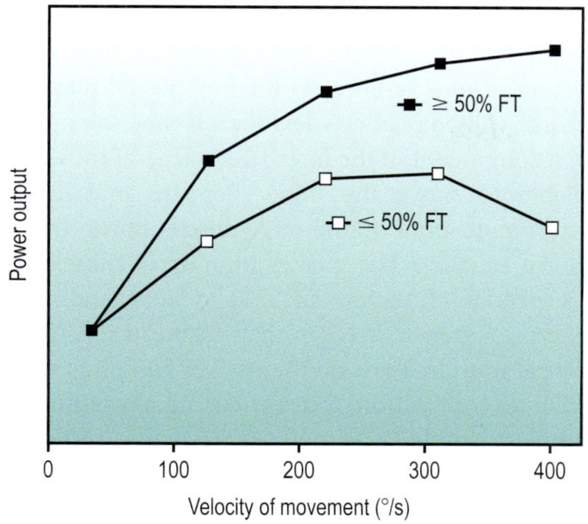

Fig. 4.18 Difference in muscle power and velocity between muscles with predominantly fast twitch *(FT)* and slow-twitch muscle fibres. (From Powers & Howley, 1997, with permission.)

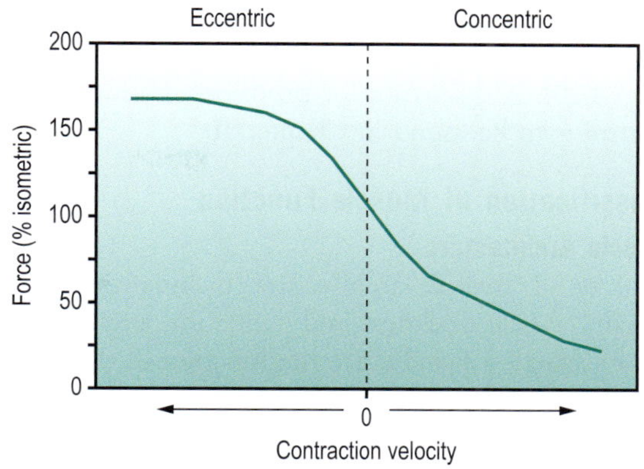

Fig. 4.19 Force–velocity relationship for skeletal muscle (From Newham, 1993, with permission.)

production directly influences velocity of movement. If force applied to an object increases within the same given epoch, acceleration increases (force = mass × acceleration); if acceleration increases, the velocity of movement must also increase. In this case as both force and velocity have increased, there is a subsequent increase in power (power = force × velocity). Researchers have reported that strength training is more beneficial than power training in individuals who are not already strong, likely due to the increase force increasing both components of the power equations as described earlier (Cormie et al., 2010, 2011; Turner et al., 2020). This is an important consideration for sedentary and older individuals, where strength training may enhance power more effectively than training modalities traditionally used to develop power.

In vitro muscle studies have demonstrated that the type of muscle action affects the force generated by a muscle. The greatest force is produced by an eccentric muscle action, the least force by a concentric muscle action; an isometric muscle action lies somewhere between the two. During single joint tasks, increased velocity of an eccentric action increases the force generated, whereas increased velocity of a concentric action reduces the force generated (Fig. 4.19).

Muscle Endurance

Muscle endurance is the ability of a muscle to continue an activity over time. It includes all types of muscle action and so may include repetitive movement (e.g. walking), or it may involve holding an isometric muscle action over a period (e.g. using the rings in gymnastics). Muscle strength is positively associated with the endurance capacity of a muscle. A muscle that is relatively weak, when required to generate force during a functional activity, will do so at a proportionally greater level of maximum capacity than a muscle that is relatively strong. Other factors affecting muscle endurance include the energy store and blood circulation within the muscle (De Vries & Housh, 1994).

There are a variety of ways to measure muscle endurance, and they depend on what specific type of muscle action is being tested. Measuring muscle endurance involves measuring the resultant muscle fatigue, or the number of repetitions performed to failure (when insufficient force can be produced to perform another repetition). Holding an isometric contraction at 60% maximum voluntary contraction (MVC) will increase the pressure within the muscle such that there will be no blood flowing into the muscle. The ability then to continue holding the contraction will depend on accumulation of hydrogen ions and how quickly this inhibits enzyme function within the muscle.

Normal control of movement occurs because of incoming sensory information of position and movement and is integrated at all levels of the nervous system. Automatic and simple reflex movements occur in the spinal cord. Postural and balance reactions occur at the level of the brainstem and basal ganglia. More complicated movements are initiated and controlled at the motor/sensory cortices, and the cerebellum controls and coordinates movement (Crow & Haas, 2001) (Fig. 4.20). A discussion of proprioception and motor control is to be found in Chapter 10.

Classification of Muscle Function

Muscle Architecture

Aspects of muscle architecture include the fascicle length, fascicle thickness and pennation angle. Each of these aspects will influence the function of the muscle. Each muscle fibre can shorten to approximately half its total length (Norkin & Levangie, 1992). Thus a longer muscle shortens over a greater distance than a shorter fascicle, resulting in the potential for higher shortening velocities and therefore higher movement velocities.

The direction of the muscle fibres (pennation angle) differs with each muscle shape and so affects the direction of force during muscle action, but this does alter with training, especially in superficial muscles (Blazevich, 2006) (Fig. 4.21). A quadrilateral muscle, as the name suggests, is flat and square. The muscle fibres run parallel and extend the length of the muscle. Muscles of this shape, such as pronator quadratus and quadratus lumborum, are well designed to support and stabilize underlying bones and joints.

Strap muscles are long and rectangular in shape, with fibres running the full length of the muscle. They produce movement through a large range (e.g. sartorius). Rectus abdominis is a strap muscle but is unusual in that it has three fibrous bands running across it.

Fusiform muscles are in the shape of a spindle with fibres running almost parallel to the line of pull. The two ends of the muscle converge on to a tendon. Biceps brachii consists of two fusiform-shaped muscles, whereas triceps brachii has three fusiform-shaped muscles.

Triangular muscles have a tendon at one end, and at the other end the muscle attaches to bone via either a flat tendon or an aponeurosis. The shape of the muscle means that some muscle fibres run at quite an oblique angle to the line of pull of the tendon, thus reducing its potential force of contraction. However, at its flat attachment, the force of pull is across a broad area. Lower trapezius is an example of a triangular muscle.

Pennate muscles appear like a feather and may be unipennate (fibres attach to only one side of the tendon), bipennate (to both sides of the tendon) or multipennate (several bipennate arranged fibres). Examples include flexor pollicis longus (unipennate), rectus femoris (bipennate) and deltoid (multipennate). The oblique direction of muscle fibres to the line of pull means that the force will be relatively less than if they were parallel; only a component of the force (the cosine of the angle) is available to move the bone. Pennate muscles have shorter and more numerous muscle fibres than do fusiform muscles. The greater number of muscle fibres gives pennate muscles, such as deltoid and gluteus maximus, a greater strength than fusiform muscles.

Spiral muscles twist on themselves and often untwist on muscle contraction, thus producing a rotation force. Examples include latissimus dorsi twisting 180 degrees through its length to rotate the humerus medially (Lockwood, 1998).

These architectural arrangements provide valuable insight into the function of a muscle and have been shown to have more effect on the force-generating capability of a muscle than its fibre-type composition (Sacks & Roy, 1982; Burkholder et al., 1994).

Monoarticular and Polyarticular

Monoarticular muscles cross only one joint, whereas polyarticular muscles cross more than one joint. This classification system describes the relationship of muscle to joint and so provides insight into the movement that will be produced by the muscle. For example, the rectus femoris is a polyarticular muscle crossing the anterior aspect of the hip and knee (biarticular as it crosses two joints) and therefore causing hip flexion and knee extension on concentric contraction. Muscles crossing more than one joint will be longer and will produce more movement than a muscle crossing just one joint.

Prime Mover, Antagonist, Fixator and Synergist

This classification system describes the way in which a muscle functions in relation to a specific movement (Fig. 4.22). Any one muscle may act as a prime mover (or agonist), antagonist, fixator or synergist. The way in which a muscle acts depends on several factors which include the start position, the direction and speed of the movement, the phase of the movement and the resistance to movement.

Prime Mover and Antagonist

When a muscle is active in initiating and maintaining a movement, it is acting as a prime mover (agonist). A

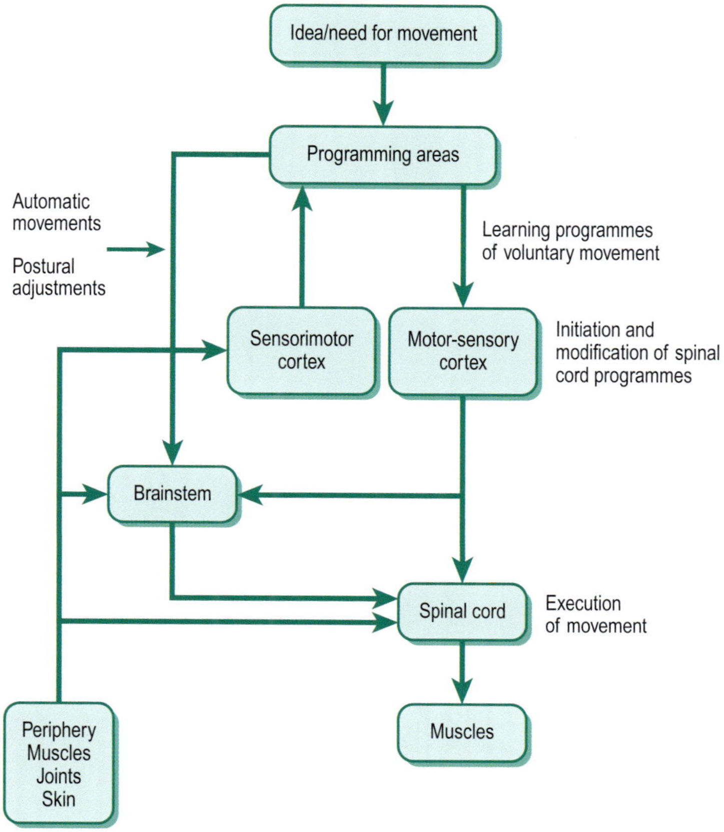

Fig. 4.20 Schematic diagram of the control of movement. (After Kidd et al., 1992, with permission.)

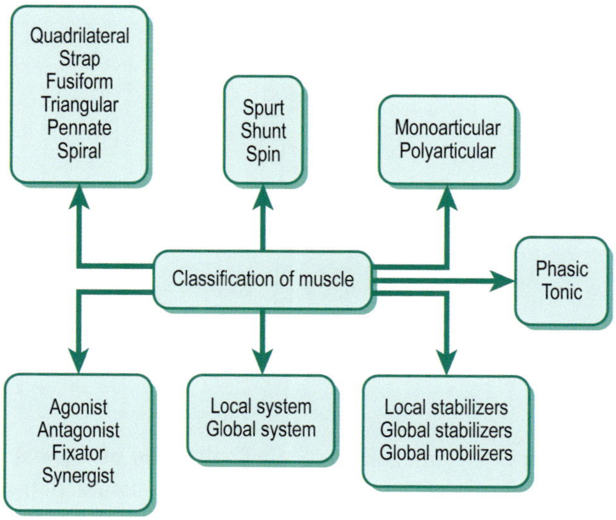

Fig. 4.21 Classification systems for muscle.

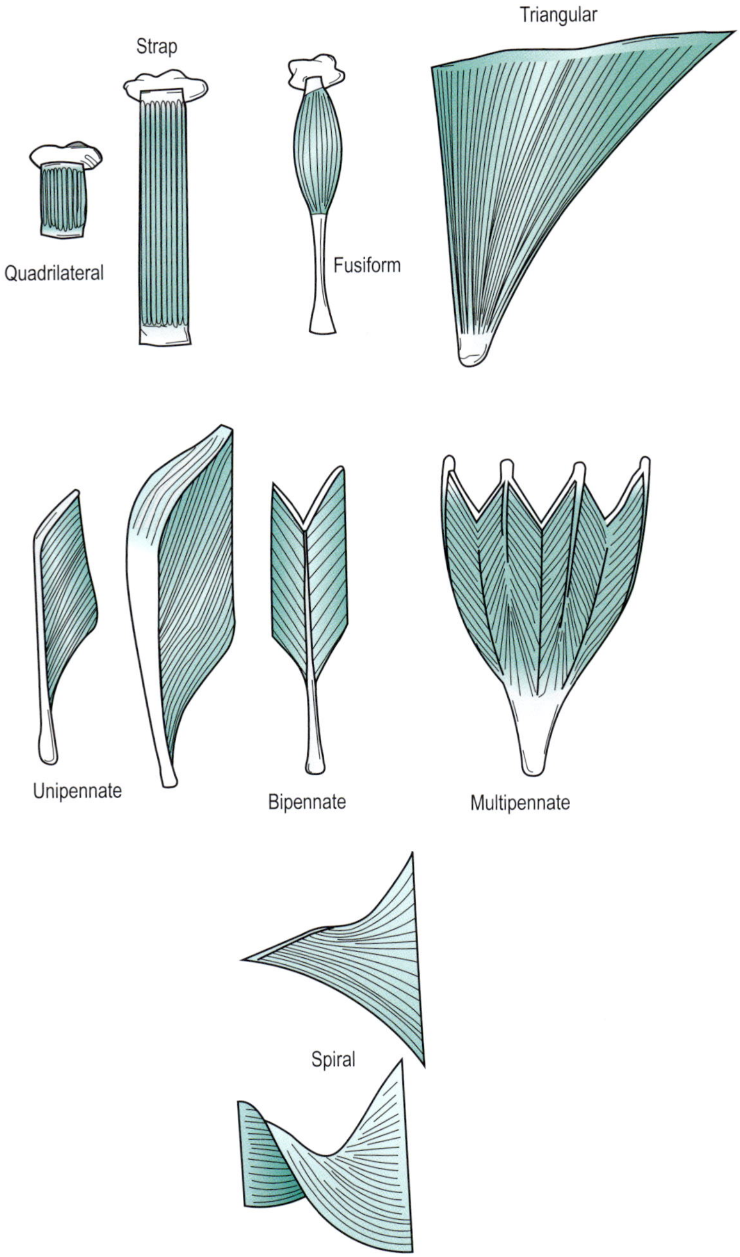

Fig. 4.22 Shapes of muscles: quadrilateral, strap, fusiform, triangular, pennate and spiral. (From Williams et al., 1995.)

muscle that opposes the prime mover is the antagonist. For example, during a knee extension exercise, the quadriceps are the prime mover (agonist), while the hamstring muscles co-contract to stabilize the knee joint (antagonist); this reverses during the knee flexion exercise.

Co-Contraction of Agonist and Antagonist

It might be assumed that when the prime mover is contracting, the antagonist is silent; however, there are numerous examples of co-contraction of agonist and antagonist. During maximal voluntary knee extension, the flexors of the knee are also contracting, albeit to a lesser degree (Baratta et al., 1988). When maintaining trunk extension during a lifting task, there is co-contraction of the trunk flexors and extensors (Granata & Marras, 1995), with these muscles performing isometric actions to maintain spinal alignment. With a rapid voluntary movement, there is a triphasic pattern of muscle activity, with bursts of activity initially in the agonist, then the antagonist and then the agonist (Friedli et al., 1984). The effect of co-contraction is to increase stiffness and thus stability of a joint, which is likely to be needed in stressful and complex movements (Fig. 4.23). There is therefore activity of the agonist and antagonist muscles during active movements.

Interestingly, the amount of co-contraction can be altered by activity. Athletes who strongly exercised the quadriceps and not the hamstrings had reduced co-contraction of the hamstrings on active knee extension compared with those who exercised both groups of muscles (Baratta et al., 1988). The amount of co-contraction is related to motor control; co-contraction is greater when motor skill is poor and reduces when motor skill is improved (Osu et al., 2002).

Increased levels of co-contraction of the hamstrings and quadriceps during gait appear to be related to increased severity of knee osteoarthritis (OA) (Mills et al., 2013) and decreasing levels of co-contraction reduces knee OA symptoms (Al-Khaifat et al., 2016), whereas co-contraction of the latissimus dorsi muscle during tackling tasks appears to stabilize the shoulder in the presence of superior labrum from anterior to posterior tear (SLAP) lesions (Horsley et al., 2010).

The amount of co-contraction increases with age: elderly women compared with young women were found to have more than 100% greater activity of hamstring muscles just before and during a step-down movement (Hortobagyi & DeVita, 2000), and both men and women were found to have greater co-contraction of biceps femoris during a maximum isometric contraction and 1RM of quadriceps femoris muscle (Tracy & Enoka, 2002). This increased co-contraction functions to increase joint stiffness and is thought to compensate for the neuromotor impairments (atrophy/sarcopenia, reduced strength and proprioception) associated with the elderly (Hortobagyi & DeVita, 2000).

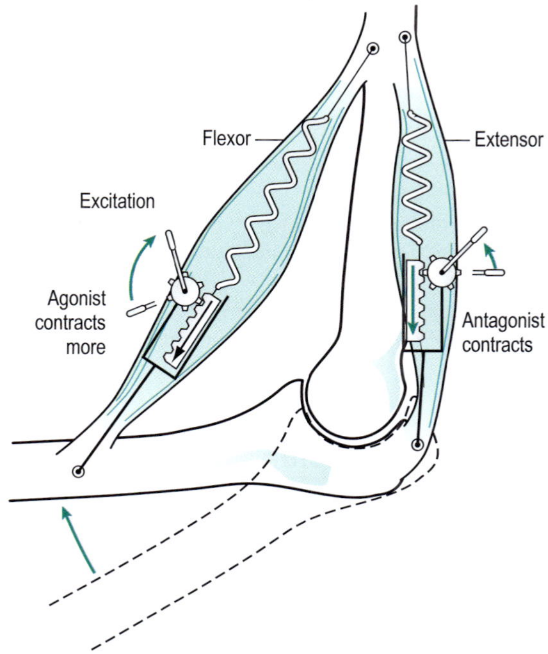

Fig. 4.23 Co-contraction of elbow flexors and extensors to increase joint stiffness and stability. (From Ghez, 1991, with permission.)

Fixators

This is when muscles contract to fix a bone. Muscles on either side of a joint sometimes contract together to create a fixed base on which another muscle can contract. For example, the muscles acting around the wrist contract together to fix the wrist when a strong fist is made.

Synergists

When a muscle acts over two or more joints but the required movement is only over one joint, other muscles contract to eliminate the movement. When a muscle acts in this way, it is said to act as a synergist (derived from *syn*, together, and *ergon*, work). Contraction of the finger flexors would produce flexion at both the wrist and fingers. The wrist extensors contract to eliminate the wrist flexion during a power grip and thus act as a synergist. Similarly, during elbow flexion with a pronated forearm, the contraction of biceps brachii will produce both elbow flexion and supination. When muscles around the shoulder contract to produce movement at the glenohumeral joint, muscles around the cervical spine, thoracic spine and scapula must contract to prevent unwanted movement and are therefore acting as synergists.

Any clinician attempting to analyse muscle activity during movement will immediately appreciate the difficulty in doing this. Visual and palpatory cues are simply inadequate to sense whether a particular muscle is active and in what way it is active.

KNOWLEDGE CHECK

1. What factors can influence muscle force output?
2. How would you define muscle endurance?
3. How do muscle spindles and Golgi tendon organs function to understand muscle force?

MUSCLE DYSFUNCTION

Just as the function of muscles depends on the function of joints and nerves, so dysfunction of muscles can lead to dysfunction of joints and nerves. They are dependent on each other in both normal and abnormal conditions (Fig. 4.24).

Dysfunction in muscles and joints often occur together. For example, abnormality of the eccentric muscle force of the quadriceps muscle may be a contributing factor in anterior knee pain (Bennett & Stauber, 1986), and lateral epicondylitis is associated with tears of the lateral collateral ligament of the elbow (Bredella et al., 1999). This evidence highlights the close relationship of muscle and joint dysfunction.

There is overwhelming evidence that weakness of a muscle occurs with joint pathology and dysfunction. This has been demonstrated in the knee in the presence of a variety of pathologies: rheumatoid arthritis and OA (Hurley & Newham, 1993), ligamentous knee injuries (DeVita et al., 1997; Urbach & Awiszus, 2002) and following meniscectomy (Hurley et al., 1994; Suter et al., 1998a) and in the glenohumeral joint in the presence of anterior dislocation (Keating & Crossan, 1992). The inhibition of muscle is thought to be due to inhibitory input (Suter & Herzog, 2000; Torry et al., 2000) or abnormal input from joint afferents (Hurley et al., 1991; Hurley & Newham, 1993). Thus joint pathology leads to altered neural activity, which alters muscle activity. A muscle that is inhibited will, over time, atrophy and weaken, and this may make the joint vulnerable to further injury (Stokes & Young, 1984). For example, it is thought that weakness of the posterior rotator cuff muscles may make the glenohumeral joint vulnerable to recurrent anterior dislocation (Keating & Crossan, 1992) (Fig. 4.25).

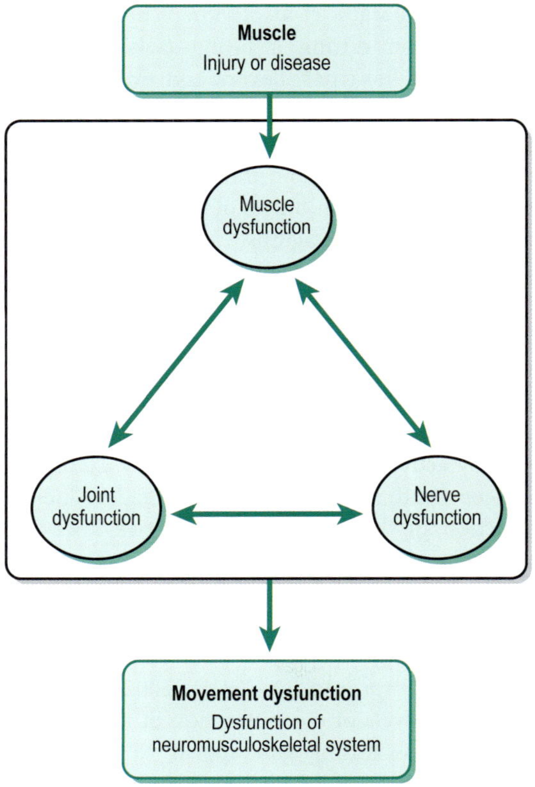

Fig. 4.24 Dysfunction of muscle can produce joint and/or nerve dysfunction and can lead to movement dysfunction.

Muscle activity around a joint is altered in the presence of ligament insufficiency and joint instability. During throwing, electromyography (EMG) activity of the elbow muscles is altered with ligament insufficiency of the elbow (Glousman et al., 1992). Similarly, during throwing, the EMG activity around the shoulder region is altered with shoulder instability (Glousman et al., 1988). In the lower limb, the EMG activity of quadriceps and hamstring muscle groups is altered with ACL deficiency during knee movement and during gait and functional activities (Frank et al., 2016). Fig. 4.26 identifies a proposed cycle of events of progressive knee instability following an initial ligament injury (Kennedy et al., 1982).

Muscle activity is directly affected by joint nociceptor activity. Pain around the knee causes a nociceptive flexor withdrawal response: hip and knee flexion and ankle dorsiflexion. There is increased α motor neurone excitability of the muscles to produce this movement and

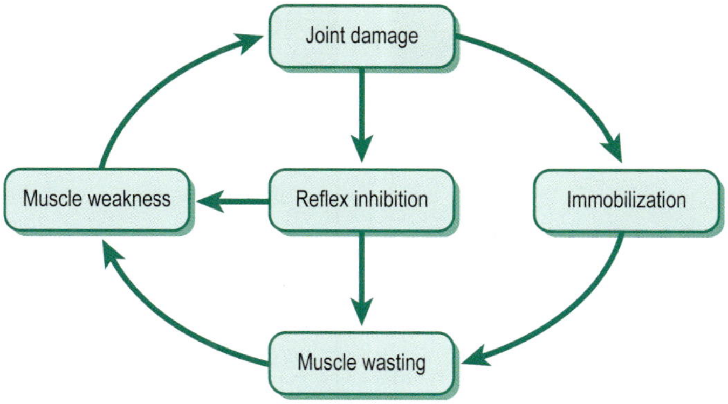

Fig. 4.25 Effect of joint damage and/or immobilization on muscle and nerve tissues. (Reproduced with permission, from Stokes, M., Young, A., 1984. Clinical Science 67:7–14. © The Biochemical Society and the Medical Research Society. (http://www.clinsci.org).)

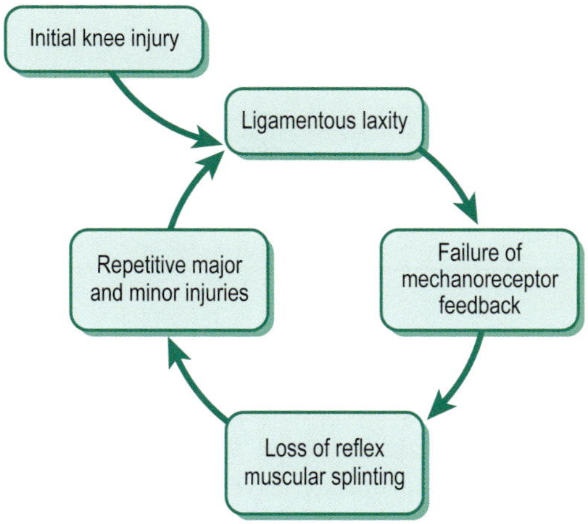

Fig. 4.26 A proposed cycle of progressive knee instability following an initial ligament injury. (From Kennedy et al., 1982, with permission.)

reciprocal inhibition of the knee extensors. For example, pressure or tension on a partially ruptured medial collateral ligament results in an increased activity of sartorius and semimembranosus (knee flexors) with inhibition of the vastus medialis (extensor), resulting in reduced external force during knee extension.

Nociceptor activity is thought to influence muscle activity via the α motor neurone (Wyke & Polacek, 1975). Nociceptor activity is thought to have a greater inhibitory effect upon the low-threshold motor units supplying type I muscle fibres than on the high-threshold motor units supplying type II fibres (Gydikov, 1976). If this is true, it might be speculated that a muscle containing a relatively higher proportion of type I fibres, such as soleus and tibialis anterior, may be more affected by nociceptor activity than a muscle that has a more equal proportion of type I and II fibres.

The functions of a muscle are essentially to produce and allow movement to occur. That is, it will contract with strength, power and endurance, it will lengthen and shorten with movement and, under the control of the central nervous system (CNS) (motor control), it will produce coordinated movement. The signs and symptoms of muscle dysfunction are related to these functions; that is, there may be one or more of the following: reduced muscle strength (which is accompanied by a reduction in both muscle power and muscle endurance), reduced muscle power, reduced muscle endurance, altered motor control, reduced muscle length or production of symptoms. Box 4.3 highlights these characteristics of muscle function and dysfunction.

Reduced Muscle Strength

Reduced muscle strength can occur because of disuse such as immobility (Berg et al., 1997), immobilization (Vaughan, 1989; Labarque et al., 2002), trauma (DeVita et al., 1997; Urbach & Awiszus, 2002), weightlessness (Fitts et al., 2000, 2001) and pathology (Zhao et al., 2000; Yoshihara et al., 2001). As will be seen later, a reduction in muscle strength will result in a reduction in muscle power (if force generation, over a specified epoch, decreases so does acceleration and therefore velocity of movement; as power = force × velocity, it is clear reduction that a in force production capability

BOX 4.3 Signs and Symptoms of Muscle Dysfunction

Reduced muscle strength
Reduced muscle power
Reduced muscle endurance
Altered motor control
Reduced muscle length
Production of symptoms

directly impacts muscle power) and a reduction in endurance.

Muscle atrophy has been found to occur with pathology. For example, in patients who underwent surgery for a chronic lumbar disc herniation, there was atrophy of the multifidus and longissimus muscles (Sirca & Kostevc, 1985). In another similar study a biopsy of multifidus at L4/5 and L5/S1 levels also revealed muscle atrophy on the side of herniation, with smaller type I and type II fibres (Zhao et al., 2000). Patients with an L4/5-disc herniation and L5 nerve root compression (identified at surgery) were found to have atrophy of multifidus with a 6.4% reduction in cross-section area of type I fibres and a 9.8% reduction in type II fibres at the level of the herniation; interestingly, no atrophy was found at the L4 level (Yoshihara et al., 2001).

It should be remembered that there are normal age-related changes in muscle strength (Piasecki et al., 2016). Between the fourth and seventh decade, there is a 14% reduction in isokinetic quadriceps strength per decade (Hughes et al., 2001). However, such decreases are associated with a reduction in activity, and the decline in strength can be slowed with appropriate and progressive training. In fact, in weak individuals' strength will noticeably increase with appropriate training.

Immobilization

Immobilization affects the contractile portion of muscle, the musculotendinous junction and the tendon. The reduced strength resulting from immobilization is primarily due to muscle atrophy and reduced neural input to the muscle (Young et al., 1982; Berg et al., 1997), although architectural changes are also likely to occur in trained individuals. The effects of immobilization on muscle depend on the length of time, the position of the muscle when immobilized and the predominant muscle fibre type within the muscle.

BOX 4.4 Effects of Immobilization on Muscle in a Shortened Position

Decrease in muscle weight and fibre size	Williams & Goldspink, 1978 Witzmann, 1988
Decrease in the number of sarcomeres	Goldspink, 1976 Tabary et al., 1972 Williams & Goldspink, 1973 Williams & Goldspink 1978
Increase in the sarcomere length	Williams & Goldspink, 1978, 1984
Increase in amount of perimysium	Williams & Goldspink, 1984
Increase in ratio of collagen concentration	Goldspink & Williams, 1979 Williams & Goldspink, 1984
Increase in ratio of connective tissue to muscle fibre tissue	Goldspink & Williams, 1979 Williams & Goldspink, 1984
Reduction in the cross-sectional area of the intrafusal fibres of the muscle spindle	Jozsa et al., 1988
Increase in the thickness of the capsule surrounding the muscle spindle	Jozsa et al., 1988

Duration of immobilization. If a muscle does not contract at all, muscle strength will decrease by approximately 5% per day. However, low levels of isometric exercise, where appropriate, have been shown to reduce this rate of decline.

Position of the muscle. The effects of immobilization on muscle depend on the position in which the muscle is held, whether it is in a shortened or lengthened position. The effects of immobilization in a shortened position are summarized in Box 4.4. The decrease in the number of sarcomeres and increase in length of each sarcomere ensure that the muscle can contract maximally in the shortened immobilized position. The connective tissue loss occurs at a lower rate than the loss of contractile tissue, resulting in a relative increase in connective tissue; this can occur as early as 2 days after immobilization (Williams & Goldspink, 1984). In addition, the connective tissue remodels during immobilization to produce a thicker perimysium and endomysium. These changes produce an increased stiffness to passive lengthening. Tendon stiffness

BOX 4.5 Effects of Immobilization on Muscle in a Lengthened Position

Increase in the number of sarcomeres in series	Goldspink, 1976 Tabary et al., 1972 Williams & Goldspink, 1973, 1976, 1978
Decrease in the length of sarcomeres	Tabary et al., 1972 Williams & Goldspink, 1978, 1984
Muscle hypertrophy that may be followed by atrophy	Williams & Goldspink, 1984

appears to decrease due to immobilization at a similar rate in both young and old men (Couppe et al., 2012). Interestingly, collagen turnover after an acute bout of exercise is not affected by a period of immobilization (Moerch et al., 2013).

The effects of immobilization of muscle in a lengthened position are summarized in Box 4.5. There is an increase in the number of sarcomeres that lie in series, thus lengthening the muscle (Goldspink, 1976; Williams & Goldspink, 1978); however, the length of individual sarcomeres is reduced (Williams & Goldspink, 1978, 1984). Functionally the muscle has a greater capacity to generate tension at longer lengths, but this will be offset by the resultant atrophy from immobilization.

Predominant type of muscle fibre within the muscle. There is some suggestion that the effect of immobilization on a muscle is affected by its proportion of type I and type II muscle fibres. The effect of immobilization in near-resting length of a guinea pig soleus (predominantly type I muscle fibres) has been compared with immobilization of gastrocnemius (predominantly type II muscle fibres) (Maier et al., 1976). This is discussed in more detail in the section on Reduced Muscle Power, later in this chapter.

Effect of Immobilization on the Musculotendinous Junction and the Tendon

Immobilization has widespread effects on the musculotendinous junction and the tendon (Box 4.6). As tendons adapt in response to the load that is applied to them via muscular actions, reduction in loading of the tendon or musculotendinous junction results in a decrease in strength and stiffness of the tendon. At the musculotendinous junction, 3 weeks of immobilization of the rat gastrocnemius–soleus–tendon unit in a shortened position resulted in more than 40% reduction in the contact area between the muscle and the tendon (Kannus et al., 1992). Other changes included an increase in scar tissue in the area, reduced glycosaminoglycans and an increase in weaker type III collagen fibres (Kannus et al., 1992).

Collectively, these changes will reduce the tensile strength of the musculotendinous junction. An experimental muscle strain and 2 days of immobilization have been shown to result in a reduction in tensile strength and stiffness at the musculotendinous junction

BOX 4.6 Effects of Immobilization on the Musculotendinous Junction and Tendon

Musculotendinous Junction	
Reduction in the contact area between muscle and tendon	Kannus et al., 1992
Increase in scar tissue	Kannus et al., 1992
Reduced glycosaminoglycans	Kannus et al., 1992
Increase in the weaker type III collagen fibres	Kannus et al., 1992
Reduced tensile strength	Almekinders & Gilbert, 1986 Kannus et al., 1992
Reduced stiffness	Almekinders & Gilbert, 1986
Reduction in blood vessels	Kvist et al., 1995
Increase in the thickness of the capsule of the Golgi tendon organ	Jozsa et al., 1988
Tendon	
Reduced collagen fibres	Nakagawa et al., 1989
Reduced energy supply, oxygen consumption and enzyme activity	Jozsa & Kannus, 1997

(Almekinders & Gilbert, 1986). In addition, a 30% reduction in blood vessels in the musculotendinous junction has been observed following immobilization (Kvist et al., 1995), along with a reduced energy supply, oxygen consumption and enzyme activity within the tendon following a period of immobilization (Jozsa & Kannus, 1997).

Measurement of Muscle Strength

Manual, subjective assessments of strength are not sufficient, and assumptions should not be made based on muscle atrophy (circumference measurements) because this does not take neurological and architectural changes into account. Force should be measured using devices such as the hand-held dynamometer for isometric strength, and isotonic force (eccentric/concentric actions) can be measured using isokinetic dynamometers (Watkins et al., 1984). In both situations only single joint actions and therefore individual groups of muscles are assessed; although this can be useful, it is limited by the fact that force assessed during such tasks do not reflect functional performance in the normal population or athletes (Augustsson et al., 1998; Blackburn and Morrissey, 1998; Ostenberg et al., 1998). Where isometric strength is measured, muscle length will affect the resultant force, and therefore the joint angle used during assessment must be consistent to ensure comparable measures; similarly during isokinetic testing the velocity of contraction will influence force measured so must be decided upon. In addition, the motivation and subsequent effort by an individual will affect the force measurement.

Muscle strength testing is further complicated by the fact that asymptomatic subjects have been found to vary the maximal voluntary contraction over different days of testing (Allen et al., 1995; Suter & Herzog, 1997), but the typical measurement error (standard error of measurement (SEM)) for an isometric test for quadriceps and gluteus medius is less than 10%. However, Mentiplay et al. (2015) concluded that hand-held dynamometry is suitably reliable for the assessment of force and rate of force development (RFD) in clinical settings.

Multijoint assessments, such as the isometric mid-thigh pull, has been shown to be highly reliable between sessions, with smallest detectable differences of 1.3% and 10.3%, for peak force and rate of force development respectively, demonstrating meaningful differences between sessions (Comfort et al., 2015). Peak force and rate of force development during the isometric mid-thigh pull have also been shown to be related to performance in athletic tasks (Winchester et al., 2010; Spiteri et al., 2014; Thomas et al., 2015) and is more commonly being used in elite sport settings as part of return to play criteria for both strength and RFD.

Other useful methods of assessing strength include repetition maximum testing, with a high reliability of 1RM testing reported in both recreationally trained individuals (Comfort & McMahon, 2015), adolescents (Faigenbaum et al., 2012) and older females (Amarante do Nascimento et al., 2013), with similarly high reliability using 8RMs (Taylor & Fletcher, 2012). For individuals not used to strength training or the specific exercises, a period of familiarization is recommended (Taylor & Fletcher, 2012; Amarante do Nascimento et al., 2013). Assessing strength via repetition maximum testing may be easier for most individuals when using a resistance machine and those not familiar with such practices; with higher repetitions (e.g. 6–12RM), it is potentially safer and more useful: for example, performance in a 6RM can be used directly to prescribe strength training loads for the exercise assessed, ideally using the 6RM loads for three sets of four to five repetitions if the aim is increased strength. It is also possible to predict 1RM performance from maximal performance during higher repetitions in some exercises (Julio et al., 2012), although the reliability tends to decrease with an increase in repetitions.

Reduced Muscle Power

Muscle power is a function of force and velocity, and if either is reduced there will be a subsequent reduction in power. Where there is a reduction in muscle strength, there will be, by definition, a reduction in power. Force applied to a mass determines its acceleration (force = mass × acceleration) and therefore its resultant velocity. It has already been identified that immobilization in a shortened position causes a reduction in strength and a reduction in length; changes in either will cause a reduction in muscle power, as fascicle length also determines fascicle shortening velocity and therefore movement velocity and power (Blazevich, 2006; Earp et al., 2010).

The velocity of a contraction is determined, in part, by the proportion of fibre types within the muscle: the greater the proportion of type II fibres, the greater the power. Any reduction in type II fibres within a muscle would potentially reduce its power. In addition, the pennation angle and fascicle length are also associated with power output and have been shown to adversely change in response to detraining, sarcopenia, injury and immobilization (Narici et al., 2016).

Researchers have investigated the effect of knee immobilization on the proportion of type I and type II fibres in vastus lateralis (MacDougall et al., 1980; Hortobagyi et al., 2000). Three weeks of knee immobilization resulted in a 13% reduction in type I fibres and a 10% reduction in type II fibres (Hortobagyi et al., 2000). Following a lower-limb fracture and knee immobilization for up to 7 weeks, there was a 46% reduction in type I fibres and a 37% reduction in type II fibres (Sargeant et al., 1977). Following knee surgery and 5 weeks of knee immobilization, there was a reduction only in the cross-sectional area of type I fibres, with no alteration in type II fibres (Haggmark et al., 1981). The results of these studies suggest that knee immobilization causes a greater atrophy of type I fibres than of type II fibres in vastus lateralis, but more importantly both force and power decrease.

Reduced Muscle Endurance

Reduced muscle endurance may be manifested by a reduced ability to repeat a muscle action or a reduced ability to hold an isometric action over time. To avoid testing/training muscle strength, it is suggested that the resistance is sufficiently low (usually 60%–70% 1RM) to allow 8–15 repetitions.

Altered Motor Control

Aspects of altered motor control include:

- muscle inhibition
- timing of onset
- increased muscle activation
- altered activation of agonist and antagonist.

Muscle Inhibition

Muscle inhibition may be identified by the clinician by visual and/or palpatory cues. While these methods are clearly practical in the clinical setting and require no special equipment, they may have questionable reliability. Some muscles are superficial and may be relatively easy to identify (e.g. sternocleidomastoid); most muscles overlap with other muscles or lie deep underneath a whole muscle, so that identification of decreased activity in these muscles is extremely difficult, if not impossible. This has led to the development of instrumentation to help the clinician identify muscle inhibition; it includes ultrasound imaging (Hides et al., 1995) and EMG biofeedback (Richardson et al., 1999). In research, voluntary muscle activity can be measured using the interpolated twitch technique (ITT) and involuntary muscle activity by a reduction in the Hoffman (H)-reflex.

The ITT involves applying a single electrical twitch to a nerve during a maximal isometric contraction and indicates the motor unit activity (Hales & Gandevia, 1988; Gandevia et al., 1998), although a high-frequency train of stimuli is a more sensitive measure than the single twitch (Kent-Braun & Le Blanc, 1996). A dynamometer measures muscle torque during the active contraction, and if there is full motor unit activity then the addition of nerve stimulation will not produce any increase in torque. Any increase in torque (referred to as 'interpolated twitch torque': Suter & Herzog, 2000) indicates muscle inhibition due to incomplete activation.

In asymptomatic subjects, the ITT will produce, on average, a 4% increase in isometric quadriceps muscle torque at 90 degrees flexion (Suter et al., 1996). It should be noted that the extent of muscle inhibition measured by the ITT is dependent on the joint angle; at 60 degrees, knee flexion muscle inhibition is three times greater than with the knee in extension (Suter & Herzog, 1997).

Involuntary muscle activity is measured by a reduction in the H-reflex, indicating an inhibition of the α motor neurone pool. The H-reflex is a small muscle contraction (via α motor neurones) in response to low-intensity stimulation of a mixed nerve (via stimulation of group Ia fibres from muscle spindles). This reflex inhibition continues to be present during active contraction of the muscle (Iles et al., 1990).

Both acute and chronic joint pathology, effusion, pain and immobilization have been found to lead to inhibition of the overlying muscle, a response sometimes referred to as arthrogenous muscle inhibition (Stokes & Young, 1984). All studies identified in Box 4.7 have been carried out on the knee, apart from those on rheumatoid arthritis of the elbow joint. The muscle inhibition of an active voluntary contraction seems to be related to the extent of the joint damage: the greater

BOX 4.7 Possible Causes of Arthrogenic Muscle Inhibition

Causes	References
Rheumatoid arthritis of the knee	deAndrade et al., 1965
Rheumatoid arthritis of the elbow	Hurley et al., 1991
Osteoarthritis (knee joint) with no pain or effusion	deAndrade et al., 1965 Hurley & Newham, 1993
Articular cartilage	Suter et al., 1998a
Degeneration of the patellar or tibial plateau	Hurley & Newham, 1993
Subperiosteal tumour of the femur	Stener, 1969
Anterior knee pain	Suter et al., 1998a, b
Muscle pain	Rutherford et al., 1986
Ligamentous knee injuries without pain or effusion	DeVita et al., 1997 Hurley et al., 1992 Newham et al., 1989 Hurley et al., 1994 Snyder-Mackler et al., 1994 Urbach & Awiszus, 2002
Postmeniscectomy (knee joint)	Hurley et al., 1994 Shakespeare et al., 1985 Stokes & Young, 1984 Suter et al., 1998a
Presence of pain	Arvidsson et al., 1986 Rutherford et al., 1986
Effusion of the knee joint	deAndrade et al., 1965 Fahrer et al., 1988 Kennedy et al., 1982 Jones et al., 1987 Iles et al., 1990 Spencer et al., 1984 Stratford, 1981 L. Wood et al., 1988
Anterior cruciate ligament	Newham et al., 1989 Hurley et al., 1994
Deficiency of the knee joint	Snyder-Mackler et al., 1994 Suter et al., 1998a, 1998b
Immobilization	Vaughan, 1989

the injury, the greater the inhibition of muscle (Urbach & Awiszus, 2002). The presence of pain can cause muscle inhibition (Arvidsson et al., 1986; Rutherford et al., 1986), although the mechanism is not fully understood. It has been suggested that muscle inhibition can be due to inhibitory input (Suter & Herzog, 2000; Torry et al., 2000) or abnormal input (Hurley & Newham, 1993) from joint afferents, which reduces the motor drive to muscles acting over the joint.

The presence of effusion can cause muscle inhibition (Fahrer et al., 1988; Torry et al., 2000), although one study found no effect on quadriceps strength or power (McNair et al., 1994). Knee joint effusion and muscle inhibition do however have a marked effect on gait (Torry et al., 2000). This inhibition is thought to be due to increased intra-articular pressure causing an increase in tension in the joint capsule that stimulates mechanoreceptors in the intracapsular receptors and causes a reflex inhibition of the α motor neurone pool (Torry et al., 2000).

In experimentally produced effusion, there is a linear relationship between the volume of the effusion and the reduction in the H-reflex amplitude (i.e. the greater the effusion the greater the muscle inhibition) (Iles et al., 1990). In chronic effusions, associated with arthritis, the degree of effusion is not related to the amount of inhibition (Jones et al., 1987). With experimentally induced knee joint effusion, aspiration reduces the muscle inhibition (Spencer et al., 1984), whereas in chronic or recurrent knee joint effusions, muscle inhibition remains the same post aspiration (Jones et al., 1987). The amount of inhibition of the muscle is related to the angle of the joint, with greater inhibition occurring with the knee in extension than in flexion (Stokes & Young, 1984; Jones et al., 1987). This is thought to be due to the difference in intraarticular pressure, which is greater in full extension than in a few degrees of flexion (Levick, 1983).

Interestingly, researchers have found that muscle inhibition is not just restricted to the local muscles but also occurs in the contralateral limb (Suter et al., 1998a, 1998b; Urbach & Awiszus, 2002). The clinician needs to be aware of this when comparing muscle function on the side of injury with the unaffected side, as the degree of inhibition may be underestimated. The reason for the change on the unaffected side is unclear: it has been suggested to be due to altered movement patterns (Berchuck et al., 1990; Frank et al., 1994). Another explanation may be the connection of nerve pathways in the spinal cord.

Timing of Onset

The timing of onset of muscle activation during movement and functional activities has been identified in patients. Patients with chronic low-back pain have exhibited delayed activation of transversus abdominis, internal oblique, external oblique and rectus abdominis muscles when asked to perform rapid arm movements (Hodges & Richardson, 1996), although the true biological significance of these differences has been challenged recently even by the authors of these papers. It should be noted that there are normal age-related changes in the activation of muscles. For example, with age, there is increased coactivation of quadriceps and hamstring muscle groups during a step-down movement (Hortobagyi & DeVita, 2000). In addition, older subjects have been found to have a delay in muscle activation in the lower limb when stepping to regain balance during a fall (Thelen et al., 2000).

Increased Muscle Activation

Increased muscle activation is brought about by an increase in the activation of the α motor neurone pool supplying the muscle. The α motor neurone pool can be activated by the CNS, as part of motor control, or by peripheral input from muscle spindles, skin, joint, nerve and muscle afferents, including nociceptors. The underlying causes are therefore wide ranging and could include the perception of pain, as well as joint, nerve or muscle dysfunction.

Baseball players with known elbow medial collateral ligament insufficiency have been found to have increased EMG activity of extensor carpi radialis longus and brevis and reduced EMG activity of triceps, flexor carpi radialis and pronator teres compared with a control group (Glousman et al., 1992). Flexor carpi radialis and pronator teres might have been expected to demonstrate increased activity to compensate for the ligamentous insufficiency, but this was not the case. In addition, baseball players with known anterior shoulder instability have been found to have reduced EMG activity of pectoralis major, subscapularis, latissimus dorsi and serratus anterior and increased activity of biceps and supraspinatus compared with a control group (Glousman et al., 1988). The authors postulate that the reduced muscle activity exacerbates the anterior shoulder instability while the increased activity of biceps and supraspinatus compensates for the anterior instability. Similarly, in rugby players with SLAP lesions in the shoulder, Horsley et al. (2010) found increased latissimus dorsi muscle activity, which appear to be compensating for poor activity elsewhere to stabilize the shoulder.

Altered Activation of Agonist and Antagonist

This alteration in the relative activation of agonist and antagonist can result from the aforementioned consequences of increased or decreased muscle activation. In addition to these dysfunctions, there is also evidence of a specific alteration in the agonist and antagonist activation patterns. Pain around the knee causes a nociceptive flexor withdrawal response: hip and knee flexion and ankle dorsiflexion. To produce this movement, there is increased α motor neurone excitability of the hip and knee flexors and ankle dorsiflexors (Stener & Peterson, 1963) and reciprocal inhibition of the knee extensors (Young et al., 1987).

Patients with chronic anterior cruciate ligament (ACL) deficiency (16 months to 21 years) have been found to have less quadriceps and gastrocnemius activity and greater hamstring activity during the stance phase, and increased hamstring activity during the swing phase of gait (Branch et al., 1989). However, in another study of patients with chronic ACL deficiency (2–3 years), horizontal walking failed to show any difference in EMG activity of quadriceps and hamstrings but on walking uphill the hamstring muscle was activated much earlier than in control subjects (Kalund et al., 1990). Patients with an ACL-deficient knee following 6 months' rehabilitation continued to exhibit increased EMG activity of vastus lateralis, biceps femoris and tibialis anterior muscles during functional movements, compared with a control group (Ciccotti et al., 1994). This indicates a change in recruitment strategy of the muscles around the knee and possible subsequent muscle atrophy from disuse.

The results of numerous studies have demonstrated that chronic ACL deficiency and reconstruction cause an alteration of the motor control around the knee (Ciccotti et al., 1994; Beard et al., 1996; DeVita et al., 1997), with patients demonstrating what has been call a quadriceps avoidance strategy. Patients who have had an ACL reconstruction were found to have an altered gait pattern such that, compared with control subjects and the uninjured limb, the knee was in more flexion at heel contact and midstance, and a greater range of extensor torque was present during the stance phase (DeVita et al., 1997). Patients with chronic ACL deficiency, longer than 6 months without repair, were found to walk with the knee in more flexion at heel contact and mid-stance, and this correlated with an increased duration of hamstring activity (Beard et al., 1996), although later studies dispute these findings (Lepley et al., 2016). Whilst during running, landing and cutting, they demonstrated decreased knee flexion, and knee extensor moments are often reported (Trigsted et al., 2015).

Altered Muscle Length

The most obvious reduction in muscle length is seen following immobilization of a joint when the muscle is held in a shortened position. In this situation the muscle will be shortened and will have an increased resistance to passive lengthening (Goldspink, 1976; Goldspink & Williams, 1979). Muscle length can be approximated by lengthening muscle fully and measuring the range of motion based on the final joint angle using a goniometer; when compared with a previous measurement, changes in musculotendinous length can be inferred. To measure muscle length (fascicle length) itself, diagnostic ultrasound is required. The passive resistance of muscle to lengthening is more difficult to measure, if not impossible to distinguish between when there is passive or active resistance to elongation; this could only truly be tested with the patient under anaesthetic.

Production of Symptoms

Symptoms from muscle dysfunction are commonly a pain or an ache. Symptoms may be felt when the muscle is at rest, when it is lengthened or when it contracts. Muscle can be a primary source of pain with both free nerve endings activated by noxious thermal, mechanical and chemical stimuli (Mense, 1996). The last two, noxious mechanical and chemical forms of irritation, are the probable causes in patients with muscle pain seen in the musculoskeletal field. The pain from muscle can therefore be classified as mechanical or chemical nociceptive pain (Gifford, 1998).

Mechanical pain occurs when certain movements stress injured tissue, increasing the mechanical deformation and activation of nociceptors; other movements may reduce the stress on injured tissue, reducing the mechanical deformation and activation of nociceptors. Thus, with mechanical pain, particular movements which aggravate and ease the pain, sometimes referred to as 'on/off' pain. The magnitude of the mechanical deformation may be directly related to the magnitude of nociceptor activity (Garell et al., 1996).

Ischaemic nociceptive pain in muscle is not yet fully understood (Mense, 1996). It may be related to chemical irritation, build-up of potassium ions or lack of oxidation of metabolic products. The underlying mechanism of ischaemic contraction causing nociceptor activity appears to be related to chemical sensitization of muscle nociceptors (Mense, 1996), although experimentally induced ischaemia of muscle activated only 10% of muscle nociceptors.

Clinical features of ischaemic pain are thought to be symptoms produced after prolonged or unusual activities, rapid ease of symptoms after a change in posture, symptoms towards the end of the day or after the accumulation of activity, a poor response to antiinflammatory medication and sometimes absence of trauma (Butler, 2000).

The sympathetic nervous system can cause pain. Increased concentrations of adrenaline (epinephrine) in muscle cause an increased discharge frequency of muscle nociceptors, and this response is enhanced with the addition of noxious mechanical stimulation (Kieschke et al., 1988). In the presence of tissue injury or inflammation, sympathetic nervous system activity can maintain the perception of pain or enhance nociception in inflamed tissue (Raja et al., 1999). Sympathetically maintained pain can occur with complex regional pain syndromes and may play a part in chronic arthritis and soft-tissue trauma (Raja et al., 1999). Thus it appears that the sympathetic nervous system can cause muscle pain.

Constant experimentally induced muscle pain in humans has been found to cause an increase in the stretch reflex of the relaxed muscle, suggesting that muscle pain increases the sensitivity of the muscle spindle to stretch (Matre et al., 1998). In the same study, muscle pain did not alter the H-reflex, suggesting that muscle pain does not directly alter the sensitivity of α motor neurone activity, although it may have an indirect effect by causing a reduction in descending inhibition on the α motor neurone activity and thus cause an increase in the stretch reflex. Inducing muscle pain also increases the stretch reflex of the antagonist muscle group; pain in tibialis anterior increases the stretch reflex of soleus (Matre et al., 1998).

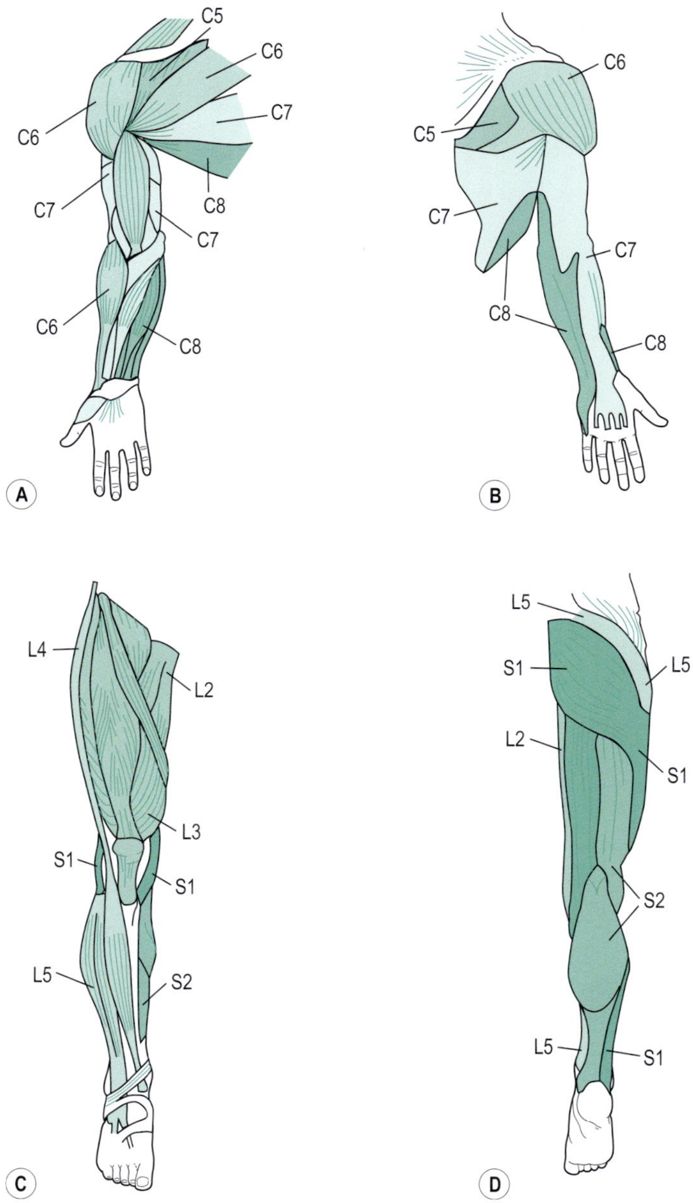

Fig. 4.27 Myotomes of (A) upper limb, anterior view, (B) upper limb, posterior view, (C) lower limb, anterior view and (D) lower limb, posterior view. (Reproduced with permission, from Kellgren, J.H., 1938. Clinical Science 3:175–190. © The Biochemical Society and the Medical Research Society (http://www.clinsci.org).)

Referral of Pain From Muscle

In the upper and lower limbs, muscle pain is often felt over the joint that the muscle moves, provided that the joint has the same segmental innervation as the muscle. The segmental distribution of muscle is given in Fig. 4.27. The chart of pain referral for various muscles is shown in Fig. 4.28. There are differences in the quality of pain from muscle, from tendon and from fascia. Fascia and tendon tend to produce sharp localized pain, whereas muscle tends to produce some localized pain and a diffuse referred pain with tenderness of structures deep to the skin. Pain from muscle appears to be referred to regions corresponding to the spinal segments from which it obtains its motor

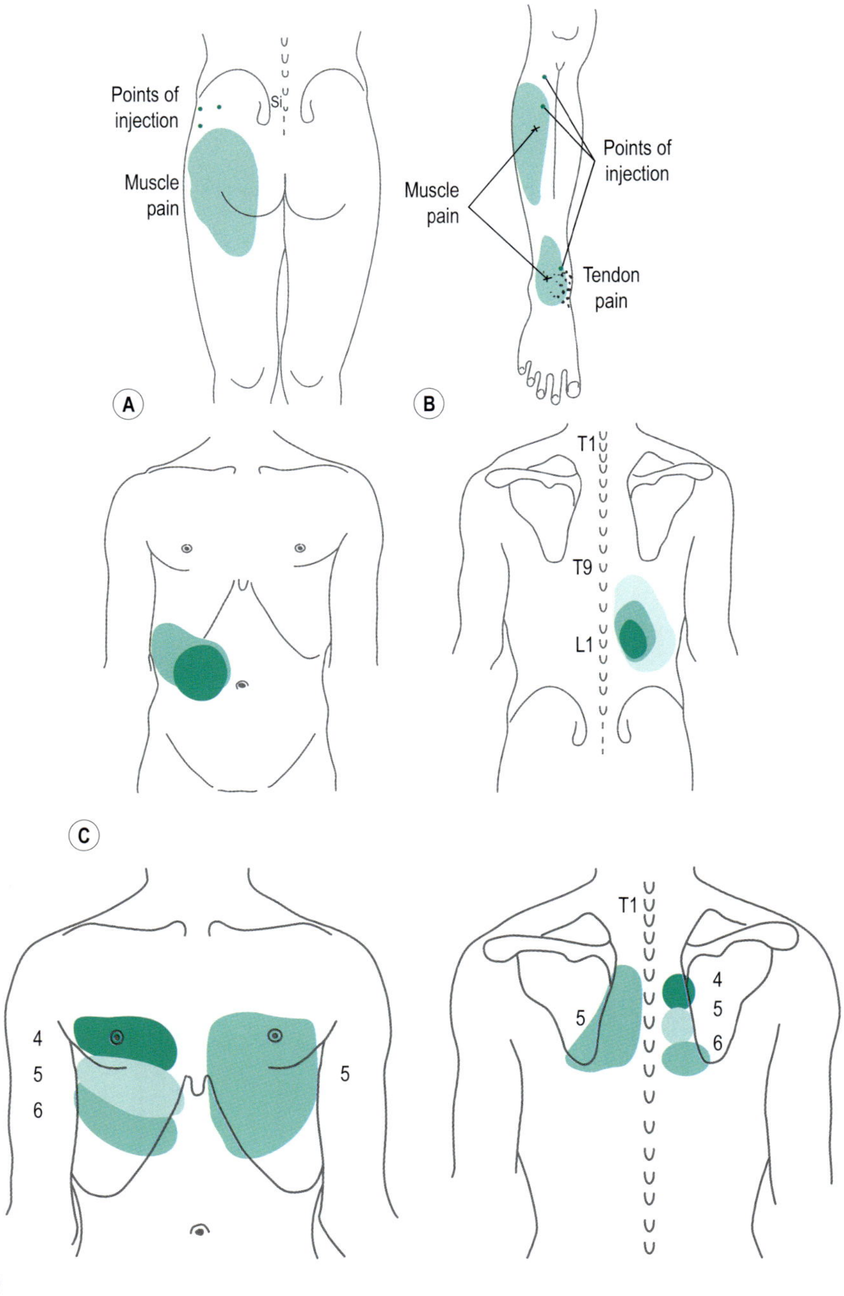

Fig. 4.28 Referred pain from muscle (Reproduced, with permission, from Kellgren (1938) © The Biochemical Society and the Medical Research Society). (A) Gluteus medius. (B) Tibialis anterior; stippling is tendon pain. (C) Horizontal hatching from multifidus, vertical hatching from intercostals and stippling from rectus abdominis. (D) From 4th, 5th and 6th intercostal muscles. (E) Vertical hatching from testis, horizontal hatching from abdominal obliques and stippling from multifidus. (F) Crosses from rhomboids, oblique hatching from flexor carpi radialis, stippling from abductor pollicis longus, vertical hatching from third dorsal interosseous, horizontal hatching from first intercostal space. (G) Vertical hatching from serratus anterior, oblique hatching from infraspinatus and stippling from latissimus dorsi. (H) Left leg with oblique hatching from adductor longus, right leg with oblique hatching from sartorius, vertical hatching from gastrocnemius, horizontal hatching from first interosseous, crosses from tensor fasciae latae and stippling from peroneus longus. (I) Vertical hatching from erector spinae and horizontal hatching from multifidus stimulated opposite T9 and L5. (J) Left figure represents anterior aspect of erector spinae and right figure posterior aspect of erector spinae at the spinal level indicated.

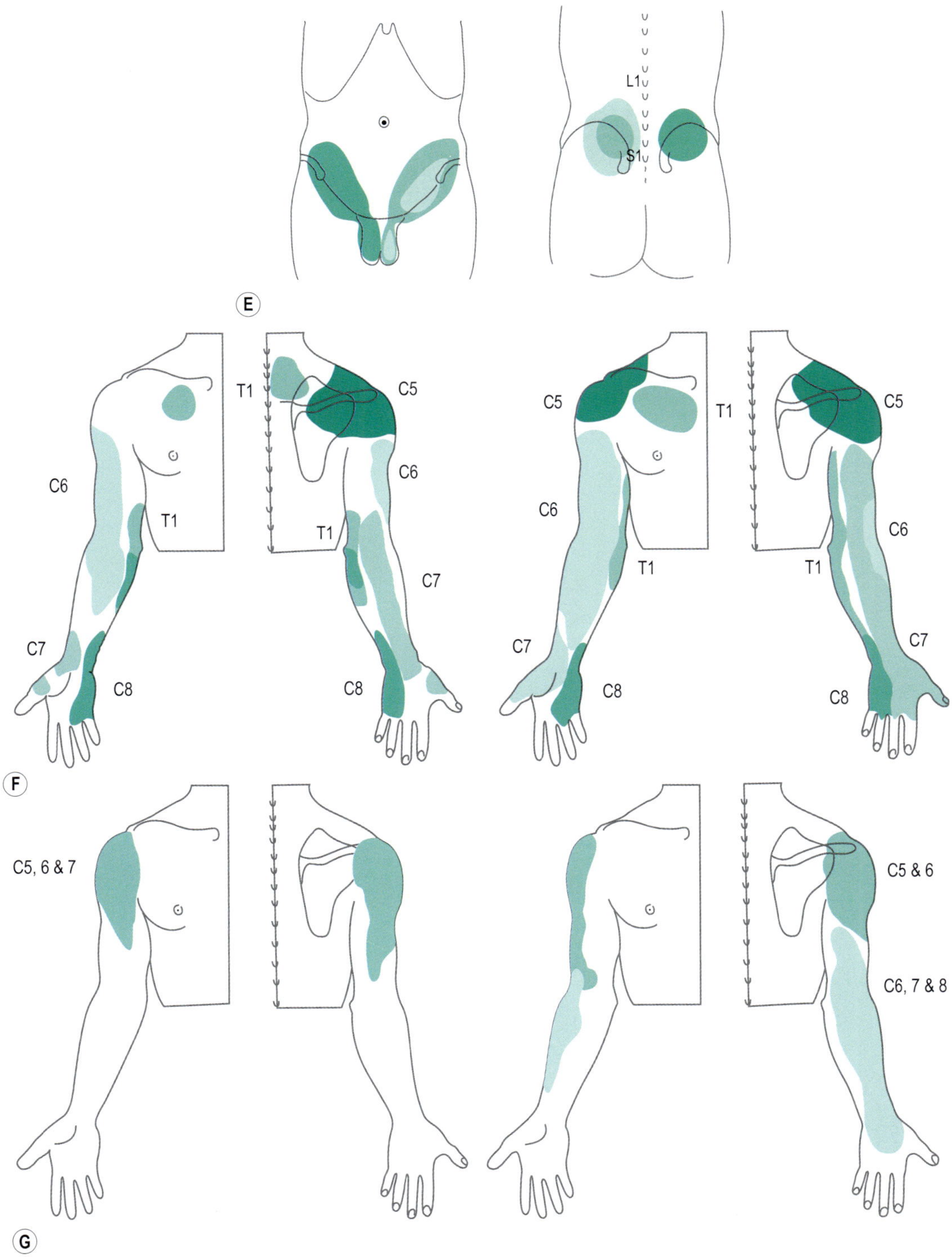

Fig. 4.28 cont'd

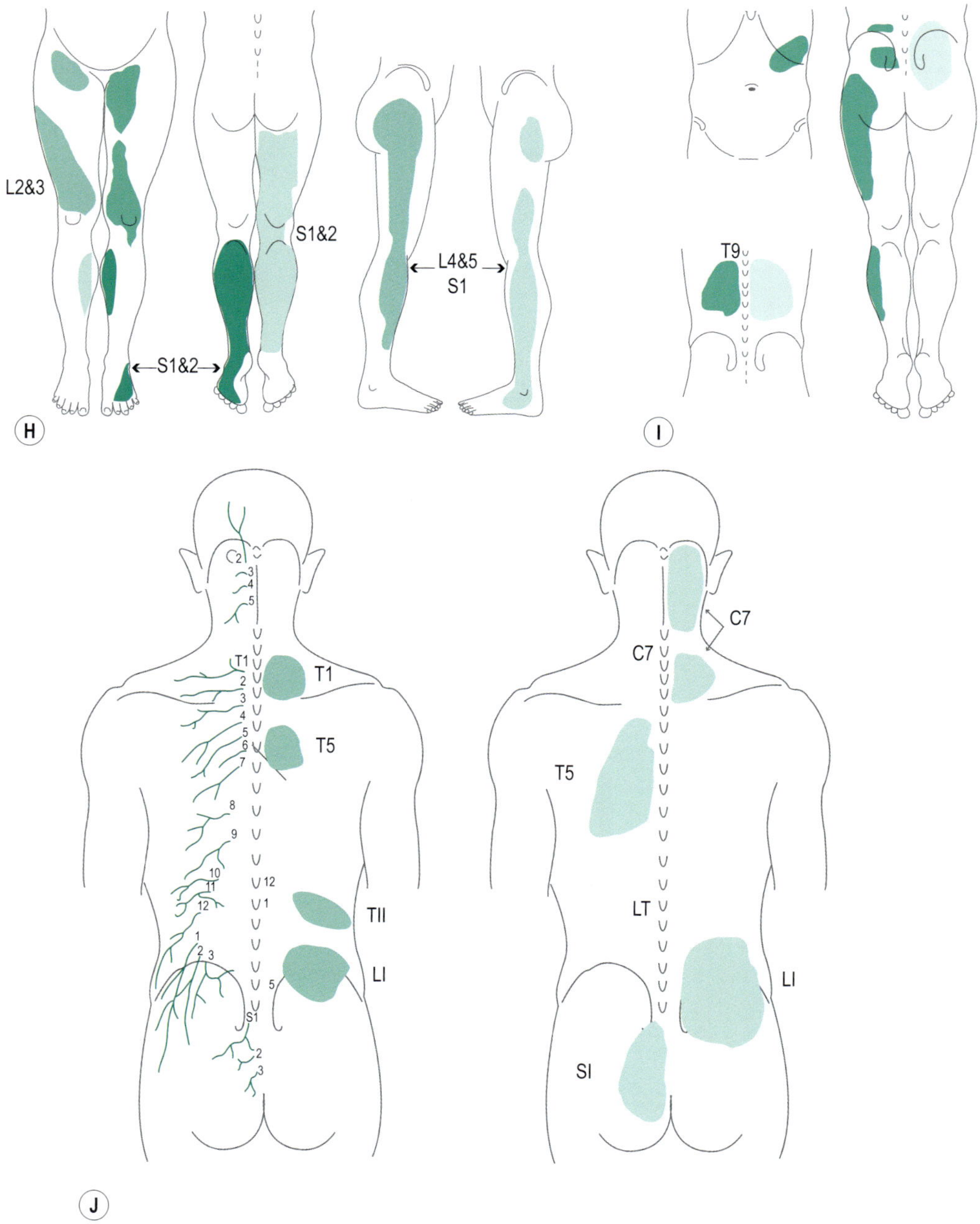

Fig. 4.28 cont'd

supply; this is clearer in the upper limb than in the lower limb.

Pain from muscle may be poorly localized to muscle. Pain from the lumbar erector spine muscle produces pain like that caused by injection of the gluteal fascia. Some muscles, such as rectus abdominis and muscles in the hand, are much more sensitive and produce more severe pain than biceps brachii and glutei muscles. In contrast, metabolic muscle disease typically causes pain that the patient can locate as 'in the muscle'; it is not vague and does not refer (Petty, 2003).

The mechanism of referred pain is thought to be due to the convergence of afferents in the periphery and in the dorsal horn (Torebjork et al., 1984). This is depicted

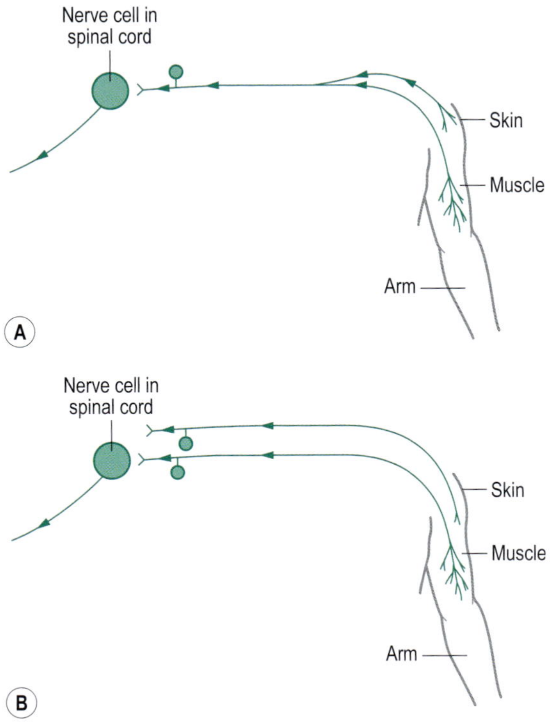

Fig. 4.29 Referred pain due to convergence of afferents (A) in the periphery and (B) in the spinal cord. (After Wells et al., 1994, with permission.)

in Fig. 4.29. In the periphery, proximal to the spinal cord, sensory neurones from skin and muscle converge (Wells et al., 1994). In the dorsal horn, there is convergence of skin afferents and group III and IV muscle afferents on to wide dynamic range cells (Foreman et al., 1979). In both cases, activation of nociceptors from the muscle, for example, is perceived by the brain to come from the skin; the brain thus misinterprets the information.

KNOWLEDGE CHECK

1. List the potential causes of decreases in muscle strength.
2. Summarize the different ways muscle strength could be measured.

Tendon Injury and Repair

The elastic properties (compliance vs. stiffness) of tendons are associated with the force production characteristics of the muscle they attach to (Muraoka et al.,

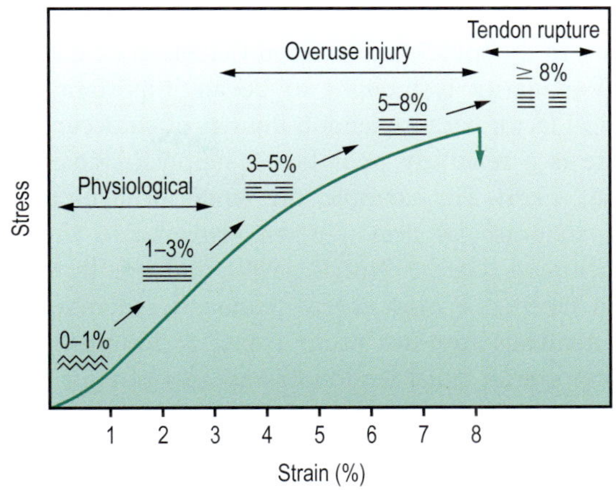

Fig. 4.30 Stress–strain curve of tendon depicting the amount of stress involved in microtrauma (3%–8%) and macrotrauma (<8%). (From Jozsa & Kannus, 1997.)

2005), as they adapt in response to the stress and strain which the muscles impart on them.

Tendons can tear in the middle region, by avulsion of bone and more rarely at the insertion site (Woo et al., 1988). Repetitive strain of a tendon can produce microtrauma and macrotrauma of the tendon. The amount of strain needed to cause microtrauma and macrotrauma is given in Fig. 4.30. Repetitive strain may alter the collagenous structure of tendon with resultant inflammation, oedema and pain (Jozsa & Kannus, 1997). Overuse injury occurs where this repetitive strain, causing tissue damage, is greater than the natural repair and healing process, and this may lead, with further strain, to partial or complete rupture of the tendon (Archambault et al., 1995; Jozsa & Kannus, 1997). Researchers suggest that very little inflammation exists within the tendon (Rees et al., 2006; Woodley et al., 2007). Often, these overuse injuries are seen in the upper extremity in occupations that require repetitive movement of the hands and forearms, and in the lower extremities (usually Achilles and patella tendons) in sports-related injuries.

The aetiology of sports-related lower-limb tendon injuries is thought to include vascularity of the tendon, malalignments, leg length discrepancy, age and weight (Jozsa & Kannus, 1997), as well as extrinsic factors such as type of sport, training errors, environmental conditions, equipment and ineffective rules (Jozsa & Kannus, 1997). Interestingly a review and meta-analysis concluded that strength training appears to be the most effective method of preventing sports-related injuries to the muscle and tendon (Lauersen et al., 2014).

Vascularity is thought to be an important aetiological factor because tendon injuries often occur where there is a relatively poor blood supply (Archambault et al., 1995). For example, the tendocalcaneus tendon has an avascular area 2–6 cm proximal to its distal attachment (Carr & Norris, 1989), and it is in this region where the most severe tendon degeneration and spontaneous ruptures occur (Jozsa & Kannus, 1997). The posterior tibial tendon has an area of poor vascularity posterior and distal to the medial malleolus, and it is in this region that it frequently ruptures (Frey et al., 1990). The supraspinatus tendon has poor vascularity where it inserts on to the humerus (Chansky & Iannotti, 1991), and, again, it is in this region where the tendon ruptures (Jozsa & Kannus, 1997). Age-related degenerative changes within the tendon can cause narrowing or obliteration of blood vessels, further reducing the vascularity of the tendon (Kannus & Jozsa, 1991).

In work-related upper-limb tendon injuries, the strain placed on tendon may not be excessive, but the repetitive nature of the task may be sufficient to cause change in the tissue. It is proposed that, initially, in the first 5 days, there is ischaemia, metabolic disturbance and cell membrane damage leading to inflammation (Jozsa & Kannus, 1997). The increase in tissue pressure further impairs the circulation and enhances the ischaemic changes.

Spontaneous tendon rupture is associated with degenerative changes (Jozsa et al., 1989b). The diameter of collagen fibres decreases in degenerative tendon, suggesting an increase in weaker type III collagen fibres (Jozsa et al., 1989a). Degenerative changes were found in 97% of ruptured tendons, which included the Achilles tendon, biceps brachii and extensor pollicis longus from nearly 900 patients, compared with 35% in a control group (Kannus & Jozsa, 1991).

Tendon Repair

Healing of tendon is like that of other soft tissues and consists of three phases: inflammation phase (1–7 days), regeneration or proliferation phase (7–21 days) and remodelling or maturation phase (21 days to 1 year) (Jozsa & Kannus, 1997). Initially type III collagen is laid down; this is replaced by type I collagen tissue during the late proliferation stage and maturation phase (Coombs et al., 1980).

Muscle Injury and Repair

Muscle strain injury can occur predominantly with eccentric exercise, producing delayed muscle soreness. Pain, weakness and muscle stiffness are felt after unaccustomed eccentric exercise. There is disruption of the Z band, predominantly of type II fibres, with repair largely completed by 6 days (Jones et al., 1986). The reason for the delayed-onset muscle soreness (DOMS) following eccentric action may be because eccentric actions produce greater force than other types of muscle action. It is important to note that DOMS reduces within a few training sessions, after the individual becomes familiar with a new mode of exercise and should not be considered a 'real' injury. The myotendinous region is the weakest part of the tendon–muscle unit and is the region most susceptible to true strain injuries (Garrett, 1990; Tidball, 1991).

Muscle Repair

Repair of muscle injury follows the typical healing process of all soft tissues: the lag phase, regeneration and remodelling. There is initially the development of a necrotic zone at the site of damage, and the adjacent uninjured myofibrils retract and begin the repair process, with activation of satellite cells (McComas, 1996). The satellite cells migrate into the necrotic area and differentiate into myotubes, which begin to bridge the gap between the retracted uninjured myofibrils.

REVIEW AND REVISE QUESTIONS

1. Describe the constituent parts of the muscle.
2. Define the contractile components of a muscle.
3. Describe the three primary muscle actions.
4. Explain the role of the muscle spindle during stretch shortening cycle actions.
5. Explain the role of the Golgi tendon organ during stretching.

6. Define muscle strength, muscle endurance and muscle power and explain the differences between them.
7. Discuss the effects of ageing, injury and immobilization on muscle and tendon function.
8. Explain how ageing, injury and immobilization affect muscle mass and force production capability.
9. Outline the key features of (i) tendon repair and (ii) muscle repair.

REFERENCES

Aagaard, P., Andersen, J.L., Dyhre-Poulsen, P., et al., 2001. A mechanism for increased contractile strength of human pennate muscle in response to strength training: changes in muscle architecture. J. Physiol. 534, 613–623.

Al-Khaifat, L., Herrington, L., Hammond, A., et al., 2016. The effectiveness of an exercise programme on knee loading, muscle co-contraction, and pain in patients with medial knee osteoarthritis. The Knee 23, 63–69.

Allen, G.M., Gandevia, S.C., McKenzie, D.K., 1995. Reliability of measurements of muscle strength and voluntary activation using twitch interpolation. Muscle Nerve 18, 593–600.

Almekinders, L.C., Gilbert, J.A., 1986. Healing of experimental muscle strains and the effects of nonsteroidal antiinflammatory medication. Am. J. Sports Med. 14 (4), 303–308.

Amarante do Nascimento, M., Januario, R.S., Gerage, A.M., et al., 2013. Familiarization and reliability of one repetition maximum strength testing in older women. J. Strength Cond. Res. 27 (6), 1636–1642.

Archambault, J.M., Wiley, J.P., Bray, R.C., 1995. Exercise loading of tendons and the development of overuse injuries, a review of current literature. Sports Med. 20 (2), 77–89.

Arvidsson, I., Eriksson, E., Knutsson, E., et al., 1986. Reduction of pain inhibition on voluntary muscle activation by epidural analgesia. Orthopaedics 9 (10), 1415–1419.

Augustsson, J., Esko, A., Thomee, R., et al., 1998. Weight training of the thigh muscles using closed vs open kinetic chain exercises: a comparison of performance enhancement. J. Orthop. Sports Phys. Ther. 27, 3–8.

Baratta, R., Solomonow, M., Zhou, B.H., et al., 1988. Muscular coactivation. The role of the antagonist musculature in maintaining knee stability. Am. J. Sports Med. 16 (2), 113–122.

Beard, D.J., Soundarapandian, R.S., O'Connor, J.J., et al., 1996. Gait and electromyographic analysis of anterior cruciate ligament deficient subjects. Gait Posture 4, 83–88.

Bennett, J.G., Stauber, W.T., 1986. Evaluation and treatment of anterior knee pain using eccentric exercise. Med. Sci. Sports Exerc. 18 (5), 526–530.

Berchuck, M., Andriacchi, T.P., Bach, B.R., et al., 1990. Gait adaptations by patients who have a deficient anterior cruciate ligament. J. Bone Joint Surg. 72A (6), 871–877.

Berg, H.E., Larsson, L., Tesch, P.A., 1997. Lower limb skeletal muscle function after 6 wk of bed rest. J. Appl. Physiol. 82, 182–188.

Blackburn, J.R., Morrissey, M.C., 1998. The relationship between open and closed kinetic chain strength of the lower limb and jumping performance. J. Orthop. Sports Phys. Ther. 27 (6), 430–435.

Blazevich, A.J., 2006. Effects of physical training and detraining, immobilisation, growth and aging on human fascicle geometry. Sports Med. 36, 1003–1017.

Bouchonville, M.F., Villareal, D.T., 2013. Sarcopenic obesity – How do we treat it? Curr. Opin. Endocrinol. Diabetes Obes. 20, 412–419.

Boyd, I.A., 1976. The mechanical properties of dynamic nuclear bag fibres, static nuclear bag fibres and nuclear chain fibres in isolated cat muscle spindles. Prog. Brain Res. 44, 33–50.

Branch, T.P., Hunter, R., Donath, M., 1989. Dynamic EMG analysis of anterior cruciate deficient legs with and without bracing during cutting. Am. J. Sports Med. 17 (1), 35–41.

Bredella, M.A., Tirman, P.F.J., Fritz, R.C., et al., 1999. MR imaging findings of lateral ulnar collateral ligament abnormalities in patients with lateral epicondylitis. Am. J. Roentgenol. 173, 1379–1382.

Brumitt, J., Cuddeford, T., 2015. Current concepts of muscle and tendon adaptation to strength and conditioning. Int. J. Sports Phys. Ther. 10, 748–759.

Burkholder, T.J., Fingado, B., Baron, S., et al., 1994. Relationship between muscle fiber types and sizes and muscle architectural properties in the mouse hindlimb. J. Morphol. 221, 177–190.

Butler, D.S., 2000. The Sensitive Nervous System. Noigroup, Adelaide.

Carr, A.J., Norris, S.H., 1989. The blood supply of the calcaneal tendon. J. Bone Joint Surg. 71B (1), 100–101.

Chalmers, G., 2002. Do golgi tendon organs really inhibit muscle activity at high force levels to save muscles from injury, and adapt with strength training. Sports Biomech. 1, 239.

Chalmers, G., 2004. Re-examination of the possible role of Golgi tendon organ and muscle spindle reflexes in proprioceptive neuromuscular facilitation. Sports Biomech. 3, 159–183.

Chansky, H.A., Iannottti, J.P., 1991. The vascularity of the rotator cuff. Clin. Sports Med. 10 (4), 807–822.

Ciccotti, M.G., Kerlan, R.K., Perry, J., et al., 1994. An electromyographic analysis of the knee during functional activities. II. The anterior cruciate ligament-deficient and -reconstructed profiles. Am. J. Sports Med. 22 (5), 651–658.

Comfort, P., Jones, P.A., McMahon, J.J., et al., 2015. Effect of knee and trunk angle on kinetic variables during the isometric midthigh pull: test-retest reliability. Int. J. Sports Physiol. Perform. 10, 58–63.

Comfort, P., McMahon, J.J., 2015. Reliability of maximal back squat and power clean performances in inexperienced athletes. J. Strength Cond. Res. 29, 3089–3096.

Coombs, R.R.H., Klenerman, L., Narcisi, P., et al., 1980. Collagen typing in Achilles tendon rupture. J. Bone Joint Surg. 62B (2), 258.

Cormie, P., McBride, J.M., McCaulley, G.O., 2007. Validation of power measurement techniques in dynamic lower body resistance exercises. J. Appl. Biomech. 23, 103–118.

Cormie, P., McGuigan, M.R., Newton, R.U., 2010. Influence of strength on magnitude and mechanisms of adaptation to power training. Med. Sci. Sports Exerc. 42, 1566–1581.

Cormie, P., McGuigan, M.R., Newton, R.U., 2011. Developing maximal neuromuscular power: part 2 – training considerations for improving maximal power production. Sports Med. 41, 125–146.

Couppe, C., Suetta, C., Kongsgaard, M., et al., 2012. The effects of immobilization on the mechanical properties of the patellar tendon in younger and older men. Clin. Biomech. (Bristol, Avon) 27 (9), 949–954.

Crow, J.L., Haas, B.M., 2001. The neural control of human movement. In: Trew, M., Everett, T. (Eds.), Human Movement: An Introductory Text, fourth ed. Churchill Livingstone, Edinburgh.

deAndrade, J.R., Grant, C., DixonSt, A.J., 1965. Joint distension and reflex muscle inhibition in the knee. J. Bone Joint Surg. 47A (2), 313–322.

de Brito Fontana, H., Roesler, H., Herzog, W., 2014. In vivo vastus lateralis force-velocity relationship at the fascicle and muscle tendon unit level. J. Electromyogr. Kinesiol. 24, 934–940.

DeVita, P., Hortobagyi, T., Barrier, J., et al., 1997. Gait adaptations before and after anterior cruciate ligament reconstruction surgery. Med. Sci. Sports Exerc. 29 (7), 853–859.

De Vries, H.A., Housh, T.J., 1994. Physiology of Exercise for Physical Education, Athletics and Sports Science, fifth ed. Brown & Benchmark, Madison, Wisconsin.

Earp, J.E., Kraemer, W.J., Newton, R.U., et al., 2010. Lower-body muscle structure and its role in jump performance during squat, countermovement, and depth drop jumps. J. Strength Cond. Res. 24, 722–729.

Fahrer, H., Rentsch, H.U., Gerber, N.J., et al., 1988. Knee effusion and reflex inhibition of the quadriceps – a bar to effective retraining. J. Bone Joint Surg. 70B (4), 635–638.

Faigenbaum, A.D., McFarland, J.E., Herman, R.E., et al., 2012. Reliability of the one-repetition-maximum power clean test in adolescent athletes. J. Strength Cond. Res. 26, 432–437.

Fitts, R.H., Riley, D.R., Widrick, J.J., 2000. Microgravity and skeletal muscle. J. Appl. Physiol. 89, 823–839.

Fitts, R.H., Riley, D.R., Widrick, J.J., 2001. Functional and structural adaptations of skeletal muscle to microgravity. J. Exp. Biol. 204, 3201–3208.

Foreman, R.D., Schmidt, R.F., Willis, W.D., 1979. Effects of mechanical and chemical stimulation of fine muscle afferents upon primate spinothalamic tract cells. J. Physiol. (Lond.) 286, 215–231.

Frank, C.B., Loitz, B., Bray, R., et al., 1994. Abnormality of the contralateral ligament after injuries of the medial collateral ligament – an experimental study in rabbits. J. Bone Joint Surg. 76A (3), 403–412.

Frank, R.M., Lundberg, H., Wimmer, M.A., et al., 2016. Hamstring activity in the anterior cruciate ligament injured patient: injury implications and comparison with quadriceps activity. Arthroscopy 32 (8), 1651–1659. E-pub ahead of print.

Franz, M., Mense, S., 1975. Muscle receptors with group IV afferent fibres responding to application of bradykinin. Brain Res. 92, 369–383.

Frey, C., Shereff, M., Greenidge, N., 1990. Vascularity of the posterior tibial tendon. J. Bone Joint Surg. 72A (6), 884–888.

Friedli, W.G., Hallett, M., Simon, S.R., 1984. Postural adjustments associated with rapid voluntary arm movements. 1. Electromyographic data. J. Neurol. Neurosurg. Psychiatry 47, 611–622.

Fung, Y.C., 1993. Biomechanics, Biomechanical Properties of Living Tissues, second ed. Springer-Verlag, New York.

Gajdosik, R.L., Linden, D.W.V., Williams, A.K., 1996. Influence of age on concentric isokinetic torque and passive extensibility variables of the calf muscles of women. Eur. J. Appl. Physiol. 74, 279–286.

Gandevia, S.C., Herbert, R.D., Leeper, J.B., 1998. Voluntary activation of human elbow flexor muscles during maximal concentric contractions. J. Physiol. 512 (2), 595–602.

Garell, P.C., McGillis, S.L.B., Greenspan, J.D., 1996. Mechanical response properties of nociceptors innervating feline hairy skin. J. Neurophysiol. 75 (3), 1177–1189.

Garrett, W.E., 1990. Muscle strain injuries: clinical and basic aspects. Med. Sci. Sports Exerc. 22 (4), 436–443.

Ghez, C., 1991. Muscles: effectors of the motor systems. In: Kandel, E.R., Schwartz, J.H., Jessell, T.M. (Eds.), Principles of Neural Science, third ed. Elsevier, New York, pp. 548–563.

Gifford, L., 1998. Pain. In: Pitt-Brooke, J., Reid, H., Lockwood, J., Kerr, K. (Eds.), Rehabilitation of Movement, Theoretical Basis of Clinical Practice. W B Saunders, London, pp. 196–232.

Glousman, R., Jobe, F., Tibone, J., et al., 1988. Dynamic electromyographic analysis of the throwing shoulder with glenohumeral instability. J. Bone Joint Surg. 70A (2), 220–226.

Glousman, R.E., Barron, J., Jobe, F.W., et al., 1992. An electromyographic analysis of the elbow in normal and injured pitchers with medial collateral ligament insufficiency. Am. J. Sports Med. 20 (3), 311–317.

Goldspink, G., 1976. The adaptation of muscle to a new functional length. In: Anderson, D.J., Matthews, B. (Eds.), Mastication. Wright, Bristol, pp. 90–99.

Goldspink, G., Williams, P.E., 1979. The nature of the increased passive resistance in muscle following immobilization of the mouse soleus muscle. J. Physiol. 289, 55. Proceedings of the Physiological Society December 15/16th 1978).

Granata, K.P., Marras, W.S., 1995. The influence of trunk muscle coactivity on dynamic spinal loads. Spine 20 (8), 913–919.

Grimby, G., 1995. Muscle performance and structure in the elderly as studied cross-sectionally and longitudinally. J. Gerontol. 50A, 17–22 (special issue).

Gydikov, A.A., 1976. Pattern of discharge of different types of alpha motoneurones and motor units during voluntary and reflex activities under normal physiological conditions. In: Komi, P.V. (Ed.), Biomechanics V-A. University Park, Baltimore, pp. 45–57.

Haggmark, T., Jansson, E., Eriksson, E., 1981. Fibre type area and metabolic potential of the thigh muscle in man after knee surgery and immobilization. Int. J. Sports Med. 2, 12–17.

Hales, J.P., Gandevia, S.C., 1988. Assessment of maximal voluntary contraction with twitch interpolation: an instrument to measure twitch responses. J. Neurosci. Methods 25, 97–102.

Hauraix, H., Nordez, A., Guilhem, G.I., Rabita, G., Dorel, S., 2015. In vivo maximal fascicle-shortening velocity during plantar flexion in humans. J. Appl. Physiol. 119 (11), 1262–1271.

Henneman, E., Olson, C.B., 1965. Relations between structure and function in the design of skeletal muscles. J. Neurophysiol. 28, 581–598.

Henneman, E., Somjen, G., Carpenter, D.O., 1965. Functional significance of cell size in spinal motoneurons. J. Neurophysiol. 28, 560–580.

Herzog, W., Gal, J., 1999. Tendon. In: Nigg, B.M., Herzog, W. (Eds.), Biomechanics of the Musculo-Skeletal System, second ed. John Wiley, Chichester, pp. 127–147.

Herzog, W., Gal, J., 2007. Tendon. In: Nigg, B.M., Herzog, W. (Eds.), Biomechanics of the Musculo-Skeletal System, third ed. John Wiley, Chichester, pp. 127–147.

Hess, G.P., Cappiello, W.L., Poole, R.M., et al., 1989. Prevention and treatment of overuse tendon injuries. Sports Med. 8 (6), 371–384.

Heyley, M.V., Rees, J., Newham, D.J., 1998. Quadriceps function, proprioceptive acuity and functional performance in healthy young, middle-aged and elderly subjects. Age Ageing 27 (1), 55–62.

Hides, J., Richardson, C., Jull, G., et al., 1995. Ultrasound imaging in rehabilitation. Aust. J. Physiother. 41 (3), 187–193.

Hirsch, C., 1974. Tensile properties during tendon healing. A comparative study of intact and sutured rabbit peroneus brevis tendons. Acta Orthop. Scand. 153 (Suppl.), 11.

Horowits, R., Maruyama, K., Podolsky, R.J., 1989. Elastic behavior of connectin filaments during thick filament movement in activated skeletal muscle. J. Cell Biol. 109, 2169–2176.

Horsley, I., Herrington, L.C., Rolf, C., 2010. Does SLAP lesion affect muscle recruitment as measured by EMG activity during a rugby tackle? J. Orthop. Surg. Res. 5 (12), 67–71.

Hortobagyi, T., Dempsey, L., Fraser, D., et al., 2000. Changes in muscle strength, muscle fibre size and myofibrillar gene expression after immobilization and retraining in humans. J. Physiol. 524 (1), 293–304.

Hortobagyi, T., DeVita, P., 2000. Muscle pre- and coactivity during downward stepping are associated with leg stiffness in aging. J. Electromyogr. Kinesiol. 10, 117–126.

Houk, J., Henneman, E., 1967. Responses of Golgi tendon organs to active contractions of the soleus muscle of the cat. J. Neurophysiol. 30, 466–481.

Hughes, V.A., Frontera, W.R., Wood, M., et al., 2001. Longitudinal muscle strength changes in older adults: influence of muscle mass, physical activity, and health. J. Gerontol. 56A (5), B209B217.

Hunt, C.C., 1990. Mammalian muscle spindle: peripheral mechanisms. Physiol. Rev. 70 (3), 643–663.

Hurley, M.V., Jones, D.W., Wilson, D., et al., 1992. Rehabilitation of quadriceps inhibited due to isolated rupture of the anterior cruciate ligament. J. Orthop. Rheumatol. 5, 145–154.

Hurley, M.V., Jones, D.W., Newham, D.J., 1994. Arthrogenic quadriceps inhibition and rehabilitation of patients with extensive traumatic knee injuries. Clin. Sci. 86, 305–310.

Hurley, M.V., Newham, D.J., 1993. The influence of arthrogenous muscle inhibition on quadriceps rehabilitation of patients with early, unilateral osteoarthritic knees. Br. J. Rheumatol. 32, 127–131.

Hurley, M.V., O'Flanagan, S.J., Newham, D.J., 1991. Isokinetic and isometric muscle strength and inhibition after elbow arthroplasty. J. Orthop. Rheumatol. 4, 83–95.

Huxley, A.F., 2000. Cross-bridge action: present views, prospects, and unknowns. In: Herzog, W. (Ed.), Skeletal Muscle Mechanics: From Mechanisms to Function. John Wiley, Chichester, pp. 7–31.

Hodges, P.W., Richardson, C.A., 1996. Inefficient muscular stabilization of the lumbar spine associated with low back pain. A motor control evaluation of transverse abdominis. Spine 21 (22), 2640–2650.

Iles, J.F., Stokes, M., Young, A., 1990. Reflex actions of knee joint afferents during contraction of the human quadriceps. Clin. Physiol. 10, 489–500.

Jami, L., 1992. Golgi tendon organs in mammalian skeletal muscle: functional properties and central actions. Physiol. Rev. 72 (3), 623–666.

Jones, D.A., Newham, D.J., Round, J.M., et al., 1986. Experimental human muscle damage: morphological changes in relation to other indices of damage. J. Physiol. 375, 435–448.

Jones, D.W., Jones, D.A., Newham, D.J., 1987. Chronic knee effusion and aspiration: the effect on quadriceps inhibition. Br. J. Rheumatol. 26, 370–374.

Jozsa, L., Kannus, P., 1997. Human tendons: anatomy, physiology and pathology. Human Kinetics, Champaign, Illinois.

Jozsa, L., Kvist, M., Balint, B.J., et al., 1989b. The role of recreational sport activity in Achilles tendon rupture, a clinical, pathoanatomical, and sociological study of 292 cases. Am. J. Sports Med. 17 (3), 338–343.

Jozsa, L., Kvist, M., Kannus, P., et al., 1988. The effect of tenotomy and immobilization on muscle spindles and tendon organs of the rat calf muscles. Acta Neuropathol. (Berl.) 76, 465–470.

Jozsa, L., Lehto, M., Kvist, M., et al., 1989a. Alterations in dry mass content of collagen fibers in degenerative tendinopathy and tendon-rupture. Matrix 9, 140–146.

Julio, U.F., Panissa, V.L.G., Franchini, E., 2012. Prediction of one repetition maximum from the maximum number of repetitions with submaximal loads in recreationally strength-trained men. Sci. Sports 27, e69–e76.

Kalund, S., Sinkjaer, T., Arendt-Nielsen, L., et al., 1990. Altered timing of hamstring muscle action in anterior cruciate ligament deficient patients. Am. J. Sports Med. 18 (3), 245–248.

Kannus, P., Jozsa, L., 1991. Histopathological changes preceding spontaneous rupture of a tendon. J. Bone Joint Surg. 73A (10), 1507–1525.

Kannus, P., Jozsa, L., Kvist, M., et al., 1992. The effect of immobilization on myotendinous junction: an ultrastructural, histochemical and immunohistochemical study. Acta Physiol. Scand. 144, 387–394.

Kaufman, M.P., Iwamoto, G.A., Longhurst, J.C., et al., 1982. Effects of capsaicin and bradykinin on afferent fibers with endings in skeletal muscle. Circ. Res. 50, 133–139.

Kaufman, M.P., Longhurst, J.C., Rybicki, K.J., et al., 1983. Effects of static muscular contraction on impulse activity of groups III and IV afferents in cats. J. Appl. Physiol. 55, 105–112.

Kaufman, M.P., Waldrop, T.G., Rybicki, K.J., et al., 1984. Effects of static and rhythmic twitch contractions on the discharge of group III and IV muscle afferents. Cardiovasc. Res. 18, 663–668.

Keating, J.F., Crossan, J.F., 1992. Evaluation of rotator cuff function following anterior dislocation of the shoulder. J. Orthop. Rheumatol. 5, 135–140.

Kellgren, J.H., 1938. Observations on referred pain arising from muscle. Clin. Sci. 3, 175–190.

Kennedy, J.C., Alexander, I.J., Hayes, K.C., 1982. Nerve supply of the human knee and its functional importance. Am. J. Sports Med. 10 (6), 329–335.

Kent-Braun, J.A., Le Blanc, R., 1996. Quantification of central activation failure during maximal voluntary contractions in humans. Muscle Nerve 19, 861–869.

Kerr, K., 1998. Exercise in rehabilitation. In: Pitt-Brooke, J., Reid, H., Lockwood, J. (Eds.), Rehabilitation of Movement, Theoretical Basis of Clinical Practice. W B Saunders, London, pp. 423–457.

Kidd, G., Lawes, N., Musa, I., 1992. Understanding Neuromuscular Plasticity a Basis for Clinical Rehabilitation. Edward Arnold, London.

Kieschke, J., Mense, S., Prabhakar, N.R., 1988. Influence of adrenaline and hypoxia on rat muscle receptors in vitro. In: Hamann, W., Iggo, A. (Eds.), Progress in Brain Research. Elsevier, Amsterdam, pp. 91–97.

Kojima, T., 1991. Force–velocity relationship of human elbow flexors in voluntary isotonic contraction under heavy loads. Int. J. Sports Med. 12, 208–213.

Kolz, C.W., Suter, T., Henninger, H.B., 2015. Regional mechanical properties of the long head of the biceps tendon. Clin. Biomech. 30, 940–945.

Kvist, M., Hurme, T., Kannus, P., et al., 1995. Vascular density at the myotendinous junction of the rat gastrocnemius muscle after immobilization and remobilization. Am. J. Sports Med. 23 (3), 359–364.

Kvist, M., Jozsa, L., Kannus, P., et al., 1991. Morphology and histochemistry of the myotendineal junction of the rat calf muscles. Histochemical, immunohistochemical and electron-microscopic study. Acta Anat. (Basel) 141, 199–205.

Labarque, V.L., EijndeOp't, B., Van Leemputte, M., 2002. Effect of immobilization and retraining on torque–velocity relationship of human knee flexor and extensor muscles. Eur. J. Appl. Physiol. 86, 251–257.
Lauersen, J.B., Bertelsen, D.M., Andersen, L.B., 2014. The effectiveness of exercise interventions to prevent sports injuries: a systematic review and meta-analysis of randomised controlled trials. Br. J. Sports Med. 48 (11), 871–877.
Laughlin, M.H., Korthuis, R.J., 1987. Control of muscle blood flow during sustained physiological exercise. Can. J. Sport Sci. 12 (Suppl.), 77S, 83S.
Lepley, A., Gribble, P., Thomas, A., et al., 2016. Longitudinal evaluation of stair walking in patients with ACL injury. Med. Sci. Sports Exerc. 48, 7–15.
Levick, J.R., 1983. Joint pressure–volume studies: their importance, design and interpretation. J. Rheumatol. 10, 353–357.
Lockwood, J., 1998. Musculoskeletal requirements for normal movement. In: Pitt-Brooke, J., Reid, H., Lockwood, J. (Eds.), Rehabilitation of Movement, Theoretical Basis of Clinical Practice. W B Saunders, London.
Lomo, T., Westgaard, R.H., Engebretsen, L., 1980. Different stimulation patterns affect contractile properties of denervated rat soleus muscles. In: Pette, D. (Ed.), Plasticity of Muscle. Walter de Gruyter, Berlin.
MacDougall, J.D., Elder, G.C.B., Sale, D.G., et al., 1980. Effects of strength training and immobilisation on human muscle fibres. Eur. J. Appl. Physiol. Occup. Physiol. 43, 25–34.
Maier, A., Crockett, J.L., Simpson, D.R., et al., 1976. Properties of immobilized guinea pig hindlimb muscles. Am. J. Physiol. 231 (5), 1520–1526.
Manal, K., Roberts, D.P., Buchanan, T.S., 2006. Optimal pennation angle of the primary ankle plantar and dorsiflexors: variations with sex, contraction intensity, and limb. J. Appl. Biomech. 22, 255–263.
Matre, D.A., Sinkjaer, T., Svensson, P., et al., 1998. Experimental muscle pain increases the human stretch reflex. Pain 75, 331–339.
Mayer, F., Scharhag-Rosenberger, F., Carlsohn, A., et al., 2011. The Intensity and Effects of Strength Training in the Elderly. Dtsch. Arztebl. Int. 108, 359–364.
McBryde, A.M., Anderson, R.B., 1988. Sesamoid foot problems in the athlete. Clin. Sports Med. 7 (1), 51–60.
McComas, A.J., 1996. Skeletal muscle: form and function. Human Kinetics, Champaign, Illinois.
McNair, P.J., Marshall, R.N., Maguire, K., 1994. Knee effusion and quadriceps muscle strength. Clin. Biomech. 9 (6), 331–334.
Mense, S., 1996. Group III and IV receptors in skeletal muscle: are they specific or polymodal? In: Kumazawa, T., Kruger, L., Mizumura, K. (Eds.), Progress in Brain Research, 113. Elsevier Science, Amsterdam, pp. 83–100.
Mense, S., Meyer, H., 1985. Different types of slowly conducting afferent units in cat skeletal muscle and tendon. J. Physiol. 363, 403–417.
Mense, S., Stahnke, M., 1983. Responses in muscle afferent fibres of slow conduction velocity to contractions and ischaemia in the cat. J. Physiol. 342, 383–397.
Mentiplay, B.F., Perraton, L.G., Bower, K.J., et al., 2015. Assessment of lower limb muscle strength and power using hand-held and fixed dynamometry: a reliability and validity study. PloS One 10 (10), e0140822.
Mills, K., Hunt, M., Leigh, R., et al., 2013. A systematic review and meta-analysis of lower limb neuromuscular alterations associated with knee osteoarthritis during level walking. Clin. Biomech. 28, 713–724.
Milner-Brown, H.S., Stein, R.B., Yemm, R., 1973. The orderly recruitment of human motor units during voluntary isometric contractions. J. Physiol. (Lond.) 230, 359–370.
Moerch, L., Pingel, J., Boesen, M., et al., 2013. The effect of acute exercise on collagen turnover in human tendons: influence of prior immobilization period. Eur. J. Appl. Physiol. 113 (2), 449–455.
Muraoka, T., Muramatsu, T., Fukunaga, T., et al., 2005. Elastic properties of human Achilles tendon are correlated to muscle strength. J. Appl. Physiol. 99 (2), 665–669.
Nakagawa, Y., Totsuka, M., Sato, T., et al., 1989. Effect of disuse on the ultrastructure of the achilles tendon in rats. Eur. J. Appl. Physiol. 59, 239–242.
Narici, M., Franchi, M., Maganaris, C., 2016. Muscle structural assembly and functional consequences. J. Exp. Biol. 219 (2), 276–284.
Newham, D.J., 1993. Eccentric muscle activity in theory and practice. In: Harms-Ringdahl, K. (Ed.), Muscle Strength. Churchill Livingstone, Edinburgh, p. 63.
Newham, D.J., Ainscough-Potts, A.-M., 2001. Musculoskeletal basis for movement. In: Trew, M., Everett, T. (Eds.), Human Movement, fourth ed. Churchill Livingstone, Edinburgh, pp. 105–128.
Newham, D.J., Hurley, M.V., Jones, D.W., 1989. Ligamentous knee injuries and muscle inhibition. J. Orthop. Rheumatol. 2, 163–173.
Nordin, M., Frankel, V.H., 1989. Basic Biomechanics of the Musculoskeletal System, second ed. Lea & Febiger, Philadelphia.
Norkin, C.C., Levangie, P.K., 1992. Joint Structure and Function: A Comprehensive Analysis, second ed. F A Davis, Philadelphia, pp. 101–115.
Ostenberg, A., Roos, E., Ekdahl, C., et al., 1998. Isokinetic knee extensor strength and functional performance in healthy female soccer players. Scand. J. Med. Sci. Sports. 8, 275–264.

Osu, R., Franklin, D.W., Kato, H., et al., 2002. Short- and long-term changes in joint co-contraction associated with motor learning as revealed from surface EMG. J. Neurophysiol. 88 (8), 991–1004.

Panjabi, M.M., 1992. The stabilizing system of the spine. Part 1. Function, dysfunction, adaptation, and enhancement. J. Spinal Disord. 5 (4), 383–389.

Panjabi, M.M., White, A.A., 2001. Biomechanics in the Musculoskeletal System. Churchill Livingstone, New York.

Pearson, S.J., Hussain, S.R., 2014. Region-specific tendon properties and patellar tendinopathy: a wider understanding. Sports Med. 44 (8), 1101–1112.

Pedrero-Chamizo, R., Gomez-Cabello, A., Melendez, A., et al., 2015. Higher levels of physical fitness are associated with a reduced risk of suffering sarcopenic obesity and better perceived health among the elderly: the EXERNET multi-center study. J. Nutr. Health Aging 19, 211–217.

Pette, D., Peuker, H., Staron, R.S., 1999. The impact of biochemical methods for single muscle fibre analysis. Acta Physiol. Scand. 166, 261–277.

Pette, D., Staron, R.S., 1990. Cellular and molecular diversities of mammalian skeletal muscle fibres. Rev. Physiol. Biochem. Pharmacol. 116, 1–76.

Petty, R., 2003. Evaluating muscle symptoms. J. Neurol. Neurosurg. Psychiatry 74 (Suppl. 11), ii38–ii42.

Piasecki, M., Ireland, A., Jones, D.A., et al., 2016. Age-dependent motor unit remodelling in human limb muscles. Biogerontology 17 (3), 485–496.

Powers, S.K., Howley, E.T., 1997. Exercise Physiology: Theory and Application to Fitness and Performance, third ed. McGraw-Hill, Boston.

Raja, S.N., Meyer, R.A., Ringkamp, M., et al., 1999. Peripheral neural mechanisms of nociception. In: Wall, P.D., Melzack, R. (Eds.), Textbook of Pain, fourth ed. Churchill Livingstone, Edinburgh.

Rees, J.D., Wilson, A.M., Wolman, R.L., 2006. Current concepts in the management of tendon disorders. Rheumatology 45, 508–521.

Reinert, A., Mense, S., 1992. Free nerve endings in the skeletal muscle of the rat exhibiting immunoreactivity to substance P and calcitonin gene-related peptide. Pflügers Arch. 420 (Suppl. 1), R54.

Richardson, C., Jull, G., Hodges, P., et al., 1999. Therapeutic Exercise for Spinal Segmental Stabilization in Low Back Pain, Scientific Basis and Clinical Approach. Churchill Livingstone, Edinburgh.

Rutherford, O.M., Jones, D.A., Newham, D.J., 1986. Clinical and experimental application of the percutaneous twitch superimposition technique for the study of human muscle activation. J. Neurol. Neurosurg. Psychiatry 49, 1288–1291.

Sacks, R.D., Roy, R.R., 1982. Architecture of the hind limb muscles of cats: functional significance. J. Morphol. 173, 185–195.

Sargeant, A.J., Davies, C.T.M., Edwards, R.H.T., et al., 1977. Functional and structural changes after disuse of human muscle. Clin. Sci. Mol. Med. 52, 337–342.

Scott, W., Stevens, J., Binder-Macleod, S.A., 2001. Human skeletal muscle fiber type classifications. Phys. Ther. 81 (11), 1810–1816.

Seitz, L.B., Trajano, G.S., Haff, G.G., et al., 2016. Relationships between maximal strength, muscle size, and myosin heavy chain isoform composition and postactivation potentiation. Appl. Physiol. Nutr. Metab. 41 (5), 491–497. Epub ahead of print.

Shakespeare, D.T., Stokes, M., Sherman, K.P., et al., 1985. Reflex inhibition of the quadriceps after meniscectomy: lack of association with pain. Clin. Physiol. 5, 137–144.

Shumway-Cook, A., Woollacott, M.H., 1995. Motor Control, Theory and Practical Applications. Williams & Wilkins, Baltimore.

Sirca, A., Kostevc, V., 1985. The fibre type composition of thoracic and lumbar paravertebral muscles in man. J. Anat. 141, 131–137.

Snyder-Mackler, L., De Luca, P.F., Williams, P.R., et al., 1994. Reflex inhibition of the quadriceps femoris muscle after injury or reconstruction of the anterior cruciate ligament. J. Bone Joint Surg. 76-A (4), 555–560.

Solomonow, M., Baratta, R., Zhou, B.-H., et al., 1987. The synergistic action of the anterior cruciate ligament and thigh muscles in maintaining joint stability. Am. J. Sports Med. 15 (3), 207–213.

Spencer, J.D., Hayes, K.C., Alexander, I.J., 1984. Knee joint effusion and quadriceps reflex inhibition in man. Arch. Phys. Med. Rehabil. 65, 171–177.

Spiteri, T., Nimphius, S., Hart, N.H., et al., 2014. Contribution of strength characteristics to change of direction and agility performance in female basketball athletes. J. Strength. Cond. Res. 28, 2415–2423.

Staron, R.S., 1997. Human skeletal muscle fiber types: delineation, development, and distribution. Can. J. Appl. Physiol. 22 (4), 307–327.

Stener, B., 1969. Reflex inhibition of the quadriceps elicited from a subperiosteal tumour of the femur. Acta Orthop. Scand. 40, 86–91.

Stener, B., Petersen, I., 1963. Excitatory and inhibitory reflex motor effects from the partially ruptured medial collateral ligament of the knee joint. Acta Orthop. Scand. 33, 359.

Stokes, M., Young, A., 1984. The contribution of reflex inhibition to arthrogenous muscle weakness. Clin. Sci. 67, 7–14.

Suter, E., Herzog, W., 1997. Extent of muscle inhibition as a function of knee angle. J. Electromyogr. Kinesiol. 7 (2), 123–130.

Suter, E., Herzog, W., 2000. Muscle inhibition and functional deficiencies associated with knee pathologies. In: Herzog, W. (Ed.), Skeletal Muscle Mechanics, From Mechanisms to Function. Wiley, Chichester, p. 365.

Suter, E., Herzog, W., Bray, R.C., 1998a. Quadriceps inhibition following arthroscopy in patients with anterior knee pain. Clin. Biomech. 13, 314–319.

Suter, E., Herzog, W., De Souza, K.D., et al., 1998b. Inhibition of the quadriceps muscles in patients with anterior knee pain. J. Appl. Biomech. 14, 360–373.

Suter, E., Herzog, W., Huber, A., 1996. Extent of motor unit activation in the quadriceps muscles of healthy subjects. Muscle Nerve 19, 1046–1048.

Tabary, J.C., Tabary, C., Tardieu, C., et al., 1972. Physiological and structural changes in the cat's soleus muscle due to immobilization at different lengths by plaster casts. J. Physiol. 224 (1), 231–244.

Taylor, D.C., Dalton, J.D., Seaber, A.V., et al., 1990. Viscoelastic properties of muscle–tendon units, the biomechanical effects of stretching. Am. J. Sports Med. 18 (3), 300–309.

Taylor, J.D., Fletcher, J.P., 2012. Reliability of the 8-repetition maximum test in men and women. J. Sports Sci. Med. 15, 69–73.

Thelen, D.G., Muriuki, M., James, J., et al., 2000. Muscle activities used by young and old adults when stepping to regain balance during a forward fall. J. Electromyogr. Kinesiol. 10, 93–101.

Thomas, C., Jones, P.A., Rothwell, J., et al., 2015. An investigation into the relationship between maximum isometric strength and vertical jump performance. J. Strength Cond. Res. 29, 2176–2185.

Threlkeld, A.J., 1992. The effects of manual therapy on connective tissue. Phys. Ther. 72 (12), 893–902.

Tidball, J.G., 1991. Myotendinous junction injury in relation to junction structure and molecular composition. Exerc. Sport Sci. Rev. 19, 419–445.

Torebjork, H.E., Ochoa, J.L., Schady, W., 1984. Referred pain from intraneural stimulation of muscle fascicles in the median nerve. Pain 18, 145–156.

Torry, M.R., Decker, M.J., Viola, R.W., et al., 2000. Intra-articular knee joint effusion induces quadriceps avoidance gait patterns. Clin. Biomech. 15, 147–159.

Tracy, B.L., Enoka, R.M., 2002. Older adults are less steady during submaximal isometric contractions with the knee extensor muscles. J. Appl. Physiol. 92, 1004–1012.

Trigsted, S.M., Post, E.G., Bell, D.R., 2015. Landing mechanics during single hop for distance in females following anterior cruciate ligament reconstruction compared to healthy controls. Knee surgery, sports traumatology. Arthroscopy 25 (5), 1395–1402.

Turner, A.N., Comfort, P., McMahon, J., et al., 2020. Developing Powerful Athletes, Part 1: Mechanical Underpinnings. Strength Cond. J 42 (3), 30–39.

Urbach, D., Awiszus, F., 2002. Impaired ability of voluntary quadriceps activation bilaterally interferes with function testing after knee injuries. A twitch interpolation study. Int. J. Sports Med. 23 (4), 231–236.

Vaughan, V.G., 1989. Effects of upper limb immobilization on isometric muscle strength, movement time, and triphasic electromyographic characteristics. Phys. Ther. 69 (2), 36–46.

Wainright, S.A., Biggs, W.D., Currey, J.D., et al., 1982. Mechanical design in organisms. Princeton University Press, Princeton, New Jersey.

Watkins, M.P., Harris, B.A., Kozlowski, B.A., 1984. Isokinetic testing in patients with hemiparesis - a pilot study. Phys. Ther. 64 (2), 184–189.

Wells, P.E., Frampton, V., Bowsher, D., 1994. Pain Management by Physiotherapy, second ed. Butterworth-Heinemann, Oxford.

Williams, P.E., Goldspink, G., 1973. The effect of immobilization on the longitudinal growth of striated muscle fibres. J. Anat. 116 (1), 45–55.

Williams, P.E., Goldspink, G., 1978. Changes in sarcomere length and physiological properties in immobilized muscle. J. Anat. 127 (3), 459–468.

Williams, P.E., Goldspink, G., 1984. Connective tissue changes in immobilized muscle. J. Anat. 138 (2), 343–350.

Williams, P.L., Bannister, L.H., Berry, M.M., et al., 1995. Gray's Anatomy, thirty-eighth ed. Churchill Livingstone, New York.

Winchester, J., McGuigan, M.R., Nelson, A.G., et al., 2010. The relationship between isometric and dynamic strength in college aged males. J. Strength Cond. Res. 24, 1.

Witzmann, F.A., 1988. Soleus muscle atrophy in rats induced by cast immobilization: lack of effect by anabolic steroids. Arch. Phys. Med. Rehabil. 69 (2), 81–85.

Woo, S., Maynard, J., Butler, D., et al., 1988. Ligament, tendon, and joint capsule insertions to bone. In: Woo, S.L.Y., Buckwalter, J. (Eds.), Injury and Repair of the Musculoskeletal Soft Tissues. American Academy of Orthopaedic Surgeons, Park Ridge, Illinois, pp. 133–166.

Wood, L., Ferrell, W.R., Baxendale, R.H., 1988a. Pressures in normal and acutely distended human knee joints and effects on quadriceps maximal voluntary contractions. Q. J. Exp. Physiol. 73, 305–314.

Wood, T.O., Cooke, P.H., Goodship, A.E., 1988b. The effect of exercise and anabolic steroids on the mechanical properties and crimp morphology of the rat tendon. Am. J. Sports Med. 16 (2), 153–158.

Woodley, B.L., Newsham-West, R.J., Baxter, D., et al., 2007. Chronic tendinopathy: effectiveness of eccentric exercise. Br. J. Sports Med. 41, 188–198.

Wyke, B.D., Polacek, P., 1975. Articular neurology: the present position. J. Bone Joint Surg. 57B (3), 401.

Yoshihara, K., Shirai, Y., Nakayama, Y., et al., 2001. Histochemical changes in the multifidus muscle in patients with lumbar intervertebral disc herniation. Spine 26 (6), 622–626.
Young, A., Hughes, I., Round, J.M., et al., 1982. The effect of knee injury on the number of muscle fibres in the human quadriceps femoris. Clin. Sci. 62, 227–234.
Young, A., Stokes, M., Iles, J.F., 1987. Effects of joint pathology on muscle. Clin. Orthop. Relat. Res. 219, 21–27.
Zhao, W.P., Kawaguchi, Y., Matsui, H., et al., 2000. Histochemistry and morphology of the multifidus muscle in lumbar disc herniation comparative study between diseased and normal sides. Spine 25 (17), 2191–2199.

5

Principles of Muscle and Tendon Treatment

Paul Comfort and Lee Herrington

LEARNING OUTCOMES

After studying this chapter, you should be able to:

- Understand the basic principles of training, including progressive overload
- Understand how to appropriately apply these principles to ensure improvements in specific muscular qualities (e.g. muscular strength, muscular power, muscular endurance, hypertrophy)
- Understand tendon injury and repair

CHAPTER CONTENTS

It is not possible to treat muscle tissue in isolation; any management approaches applied to muscle will always affect tendons, joint and/or nerve tissue. In this text a 'muscle treatment' is defined as a 'treatment to effect a change in muscle'; that is, the intention of the clinician is to produce a change in muscle structure and/or function, and therefore it is described as a muscle treatment. Similarly, where a technique is used to effect a change in a joint, it will be referred to as a 'joint treatment', and where a technique is used to effect a

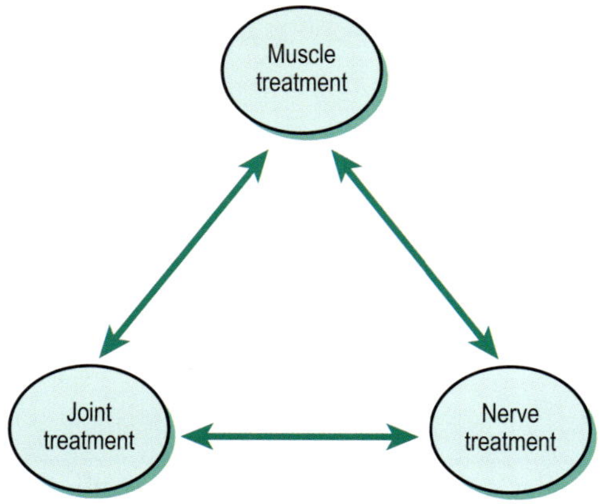

Fig. 5.1 Relationship of treatment techniques of muscle, joint and nerve. Treatment of muscle will also affect joint and nerve.

change in nerve, it will be referred to as a 'nerve treatment'. Thus treatments are classified according to which tissue the clinician is predominantly attempting to affect. This relationship of treatment of muscle, joint and nerve is depicted in Fig. 5.1.

There are a variety of muscle treatments, categorized in this text from the dysfunctions identified in the previous chapter, namely, reduced muscular strength, power and endurance, altered motor control, reduced length and production of symptoms (Table 5.1). From this, a classification of muscle treatment can be identified: to increase muscle strength, power and endurance, alter motor control (increase or decrease muscle activation, change timing of onset, alter activation of agonist and antagonist), increase muscle length and reduce muscle-related symptoms.

PRINCIPLES OF INCREASING MUSCLE STRENGTH, POWER AND ENDURANCE

There are a variety of exercise regimes used to increase muscle strength, power and endurance, and the reader is referred to the numerous exercise physiology and strength and conditioning textbooks for further details on these.

This text reviews the principles involved in increasing muscle strength, power and endurance. The principles are overload, specificity, individuality, motivation, learning, reversibility and diminishing returns (Box 5.1).

TABLE 5.1 Muscle Dysfunction, Aims of Muscle Treatment and Treatment Techniques

Muscle Dysfunction	Aims of Muscle Treatment	Treatment Techniques
Reduced strength, power and endurance	Increase strength, power and endurance	Training regimes using free weights, springs, pulleys, TheraBand, dynamometers, PNF
Altered motor control	Increase muscle activation	Active assisted movements, rapid stretch mechanical vibration, PNF, touch, use of overflow, ice and taping
Muscle inhibition delayed timing of onset	Increase time of onset	Challenge posture and balance using, for example, SitFit, gym ball
Increased muscle activation	Reduce muscle activation	Made aware of the unwanted muscle activity using a mirror, verbal feedback, touch, electromyogram feedback. Positioning, PNF, trigger points, deep inhibitory massage and taping
Reduced length	Increase length	Stretching: ballistic or static, passively by clinician or actively by patient PNF
Symptom production	Reduce symptoms	Soft-tissue mobilization: massage, connective tissue massage, specific soft-tissue mobilizations, trigger points, frictions Joint mobilizations Taping Electrotherapy

PNF, Proprioceptive neuromuscular facilitation.

BOX 5.1 Principles of Increasing Muscle Strength, Power and Endurance

- Overload
- Specificity
- Individuality
- Motivation
- Learning
- Reversibility
- Diminishing returns

Overload

For any of the systems within the body to adapt, the stimuli must be sufficient to create overload (i.e., expose the tissue to a load greater than it is currently experiencing). To improve the strength, power or endurance of a muscle, it must be *progressively* and appropriately overloaded. To create overload when strengthening a muscle, the resistance (load) must be greater than the muscles are accustomed to during everyday activities, and as the muscle gains strength the resistance must be progressively increased. Overload in this case can be achieved initially through a slight increase in repetitions (2–6) or sets (3–6), but once the maximum number of repetitions is achieved at a given resistance, the resistance (external load) must be increased. To further increase repetitions would alter the focus from muscular strength to hypertrophy or endurance. When increasing muscle endurance, there must be a progressive increase in volume of exercise, again via an increase in repetitions (10–15) of sets (3–4), although as with strength, if the maximum number of repetitions can be achieved with a given resistance the resistance must be increased. It is this progressive nature which ensures that overload continues across rehabilitation/training session. It should be noted that Schoenfeld et al. (2021) provided updated loading recommendations for muscle strength, hypertrophy and endurance, suggesting that each of these characteristics can be improved using loads as low as 30% of one repetition maximum (RM). However, what is clear is that, while strength can be increased with lower loads and endurance can be increased with higher loads, higher loads result in greater increases in strength adaptations and lower loads result in greater increases in muscular endurance. If aiming to optimize a specific adaptation to the imposed demands of exercise, it is essential that the demands of the task elicit the greatest adaptations required to enhance a specific physical characteristic, which is predominantly determined using appropriate loading paradigms.

Specificity

This relates to the specific adaptation (of muscle) to the imposed demands (DiNubile, 1991), referred to as the SAID principle. The effect on muscle is specific to the nature of the exercise:

1. High resistance and low repetition (usually 2–6 repetitions) will result in an increase in muscle strength (Staron et al., 1994; Hakkinen et al., 1998). It is also worth noting that increasing strength also increases muscular endurance, as the relative effort required to move a submaximal load multiple times decreases with an increase in strength, meaning additional repetitions can be performed. Training to the point of momentary muscle failure (no further repetitions can be performed within the set) is not necessary (Izquierdo et al., 2006), if exercise is performed in sufficient load (usually ≥80% 1 RM).
2. Low resistance (60%–75% 1 RM) and high repetition 10–15 repetitions) will result in an increase in muscle endurance, with only small increases in strength associated with the hypertrophic response to muscular endurance training resulting in an increased cross-sectional area of a muscle. Training to momentary muscle failure appears advantageous (Izquierdo et al., 2006).
3. Low resistances (≤40% 1 RM) moved at a high velocity will increase muscle power (i.e. an increase in fascicle shortening velocity). Power can also be increased with higher loads (≥60% 1 RM) if the intention is to move quickly, even if the level of resistance results in a relatively low movement velocity (Behm & Sale, 1993). In addition, increasing strength also increases power output because of increased force production and therefore greater acceleration, if greater force can be produced over the same epoch (Cormie et al., 2011; Haff & Nimphius, 2012).

The implication of specificity is that the prescribed exercise does not need to mirror the movement pattern of the functional activity it aims to improve; that is, it does not need to look like the movement in terms of its kinematics. The activity needs to target the appropriate musculature, and the loading and/or velocity of movement need to be specific to the aim; for example, strength for the quadriceps should be high resistance and low repetition, but the exercise could be a squat or lunge variation or a simple knee extension exercise, although the transfer from knee extension to sit to stand will be less effective than from a squat or lunge variation (Augustsson et al., 1998; Blackburn & Morrissey, 1998). If hypertrophy is the aim, due to the individual suffering from atrophy, then moderate loads, generally using repetition ranges greater than eight should be implemented. If the atrophy is to a specific muscle, then single joint exercises may be most appropriate, whereas if the atrophy affects a group of muscles/entire limb multijoint tasks are likely to be most beneficial.

Individuality

Individuals will respond differently to the same exercise; this response is determined by genetics, cellular growth rates, metabolism, and neural and endocrine regulation. For example, older than the age of 60 years, the number of fast-twitch fibres diminishes; therefore an exercise given to an 80-year-old and a 26-year-old will have different effects. Differences in strength levels between middle aged and older men are partly explained by the decrease in anabolic hormones associated with aging (Izquierdo et al., 2001), although these decreases in strength are somewhat reversible with appropriate strength training (Suetta et al., 2004). Training status, based on strength levels, also determines the response to subsequent training, with individuals who are already strong progressing at a slower rate due to the law of diminishing returns (Cormie et al., 2010; Suchomel et al., 2016).

Motivation

Only those motivated enough will make the physical and mental effort of following a training program. The clinician can help to motivate the patient using explanation and enthusiasm. During prolonged and frequent periods of rehabilitation, variety is also required. Improving compliance can also be aided by educating the patient as to the relevance and importance of the exercises program and by clear goal setting.

Learning

The clinician educates the patient about the required exercise so that it is carried out effectively. Where the movement is unfamiliar, motor learning will have to occur prior to progressing load. Motor learning also benefits from frequent repetition of the task, so in the early stage, progression could simply be performing the task more frequently; however, when increased load is required to emphasize increases in strength, frequency must be reduced to approximately 3 × week.

Diminishing Returns

An exercise regime will produce a greater improvement in people in poor physical condition than in those already in a good physical condition. However, even in athletic populations, many individuals may not have reached such high levels of development, especially in terms of strength, where diminishing returns have only been reported once the athlete can squat to 90-degree internal knee angle with an external load of greater than 2 × body mass (Cormie et al., 2010; Suchomel et al., 2016). Strength endurance and hypertrophy training adaptations take longer to have an effect but are longer-lasting, whereas power can be achieved more quickly but tends to diminish faster if high-velocity movements are ceased for greater than 2 weeks.

Reversibility

This rather disappointing principle states that, when specific training stops, any strength or endurance adaptations will be progressively lost (Bruton, 2002), as can be clearly observed when a limb is immobilized. However, it is possible to maintain such adaptations via regular physical activity in the 'normal' population and via applying the minimum effective dose in more athletic individuals, which in terms of resistance exercise can be 2 × week for approximately 20 minutes, performing 2–3 sets per muscle group (Spiering et al., 2021).

Increasing Muscle Strength

The aforementioned principles need to be applied when attempting to increase muscle strength. The resistance to a muscle contraction needed to strengthen a muscle can be provided by gravity, the clinician, the patient, free weights, pulleys, springs, elastic resistance bands and isokinetic dynamometers. Interestingly, an isotonic exercise program using free weights has been found to be as effective in strengthening the quadricep femoris muscle as the more expensive dynamometers machine (DeLateur et al., 1972). One benefit of free weights is the versatility and greater transference of the adaptive responses to activities of daily living and athletic tasks. In addition, the ability to easily add resistance to achieve progressive overload in a quantifiable and planned manner, which can be included in goal setting for the individual, makes resistance training with free weights the easiest method to implement.

Recommended strengthening regimes for sedentary adults have been advocated by the American College of Sports Medicine (ACSM), but it is important to be aware that these are recommendations for strengthening (resulting in an increase in muscular endurance, muscle mass and some increase in strength), not strength training where the primary focus is increasing muscular strength. Such programs recommend three sets of 8–10 repetitions at least twice a week using the major muscle groups, using a 10 RM load. A 10 RM would be the maximum amount of weight that could be lifted 10 times before fatigue or loss of technique occurs. This type of training has been implemented by practitioners and researched extensively for more than 60 years, since it was first formally introduced by DeLorme in the 1940s (Delorme, 1945; Delorme & Watkins, 1948; Delorme et al., 1950; Todd et al., 2012).

The Daily Adjustable Progressive Resistance Exercise (DAPRE) system was introduced nearly 30 years ago as a simple tool to take the guesswork out of prescribing training loads and 1 RM numbers. Although there have been many advances in programming and periodization models for athletes, the DAPRE method has stood the test of time as an effective method to strengthen novice weight trainers and in rehabilitation (Knight, 1985). Table 5.2 explains the basic principles of application.

The optimum frequency of exercise has also been investigated by numerous researchers with varying results. An optimum frequency for strengthening the muscles has been found to be 3 times a week (Leggett et al., 1991; Pollock et al., 1993; DeMichele et al., 1997). A reasonable guideline for frequency would be a minimum of twice per week (Feigenbaum & Pollock, 1999), although if motor learning is the goal and the intensity of the exercise is low, more frequent performance of the task will result in greater improvements in motor control, as already mentioned.

A strengthening regime would normally start slowly with a low intensity of exercise (ACSM, 2013; Feigenbaum & Pollock, 1999). Initially, loads that permit three sets of 10 repetitions, without reaching momentary muscle failure, should be used. Once 3 sets of 12 repetitions can be performed (with a rating of perceived exertion (RPE) of 12–14 RPE (Borg, 1982)), a 5% increase in load can be added to the next training session (Fig. 5.2). Exercising near to maximal effort (i.e. to ~19 RPE) produces the greatest gains in strength (ACSM, 1998), with progression of weight every 1–2 weeks. However, such intensities tend to, initially, result in additional delayed-onset muscle soreness (DOMS), which can discourage unaccustomed individuals from further participation; therefore a progressive and gradual approach to load and intensity should be used.

It is recommended that, for the elderly and those with clinically significant chronic conditions, the intensity be reduced to one set of 10–15 RM, increasing the weight every 2–4 weeks (Feigenbaum & Pollock, 1999; Nelson et al., 2007). Using 1 RM to assess strength in those with musculoskeletal injuries and chronic diseases can increase injury risk, so a 10 RM is a

TABLE 5.2 Progressive Resistance Exercise (PRE) Programme[a]

Number of Repetitions	Adjustment for Set 3	Adjustment for Next Day
0–2	Decrease by 2.5–5 kg; repeat set	Decrease by 2.5–5 kg
3–4	Decrease by 2.5–5 kg	Keep weight the same
5–7	Keep weight the same	Increase by 2.5–5 kg
8–12	Increase by 2.5–5 kg	Increase by 2.5–7.5 kg
13+	Increase by 2.5–7.5 kg	Increase by 7.5–10 kg

[a]Adjustment of the weight for the exercise programme using the daily adjustable progressive resistive exercise (DAPRE) technique. The number of repetitions during set #2 is used to adjust weight for set #3. The number of repetitions during set #4 is used to adjust the weight for the next session.

6	
7	Very very light
8	
9	Very light
10	
11	Fairly light
12	
13	Somewhat hard
14	
15	Hard
16	
17	Very hard
18	
19	Very very hard
20	

Fig. 5.2 Fifteen-point scale for ratings of perceived exertion, the rating of perceived exertion (RPE) scale. (Reproduced from Borg 1982, with permission).

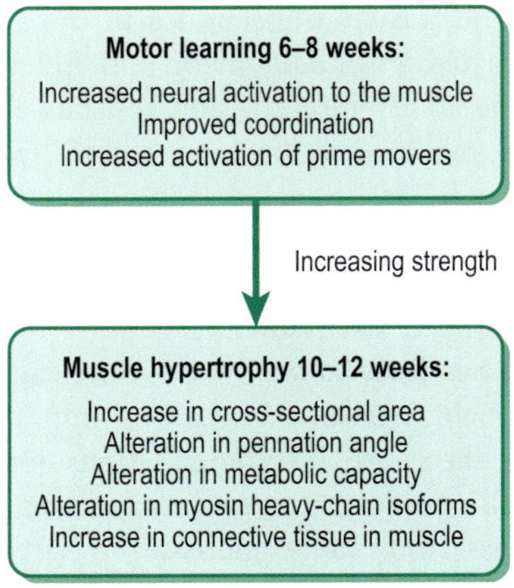

Fig. 5.3 The underlying effects of strengthening muscle.

more appropriate estimation. While muscle strength is less in the older person, the potential to strengthen muscle with a training program is much the same as with a young person (Grimby, 1995; Hakkinen et al., 1998; Newton et al., 2002; Grgic et al., 2020).

In alignment with the principle of specificity, the type of muscle contraction used in an exercise regime affects the change in muscle strength. Eccentric muscle actions appear to be more effective and efficient in increasing muscle strength. Eccentric exercises have been found to cause a greater increase in eccentric, isometric and concentric muscle strength than either concentric exercises or a mixed exercise regime (Hortobagyi et al., 2000). Eccentric exercise performed three times a week for 12 weeks has been found to increase eccentric strength three and a half times more than concentric exercises (Hortobagyi et al., 1996). However, such exercise is associated with pronounced DOMS due to the associated muscle damage, in those unaccustomed to eccentric muscle loading (Hody et al., 2019), which may reduce adherence and therefore the desired benefits. If eccentric exercise is being used then a conservative approach should be implemented in the early stages, with the initial bouts of eccentric exercise providing a protective effect for subsequent bouts (known as the repeated bout effect), thereby reducing the level of DOMS associated with the subsequent bouts of exercise (Hody et al., 2019).

Underlying Effect of Strengthening a Muscle

A low number of repetitions performed using a relatively high resistance (>80% 1 RM) will strengthen muscle (Staron et al., 1994; Hakkinen et al., 1998). The underlying effects are, first, neural adaptations including increased recruitment and synchronization of motor units along with reduced activation of antagonists, as part of improved motor learning, and second, a change in muscle tissue, including hypertrophy, although this is preceded by architectural adaptations (e.g., alterations is fascicle length, pennation angle) (Seynnes et al., 2007) (Fig. 5.3). The stimulus for a strength change is the force of muscle action determined by the load applied, and this is reflected in the nature of the adaptations.

Motor Learning

The first stage, which lasts for 6–8 weeks (if the individual is not familiar with the task exercise), is where motor learning occurs; performance improves, but strength remains the same. However, although the force-generating capacity of the muscle may not change, the load lifted or the speed in which it is lifted may increase due to improved efficiency and decreased antagonist activation. The changes include:

- Increased neural activation to the muscle (Sale et al., 1983; Komi, 1986) which parallels the increase in muscle strength
- Increased activation of prime movers (Sale, 1988)
- Improved coordination (Sale, 1988)
- Decreased activation of antagonists

These neural changes alone can produce an increase in force production (Enoka, 1988). During an 8-week training program, neural changes were responsible for almost all the strength gains in older subjects (~70 years), whereas in younger subjects (~22 years), neural changes were responsible for most of the increased strength in the first 4 weeks, with muscle hypertrophy after 4–6 weeks (Moritani & DeVries, 1979). These differences are likely to be related to activity levels and initial muscle strength.

In symptomatic individuals, changes in neural activation may be responsible for improved strength and endurance beyond the suggested 6–8 weeks (Kaser et al., 2001; Mannion et al., 2001). Patients with chronic low-back pain followed a 3-month back exercise programme (Mannion et al., 2001), and, although activation, strength and endurance improved, this was not accompanied by any change in the size of the muscle fibres or proportion of muscle fibre type (Kaser et al., 2001). It is likely that in such cases that neural activation was initially impaired due to neural inhibition of the muscle.

Muscle Hypertrophy

After the initial neurological adaptations, subsequent increases in strength are attributable to muscle architectural adaptations and increases in cross-sectional area (hypertrophy). The changes are:

1. An increase in the cross-sectional area of the muscle (Housh et al., 1992; Narici et al., 1996) and muscle fibres (Melissa et al., 1997; Andersen & Aagaard, 2000) visible after a few weeks of training. The increase in cross-sectional area of the muscle is due to hypertrophy of muscle fibres (see later) and an increase in the connective tissue in muscle. In addition, where the strength training involves a group of muscles, the increase in cross-sectional area is not equal in each muscle (Housh et al., 1992; Narici et al., 1996). For example, with quadriceps strength training, using the knee extension, greatest hypertrophy was seen in rectus femoris and least hypertrophy in vastus intermedius (Narici et al., 1996). In contrast, the rectus femoris was the only muscle to show no adaptation after 8 weeks of heavy squat or squat jump training (Earp et al., 2015). Such findings demonstrating differential adaptations to specific exercises highlight the importance of appropriate selection of exercises.
2. Alteration in muscle fibre types. Some researchers have found no change in proportion of type I or type II fibres (Terrados et al., 1990; Labarque et al., 2002), whereas other researchers have found an increase in the proportion of type IIa fibres and a decrease in type IIb fibres following strength training (Hortobagyi et al., 1996; Andersen & Aagaard, 2000). These differences may be attributable to differences in loading during the exercises and the volume of additional exercise performed.
3. An alteration in pennation angles (Kawakami et al., 1993, 1995).
4. An alteration in metabolic capacity of muscle has been demonstrated; this effect appears to be genetically determined (Simoneau et al., 1986).
5. An alteration in myosin heavy-chain (MHC) isoforms (Gea, 1997; Andersen & Aagaard, 2000). The myosin head, which binds with actin during a muscle contraction, contains the MHC isoforms (Scott et al., 2001).
6. An increase in the connective tissue found in muscle structures proportional to muscle hypertrophy.

Increasing Muscle Power

Muscle power is a function of muscle force and movement velocity; improvement in either or both aspects will result in an increase in muscle power. In addition, repeated practice of the movement, or a component of the movement, at speed, is thought to produce an improvement in muscle power likely due to increased efficiency of movement and decreased antagonist activation (deVries & Housh, 1994).

Force production (strength) is the key determinant of power, with an increase in force production resulting in an increased ability to accelerate an object ($F = M \times A$). If acceleration of an object increases from an increase in force production, there is a resultant increase in velocity of movement; therefore increasing both force and velocity results in a greater improvement in power ($P = F \times V$) (Cormie et al., 2010; Suchomel et al. 2016; Turner et al., 2020a, 2020b).

It has been suggested that movement should be carried out as fast as possible against a resistance of 30% maximal voluntary isometric contraction (MVIC) force, although exercises performed with low loads result in improvement in power at low loads, whereas exercises using moderate or heavy loads increased power at across all loads (Kaneko et al., 1983; Toji & Kaneko,

2004). In line with the principle of specificity, the load and resultant velocity result in the greatest increases in power at those loads and velocities; however, the heavier load training results in greater improvements in power across a range of loads (Kaneko et al., 1983; Toji et al., 1997; Toji & Kaneko, 2004; Harris et al., 2008). The key factor in power development appears to be the ability to rapidly produce force, which is best training with a focus on strength development rather than power, unless the individual is already strong (Cormie et al., 2010; Turner et al., 2020a, 2020b).

Increasing Muscle Endurance

Muscle endurance refers to the ability of a muscle to produce a specific force repetitively or to sustain an isometric action for a prolonged duration (Bruton, 2002). To increase muscle endurance, a muscle must contract at 50% to 70% of its maximum force, for 8–20 repetitions, for 3–4 sets during each session, ideally 2–3 times per week. It is worth noting that such intensity and repetition ranges helps to increase work capacity of the muscles, but due to the high volume of exercise associated with such training this is most likely to result in a hypertrophic response and residual fatigue, lasting up to 48 hours. In addition, for individuals who are weak initially, increasing strength increases endurance of the muscles purely by ensuring that activities of daily living are no longer near maximal intensity.

Underlying Effects of Increasing Muscle Endurance

A high number of repetitions of muscle actions against a moderate resistance will increase muscle endurance by effecting a change in the muscle (increased cross-sectional area, increased glycolytic enzymes and increased glycogen storage). The stimulus is the metabolic demand and tensile stress on the muscle, and this is reflected in the nature of the changes (Box 5.2) and includes:

- An increase in the number of type I and IIa fibres and a decrease in type IIb fibres (Ingjer, 1979; Demirel et al., 1999)
- An increase in the cross-sectional area of type I and IIb fibres (Ingjer, 1979)
- An increase in number of capillaries surrounding each muscle fibre (Ingjer, 1979)
- An increase in blood flow in muscle (Vanderhoof et al., 1961; Rohter et al., 1963)
- An increase in myoglobin content (Holloszy, 1976)

BOX 5.2 Underlying Effect of Increasing Muscle Endurance

- Increase in number of I and IIa fibres and a decrease in type IIb fibres
- Increase in cross-sectional area of type I fibres
- Increase in number of capillaries
- Increase in myoglobin content
- Increase in oxidative power and enzyme activity of mitochondria
- Increase in oxidative enzymes
- Increased store of muscle glycogen and fat
- Increased activity of enzymes
- Higher threshold level of lactate
- Altered myosin heavy-chain isoforms

Aerobic Endurance

Where endurance training incorporates general cardiorespiratory exercises, such as walking, running, swimming and cycling, the ACSM provides guidance for healthy adults, recommending moderate exercise intensity sufficient to raise the heart rate to 60% to 90% of maximum, and it should be carried out for 30 minutes five times a week, or 20 minutes of vigorous intensity (80% to 90% maximum heart rate) three times per week (Haskell et al., 2007). For the older adult and those with clinically significant chronic conditions, the recommendations are similar except the heart rate should be raised to 50% to 85%, where 5–6 is moderate (50%) and 7–8 (80%) is vigorous intensity on a 10-point scale (or 10–12 and 14–16 based on the Borg scale (see Fig. 5.2)).

Clinical Implications of Strength Power and Endurance Training

Exercise prescription is a core skill of therapists that combines management of disorders of movement, knowledge of exercise regimens and clinical reasoning skills to ensure that the exercises prescribed are appropriate for the individual (Taylor et al., 2007). For example, there is strong evidence that strengthening and aerobic exercises reduce pain and improve activity level in people with osteoarthritis of the knee (Brosseau et al., 2004; Hurley et al. 2007). The implementation of resistance exercise also has clear benefits for individuals suffering from multiple common health conditions (e.g. cancer, metabolic and cardiovascular disease, dementia, depression), in addition to reducing age related deterioration in physical capacity (Maestroni et al., 2020). A patient with osteoarthritis of the knee is likely to have weak quadriceps and pain and may be unable to perform a functional activity such as sit to stand, stair-climbing and walking for more than 10 minutes. Therefore a training program needs to reflect each of these elements. It requires strength training to enable the patient to carry out sit to stand, improvements in muscular endurance to climb stairs and cardiovascular endurance to enable the patient to walk for extended periods of time. Consideration needs to be taken for the load, repetition, rest period and order of exercise. As with any exercise regimen, the most complex and fatiguing tasks should be performed at the start of the session, with adequate rest between sets (usually 2–3 minutes) to ensure that the subsequent set does not commence when the muscles are still fatigued.

Altering Motor Control

Signs of altered motor control, such as muscle inhibition, delayed timing of onset of muscle activation, increased muscle activation and altered relative activation of agonist and antagonist, have been considered in the previous chapter. The aim of treatment, in this case, would therefore be to increase muscle activation (if inhibited), increase the speed of onset of muscle contraction, reduce muscle activation (to increase efficiency, which occurs with an increase in strength) or alter relative activation of agonist and antagonist (increasing movement efficiency via a reduction in co-contraction, if this does not reduce joint stability). The common theme for each of these aims is to alter the pattern of muscle activation, which is to alter motor control. Aspects of motor learning will be covered in Chapter 10 of this book.

To Increase Muscle Activation

Methods for increasing muscle activation (i.e. for facilitating muscle contraction) include active assisted movements, rapid stretch, mechanical vibration, proprioceptive neuromuscular facilitation (PNF), touch, use of overflow, ice and taping (Box 5.3). Electrical stimulation of muscle is also available and has been shown to be very successful, especially in combination with a volitional muscle contraction being undertaken at the same time. With the muscle contracting and in a lengthened position, a rapid stretch is applied to the muscle; this stimulates the muscle spindles to facilitate extrafusal muscle contraction. Vibration similarly stimulates the muscle spindles such as using vibration platforms. PNF may also prove helpful in facilitating muscle contraction. Touch can be used to facilitate muscle contraction; stimulation of the skin has been shown to enhance α and γ motor neurone activity in the underlying muscles and cause inhibition of more distal muscles (Eldred & Hagbarth, 1954). Taping is thought to increase activation of the underlying muscle (Gilleard et al., 1998; Cowan et al., 2002) dependent on it being appropriately applied.

BOX 5.3 Treatment to Increase Muscle Activation

- Active assisted movements
- Rapid stretch
- Proprioceptive neuromuscular facilitation
- Touch
- Use of overflow
- Mechanical vibration
- Ice
- Taping

Inhibition of an active voluntary contraction was eliminated with a high-velocity isotonic contraction (Newham et al., 1989). This can be explained by the relationship of force and speed, where increased speed of concentric contraction (increased fascicle shortening velocity) reduces the force generated (Hill, 1938).

Increased Speed of Onset

Using the principles of motor learning, it would seem reasonable to suggest that, to increase the speed of onset of muscle action, treatment needs to use normal functional activities that will produce a need for the muscle to contract. With delayed activation of transversus abdominis in patients with low-back pain (Hodges & Richardson, 1996), treatment would include functional postures and movements that challenge postural stability, and this would need to be continued repetitively over time. In patients with anterior knee pain, a combination of specific muscle exercise with biofeedback, muscle stretches, taping and patellofemoral accessory movements has been shown, over a 6-week period, to improve the timing of muscle onset of vastus medialis, when going up and down stairs (Gilleard et al., 1998; Cowan et al., 2002). The mechanism by which the tape increased the onset of vastus medialis is unclear. Cutaneous stimulation has been shown to alter recruitment threshold and recruitment order of motor units (Garnett & Stephens, 1981; Jenner & Stephens, 1982).

To Reduce Muscle Activation

This may be needed where the clinician feels there is overactivity of muscles. For example, in the early stages of motor learning, there is co-contraction of the agonist and antagonist when carrying out a movement (Moore & Marteniuk, 1986). Similarly, there may be unwanted muscle activity as a patient attempts to produce a specific muscle contraction (e.g. flexion of the lumbar spine) while trying to isolate contraction of the transversus abdominis and lumbar multifidus. The patient may have overactivity of muscles because of pain, which may be sufficient to produce muscle spasm, in which case the clinician may need to reduce the muscle activity. To do this the patient may need to be made aware of the unwanted muscle activity using a mirror, verbal feedback, touch or electromyography (EMG) feedback. Other methods for reducing muscle activation include positioning, PNF, massage, relaxation techniques and taping (Box 5.4). It has been speculated that tape to the posterior thigh inhibits overactive hamstring muscles (Tobin & Robinson, 2000; McConnell, 2002). Tape over the lower fibres of the trapezius of asymptomatic subjects was found to inhibit the muscle by as much as 22% when measured using the H reflex (Alexander et al., 2003). The underlying mechanism is not known; it has been postulated that it could be due to an alteration in muscle length and/or stimulation of cutaneous afferents, leading to inhibition of the underlying muscle and/or decrease in descending drive of the motor neurone pool (Alexander et al. 2003).

BOX 5.4 Treatment to Reduce Muscle Activity

- Mirror
- Verbal feedback
- Touch
- Electromyogram feedback
- Positioning
- Proprioceptive neuromuscular facilitation
- Trigger points
- Deep inhibitory massage
- Taping

Altering Muscle Length

The aim of a treatment may be to decrease or increase muscle length. The reason a muscle may be considered long, and why treatment should be aimed at reducing its length, is likely to be associated with reduced muscle tone or hypermobility. Where the clinician identifies reduced tone, treatment would be directed at increasing the strength of the muscle, which has been discussed earlier.

Increasing Muscle Length

When considering muscle stretching, it can be helpful to categorize muscle into the active contractile unit and the noncontractile connective tissue, within the muscle belly and tendon. Treatment can be classified according to which effect the clinician is attempting to have on the muscle. Increasing the length of a muscle can be achieved by passively lengthening the connective tissue such that there is a permanent increase in length, or by attempting to produce physiological relaxation of the active contractile unit of the muscle belly using, for example, PNF (autogenic or reciprocal inhibitory techniques). Clearly, the contractile and noncontractile elements are inseparable, and what is not being stated here is that treatment to lengthen the connective tissue affects the connective tissue alone and has no effect on the contractile unit, or vice versa. The classification of treatment is used simply to aid communication between clinicians and is not attempting to describe the effect of the treatment. Muscle can be stretched passively with the aim of treatment to produce a permanent lengthening the muscle–tendon unit. It is also worth noting that eccentric exercise has been shown to result in longer muscle fascicles (Franchi et al., 2014), which also likely increase the length of the entire muscle.

Passive Muscle Stretching

An effective passive stretch is produced when a force moves the proximal and distal muscle attachments further apart; often, this involves fixing the proximal attachment while passively moving the distal attachment away. Positioning can often be used to help fix the proximal attachment; for example, supine with one leg flexed on to the chest helps to fix the pelvis as the other hip is moved into extension to lengthen the iliopsoas muscle.

Direction of movement. There is no single direction of movement that will stretch all parts of a muscle because the muscle line of action often lies across multiple planes; the clinician needs to explore fully and treat all aspects of muscle length by combining movements (Hunter, 1998). The muscle attachments, direction of its fibres, position of the muscle and the relationship of the muscle to other structures enable the clinician to decide how to combine movements for any muscle. For example, to lengthen biceps femoris fully, a combination of hip flexion, medial rotation and adduction with knee extension and medial tibial rotation needs to be used. Similarly, to lengthen extensor carpi radialis brevis fully, elbow extension with forearm pronation, wrist flexion, ulna deviation and individual finger flexion need to be combined (Hunter, 1998).

Magnitude of force. When a muscle is stretched, the force is distributed throughout the connective tissue framework of the muscle (Hill, 1950). Whenever a permanent lengthening is achieved, there is initially some degree of mechanical weakening. Interestingly, the amount of weakening depends on the way the muscle has been lengthened as well as how much it has been lengthened. A small force for a long duration will induce less weakening than a large force for a short duration (Sapega et al., 1981; Taylor et al., 1990).

Speed of movement. The speed of the movement can be described as slow or fast, and the rhythm should be smooth. The connective tissue in muscle is viscoelastic and is therefore sensitive to the speed of the applied force. A force applied quickly will produce less movement, provoking a greater stiffness; that is, the gradient of the resistance curve will increase; in contrast, a force applied more slowly will cause more movement as the stiffness is relatively less. If the intention of treatment is to maximize range of movement by lengthening connective tissue, then low speeds would seem preferable.

In addition, as the muscle spindles detect both the magnitude and rate of change in length, rapidly moving the limb into a position where the muscle is stretched results in early stimulation of this sensory receptor. Such stimulation results in reflex stimulation of the muscle, creating a shortening rather than a lengthening of the muscle fascicles and therefore a less effective stretch, highlighting the importance of the stretch being performed in a slow and controlled manner if the aim is to increase muscle length.

Duration. In terms of treatment dose, time relates to the duration of the stretch, the number of times this is repeated and the frequency of the appointments. Hamstring muscle length has been found to be as effectively lengthened with daily static stretches using a 30-second stretch as with three repetitions of 1-minute stretches (Bandy et al., 1997). Reassessment after each repetition enables the clinician to determine the effect of treatment on the patient's signs and symptoms. Depending on this change (better, same or worse), the clinician may alter the time and number of repetitions within a treatment session. A permanent (plastic) lengthening of the connective tissue of muscle and tendon with minimal structural weakness is enhanced by a long duration stretch (Sapega et al., 1981).

Temperature. Temperature influences the mechanical behaviour of connective tissue under tensile load. As temperature rises to approximately 40°C to 45°C, stiffness decreases and extensibility increases (Rigby, 1964; Lehmann et al., 1970). At approximately 40°C, a change in the microstructure of collagen occurs, which significantly enhances the extensibility and potential for a permanent (plastic) change in length (Rigby, 1964). The viscoelastic properties can be increased by as much as 170% when muscle temperature is raised to 43°C, and a higher temperature will induce less weakening than a lower temperature (Sapega et al., 1981). Once the heat is removed, it has been found that maintaining the tension as the tissue cools enhances the plastic deformation (Lehmann et al., 1970; Sapega et al., 1981).

Symptom response. The clinician decides which symptom, and to what extent, is to be provoked during treatment. Choices include:

- no provocation
- provocation to the point of onset or increase in resting symptoms
- partial reproduction
- total reproduction.

The decision as to what extent symptoms are provoked during treatment depends on the severity and irritability of the symptom(s) and the nature of the condition. If the symptoms are severe (i.e. the patient is unable to tolerate the symptom being produced), the clinician would choose not to provoke the symptoms. The clinician may also choose not to provoke symptoms if they are irritable; that is, once symptoms are provoked, they take some time to ease. However, if the symptoms are not severe and not irritable, then the clinician is able to reproduce the patient's symptoms during treatment, and the extent to which symptoms are reproduced will depend on the tolerance of the patient. The nature of the condition may limit the extent to which symptoms are produced, such as a recent traumatic injury. Treatment is progressed or regressed by altering appropriate aspects of the treatment dose: patient position, movement, direction of force, magnitude of force, amplitude of oscillation, speed, rhythm, time or symptom response. Table 5.3 highlights the ways in which each aspect of the treatment dose can be progressed and regressed.

Table 5.4 provides an example of how a treatment dose for lengthening the upper fibres of trapezius may be progressed and regressed. An increase in time from 30 seconds to 1 minute provides a progression of the treatment dose, and a reduction in the amount of symptoms accounts for the regression. Other aspects of treatment dose which are closely linked are the length of time for each repetition and the number of repetitions; these, together, provide a dose of time, and so each can be altered at the same time.

In sports medicine, two types of stretching are advocated: ballistic and static stretching. Ballistic stretching involves the person performing bouncing, rhythmic end-range movements. While such stretching may be beneficial during a warm-up in preparation for participation in sport, due to the rate of lengthening, the muscle spindle is stimulated resulting in a less effective stretch. Static stretching involves a

TABLE 5.3 Progression and Regression of Treatment Dose

Treatment Dose	Progression	Regression
Position	Muscle towards end of available range	Muscle towards beginning of available range
Direction of force	More provocative	Less provocative
Magnitude of force	Increased	Decreased
Amplitude of oscillation	Decreased	Increased
Rhythm	Staccato	Smoother
Time	Longer	Shorter
Speed	Slower or faster	Slower
Symptom response	Allowing more symptoms to be provoked	Allowing fewer symptoms to be provoked

TABLE 5.4 Example of How a Treatment Dose for Increasing the Passive Length of the Upper Fibres of Trapezius Can Be Progressed and Regressed

Regression	Dose	Progression
In full cervical flexion and ½ range contralateral flexion, static hold for 30 s to partial reproduction of patient's neck pain	In full cervical flexion and ½ range contralateral flexion, static hold for 30 s to full reproduction of patient's neck pain	In full cervical flexion and ½ range contralateral flexion, static hold for 1 min to full reproduction of patient's neck pain

simple hold at the end of range. Controversy exists over the effectiveness of each type of stretching in producing an increase in muscle length; however, based on the underpinning physiology of the muscle (including the muscle spindle and associated stretch reflex), it makes sense that static stretching, performed in a controlled manner, held for approximately 30 seconds per repetition, would be most effective.

Increasing Length via the Contractile Unit of Muscle

The aim of this type of treatment is to cause a relaxation of the contractile unit of muscle to increase muscle length. Muscle energy techniques and positional release techniques can also be used to cause muscle relaxation (Chaitow, 2013, 2015). PNF is advocated to achieve this muscle relaxation. These are rotational movement patterns through full range of movement, hold–relax, contract–relax and agonist–contract.

Hold–Relax. The muscle is positioned in its stretched position, either actively or passively. A strong isometric contraction of the muscle is achieved by the clinician providing manual resistance. The muscle contraction needs to be carefully controlled by the clinician. This is achieved by saying to the patient, 'Don't let me move you' or 'Hold' and by slowly and smoothly increasing the manual resistance to maximum contraction. Following contraction, the patient is asked to relax, the clinician gradually reduces the resistance and time is allowed for muscle relaxation to occur. The clinician then moves further into range to increase the length of the muscle. The procedure of contraction followed by relaxation is then repeated until no further increase in muscle length can be achieved.

Contract–Relax

This is the same as hold–relax except that, following the isometric contraction, the patient actively contracts to lengthen the antagonistic muscle further, rather than the clinician passively lengthening the muscle. For example, to lengthen quadriceps the patient isometrically contracts the quadriceps at, for example, 60-degree flexion for 3–6 seconds. The patient is then asked to relax and actively to contract the hamstrings to increase knee flexion and stretch the quadriceps muscle group. As in hold–relax, the procedure is repeated in the new range of movement and repeated until no further increase in muscle length is achieved.

Agonist–Contract

The muscle is put in a position of stretch, and a contraction of the agonist attempts to increase movement and thus increase stretch of the muscle. The clinician facilitates this movement by carefully applying a passive force. For example, to lengthen quadriceps, the knee is positioned in 60-degree flexion. The patient actively contracts the hamstrings to increase knee flexion and stretch the quadriceps muscle group. The clinician applies a force to the lower leg to enhance this movement.

Reducing Symptoms

A useful premise for the clinician is to consider that the symptom is whatever patients say it is, existing whenever they say it is. This was originally used for pain but can be widened to any symptom the patient feels.

The assumption in this text is that the cause of the muscle pain is some sort of injury to the muscle and/or tendon. In this situation, the pain will be a result of mechanical and/or chemical irritation of the muscle nociceptors. The subjective information from the patient, particularly the behaviour of symptoms and mechanism of injury, may enable the clinician to identify whether it is the contractile unit of muscle and/or connective tissue of muscle that is involved in the pain. For example, an overstretch injury may affect the contractile tissue of muscle (as this elongates more than the relatively stiffer non-contractile elements) and require treatment to increase the muscle contractile ability, so control elongation and reduce pain.

Various manual therapy techniques can be used to reduce symptoms emanating from muscle, including massage, connective tissue massage trigger points and frictions. Joint mobilizations, taping and electrotherapy can also be used. The mechanism by which pain is relieved with each of these manual techniques is still unclear. Large-diameter type III afferents are distributed throughout muscle tissue and are stimulated by pressure, mechanical force caused by lengthening muscle or by muscle contraction (Mense & Meyer, 1985). It is possible that the manual techniques described previously may stimulate the type III afferents and cause a reflex inhibition of the type IV muscle nociceptors according to the pain gate theory (Melzack & Wall, 1965). Clearly, large-diameter afferents in the skin and joint may also contribute to this pain inhibition. The pain may also be reduced via a descending inhibitory system explained later and expanded rather more in Chapter 7 on nerve treatment.

Descending Inhibition of Pain

The periaqueductal grey (PAG) area has been found to be important in the control of nociception. PAG projects to the dorsal horn and has a descending control of nociception. It also projects upwards to the medial thalamus and orbital frontal cortex and so may have an ascending control of nociception (Heinricher & Fields, 2013). The PAG has two distinct regions, the dorsolateral PAG (dPAG) and the ventrolateral PAG (vPAG).

dPAG

Noxious stimuli can cause activation of the descending control system (Yaksh & Elde, 1981; Heinricher & Fields, 2013), which may reduce nociceptive transmission. Noxious stimulation has been found to cause release of enkephalins at the supraspinal and spinal levels (Yaksh & Elde, 1981). It has also been found that stimulation of the spinothalamic tract, transmitting nociceptive information from one foot, can be inhibited by noxious input from the contralateral foot, hand, face or trunk (Gerhart et al., 1981). It has been suggested that this may explain the relief of pain with acupuncture, and pain behaviours such as 'biting your lip' (Melzack, 1975). Painful treatment of muscle may also activate the descending control system.

Addressing the Biopsychosocial Aspects of Symptoms

Injury, or the perception of injury, produces anxiety and fear (Craig, 1999). Who has ever injured themselves, however minimally, and not experienced an emotional reaction? We all will have a cognitive and emotional response to injury because injury interrupts our lives. It seems reasonable to suggest, therefore, that all patients with neuromusculoskeletal dysfunction will have thoughts and feelings about their problem, and it would be an oversight on the part of the clinician not to enquire about these. This enquiry involves the clinician understanding the patient's thoughts and feelings. This is no easy task, and to do it well requires a high level of skill in active listening. Active listening involves putting our own thoughts, beliefs and feelings to one side and choosing, instead, to hear what the patient has to say. It involves trying to understand patients and their world, through their eyes, and avoiding the all-too-easy error of reinterpreting through our eyes. It requires the clinician to listen with compassion and patience and without judgement. It involves the clinician using words carefully and meaningfully and using open-ended questions to search for information, until understanding is reached. It involves sensitive verbal and nonverbal communication, encouraging safe and open communication. Following the enquiry of patients as to their thoughts and feelings, two further steps are recommended: education and exposure (Vlaeyen & Crombez, 1999). Education involves the clinician carefully facilitating the patient's understanding of his or her problem. How this is carried out with patients will vary based on several factors, including their prior knowledge, thoughts and beliefs and how they feel about the problem. All the listening skills discussed earlier will be essential in this process. The ability of the clinician to be honest is important. The clinician needs to explain the problem to the patient in a careful way. There is a world of difference between 'The pain in your back is from the disc' and 'I think the pain in your back could be coming from the disc'. The former explanation suggests that you know that the pain is coming from the disc, and yet there is overwhelming evidence that you cannot make such claims; it has been estimated that a definite diagnosis of pathology can be made in about only 15% of cases (Waddell, 2004). Furthermore, there is a long-term problem with being so confident as the patient may, in the future, have a recurrence of the same pain and may see another clinician who may say 'The pain in your back is from your sacroiliac joint'. The patient is aware that this is a repeat episode and now, quite rightly, begins to have doubts about the ability of these two clinicians. This will be a familiar story to experienced clinicians, who will have come across patients who may have received three, four or even more confident 'diagnoses' of the same problem, and who come to you depressed, cynical and disillusioned with the medical profession.

The final aspect is exposure, which involves careful and graded exposure to the movements or postures that provoke pain (Vlaeyen & Crombez, 1999). While this is designed for chronic pain patients who learn to avoid movements and posture through fear (Waddell & Main, 2004), it may also be an important part of the treatment of acute tissue damage. Using movements and postures in a careful, controlled and graded way may help to avoid long-term movement dysfunctions; the principles of graded exposure and reloading are further explored in Chapter 10.

Muscle Injury and Repair

Muscle can be damaged by a direct injury, such as a laceration or contusion, or indirectly by a sudden forceful contraction causing a muscle or tendon tear; damage may also be due to a chronic overuse injury (Kellett, 1986). Whatever the mechanism of injury, the effect on muscle tissue is similar (Hurme et al., 1991) and can be considered in three phases: inflammatory or lag phase, regeneration phase and remodelling phase (Jarvinen & Lehto, 1993).

The inflammatory or lag phase is characterized by hematoma formation, tissue necrosis and an inflammatory reaction. Necrosis of muscle tissue occurs with retraction of the muscle fibres on either side of the necrotic zone. It is generally accepted that treatment for the first 48–72 hours of a muscle injury is summarized by RICE: rest, ice, compression and elevation (Evans, 1980; Kellett, 1986). This has more recently been revised to the acronym POLICE (Bleakley et al., 2012), which stands for Protection, Optimal Loading, Ice, Compression, Elevation, with the emphasis now being more on returning the injury to loading in a controlled manner (see Chapter 10).

During the regeneration phase, there is phagocytosis of damaged tissue and production of connective scar tissue. Capillary growth satellite cells migrate into the necrotic area. Muscle fibres regenerate by differentiation into myoblasts and then into myotubes, which link the two stumps on either side of the necrotic region. The connective tissue within muscle is also damaged and undergoes healing with subsequent scar formation (Jarvinen & Lehto, 1993). Following a short period of immobilization—more than 3–5 days for rats (Jarvinen & Lehto, 1993)—it is considered beneficial to mobilize the muscle, within the limits of symptoms. Early mobilization is thought to enhance tensile strength, orientation of the regenerating muscle fibres, resorption of connective scar tissue and blood flow to the damaged area and to avoid atrophy brought about by immobilization (Jarvinen & Lehto, 1993). The tensile strength of a tendon has been found to increase as a result of 60 repetitions per day of manual wrist and finger flexion/extension following a primary repair (Takai et al., 1991).

The remodelling phase is characterized by the maturation of regenerated muscle (Jarvinen & Lehto, 1993). There is contraction and reorganization of scar tissue and a gradual recovery of the functional capacity of the muscle.

The key to managing muscle injury through each of these stages is to expose it to the appropriate level of load, which is sufficient to stimulate adaptation, whilst not provoking symptoms. In the inflammatory stage, this might be through low-intensity isometric exercises in midrange positions with short contraction durations, progressing to isometric contractions in elongated positions, then dynamic contractions (concentric and eccentric) in mid- then outer-range, followed by increasing the intensity and velocity of the contractions.

Alongside damage to muscle and connective tissue, neural tissue may also be damaged. It is worth mentioning here that a patient presenting with classical signs of a hamstring tear may, in fact, have a neurodynamic (neural) component to the problem. In Australian Rules football, players with signs of a hamstring tear had a positive slump test, and when this was addressed in treatment there was a better result than with more traditional muscle treatment techniques (Kornberg & Lew, 1989). This highlights the need for a full and comprehensive examination of a patient.

Delayed-Onset Muscle Soreness

Muscle strain injury occurs with eccentric exercise, producing DOMS (Friden et al., 1983; Jones et al., 1986). Pain, weakness and muscle stiffness are felt after unaccustomed eccentric exercise (Hody et al., 2019). There is breakdown of collagen (Brown et al., 1997) and disruption of the Z band, predominantly in type II fibres, with repair largely completed by 6 days (Friden et al., 1983; Jones et al., 1986). The reason for DOMS following eccentric contraction may be that eccentric actions produce more force within the muscle than other muscle action, resulting in greater damage and inflammation (Kanda et al., 2013). It is worth noting that a single bout of eccentric exercise, even of low volume, provides a protective effect for subsequent exercises known as the repeated bout effect (Hody et al., 2019). As such, a conservative approach to eccentric training should be adopted during the initial sessions, to avoid excessive DOMS, which should improve adherence and permit the manifestation of the repeated bout effect for more progressive eccentric exercise in subsequent sessions.

Tendon Injury and Repair

Tendons can tear in the middle region, by avulsion of bone and, more rarely, at the insertion site. The myotendinous region is the weakest part of the tendon–muscle unit and is the region most susceptible to strain injuries (Garrett et al. 1989; Garrett, 1990; Tidball, 1991). Healing of tendon is like that of other soft tissues and consists of three phases: lag or inflammation phase (1–7 days), regeneration or proliferation phase (7–21 days) and remodelling or maturation phase (21 days to 1 year) (Jozsa & Kannus, 1997).

Repetitive strain may alter the collagenous structure of tendon with resultant inflammation, oedema and pain (Jozsa & Kannus, 1997). Overuse injury occurs where this repetitive strain causing tissue damage is greater than the natural repair and healing process (Archambault et al., 1995; Jozsa & Kannus, 1997). Conditions including tendinopathies may lead, with further strain, to partial or complete rupture of the tendon. Eccentric exercises have been advocated for chronic Achilles tendinopathy (Alfredson et al., 1998); however, it is the high load and time under tension (i.e. duration of muscle action) which are important here as the tendon cannot differentiate between types of muscle action.

In work-related upper-limb tendon injuries, the repetitive nature of the task may be sufficient to cause change in the tissue. It is proposed that, initially, in the first 5 days, there is ischaemia, metabolic disturbance and cell membrane damage leading to inflammation (Jozsa & Kannus, 1997). The increase in tissue pressure further impairs the circulation and enhances the ischaemic changes. In the proliferation phase (5–21 days), there is fibrin clotting, and fibroblast, synovial cell and capillary proliferation followed by the maturation phase (<21 days) in which adhesions and thickening of the tenosynovium and paratenon occur (Kvist & Kvist, 1980; Jozsa & Kannus, 1997).

Treatment of a tendon injury may include soft-tissue mobilization, frictions, controlled exercises, lengthening, tape and electrotherapy. The reader is directed to relevant texts for further information.

Choice of Muscle Treatment

The choice of treatment depends on the assessment of the patient, whether the patient has a dysfunction of muscle and, if so, what that dysfunction is. Treatment may be to increase muscle strength, power and/or endurance, increase muscle length or alter motor control (increase muscle activation, reduce muscle activation, increase time of onset), depending on the nature of the forces provoking symptoms. The overall aim of treatment is to normalize a dysfunction (i.e. to eradicate the abnormal signs and symptoms).

Modification, Progression and Regression of Treatment

The continuous monitoring of the patient's subjective and physical status guides the entire treatment and management program of the patient. The clinician judges the degree of change with treatment and relates this to the expected rate of change from the prognosis and normal physiological responses and decides whether a treatment needs to be altered in some way. The nature of this alteration can be to modify the technique in some way, to progress or regress the treatment. Regardless of which alteration is made, the clinician makes every effort to determine what effect this alteration has on the patient's subjective and physical status. To do this, the clinician alters one aspect of treatment at a time and reassesses immediately to determine the value of the alteration.

Modification of Treatment

The clinician may modify the treatment given to a patient by altering an existing treatment, adding a new treatment or stopping a treatment. At all times, the treatment should have the functional goals of the patient in mind. Altering an existing treatment involves altering some aspect of the treatment dose (outlined earlier). The immediate and more long-term effect of the alteration is then evaluated by reassessment of the subjective and physical markers (Fig. 5.4). The clinician then decides whether, overall, the patient is better, the same or worse, relating this to the prognosis. For instance, if a quick improvement was expected but only some improvement occurred, the clinician may progress treatment. If the patient is worse after treatment, the dose may be regressed in some way, and if the treatment made no difference at all, then a more substantial modification may be made. Before discarding a treatment, it is worth making sure that it has been fully utilized, as it may be that a much stronger or much weaker treatment dose may be effective.

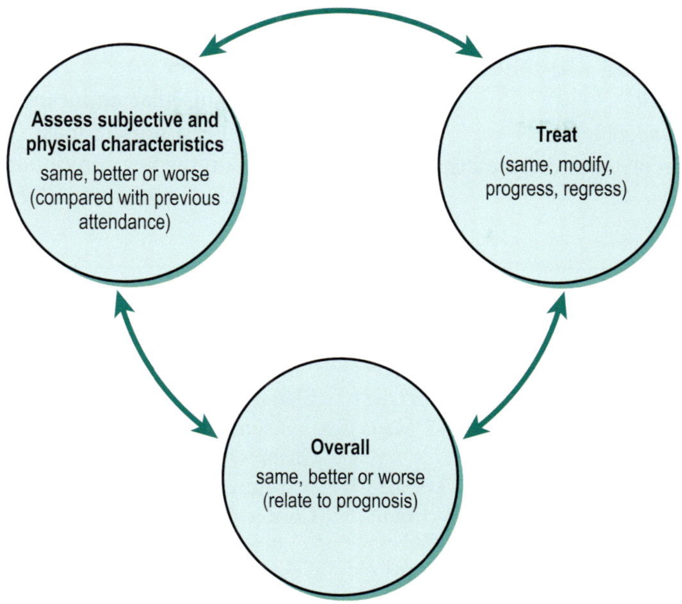

Fig. 5.4 Modification, progression and regression of treatment.

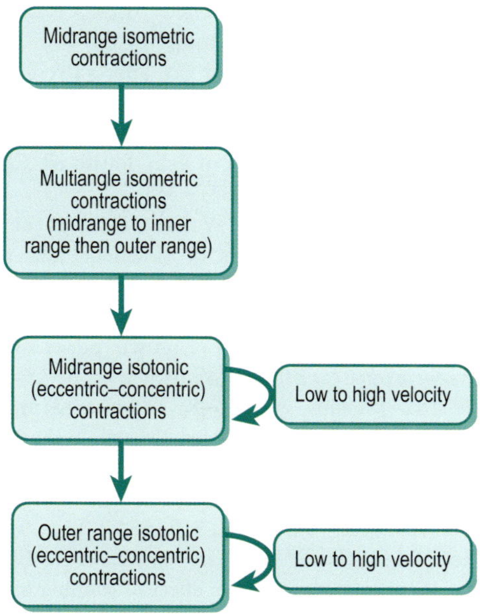

Fig. 5.5 Progressive loading paradigm for a muscle injury.

Progression and Regression of Treatment

A treatment is progressed or regressed by altering appropriate aspects of the treatment dose in such a way that more treatment, or less treatment, is applied to the tissues.

Fig. 5.5 shows typical load progression for a muscle injury.

It starts with midrange isometric contractions (once performing those without symptoms and with symmetrical strength (within 10%)) and progresses to multiangle isometric contractions (mid to inner to outer range). From there, eccentric concentric contractions would be performed in the midrange, before progressing (once performing those without symptoms and with symmetrical strength (within 10%)) to outer range eccentric and concentric contractions. When undertaking eccentric and concentric contractions, the velocity of contraction along the rate of force development would need to be considered and progressively applied.

SUMMARY

This chapter has outlined the principles of muscle treatment. Treatment is only a part of the overall management of a patient; the reader is therefore encouraged to go now to Chapter 10, where the principles of management are discussed.

REVIEW AND REVISE QUESTIONS

1. Describe progressive overload and the key training variables used to achieve it.
2. Explain the principle of specificity.
3. Describe the principle involved in the prescription of exercise to develop:
   A — Strength
   B — Power
   C — Muscular endurance
   D — Lean muscle mass
4. Explain the key components of Alfredson's approach to Achilles tendinopathy.

REFERENCES

Alexander, C.M., Stynes, S., Thomas, A., et al., 2003. Does tape facilitate or inhibit the lower fibres of trapezius? Man. Ther. 8 (1), 37—41.

Alfredson, H., Pietila, T., Jonsson, P., et al., 1998. Heavy load eccentric calf muscle training for the treatment of chronic Achilles tendinosis. Am. J. Sports Med. 26, 360—366.

American College of Sports Medicine (ACSM), 2013. Resource Manual for Guidelines for Exercise Testing and Prescription, seventh ed. Williams & Wilkins, Baltimore.

Andersen, J.L., Aagaard, P., 2000. Myosin heavy chain IIX overshoot in human skeletal muscle. Muscle Nerve 23 (7), 1095—1104.

Archambault, J.M., Wiley, J.P., Bray, R.C., 1995. Exercise loading of tendons and the development of overuse injuries. A review of current literature. Sports Med. 20 (2), 77—89.

Augustsson, J., Esko, A., Thomee, R., et al., 1998. Weight training of the thigh muscles using closed vs open kinetic chain exercises: a comparison of performance enhancement. J. Orthop. Sports Phys. Ther. 27, 3—8.

Bandy, W.D., Irion, J.M., Briggler, M., 1997. The effect of time and frequency of static stretching on flexibility of the hamstring muscles. Phys. Ther. 77 (10), 1090—1096.

Behm, D.G., Sale, D.G., 1993. Intended rather than actual movement velocity determines velocity-specific training response. J. Appl. Physiol. 74, 359—368.

Blackburn, J.R., Morrissey, M.C., 1998. The relationship between open and closed kinetic chain strength of the lower limb and jumping performance. J. Orthop. Sports Phys. Ther. 27 (6), 430—435.

Bleakley, C., Glasgow, P., MacAuley, D., 2012. Price needs updating should we call the police? BJSM. 46, 220—221.

Borg, G.A.V., 1982. Psychophysical bases of perceived exertion. Med. Sci. Sports Exerc. 14 (5), 377—381.

Brosseau, L., Pelland, L., Wells, G., et al., 2004. Efficacy of aerobic exercises for osteoarthritis (part II): a meta-analysis. Phys. Ther. Rev. 9, 125—145.

Brown, S.J., Child, R.B., Day, S.H., et al., 1997. Indices of skeletal muscle damage and connective tissue breakdown following eccentric muscle contractions. Eur. J. Appl. Physiol. 75, 369—374.

Chaitow, L., 2013. Muscle Energy Techniques, fourth ed. Churchill Livingstone, Edinburgh.

Chaitow, L., 2015. Positional Release Techniques, fourth ed. Churchill Livingstone, Edinburgh.

Cormie, P., McGuigan, M.R., Newton, R.U., 2010. Influence of strength on magnitude and mechanisms of adaptation to power training. Med. Sci. Sports Exerc. 42, 1566—1581.

Cormie, P., McGuigan, M.R., Newton, R.U., 2011. Developing maximal neuromuscular power: part 2 — training considerations for improving maximal power production. Sports Med. 41, 125—146.

Cowan, S.M., Bennell, K.L., Crossley, K.M., et al., 2002. Physical therapy alters recruitment of the vasti in patellofemoral pain syndrome. Med. Sci. Sports Exerc. 34 (12), 1879—1885.

Craig, K.D., 1999. Emotions and psychobiology. In: Wall, P.D., Melzack, R. (Eds.), Textbook of Pain, fourth ed. Churchill Livingstone, Edinburgh, pp. 331—343.

DeLateur, B., Lehmann, J.F., Warren, C.G., et al., 1972. Comparison of effectiveness of isokinetic and isotonic exercise in quadriceps strengthening. Arch. Phys. Med. Rehabil. 53, 60—64.

Delorme, T.L., 1945. Restoration of muscle power by heavy-resistance exercises. JBJS 27 (4), 645—667.

Delorme, T.L., Watkins, A.L., 1948. Technics of progressive resistance exercise. Arch. Phys. Med. Rehabil. 29 (5), 263—273.

Delorme, T.L., West, F.E., Shriber, W.J., 1950. Influence of progressive-resistance exercises on knee function following femoral fractures. JBJS 32 (4), 910—924.

DeMichele, P.L., Pollock, M.L., Graves, J.E., et al., 1997. Isometric torso rotation strength: effect of training frequency on its development. Arch. Phys. Med. Rehabil. 78, 64—69.

Demirel, H.A., Powers, S.K., Naito, H., et al., 1999. Exercise-induced alterations in skeletal muscle myosin heavy chain phenotype: dose—response relationship. J. Appl. Physiol. 86, 1002—1008.

deVries, H.A., Housh, T.J., 1994. In: Physiology of Exercise for Physical Education, Athletics and Exercise Science, fifth ed. Brown & Benchmark, Madison, Wisconsin.

DiNubile, N.A., 1991. Strength training. Clin. Sports Med. 10 (1), 33–62.

Earp, J.E., Newton, R.U., Cormie, P., et al., 2015. Inhomogeneous quadriceps femoris hypertrophy in response to strength and power training. Med. Sci. Sports Exerc. 47, 2389–2397.

Eldred, E., Hagbarth, K.E., 1954. Facilitation and inhibition of gamma efferents by stimulation of certain skin areas. J. Neurophysiol. 17, 59–65.

Enoka, R.M., 1988. Muscle strength and its development: new perspectives. Sports Med. 6, 146–168.

Evans, P., 1980. The healing process at cellular level: a review. Physiotherapy 66 (8), 256–259.

Feigenbaum, M.S., Pollock, M.L., 1999. Prescription of resistance training for health and disease. Med. Sci. Sports Exerc. 31 (1), 38–45.

Franchi, M.V., et al., 2014. Architectural, functional and molecular responses to concentric and eccentric loading in human skeletal muscle. Acta Physiol. 210 (3), 642–654.

Friden, J., Sjostrom, M., Ekblom, B., 1983. Myofibrillar damage following intense eccentric exercise in man. Int. J. Sports Med. 4, 170–176.

Garnett, R., Stephens, J.A., 1981. Changes in the recruitment threshold of motor units produced by cutaneous stimulation in man. J. Physiol. (Lond) 311, 463–473.

Garrett, W.E., 1990. Muscle strain injuries: clinical and basic aspects. Med. Sci. Sports Exerc. 22 (4), 436–443.

Garrett, W.E., Rich, F.R., Nikolaou, P.K., et al., 1989. Computed tomography of hamstring muscle strains. Med. Sci. Sports Exerc. 21 (5), 506–514.

Gea, J.G., 1997. Myosin gene expression in the respiratory muscles. Eur. Respir. J. 10, 2404–2410.

Gerhart, K.D., Yezierski, R.P., Giesler, G.J., et al., 1981. Inhibitory receptive fields of primate spinothalamic tract cells. J. Neurophysiol. 46 (6), 1309–1325.

Gilleard, W., McConnell, J., Parsons, D., 1998. The effect of patellar taping on the onset of vastus medialis obliquus and vastus lateralis muscle activity in persons with patellofemoral pain. Phys. Ther. 78 (1), 25–32.

Grimby, G., 1995. Muscle performance and structure in the elderly as studied cross-sectionally and longitudinally. J. Gerontol. 50A, 17–22 (special issue).

Grgic, J., Garofolini, A., Orazem, J., et al., 2020. Effects of resistance training on muscle size and strength in very elderly adults: a systematic review and meta-analysis of randomized controlled trials. Sports Med. 50 (11), 1983–1999.

Haff, G.G., Nimphius, S., 2012. Training principles for power. Strength Cond. J. 34, 2–12.

Hakkinen, K., Newton, R.U., Gordon, S.E., et al., 1998. Changes in muscle morphology, electromyographic activity, and force production characteristics during progressive strength training in young and older men. J. Gerontol. 53A (6), B415B423.

Harris, N.K., Cronin, J.B., Hopkins, W.G., et al., 2008. Squat jump training at maximal power loads vs. heavy loads: effect on sprint ability. J. Strength Cond. Res. 22, 1742–1749.

Haskell, W.L., Lee, I.M., Pate, R.R., et al., 2007. Physical activity and public health: updated recommendation for adults from the American College of Sports Medicine and the American Heart Association. Med. Sci. Sports Exerc. 39 (8), 1423–1434.

Heinricher, M.M., Fields, H.L., 2013. Central nervous system mechanisms of pain modulation. In: Wall, P.D., Melzack, R. (Eds.), Textbook of Pain, sixth ed. Churchill Livingstone, Edinburgh, pp. 129–142.

Hill, A.V., 1938. The heat of shortening and the dynamic constants of muscle. Proc. R. Soc. Lond. (Biology) 126, 136–195.

Hill, A.V., 1950. The series elastic component of muscle. Proc. R. Soc. B137, 273–280.

Hodges, P.W., Richardson, C.A., 1996. Inefficient muscular stabilization of the lumbar spine associated with low back pain. A motor control evaluation of transversus abdominis. Spine 21 (22), 2640–2650.

Hody, S., Croisier, J.L., Bury, T., et al., 2019. Eccentric muscle contractions: risks and benefits. Front. Physiol. 10, 536.

Holloszy, J.O., 1976. Adaptations of muscular tissue to training. Prog. Cardiovasc. Dis. 18 (6), 445–458.

Hortobagyi, T., Dempsey, L., Fraser, D., et al., 2000. Changes in muscle strength, muscle fibre size and myofibrillar gene expression after immobilization and retraining in humans. J. Physiol. 524 (1), 293–304.

Hortobagyi, T., Hill, J.P., Houmard, J.A., et al., 1996. Adaptive responses to muscle lengthening and shortening in humans. J. Appl. Physiol. 80 (3), 765–772.

Housh, D.J., Housh, T.J., Johnson, G.O., et al., 1992. Hypertrophic response to unilateral concentric isokinetic resistance training. J. Appl. Physiol. 73, 65–70.

Hunter, G., 1998. Specific soft tissue mobilization in the management of soft tissue dysfunction. Man. Ther. 3 (1), 2–11.

Hurme, T., Kalimo, H., Lehto, M., et al., 1991. Healing of skeletal muscle injury: an ultrastructural and immunohistochemical study. Med. Sci. Sports Exerc. 23 (7), 801–810.

Ingjer, F., 1979. Capillary supply and mitochondrial content of different skeletal muscle fiber types in untrained and endurance-trained men. A histochemical and ultrastructural study. Eur. J. Appl. Physiol. Occup. Physiol. 40, 197–209.

Izquierdo, M., Hakkinen, K., Anton, A., et al., 2001. Maximal strength and power, endurance performance, and serum hormones in middle-aged and elderly men. Med. Sci. Sports Exerc. 33, 1577–1587.

Izquierdo, M., Ibanez, J., Gonzalez-Badillo, J.J., et al., 2006. Differential effects of strength training leading to failure versus not to failure on hormonal responses, strength, and muscle power gains. J. Appl. Physiol. 100, 1647–1656.

Jarvinen, M.J., Lehto, M.U.K., 1993. The effects of early mobilisation and immobilisation on the healing process following muscle injuries. Sports Med. 15 (2), 78–89.

Jenner, J.R., Stephens, J.A., 1982. Cutaneous reflex responses and their central nervous system pathways studied in man. J. Physiol. (Lond.) 333, 405–419.

Jones, D.A., Newham, D.J., Round, J.M., et al., 1986. Experimental human muscle damage: morphological changes in relation to other indices of damage. J. Physiol. 375, 435–448.

Jozsa, L., Kannus, P., 1997. Human Tendons: Anatomy, Physiology and Pathology. Human Kinetics, Champaign, IL.

Kanda, K., Sugama, K., Hayashida, H., et al., 2013. Eccentric exercise-induced delayed-onset muscle soreness and changes in markers of muscle damage and inflammation. Exerc. Immunol. Rev. 19, 72–85.

Kaneko, M., Fuchimoto, T., Toji, H., et al., 1983. Training effect of different loads on the force-velocity relationship and mechanical power output in human muscle. Scand. J. Med. Sci. Sports 5, 50–55.

Kaser, L., Mannion, A.F., Rhyner, A., et al., 2001. Active therapy for chronic low back pain part 2. Effects on paraspinal muscle cross-sectional area, fiber type size, and distribution. Spine 26 (8), 909–919.

Kawakami, Y., Abe, T., Fukunaga, T., 1993. Muscle-fiber pennation angles are greater in hypertrophied than in normal muscles. J. Appl. Physiol. 74 (6), 2740–2744.

Kawakami, Y., Abe, T., Kuno, S.-Y., et al., 1995. Training-induced changes in muscle architecture and specific tension. Eur. J. Appl. Physiol. 72, 37–43.

Kellett, J., 1986. Acute soft tissue injuries – a review of the literature. Med. Sci. Sports Exerc. 18 (5), 489–500.

Knight, K.L., 1985. Guidelines for rehabilitation of sports injuries. Clin. Sports Med. 4 (3), 405–416.

Komi, P.V., 1986. Training of muscle strength and power: interaction of neuromotoric, hypertrophic, and mechanical factors. Int. J. Sports Med. 7 (Suppl), 10–15.

Kornberg, C., Lew, P., 1989. The effect of stretching neural structures on grade one hamstring injuries. J. Orthop. Sports Phys. Ther. 6, 481–487.

Kvist, H., Kvist, M., 1980. The operative treatment of chronic calcaneal paratenonitis. J. Bone Joint Surg. 62B (3), 353–357.

Labarque, V.L., Eijnde, B., Van Leemputte, M., 2002. Effect of immobilization and retraining on torque–velocity relationship of human knee flexor and extensor muscles. Eur. J. Appl. Physiol. 86, 251–257.

Leggett, S.H., Graves, J.E., Pollock, M.L., et al., 1991. Quantitative assessment and training of isometric cervical extension strength. Am. J. Sports Med. 19 (6), 653–659.

Lehmann, J.F., Masock, A.J., Warren, C.G., et al., 1970. Effect of therapeutic temperature on tendon extensibility. Arch. Phys. Med. Rehabil. 51 (8), 481–487.

Maestroni, L., Read, P., Bishop, C., et al., 2020. The benefits of strength training on musculoskeletal system health: practical applications for interdisciplinary care. Sports Med. 50 (8), 1431–1450.

Mannion, A.F., Taimela, S., Muntener, M., et al., 2001. Active therapy for chronic low back pain. Part I. Effects on back muscle activation, fatigability, and strength. Spine 26 (8), 897–908.

McConnell, J., 2002. Recalcitrant chronic low back and leg pain – a new theory and different approach to management. Man. Ther. 7 (4), 183–192.

Melissa, L., MacDougall, J.D., Tarnopolsky, M.A., et al., 1997. Skeletal muscle adaptations to training under normobaric hypoxic versus normoxic conditions. Med. Sci. Sports Exerc. 29 (2), 238–243.

Melzack, R., 1975. Prolonged relief of pain by brief, intense transcutaneous somatic stimulation. Pain 1, 357–373.

Melzack, R., Wall, P.D., 1965. Pain mechanisms: a new theory. Science 150, 971–979.

Mense, S., Meyer, H., 1985. Different types of slowly conducting afferent units in cat skeletal muscle and tendon. J. Physiol. 363, 403–417.

Moore, S.P., Marteniuk, R.G., 1986. Kinematic and electromyographic changes that occur as a function of learning a time-constrained aiming task. J. Mot. Behav. 18 (4), 397–426.

Moritani, T., DeVries, H.A., 1979. Neural factors versus hypertrophy in the time course of muscle strength gain. Am. J. Phys. Med. 58 (3), 115–130.

Narici, M.V., Hoppeler, H., Kayser, B., et al., 1996. Human quadriceps cross-sectional area, torque and neural activation during 6 months strength training. Acta. Physiol. Scand. 157, 175–186.

Nelson, M.E., Rejeski, W.J., Blair, S.N., et al., 2007. Physical activity and public health in older adults: recommendation from the American College of Sports Medicine and the American Heart Association. Med. Sci. Sports Exerc. 39 (8), 1435–1445.

Newham, D.J., Hurley, M.V., Jones, D.W., 1989. Ligamentous knee injuries and muscle inhibition. J. Orthop. Rheumatol. 2, 163–173.

Newton, R.U., Hakkinen, K., Hakkinen, A., et al., 2002. Mixed-methods resistance training increases power and strength of young and older men. Med. Sci. Sports Exerc. 34 (8), 1367–1375.

Pollock, M.L., Graves, J.E., Bamman, M.M., et al., 1993. Frequency and volume of resistance training: effect on cervical extension strength. Arch. Phys. Med. Rehabil. 74, 1080–1086.
Rigby, B.J., 1964. The effect of mechanical extension upon the thermal stability of collagen. Biochim. Biophys. Acta. 79 (SC 43008), 634–636.
Rohter, F.D., Rochelle, R.H., Hyman, C., 1963. Exercise blood flow changes in the human forearm during physical training. J. Appl. Physiol. 18 (4), 789–793.
Sale, D.G., 1988. Neural adaptation to resistance training. Med. Sci. Sports Exerc. 20 (5), S135–S145.
Sale, D.G., MacDougall, J.D., Upton, A.R.M., et al., 1983. Effect of strength training upon motor neurone excitability in man. Med. Sci. Sports Exerc. 15 (1), 57–62.
Sapega, A.A., Quedenfield, T.C., Moyer, R.A., et al., 1981. Biophysical factors in range-of-motion exercise. Phys. Sportsmed. 9 (12), 57–65.
Schoenfeld, B.J., Grgic, J., Every, D.W.V., Plotkin, D.L., et al., 2021. Loading recommendations for muscle strength, hypertrophy, and local endurance: a re-examination of the repetition continuum. Sports 9 (2), 32.
Scott, W., Stevens, J., Binder-Macleod, S.A., 2001. Human skeletal muscle fiber type classifications. Phys. Ther. 81 (11), 1810–1816.
Seynnes, O.R., de Boer, M., Narici, M.V., 2007. Early skeletal muscle hypertrophy and architectural changes in response to high-intensity resistance training. J. Appl. Physiol. 102, 368–373.
Simoneau, J.A., Lortie, G., Boulay, M.R., et al., 1986. Inheritance of human skeletal muscle and anaerobic capacity adaptation to high-intensity intermittent training. Int. J. Sports Med. 7, 167–171.
Spiering, B.A., Mujika, I., Sharp, M.A., et al., 2021. Maintaining physical performance: the minimal dose of exercise needed to preserve endurance and strength over time. J. Strength Cond. Res. 35 (5), 1449–1458.
Staron, R.S., Karapondo, D.L., Kraemer, W.J., et al., 1994. Skeletal muscle adaptations during early phase of heavy-resistance training in men and women. J. Appl. Physiol. 76, 1247–1255.
Suchomel, T.J., Nimphius, S., Stone, M.H., et al., 2016. The importance of muscular strength in athletic performance. Sports Med 46 (10), 1419–1449.
Suetta, C., Aagaard, P., Rosted, A., et al., 2004. Training-induced changes in muscle CSA, muscle strength, EMG, and rate of force development in elderly subjects after long-term unilateral disuse. J. Appl. Physiol. (1985) 97, 1954–1961.
Takai, S., Woo, S.L.-Y., Horibe, S., et al., 1991. The effects of frequency and duration of controlled passive mobilization on tendon healing. J. Orthop. Res. 9, 705–713.
Taylor, D.C., Dalton, J.D., Seaber, A.V., et al., 1990. Viscoelastic properties of muscle–tendon units the biomechanical effects of stretching. Am. J. Sports Med. 18 (3), 300–309.
Taylor, N.F., Dodd, K.J., Shields, N., et al., 2007. Therapeutic exercise in physiotherapy practice is beneficial: a summary of systematic reviews 2002–2005. Aust. J. Physiother. 53, 7–16.
Terrados, N., Jansson, E., Sylven, C., et al., 1990. Is hypoxia a stimulus for synthesis of oxidative enzymes and myoglobin? J. Appl. Physiol. 68, 2369–2372.
Tidball, J.G., 1991. Myotendinous junction injury in relation to junction structure and molecular composition. Exerc. Sport Sci. Rev. 19, 419–445.
Tobin, S., Robinson, G., 2000. The effect of McConnell's vastus lateralis inhibition taping technique on vastus lateralis and vastus medialis obliquus activity. Physiotherapy 86 (4), 173–183.
Todd, J.S., Shurley, J.P., Todd, T.C., 2012. Thomas L. DeLorme and the science of progressive resistance exercise. J. Strength Cond. Res. 26, 2913–2923.
Toji, H., Kaneko, M., 2004. Effect of multiple-load training on the force–velocity relationship. J. Strength Cond. Res. 18, 792–795.
Toji, H., Suei, K., Kaneko, M., 1997. Effects of combined training loads on relations among force, velocity, and power development. Can. J. Appl. Physiol. 22, 328–336.
Turner, A.N., Comfort, P., McMahon, J.J., et al., 2020a. Developing powerful athletes, part 1: mechanical underpinnings. Strength Cond. J. 42 (3), 30–39.
Turner, A.N., Comfort, P., McMahon, J.J., et al., 2020b. Developing powerful athletes part 2: practical applications. Strength Cond. J. 43 (1), 23–31.
Vanderhoof, E.R., Imig, C.J., Hines, H.M., 1961. Effect of muscle strength and endurance development on blood flow. J. Appl. Physiol. 16 (5), 873–877.
Vlaeyen, J.W.S., Crombez, G., 1999. Fear of movement/(re) injury, avoidance and pain disability in chronic low back pain patients. Man. Ther. 4 (4), 187–195.
Waddell, G., 2004. Diagnostic triage. In: Waddell, G. (Ed.), The Back Pain Revolution, second ed. Churchill Livingstone, Edinburgh, p. 9.
Waddell, G., Main, C.J., 2004. Beliefs about back pain. In: Waddell, G. (Ed.), The Back Pain Revolution, second ed. Churchill Livingstone, Edinburgh, pp. 187–202.
Yaksh, T.L., Elde, R.P., 1981. Factors governing release of methionine enkephalin-like immunoreactivity from mesencephalon and spinal cord of the cat in vivo. J. Neurophysiol. 46 (5), 1056–1075.

6

Classification and Pathophysiology of Nerve-Related Musculoskeletal Pain

Colette Ridehalgh and Jennifer Ward

LEARNING OUTCOMES

After studying this chapter, you should be able to:

- Describe the overall structure of the peripheral and central nervous system.
- Understand the physiological mechanisms involved in maintaining a normal, healthy nerve environment.
- Explain how the nervous system is connected.
- Describe how the structure of the nervous system enables normal function and protects the nervous system.
- Have a better understanding of the rationale behind neurodynamic tests.
- Describe the pathophysiological mechanisms that contribute to nerve-related musculoskeletal pain.
- Explain the different pain mechanisms involved in persons with nerve-related musculoskeletal pain.
- Describe the signs, symptoms and classification of neuropathic pain.
- Be aware of the different screening tools.
- Understand how to complete a bedside clinical examination.
- Discuss the risk factors for developing neuropathic pain.

CHAPTER CONTENTS

Persons presenting with nerve-related musculoskeletal dysfunction have markedly varied presentations and pathologies, ranging from central nervous system pathology with resultant CNS neurological findings through to nerve root and peripheral nerve pathology (with or without loss of peripheral nerve function). The thoughtful clinician must clinically reason to differentiate between such presentations and establish a suitable management plan accordingly. The patient with signs and symptoms of cauda equina syndrome (CES), myelopathy or an acute flaccid foot drop, for example, needs appropriate referral onwards as a matter of urgency (see Chapter 11), whilst patients with altered sensation in a recognized territory such as a dermatome or peripheral nerve distribution will require close monitoring of their neurological status and careful evaluation of their response to treatment. In order for the clinician to manage the patient appropriately, it is important to have a thorough understanding of both normal structure and function of the nervous system and pathophysiology of nerve-related musculoskeletal conditions.

STRUCTURE AND FUNCTION OF THE NERVOUS SYSTEM

The nervous system can be broadly divided into the central nervous system (brain and spinal cord), autonomic nervous system and peripheral nervous system (cranial nerves and spinal nerves with their branches).

Anatomy and Physiology of the Spinal Cord

The human spinal cord extends from the foramen magnum to the conus medullaris around the level of the first lumbar vertebra. From the conus medullaris, the roots of the cauda equina (horse's tail) project inferiorly (Fig. 6.1). Three layers of connective tissue, collectively known as the meninges, surround and protect the delicate brain and the spinal cord; they are the dura mater, arachnoid mater and pia mater (Fig. 6.2). The main function of these layers is to protect the brain and spinal cord.

Blood is supplied to the spinal cord segmentally from the aorta and other adjacent arteries, including the vertebral, cervical, intercostal, lumbar and sacral arteries. Each segmental artery passes through the intervertebral foramina and divides into the dorsal (posterior) and ventral (anterior) radicular arteries. The ventral radicular arteries supply the anterior spinal artery, which runs in the midline down the ventral aspect of the cord. The anterior artery provides 75% of the

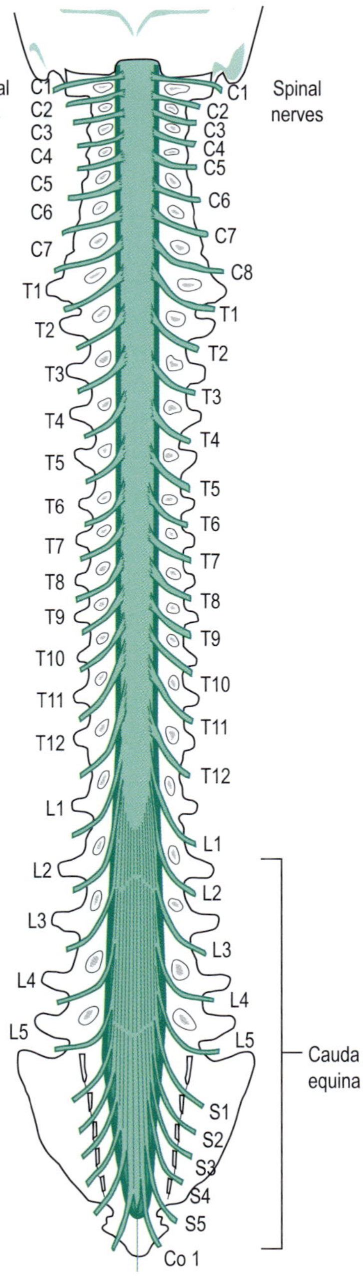

Fig. 6.1 The human spinal cord extending from the occiput to the conus medullaris, from where the roots of the cauda equina project inferiorly. *(From Palastanga & Soames 2012, with permission.)*

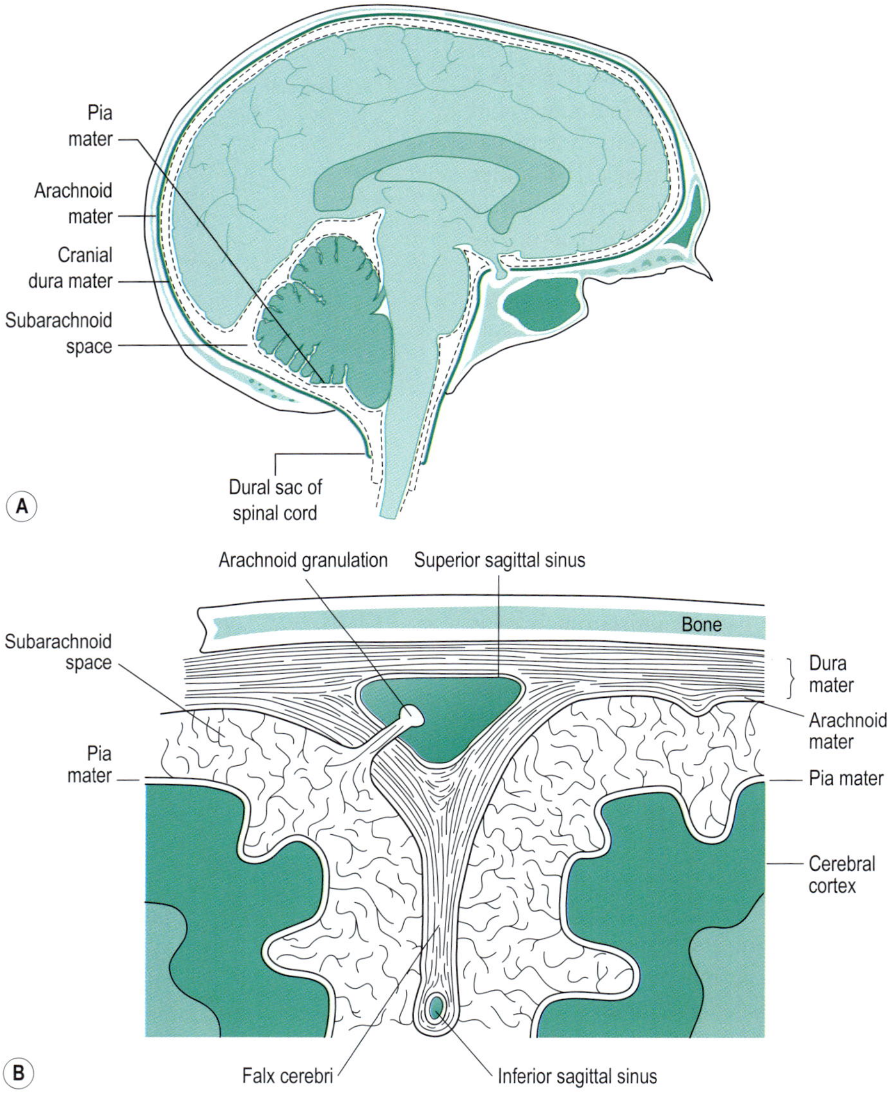

Fig. 6.2 The meninges. (A) Longitudinal section, showing the meningeal covering of the brain. (B) The meningeal covering at the falx cerebri. (*From Palastanga & Soames 2012, with permission.*)

cord's vascularity. The dorsal radicular arteries feed the two posterior spinal arteries, which supply the remainder of the cord (Fig. 6.3). As well as the arterial system, which envelops the spinal cord from the anterior and posterior arteries, venous drainage occurs via an extensive venous plexus.

Spinal rootlets project from the spinal cord both dorsally and ventrally. These rootlets unite to form the dorsal and ventral roots. The dorsal roots contain sensory fibres, whilst the ventral roots contain motor fibres (Fig. 6.4). The cell bodies of the ventral nerve axons lie in the grey matter of the ventral horn within the spinal cord, whilst the cell bodies of the dorsal axons lie outside the spinal cord in the dorsal root ganglion (DRG). The dorsal and ventral roots are enveloped by an extension of the dura mater known as the dural sleeve. The dorsal and ventral roots soon converge to form the roots of the spinal nerves, which

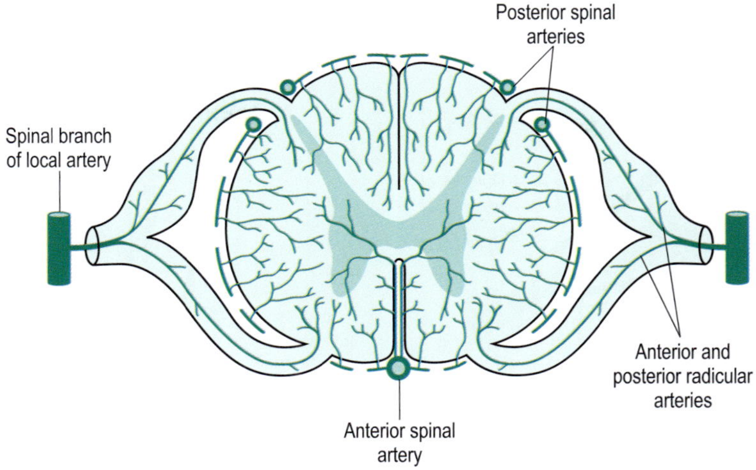

Fig. 6.3 Arterial blood supply to the spinal cord. (*From Middleditch & Oliver 2005, with permission.*)

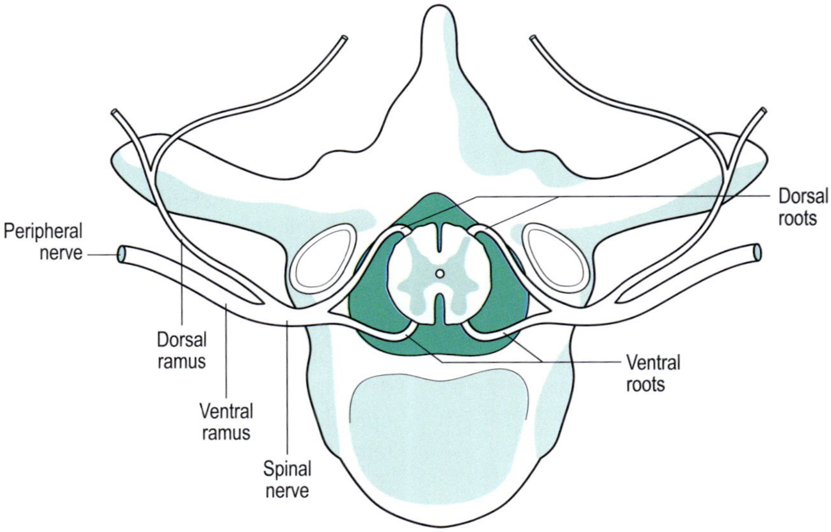

Fig. 6.4 A horizontal cross-section of the spinal cord demonstrating the dorsal and ventral roots. (*After Palastanga & Soames 2012, with permission.*)

contain the sensory and motor nerve fibres responsible for the innervation of a segment of the body. The dural sleeve becomes the epineurium (Fig. 6.5).

The spinal nerve roots descend within the spinal canal by varying amounts and then exit the intervertebral foramina, as shown in Fig. 6.1. The nerve roots are named according to the level of the spine from which they emerge. There are 8 pairs of cervical roots (the first of which emerges above the level of C1), 12 pairs of thoracic roots, 5 pairs of lumbar roots, 5 pairs of sacral roots and 1 pair of coccygeal roots. Since there are eight cervical nerve roots, this means that C1–C7 nerve roots exit above their respective vertebral level, C8 exits below C7, and from the thoracic spine caudally, the nerve roots exit from below their respective vertebral level. The sensory nerve fibres within each nerve root supply a specific segment of skin known as a dermatome. Similarly, the motor fibres within each

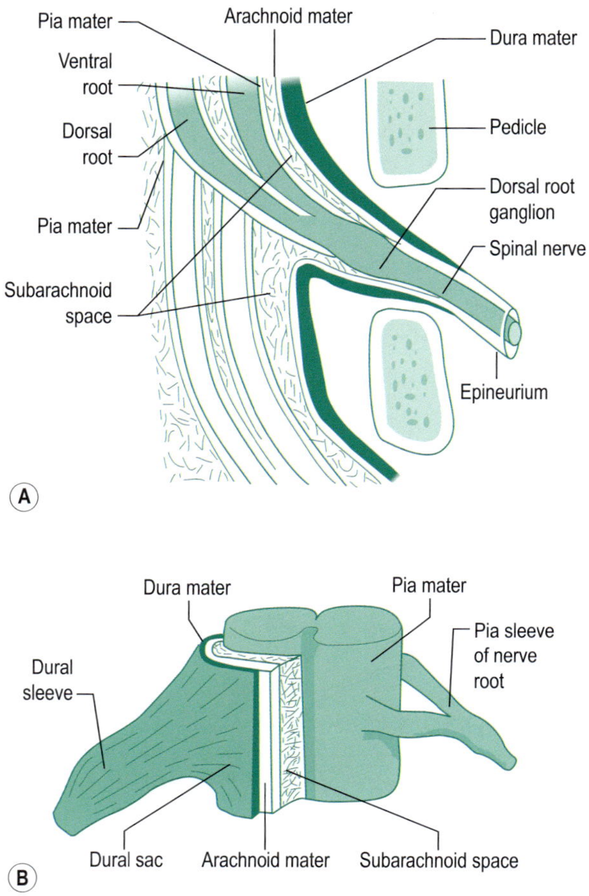

Fig. 6.5 (A) The relationship of the meningeal layers to the dorsal and ventral roots. (B) The roots are enveloped by an extension of the dura mater to form the dural sleeve. (*From Palastanga & Soames 2012, with permission.*)

nerve root supply a given muscle known as a myotome (shown in Fig. 4.27). Although dermatomal and myotomal innervation is not exact, as there is some cross-over in the dermatomal fields and muscles are typically supplied by more than one nerve root, clinically this arrangement can be very useful in determining the site of a lesion. Perhaps more accurate for skin sensation is the use of signature zones or distinctive regions (Nitta et al., 1993), which have been found to be more consistent in determining the nerve root level. These areas (Fig. 6.6) were shown to be accurate in greater than 85% of participants with lumbosacral disc herniation after selective nerve root block.

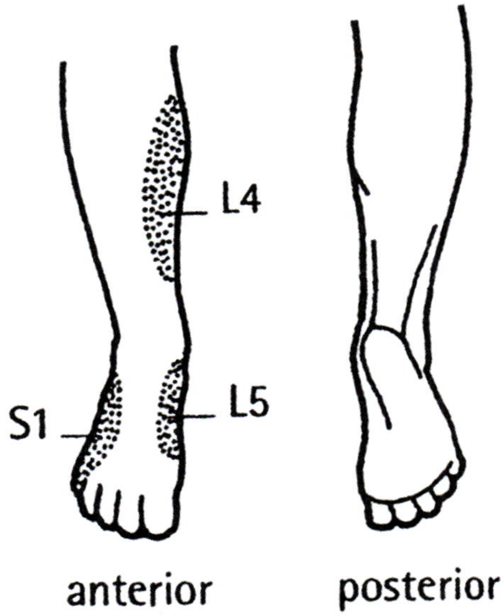

Fig. 6.6 Distinctive zones. (*From Nitta et al. 1993, with permission.*)

Because of the anatomical difference between the nerve root and a peripheral nerve, the root may be more susceptible to mechanical injury. As shown in Fig. 6.5A, the nerve sheath is relatively thin. The perineurium, which importantly acts as a diffusion barrier to protect the delicate endoneurial environment (Peltonen et al., 2013) and helps to maintain resting tension, is poorly developed, and the epineurium is also not well developed when compared to the peripheral nerve, where it tends to be thickened to provide protection when passing over bony prominences. The dura and arachnoid mater, together with the cerebrospinal fluid, are therefore almost solely responsible for protecting the nerve root as it exits the intervertebral foramen. The connective tissue covering of peripheral nerves is discussed later in this chapter.

On exiting the intervertebral foramina, the spinal nerve divides into two branches: the dorsal and ventral rami. The dorsal rami supply the zygapophyseal joints, muscles and skin overlying the head, neck and spine. The ventral rami supply the anterior and lateral trunk, and the upper and lower limbs. The ventral rami, which become the peripheral nerves, join in the cervical region to form the cervical and brachial plexi and in the lumbar and sacral regions to form the lumbar, lumbosacral and sacral plexi (Fig. 6.7). A branch from

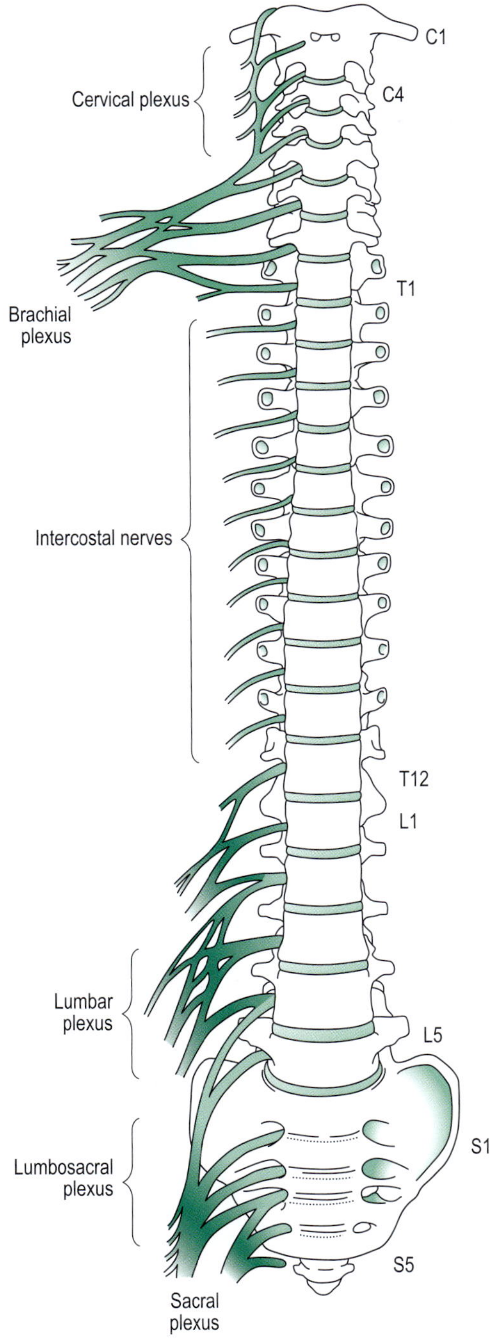

Fig. 6.7 Spinal nerves exit the intervertebral foramina to form the cervical, brachial, lumbar, lumbosacral and sacral plexi. (*From Palastanga & Soames 2012, with permission.*)

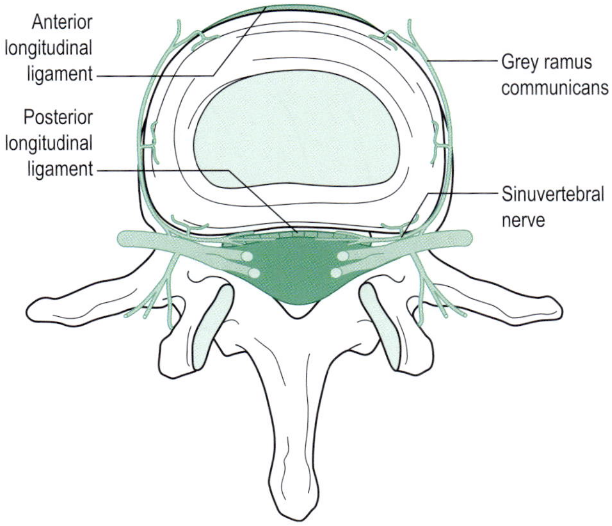

Fig. 6.8 The nerve supply of the intervertebral disc. (*From Baron et al. 2015, with permission.*)

the ventral rami, together with an autonomic branch from the grey ramus communicans, forms the sinuvertebral nerve, which passes into the intervertebral foramen. On entering the canal, the sinuvertebral nerve branches to form a complex neural network that innervates the posterior longitudinal ligament, the dura mater and outer third of the annulus fibrosus of the disc at the level of entry but also the disc one level above (Adams et al., 2006; Baron et al., 2015) (Fig. 6.8).

Tracts of the Spinal Cord

Information is continually relayed to and from the peripheries along a series of well-organized tracts within the white matter of the spinal cord. An ascending nerve signal must, however, first enter the spinal cord. This occurs via a given axon that enters the dorsal horn and terminates in the grey matter. In cross-section, the grey matter conforms to a pattern of lamination known as Rexed's laminae (Fig. 6.9). The ascending nerve signal must therefore cross one or more synapses to pass into the appropriate ascending tract within the white matter. The distinct tracts which convey ascending and descending information are represented in Fig. 6.10. A nerve signal may synapse several times en route to the cortex and may move into

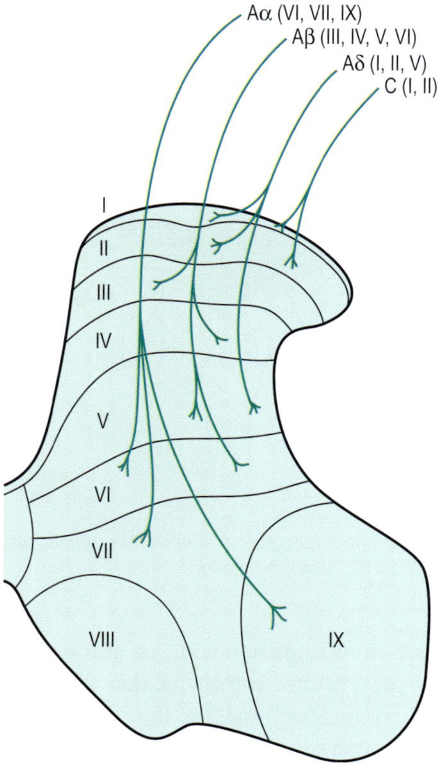

Fig. 6.9 Laminae of Rexed and the termination of afferent fibres. (*After Todd & Koerber 2006.*)

different tracts within the white matter at different stages of its journey. The ascending signal eventually reaches the thalamus, from where it is projected to the cortex. For a descending nerve signal, the converse is true. The signal travels down a descending tract within the white matter before synapsing, passing into the grey matter and exiting the spinal cord via the ventral horn.

It is outside the scope of this book to describe the ascending and descending tracts of the spinal cord in detail. For further detail, the reader is directed to Crossman and Neary (2015) and Mtui et al. (2015).

Anatomy and Physiology of Peripheral Nerves

Sensory and Motor Fibres

Peripheral nerves typically consist of sensory and motor nerve fibres surrounded by connective tissue. A typical sensory nerve fibre consists of dendrites at its distal end (peripheral axon), a cell body lying in the DRG in the intervertebral foramen and a central axon to the dorsal horn in the spinal cord (Fig. 6.11A). A typical motor nerve fibre consists of dendrites, a cell body in the ventral horn of the spinal cord and an axon (see Fig. 6.11B). Each sensory or motor nerve fibre is a single, extremely elongated cell which may run from the spinal cord as far as the toe or finger.

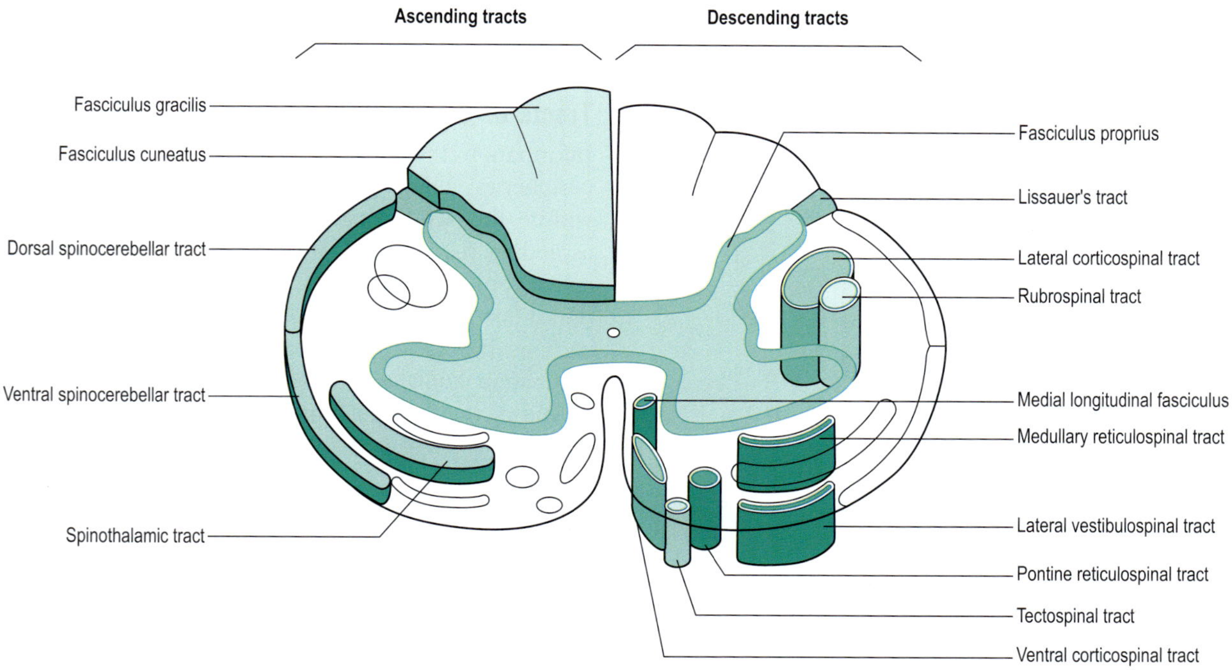

Fig. 6.10 Transverse section of the spinal cord showing the ascending and descending tracts. (*From Crossman & Neary 2015, with permission.*)

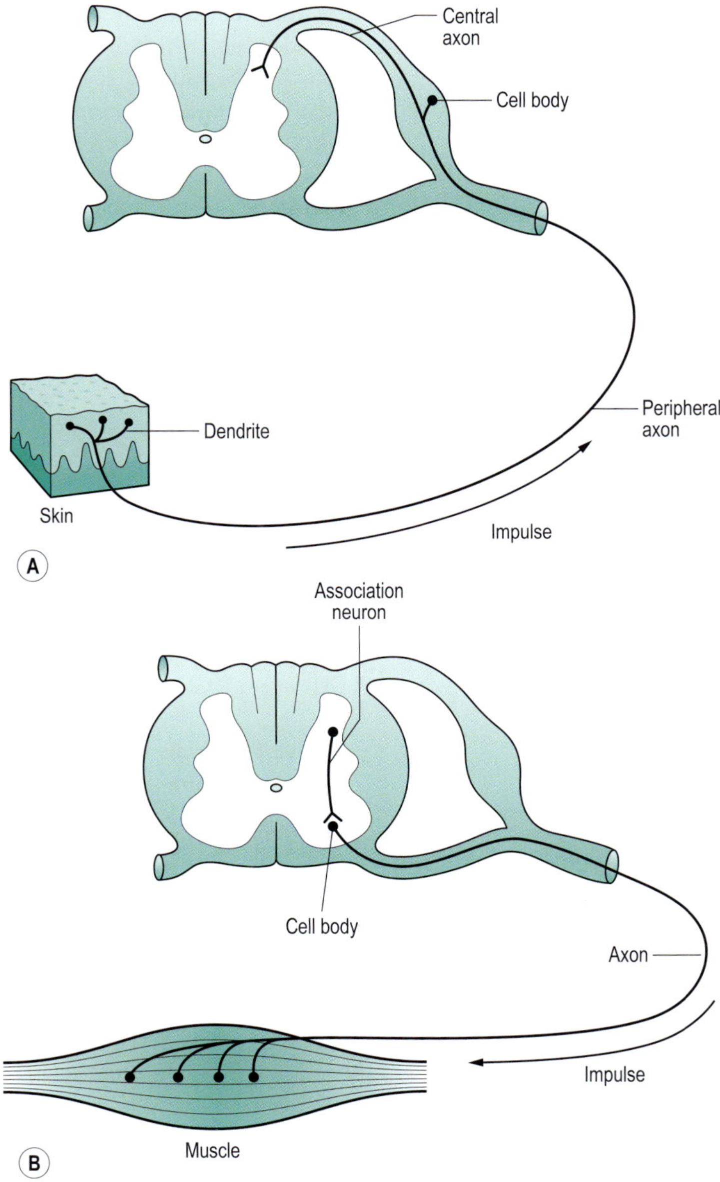

Fig. 6.11 Typical (A) sensory and (B) motor nerve fibres. (*After Marieb 1995. Copyright © 1995 by The Benjamin/Cummings Publishing Company, Inc. Reprinted by permission of Pearson Education, Inc.*)

The fascicles (nerve fibres contained within the perineurium; see later in this chapter) do not have a straight course along a nerve; rather, they repeatedly join and divide to form a complex plexus (Fig. 6.12). The number of fascicles seen in the cross-section of a nerve increases where a nerve crosses a joint, increasing its tensile strength (Sunderland, 1990).

Axons can be myelinated (i.e. surrounded by a myelin sheath) or unmyelinated. The myelin sheath (an insulated layer composed of proteins and lipids) is formed by Schwann cells wrapped a number of times

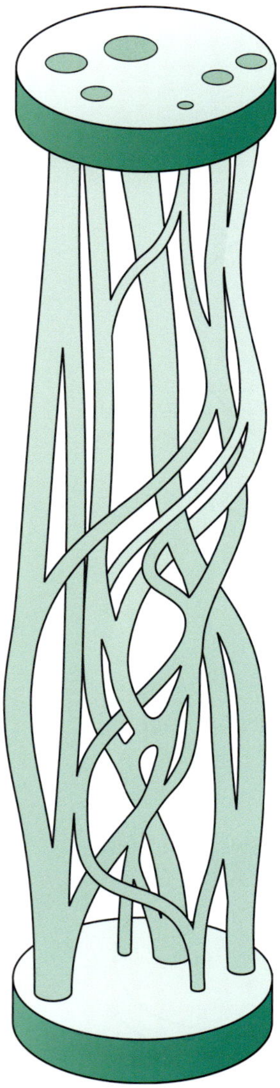

Fig. 6.12 Fascicular plexus within a nerve. (*From Sunderland 1990, with permission.*)

around part of an axon (Fig. 6.13A). By doing so, they create specific zones; the node (nodes of Ranvier), paranode, juxtaparanode and internode (Thaxton & Bhat, 2009). The nodes of Ranvier contain a large proportion of sodium ion channels, whilst the potassium channels are located in the juxtaparanode. Impulses travel along the nerve and 'jump' from one node of Ranvier to the next, a process known as saltatory conduction, which increases the speed of nerve conduction (Schmid, 2015). Unmyelinated nerve fibres are also covered in Schwann cells, but they have no myelin sheath (see Fig. 6.13B). Impulses travel in a continuous manner along an unmyelinated nerve fibre; there is no 'jumping', which reduces the speed of conduction. The nerve fibres are not only different in terms of their myelination but also on their size and function. Table 6.1 displays the different nerve fibres in mammals with their speed of conduction and function.

The sensory nerves end distally in various types of receptors in almost all the tissues of the body. The sensory receptors in joint and muscle have been covered in the relevant chapters on joint and muscle. The cutaneous sensory receptors can be seen in Fig. 6.14.

Free nerve endings responding to noxious mechanical and thermal stimuli are supplied by fast myelinated Aδ and slow unmyelinated C fibres. All the other skin receptors are supplied by fast-conducting myelinated Aβ fibres (Palastanga et al., 2002).

Action Potentials and Ion Channels

The generation of action potentials is due to the response to the stimulation of the receptors. This may be direct if the nerve has free nerve endings within the tissue or as a secondary response to the receptor due to chemical, thermal or mechanical stimuli. Briefly, the receptor must convert, or 'transduce' the input into an electrical impulse. Nociceptors are usually electrically silent, so will transmit all or none of the action potentials when stimulated (Dubin & Patapoutian, 2010). Some nociceptors are termed silent nociceptors because they only become activated after first being sensitised by inflammatory mediators. It is outside the scope of this chapter to detail the generation of action potentials, but see Fig. 6.15 for an overview of the process. When considering the development of neuropathic pain, however, it is useful to consider the ion channels responsible for the transduction of stimuli and thus the generation of action potentials. Specific ion channels such as transient receptor potential (TRP) channels seem to be important in the transduction of a variety of

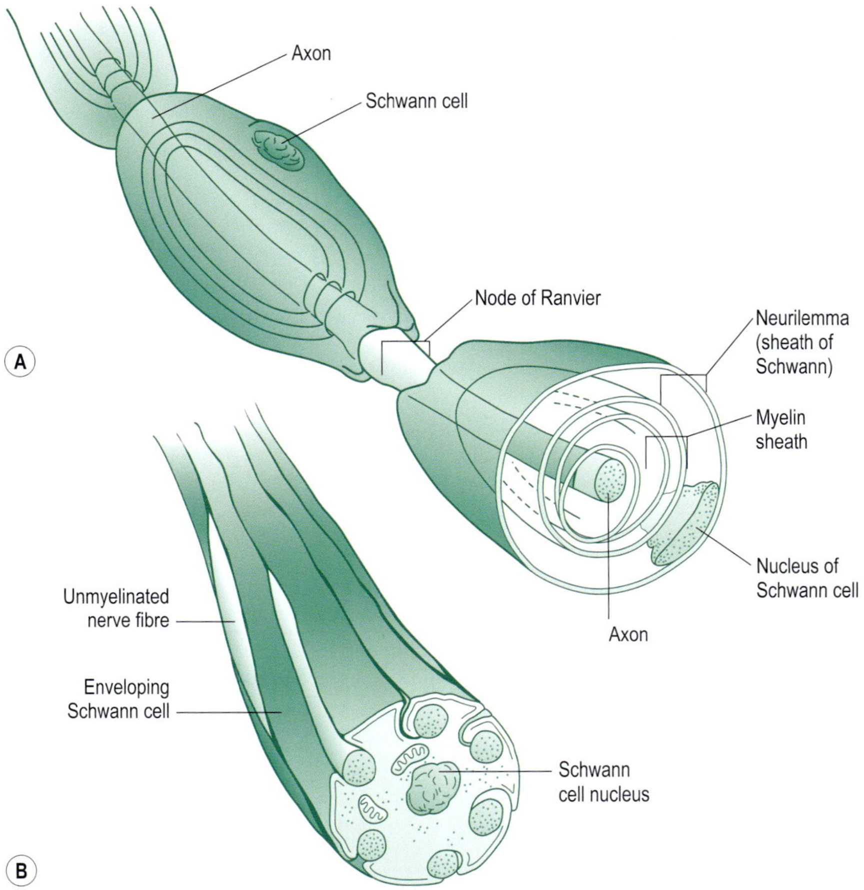

Fig. 6.13 Nerve fibres: (A) myelinated and (B) unmyelinated. (*From Marieb 1995. Copyright © 1995 by The Benjamin/Cummings Publishing Company, Inc. Reprinted by permission of Pearson Education, Inc.*)

noxious stimuli. Once transduction has occurred, voltage gated sodium channels open to amplify the TRP channels leading to the generation of action potentials (Finnerup et al., 2021). There are a variety of different types of ion channels, but genetic mutations of many of these sodium and TRP channels have been found to be involved in neuropathic pain (Finnerup et al., 2021). Such channels have been the target of some neuropathic pain medications, for example, carbamazepine, which is a sodium channel blocker (see Chapter 7).

Axonal Transport

Nerve cells contain axoplasm (synonymous with cytoplasm), which, as in all cells, plays a vital role in cell function. Nerve cells (cell body and axon) can be extremely long structures, running, for example, from the lumbar spine to the toe or from the cervical spine to the finger. Because of these long distances, a special method is required to transport substances from the cell body to the end of the axon and back (Crossman & Neary, 2015; Mtui et al., 2015; Schmid, 2015). This process is active and involves the utilisation of molecular 'motors' which drive contents along hollow

TABLE 6.1 Classification of Peripheral Nerve Fibres

Characteristics of fibre						
Type of sheath			Myelinated		Non-myelinated	
Fibre diameter	22 µm			1.5 µm	2.0–0.1 µm	
Conduction speed (metres/second)	120	60	50	30	4	0.5
Classification			A			
1. Erlanger and Gasser: All fibres				B	C	
Subclasses: Efferent	Aα Skeletomotor	Aβ Fusimotor collaterals of A fibres	Aγ Fusimotor	B Preganglionic autonomic	C Postganglionic autonomic	
Afferent	Aα and smaller. Muscle and tendon; cutaneous			Aβ Cutaneous muscle, visceral, etc.	C Cutaneous muscle, visceral, etc.	
2. Lloyd Afferent – skeletal muscle and articular	I (a) Primary spindle ending (b) Tendon ending	II Secondary spindle ending		III Free ending (nociceptor etc.), paciniform ending?	IV Free ending (nociceptor, etc.)	

It should be noted that the scale for conduction velocities is not arithmetical.
Williams, P.L., Warwick, R., 1980. Gray's Anatomy, thirty-sixth ed. Churchill Livingstone, Edinburgh.

microtubules within the axon. There are three methods of axonal transport: fast anterograde (forward moving to the end of the axon, to the periphery), slow anterograde and fast retrograde (backward moving towards the cell body) (Mtui et al., 2015).

1. Fast anterograde axonal transport moves synaptic vesicles, transmitter substances and mitochondria to the terminal of the nerve. Axonal transport occurs at a rate of approximately 300–400 mm/day (Dahlin & Lundborg, 1990; Mtui et al., 2015).
2. Slow anterograde axonal transport is the method by which the majority of axoplasm moves. Fibrous and soluble proteins and enzymes are transported slowly along the axon at a rate of 5–10 mm/day (Mtui et al., 2015).
3. Fast retrograde axonal transport moves materials from the end of the axon to the cell body. These materials can be degraded or recycled, or inform the cell body about events at the end of the axon (Bisby, 1982; Dahlin & Lundborg, 1990). For example, where nerve growth factor is released to stimulate the growth of neurons, this is transported back to inform the cell body (Schwartz, 1991). The rate of transport is about 150–200 mm/day (Mtui et al., 2015).

Immune Cells

The perineurium provides a blood–nerve diffusion barrier which protects the delicate endoneurial environment (Peltonen et al., 2013). Because of this barrier, immune cells cannot freely enter the axons to counter an attack from infectious pathogens. Thus a small number of immune cells such as lymphocytes, macrophages and mast cells reside within the endoneurium to allow an immune response (Schmid, 2015). These immune cells have an inflammatory effect once activated,

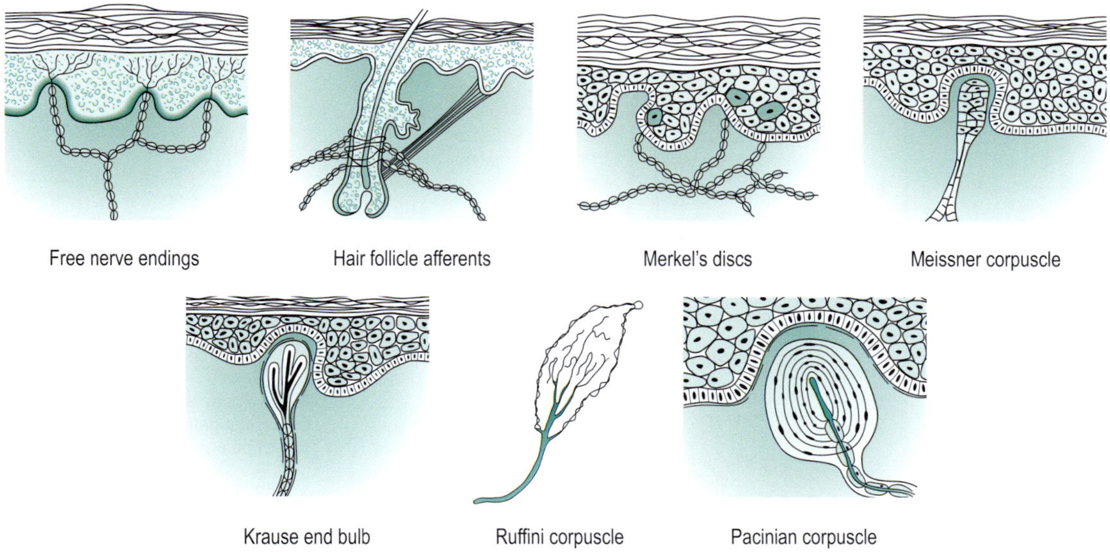

Fig. 6.14 Sensory receptors in the skin. (*From Palastanga & Soames 2012, with permission.*)

releasing inflammatory mediators such as cytokines. Furthermore, other cells such as Schwann cells within the peripheral nervous system and glial cells (microglia and astrocytes) within the dorsal horn are able to release cytokines and chemokines, sensitising the nociceptors. In particular, certain ion channels may be sensitive to certain cytokines. For example, IL-1β has been shown to sensitize TRPV1, one of the TRP family of ion channels which is sensitive to heat and chemicals (Kiguchi et al., 2012) (you will know about this channel as TRPV1 is sensitive to one such chemical called capsaicin—found in chilli pepper, and responsible for pain when you accidentally rub your eyes after chopping chillis!). The ability of these cells to produce such a strong inflammatory cascade after nerve injury is thought to be a large contribution to neuropathic pain (Kiguchi et al., 2012).

Connective Tissue Covering of Peripheral Nerves

Nerve fibres are organised into a bundle (or fascicle) and embedded in a layer of connective tissue composed of collagen and fibroblasts called the endoneurium. Each fascicle is surrounded by another layer of connective tissue called the perineurium. The perineurium acts as a diffusion barrier between the adjacent tissues (Rydevik & Lundborg, 1977; Sunderland, 1990) and is considered to be mostly responsible for providing nerves with tensile strength and elasticity (Sunderland, 1990). The outermost layer of connective tissue of a peripheral nerve is called the epineurium, consisting of loose connective tissue which helps to protect the nerve during movement (Fig. 6.16).

Blood Supply of Peripheral Nerves

Peripheral nerves are well vascularized (Fig. 6.17). Blood vessels running alongside nerves send regional feeding vessels to the epineurium which then divide and supply the deep and superficial layers of the epineurium, perineurium and endoneurium (Lundborg et al., 1987). The blood vessels are coiled, which allows a certain amount of lengthening to occur without affecting blood flow (Fig. 6.18). Vessels lie obliquely in the perineurium, and it is thought that increased endoneurial pressure will therefore close these vessels

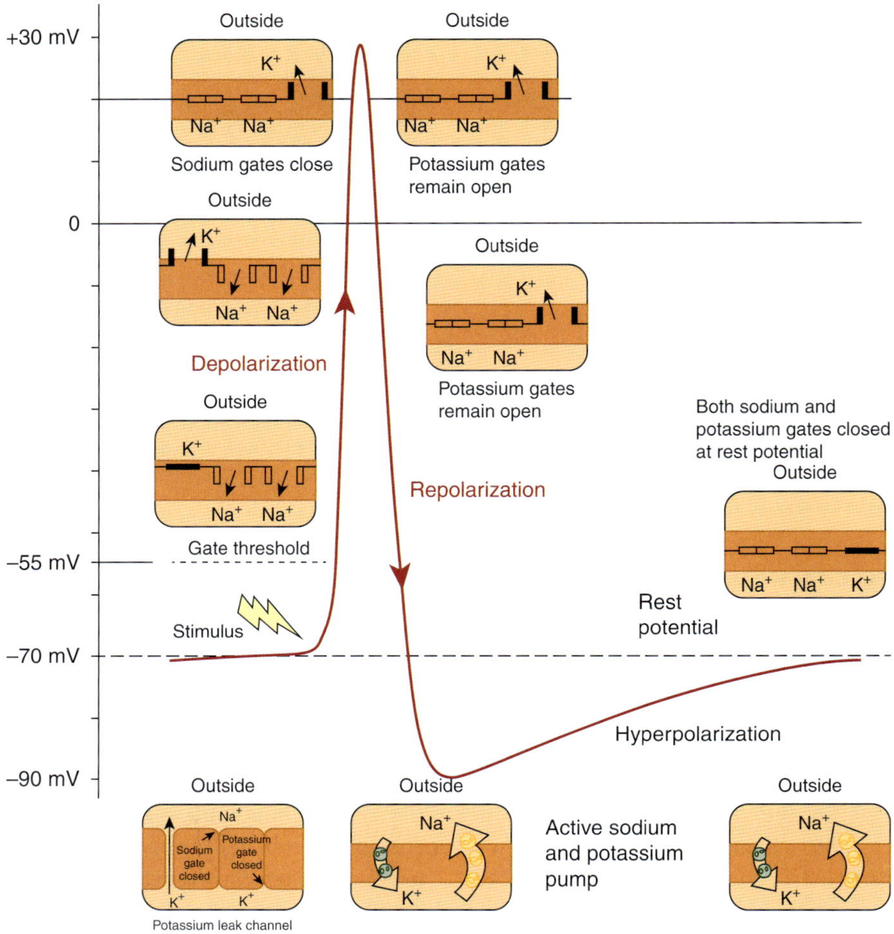

Fig. 6.15 Action potential. (*From http://hyperphysics.phy-astr.gsu.edu/hbase/Biology/actpot.html#c3 with permission.*)

(Lundborg, 1975). This is supported by the fact that a small increase in endoneurial pressure results in a reduction in blood flow within the endoneurium (Lundborg et al., 1983). Clinically, commonly encountered conditions such as carpal tunnel syndrome (CTS) or cervical or lumbosacral radiculopathy with resultant inflammation and oedema may cause elevations in endoneurial pressure resulting in ischaemia (Rydevik & Lundborg, 1977; Rydevik et al., 1981).

Nerve Supply of Peripheral Nerves

The connective tissue sheaths surrounding peripheral nerves are innervated by the nervi nervorum (Fig. 6.19) (Hromada, 1963; Bove & Light, 1995). The epineurium, perineurium and endoneurium contain both free nerve endings and encapsulated endings, and the afferent fibres are mostly unmyelinated C fibres with some thinly myelinated fibres (Hromada, 1963). The nerve supply originates from the axons within the sheath and from the blood vessels that supply the nerve (Hromada, 1963; Bahns et al., 1986; Bove & Light, 1995). The nerve endings respond to high-threshold mechanical stimuli as well as chemical stimuli (capsaicin, bradykinin, hypertonic sodium chloride or potassium chloride) and thermal stimuli, and are therefore considered to have a nociceptive function (Bahns et al., 1986; Bove & Light, 1995). The connective tissue of nerve can therefore be a direct source of pain, by mechanical deformation or chemicals released with inflammation. As such, injury to

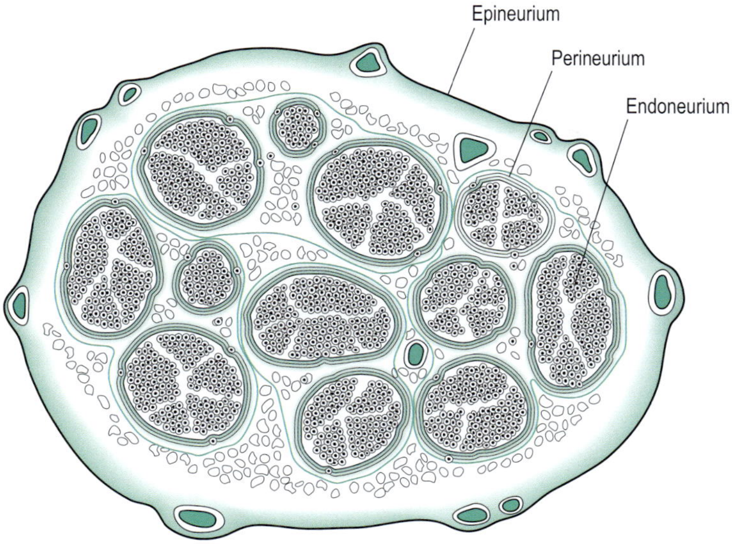

Fig. 6.16 Layers of connective tissue around nerve fibres. (*After Lundborg et al. 1987, with permission.*)

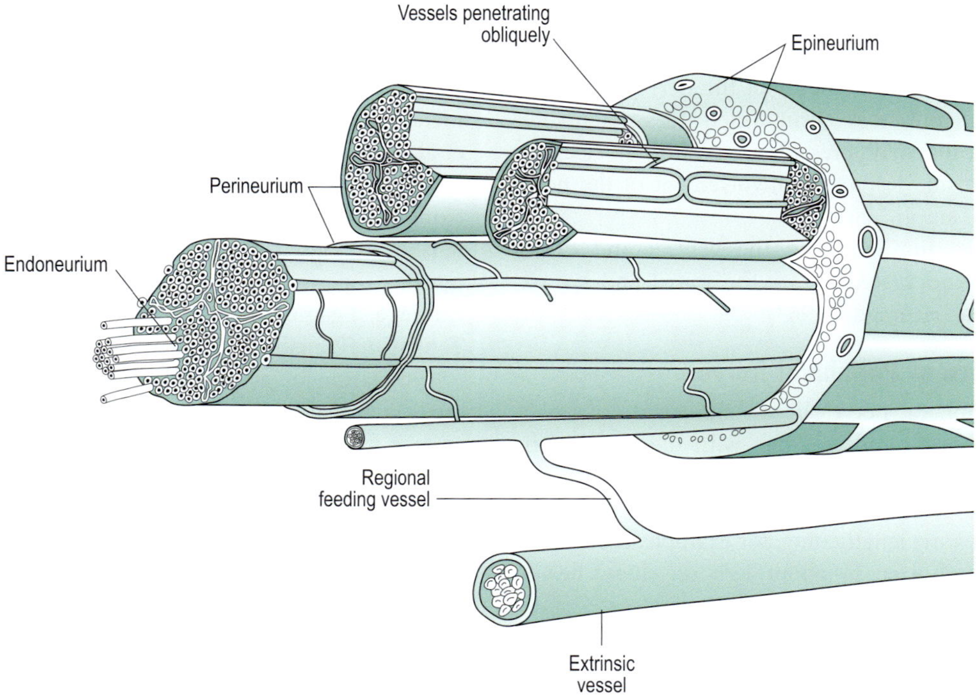

Fig. 6.17 Intraneural microcirculation. (*After Lundborg et al. 1987, with permission.*)

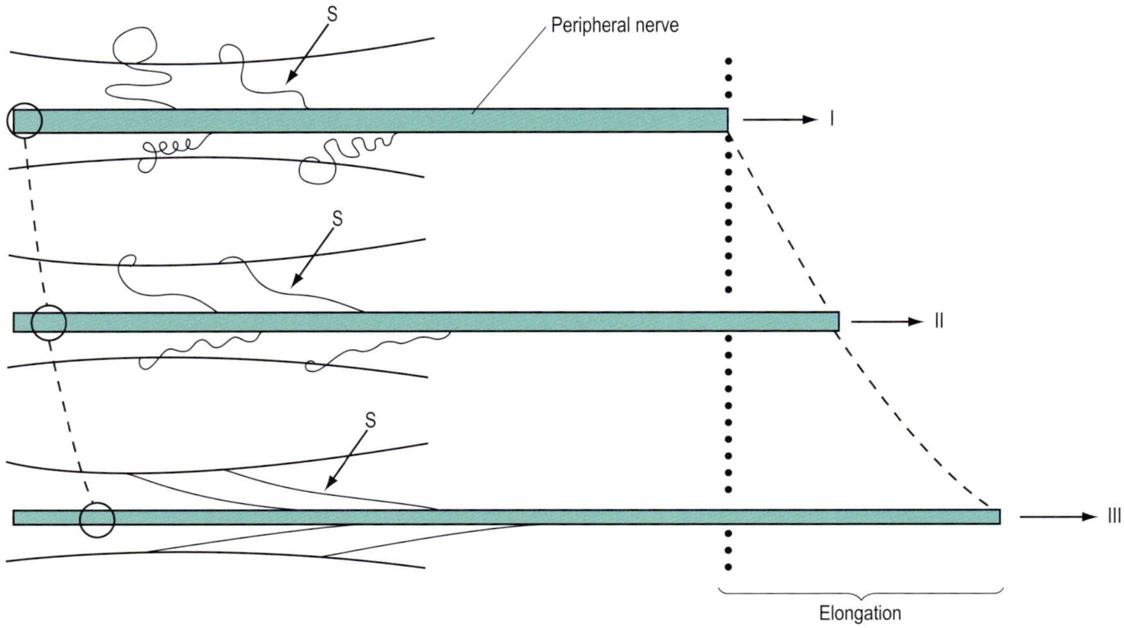

Fig. 6.18 Effect of stretching on the blood supply to the rabbit tibial nerve. Stage I is where the coiled segmental (*S*) blood vessels are unaffected by nerve lengthening. Stage II is where further increase in nerve lengthening begins to stretch the blood vessels and impair flow. Stage III is where the cross-sectional area of the nerve *(circled)* is reduced, which further impairs blood flow. (*From Rydevik et al. 1989, with permission.*)

the connective tissue elements of the nerve may result in a local inflammatory event which does not involve the axons. This may present as a more nociceptive pain mechanism, despite the involvement of the nerve (Schmid & Tampin, 2018).

The epineurium covering the ventral and dorsal roots is also innervated, as are the spinal and sympathetic ganglia (Hromada, 1963).

Biomechanics of Peripheral Nerves

Because peripheral nerves lie on either side of joints, they must shorten and lengthen with movement. The connective tissue surrounding nerves contains elastin. This therefore enables nerves to return to a shortened position following lengthening; for example, the median nerve has to shorten by about 15% on elbow flexion (Zoech et al., 1991).

There are three main mechanical events occurring with joint movement which cause the nerve bed to elongate. First of all, the nerve, which sits uncoiled in the nerve bed, starts to uncoil, followed by excursion (sliding) of the nerve with a gradual increase in nerve strain (percentage change in length) as the nerve bed continues to lengthen. The direction of nerve movement will follow the direction of the moving joint (Boyd et al., 2005; Ridehalgh et al., 2014). When lengthening occurs, a tensile (longitudinal) force is transmitted along the length of a nerve. Nerves have considerable tensile strength to withstand this tensile force. The tensile properties of nerve roots, compared with bone, cartilage, ligament, muscle and tendon, are given in Table 6.2 (Panjabi & White, 2001).

Elongation of a nerve leads to a reduction in the cross-sectional area of the nerve, with resultant increases in pressure within the fascicles (Topp & Boyd, 2006). Such compression may lead to changes in the microcirculation of the nerve (Sunderland, 1990). Hence in clinical situations where the nerve is already subject to compression, as seen in some conditions such as CTS, it is possible that movement which elongates the nerve could place further pressure on the nerve, resulting in greater ischaemic changes.

Movement of the Nervous System

The spinal arachnoid and pia mater are continuous with the perineurium of a peripheral nerve, and the

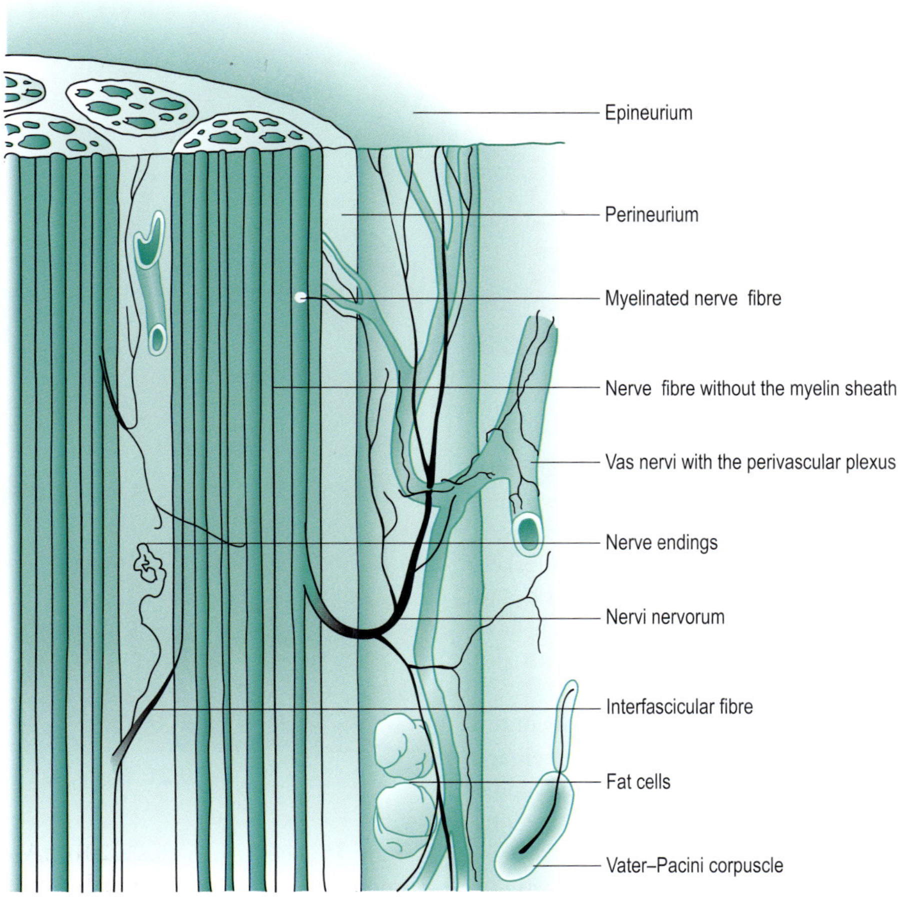

Fig. 6.19 A longitudinal schematic drawing demonstrating the nervi nervorum and nerve endings within the connective tissue sheath of a peripheral nerve. (*After Hromada 1963, with permission from the publisher, S. Karger AG, Basel.*)

TABLE 6.2 Tensile Properties of Nerve Roots Compared With Bone, Cartilage, Ligament, Muscle and Tendon

Tissue	Stress at Failure (MPa)	Strain at Failure (%)
Nerve roots	15	19
Cortical bone	100–200	1–3
Cancellous bone	10	5–7
Cartilage	10–15	80–120
Ligament	10–40	30–45
Muscle (passive)	0.17	60
Tendon	55	9–10

Panjabi, M.M., White, A.A., 2001. Biomechanics in the Musculoskeletal System. Churchill Livingstone, New York.

spinal dura mater is continuous with the epineurium of a peripheral nerve (Williams et al., 1995). Thus, the cerebral meninges, spinal meninges, and perineurium and epineurium of peripheral nerves are one continuous structure, and therefore, during normal functional movements, the nervous system moves as a continuum. As mentioned, during limb and trunk movements, the nervous system undergoes a series of biomechanical events, and an understanding of this enables the clinician to consider if the nervous system has become mechanically sensitive. For example, a person who complains of greater pain during lumbar flexion when the cervical spine is flexed than when it is extended may have heightened nerve mechanosensitivity. In addition, understanding which series of movements causes

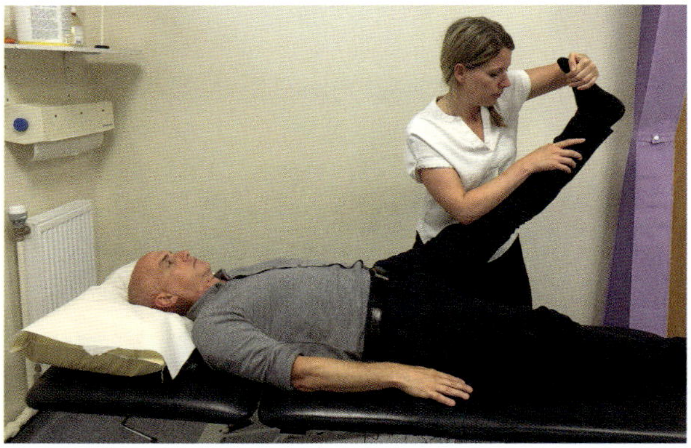

Fig. 6.20 Straight leg raise test.

greater movement and strain enables the clinician to use specific tests (commonly termed neurodynamic tests) to purposely assess heightened nerve mechanosensitivity in patients with nerve-related musculoskeletal pain. There has been an array of cadaveric and more recently, ultrasound imaging studies which have detailed these biomechanical changes during limb and trunk movements.

Early cadaveric studies noted that movements of the head and neck cause excursion and strain (percentage change in length) in the spinal dura in the cervical spine in particular, but also in the thoracic and lumbar regions (Breig & Marions, 1963; Tencer et al., 1985). However, minimal movement was found with cervical flexion at T12 spinal cord (0–2 mm, Reid, 1960) and the cauda equina (1–2 mm, Breig & Marions, 1963) than at T1 (6.8 mm, Reid, 1960). Such limited movement in the lower regions of the thoracic cord and cauda equina may have bearings on the use of cervical flexion as a structural differentiation manoeuvre during straight leg raise (SLR) test (Fig 6.20) since the trunk is not also flexed during this test. The addition of trunk with cervical flexion (such as in the slump test (Fig. 6.21)) caused greater amounts of spinal cord excursion (2–5 mm) at T12 (Reid, 1960), and trunk flexion appears to induce tensile load through the lumbosacral nerve roots (Breig, 1960; Breig & Marions, 1963).

Ultrasound imaging as well as cadaveric research has also been utilized to examine cervical spine movements. Cervical contralateral flexion and contralateral gliding resulted in a proximal movement of the median nerve in the upper limb, with the lateral glide causing a slightly greater amount of nerve excursion (mean

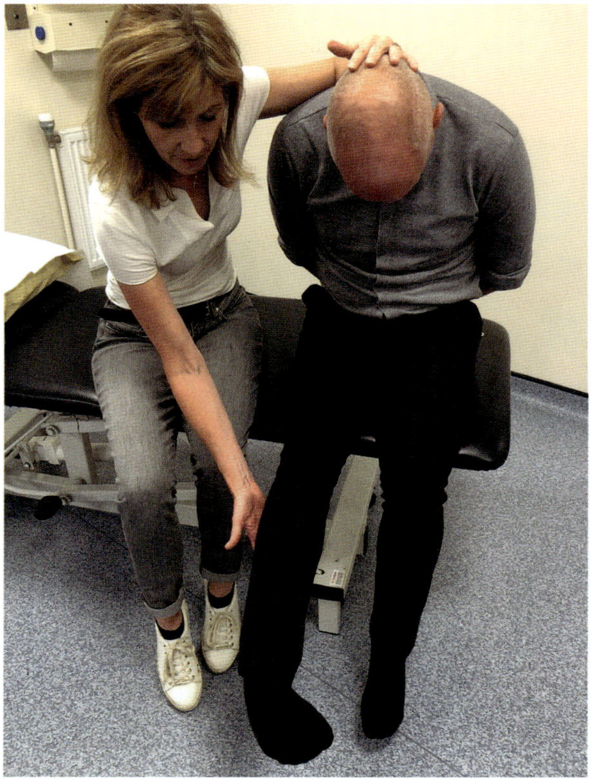

Fig. 6.21 Slump test.

1 mm, P =.005) than the lateral flexion in one study (Brochwicz et al., 2013). This may have implications when using head and neck movements to elicit symptoms during slump or upper limb neurodynamic tests or in management using nerve gliding techniques.

During SLR, excursion in the lumbosacral nerve roots has shown great variation, from 0.48 mm at L5 in older cadavers (Gilbert et al., 2007) to 5 mm in younger cadavers (Goddard & Reid, 1965). Strain values have also varied from around 3% (Goddard & Reid, 1965) to negligible strain (Gilbert et al., 2007). Such differences are likely related to variation in methods, including the use of younger (35–75 years Goddard & Reid, 1965) rather than older cadavers (>75 years Gilbert et al., 2007). The key issue to take away is that the SLR test induces excursion of the nerve roots with some accompanying strain. In addition, SLR causes excursion and strain of the sciatic and tibial nerves (Boyd et al., 2013; Coppieters et al., 2006, Goddard & Reid, 1965), and this has been replicated in in-vivo ultrasound imaging studies (Ellis et al., 2012; Coppieters et al., 2015;

Ridehalgh et al., 2012, 2014). Since the methods vary so dramatically between studies, values are not useful as they cannot be reasonably compared. However, patterns of movement and strain are consistent between studies and show that the greatest excursion and strain occur closest to and towards the moving joint (Fig. 6.22).

Upper limb movements have also demonstrated similar trends in upper limb nerve biomechanics. Even movements of the fingers alone can cause considerable excursion of the median nerve in the forearm, moving longitudinally between 1.6 and 4.5 mm from full flexion of the index finger to 30-degree extension at the interphalangeal joints (Dilley et al., 2001). It may be that this movement alone is sufficient to cause pain and symptoms in someone with CTS, and a full upper limb neurodynamic test would not be necessary. Adding wrist movement causes not only additional longitudinal excursion (Hough et al., 2000), but also movement in an ulnar direction (Greening et al., 2001).

Upper limb neurodynamic tests have also been investigated in cadavers as well as in vivo with ultrasound imaging. Manvell et al. (2015a and 2015b) examined tensile forces in the radial and ulnar nerves during the associated upper limb neurodynamic tests. Statistically significant increases in tensile force were found during the traditional ULNT2b (Fig. 6.23) with greatest changes during wrist ulnar deviation and thumb flexion (mean tension 11.32N; 95% CI 10.25, 12.29, $P < .01$), indicating that these movements may be of particular value during testing. However, ulnar nerve tensile forces were highest with the addition of internal rotation (11.86 N; 95% CI = 9.96, 13.77) rather than the traditional external rotation application during ULNT 3 (ulnar nerve bias) (Manvell et al., 2015b) (Fig 6.24), and therefore it may be useful to play with these

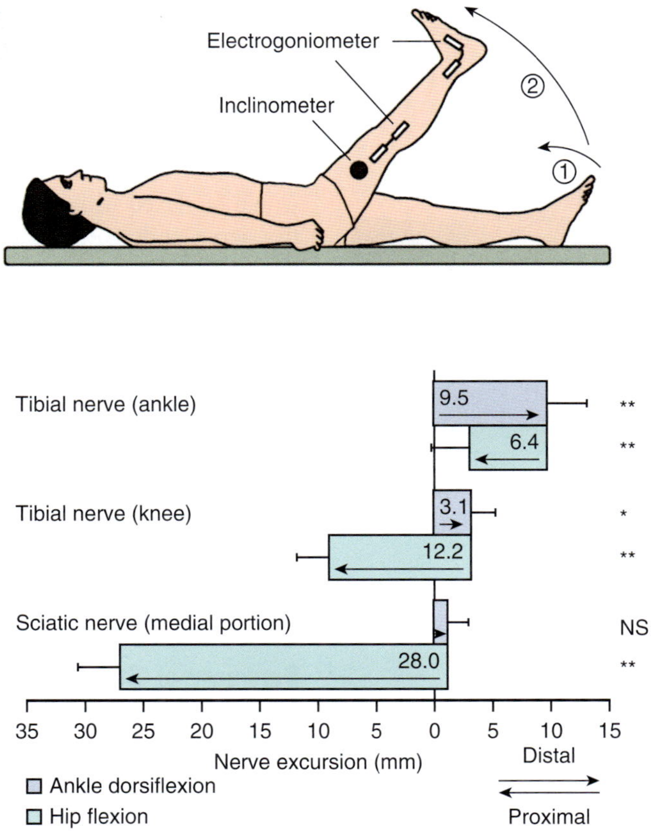

FIG. 6.22 Nerve movement during the SLR test. *(From Coppieters et al. 2006 with permission.)*

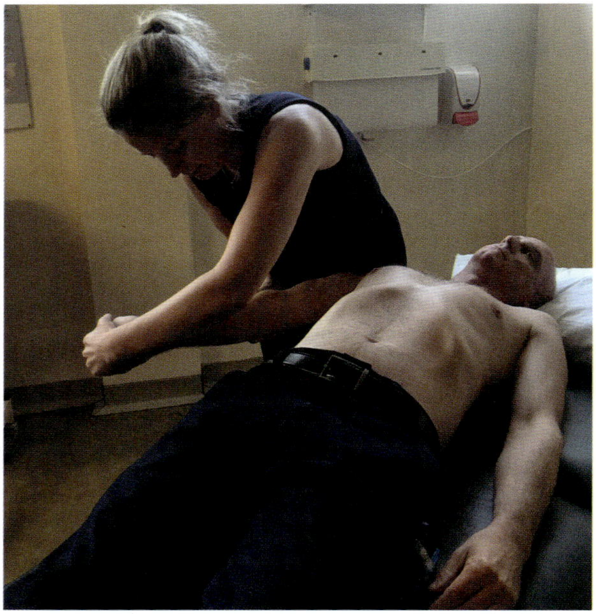

Fig. 6.23 Upper limb neurodynamic test 2b (radial nerve bias).

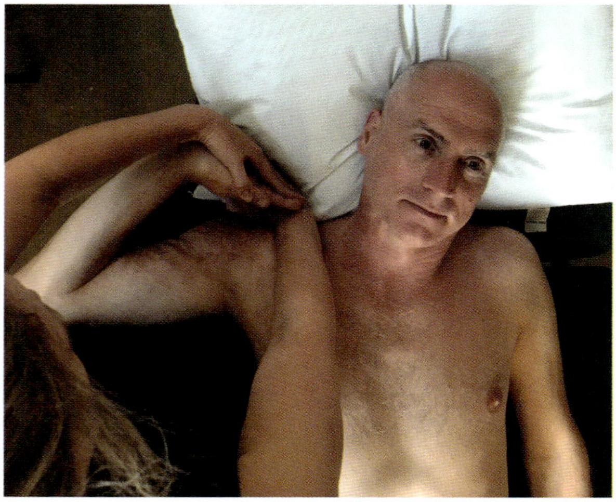

Fig. 6.24 Upper limb neurodynamic test 3 (ulnar nerve bias). (*Manvell et al. 2015b*)

two positions in people with symptoms suggestive of ulnar nerve conditions.

More recently, advances in ultrasound technology using shear wave elastography have led to a new era of biomechanical nerve-related studies to give an indication of stiffness in the nerves during limb motion (Andrade et al., 2016; Greening & Dilley, 2016; Kantarci et al., 2014). All studies indicate that with the addition of greater amounts and combinations of joint movement that increase the path the nerve has to travel, greater amounts of shear wave velocity (an indicator of stiffness) occur. For example, from position 1 (shoulder abducted to 30 degrees, elbow flexed to 90 degrees, and the wrist in maximum flexion (50–60 degrees) to position 4 (full ULNT1) the shear wave velocity increased by 236% measured in the forearm (Greening & Dilley, 2016). Such advances are useful since standard ultrasound imaging can only give an indication of nerve excursion.

One final consideration regarding biomechanical aspects of neurodynamic testing is the combinations of limb movements with respect to sliders and tensioners in the upper limbs (Coppieters & Butler, 2008; Coppieters et al., 2009) and lower limbs (Coppieters et al., 2015). The main premise is that when one end of the neurodynamic test is positioned to cause an increase in length of the nerve being tested, whilst the opposite end is positioned to cause a reduction in length (a slider), the overall amount of excursion increases, and the strain decreases compared to a tensioner technique. One example of this would be during a slump test whilst the ankle is dorsiflexed, the cervical spine is extended. In the tensioner technique the cervical spine would be flexed whilst the ankle is dorsiflexed, so that the nerve undergoes greatest amounts of lengthening (strain) with a corresponding reduction in excursion (Fig. 6.25). The choice to apply these as management techniques will be discussed in Chapter 7.

KNOWLEDGE CHECK

1. Why might inflammation be involved in nerve-related musculoskeletal pain?
2. Why could movements of the foot cause increased symptoms in the low back of someone with heightened nerve mechanosensitivity?

Summary of Structure and Function of the Nervous System

The central and peripheral nervous systems are anatomically, biomechanically and physiologically linked as part of one whole system. This highly complex

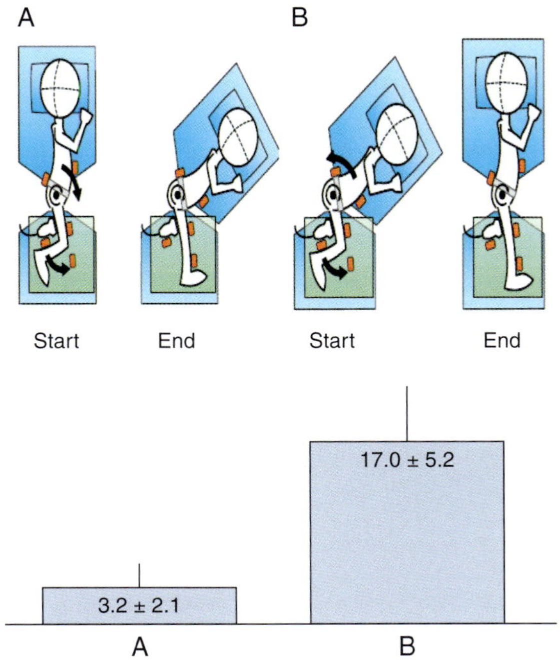

Fig. 6.25 Sliders and tensioners during SLR test. (A) Tensioner showing reduced sciatic nerve excursion. (B) Slider showing greater sciatic nerve excursion. (Modified *from Coppieters et al. 2015 with permission.*)

system not only enables normal movement to occur but also allows the continuation of normal nerve function despite considerable forces acting upon it during day-to-day movements. The continuous nature of the nervous system means that simple limb movements can be used to assess heightened responses to nerve motion utilizing tests called neurodynamic tests.

NERVE-RELATED MUSCULOSKELETAL PAIN

Pain arising from the nervous system is seen in common musculoskeletal aetiologies where nerves are more susceptible to direct pressure or constriction of blood flow. Examples of this might include radicular leg pain, where one potential mechanism involves a herniated intervertebral disc causing nerve root compromise (Caridi et al., 2011) or CTS and cubital tunnel syndrome, where the passage of the nerve through an anatomically restricted tunnel can be further restricted by changes in pressure (Lee & Lin, 2019).

Nerve-related musculoskeletal pain is complex. It is not one simple disorder that can be explained by a simple pathophysiological mechanism. A patient may present with a severe and irritable condition with significant neurological loss of function as well as heightened sensitivity to pain and touch, or may present with a nonsevere and nonirritable condition with no loss of nerve function and yet still have the involvement of a painful nerve condition. This most likely reflects the different pathophysiological mechanisms that are responsible for the resulting painful condition.

Pathophysiological Mechanisms Responsible for Nerve-Related Musculoskeletal Pain

It is well established there are local mechanisms that lead to both neuropathic pain and heightened nerve mechanosensitivity, although our understanding of these underlying mechanisms is continually evolving. This section will discuss the local pathophysiological mechanisms responsible for this, including compression and inflammatory and immunological change.

Compression

Nerves are susceptible to compression predominantly because of their superficial arrangement, their close location to other structures (e.g. bone), and their passage through narrowed tunnels (e.g. the carpal tunnel) (Sunderland, 1978; Rempel et al., 1999). The effects of such compression will depend on the magnitude and duration of the compression (Rydevik & Lundborg, 1977; Dahlin & McLean, 1986) and, to some extent, the make-up of the nerve. For example, a nerve which has fewer, larger fascicles, embedded therefore in less connective tissue, will be more vulnerable to compression than a nerve which has numerous fascicles and therefore more connective tissue (Fig. 6.26) (Sunderland, 1978; Lundborg, 2004). In addition, certain sections of the same nerve are more vulnerable to compression than others, depending on their location; nerve fibres located on the periphery of the nerve trunk are more susceptible to compressive forces than those in the middle of the nerve trunk (Lundborg, 2004).

Impact of compression to blood flow and oedema. The blood vessels within the epineurium of the nerve are the parts most susceptible to compression injuries (Rydevik

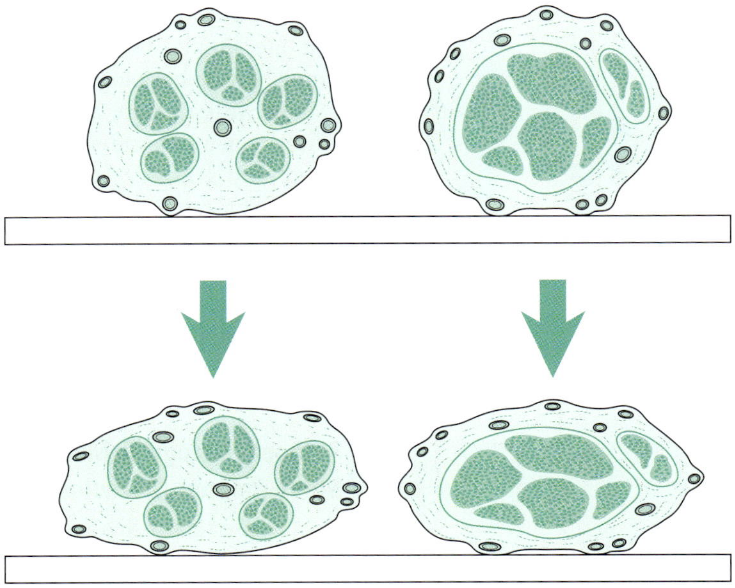

Fig. 6.26 Smaller fascicles within larger amounts of epineurium are less vulnerable than large fascicles within less epineurium. *(From Lundborg 2004 with permission.)*

& Lundborg, 1977; Lundborg et al. 1983). Pressures as low as 20–30 mmHg can reduce the blood flow to the epineurium (Rydevik et al., 1981). Since nerves are oxygen vociferous due to their high energy demands, such a loss of circulation can have devastating effects on the function and life of the nerve cells.

Compression of the blood vessels results in increased permeability of the vessel walls, resulting in the migration of proteins followed by fluid into the epineural space (Rydevik & Lundborg, 1977). The perineurium provides an important barrier to oedema, protecting the endoneurial space and therefore the nerve fibres themselves; however, more severe compression can lead to increased permeability of the endoneurial vessels, resulting in oedema within the endoneurium (Rydevik & Lundborg, 1977; Rydevik et al., 1981). It appears that much higher pressures (above 200 mmHg) are necessary for endoneurial oedema to be present (Rydevik & Lundborg, 1977), compared with 50 mmHg for epineurial oedema, and this may be related to endoneurial vessel leakage rather than failure of the perineurial barrier.

Axonal transport mechanisms. As discussed, nerves require additional resources to ensure adequate movement of intracellular substances required for homeostasis of the nerve and removal of waste products (Lundborg et al. 1983; Dahlin & McLean, 1986; Lundborg, 2004; Powell & Myers, 1986). Both slow and fast axonal transport mechanisms have been shown to be reduced at pressures sustained for 8 hours of around 30 mmHg (Dahlin & McLean, 1986). In addition, retrograde axonal transport is inhibited at pressures as low as 20 mmHg (Lundborg & Dahlin, 1992), and this results in the suspension of the provision of specific neurotrophic factors to the cell body. A depletion of these factors at the cell body has been suggested to activate the cell death programme in nerve cells (Kandel et al., 2000).

Demyelination. Direct compression to the nerve may cause disruption to Schwann cell function with resultant demyelination distal to the area of compression (Lundborg et al., 1983; Dahlin & McLean, 1986; Powell & Myers, 1986; Schmid, 2015). Pressures of 50 mmHg held for 2 minutes (Dyck et al., 1990), 30 mmHg for 2 hours (Powell & Myers, 1986) and 80 mmHg for 4 hours (Lundborg et al., 1983) have been shown to cause demyelination of nerve fibres and axonal damage. Fibrosis between the epineurium and adjacent muscles has been observed following a compression injury (Powell & Myers, 1986); such fibrosis is likely to disrupt the normal movement of the nerve through the interface.

Testing and analysing effects of compression in vivo. Experimental compression of nerves in normal subjects provides valuable information on the effect of nerve compression on clinical neurological testing. A catheter inserted into the carpal tunnel, for example, allows for controlled and accurate increases in carpal pressure to 30, 40, 50, 60, 70 and 90 mmHg (Lundborg et al., 1982; Gelberman et al., 1983; Szabo et al., 1983). The earliest signs of nerve impairment during this testing are the subjective reporting of numbness, tingling or paraesthesia in the distribution of the median nerve (Gelberman et al., 1983; Szabo et al., 1983). At 40–50 mmHg, sensation is completely blocked (Gelberman et al., 1983), and in hypertensive subjects with a higher neural arteriole pressure, sensory block occurs at 60–70 mmHg (Szabo et al., 1983). This suggests that patients with raised or lowered blood pressure may respond differently to a given amount of nerve compression (Szabo et al., 1983). In another study (Lundborg et al., 1982), compression of 90 mmHg led to paraesthesia in the hand after 20 minutes, complete sensory block after 30–50 minutes and complete motor block after a further 10–30 minutes. In people with CTS, the position of the wrist changes the amount of pressure within the carpal tunnel. In a neutral wrist position, pressures have been found to be around 30 mmHg, with an increase to 110 mmHg in wrist extension (Gelberman et al., 1981).

It is also important to relate these pressures to practice to make sense of such figures. In people undergoing discectomy for lumbosacral disc herniation, it was found that nerve root pressures before discectomy varied from 7 to 256 mmHg (mean, 53.2 ± 49.1 mmHg) (Takahashi et al., 1999). Interestingly, and perhaps not surprisingly, those with pressures greater than 50 mmHg also had neurological deficits.

In summary, nerve compression of above 20 mmHg may cause widespread mechanical and ischaemic changes to nerves. These changes may include endoneural oedema, damage to the blood–nerve barrier, disruption to conductivity and impaired axonal transportation, which in turn may impede the nerve's normal reparative processes. Whilst compression may be an important factor in many nerve-related MSK conditions seen in practice, it is also clear that compression is not required for neuropathic pain to occur. In the next section of this chapter, we will investigate inflammatory and immune cell mechanisms, ion channel changes and genetic influences which contribute to the development of neuropathic pain.

> **KNOWLEDGE CHECK**
> 1. Describe why compression may be so significant to the commencement and continuation of neuropathic pain.

Inflammatory and Immunological Change

After nerve injury, immune cells such as mast cells, neutrophils, macrophages and T cells are recruited to the area of peripheral nerve injury and release inflammatory mediators such as proinflammatory cytokines, which have been implicated in neuropathic pain by lowering the threshold at which nociceptive neurons fire and by generating ectopic impulses (Dilley et al., 2005; Thacker et al., 2007; Grossmann et al., 2009; Schmid et al., 2013). Additionally, these processes can also activate the normally silent nociceptors (Michaelis et al., 1996). Interestingly, the presence of inflammation alone can disrupt axonal transport systems, and animal studies have demonstrated that such disruption can result in axonal mechanical sensitivity in the absence of compression (Dilley & Bove, 2008) (Fig. 6.27)

The degradation of the diffusion barrier by mechanical or chemical means and the immunomodulatory role adopted by glial cells in the dorsal horn, resident satellite glial cells in the DRG and Schwann cells in the periphery may accelerate the immune response by further recruiting immune cells to the area (Schmid et al., 2013) (Fig. 6.28). Such activation of glial cells is not just local to the site of injury, but in animal models has been found to be proximal (e.g. at the DRG after sciatic nerve injury (Schmid et al., 2013), at the dorsal horn after nerve root injury (Takahata et al., 2011), the contralateral dorsal horn (Hatashita et al., 2008) and even as far as the thalamus and mid-brain after sciatic nerve ligation (Giardini et al., 2017). Such widespread changes may account for symptoms 'not fitting' in classic neuropathic pain conditions like CTS. Indeed, Nora et al. (2005) found that symptoms in people with CTS confirmed with electrophysiological studies are rarely restricted to the cutaneous distribution of the median nerve and are often felt in the fourth or fifth digits, or proximal to the wrist. From a clinical

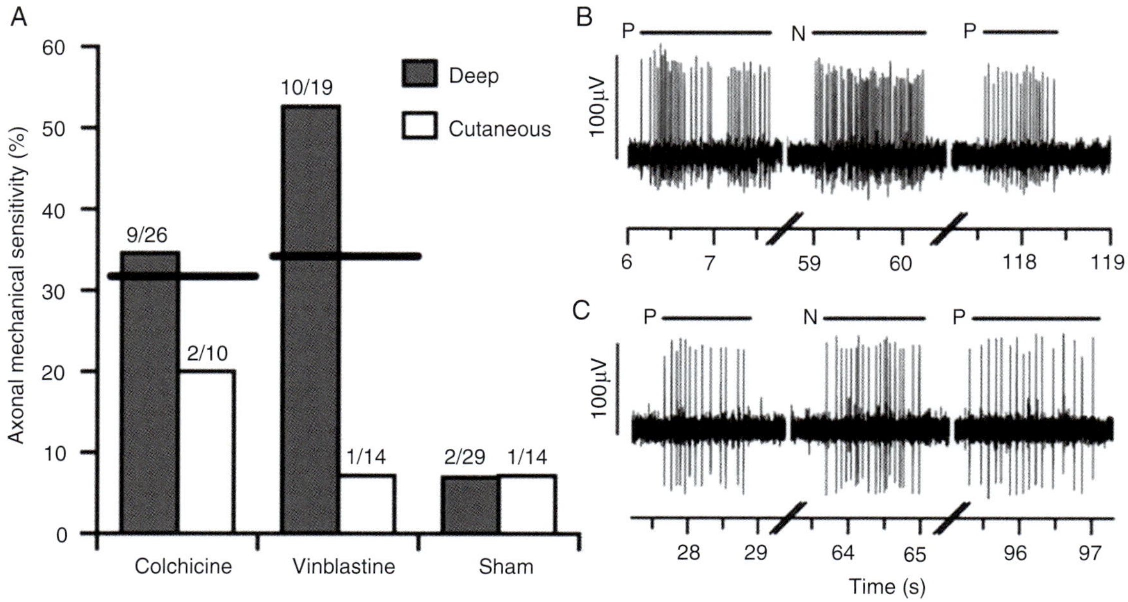

Fig. 6.27 Axonal mechanical sensitivity after inflammation. (A) Proportion of axonal mechanosensitivity in C-fibre axons following colchicine treatment, vinblastine treatment, and in sham-operated animals. The thick horizontal lines indicate the combined percentage of axons with mechanical sensitivity for cutaneous and deep-innervating neurons. The total number of neurons sampled and the number responding to mechanical stimulation at the test site are shown for each group. (B) and (C) are representative responses to mechanical stimuli of the axons of neurons with deep receptive fields following colchicine treatment (B) and vinblastine treatment (C). Short horizontal lines above the traces represent the duration of the mechanical stimuli. For each neuron, the peripheral receptive field was mechanically stimulated initially (P). This was followed by mechanical stimulation of the nerve at the test site (N). (*From Dilley et al. 2008 with permission.*)

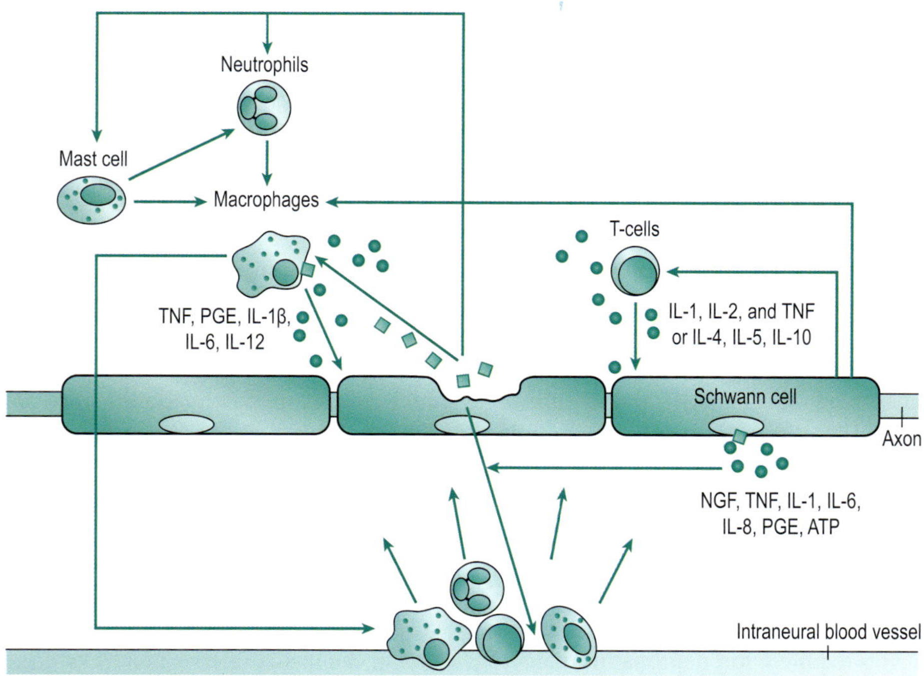

Fig. 6.28 Inflammatory and immunological change in response to peripheral nerve injury. Resident immune cells and those recruited to the area release inflammatory mediators. Schwann cells also adopt an immunomodulatory role. *ATP*, Adenosine triphosphate; *IL-1β*, interleukin-1β; *PGE*, prostaglandin E; *TNF*, tumour necrosis factor. (*From Schmid et al. 2013, with permission.*)

perspective, therefore, it is important not to discount a neuropathic pain presentation as a clinical hypothesis purely on the basis of the symptoms not conforming to a given cutaneous distribution.

There is clear acceptance in the scientific community that neuropathic pain is associated with the involvement of multiple different types of immune cells, and this occurs both close to or within the peripheral nerve cells themselves (Finnerup et al., 2021; Sommer et al., 2018). T cells, natural killer cells and macrophages appear to have a considerable role in the development of neuropathic pain. One way of assessing the role of these cells is by genetically manipulating animals so that they are deficient in certain cells. For example, in mice with experimentally induced neuropathic pain, mice without T-cells did not go on to develop neuropathic mechanical allodynia, whereas those mice with normal T cells did (Vicuna et al., 2015).

KNOWLEDGE CHECK

1. A patient presents with bilateral carpal tunnel syndrome which resolves on both sides after carpal tunnel release, Why might this be?

Ion Channel Involvement

There are a number of ways in which alteration in ion channels contributes to neuropathic pain. They may become upregulated and more densely packed along axons and increase their function (Finnerup et al., 2021). Of particular interest are voltage-gated sodium channels as well as TRP channels. Blockage of TRPV1 and TRPA1 channels has improved neuropathic pain in animal models. Genetic mutations of the Nav.1.7 channel have been linked to a number of conditions, including a painful condition called erythromelalgia and diabetic neuropathy (Finnerup et al., 2021), and a genetic loss of function of the ion channel leads to an inability to feel pain (Cox et al., 2006). However, a number of pharmacological studies targeting the channel have been discontinued due to failure to show an effect in a number of conditions including painful radiculopathy (Kingwell, 2019). This may be due to difficulties in providing a sufficient dose of medication to completely block the channel. What is clear is that future exploration of these channels will continue to be a target from pharmacological companies and the focus of research into neuropathic pain conditions.

Subcortical and Cortical Changes

As well as local mechanical and immunoinflammatory effects of nerve dysfunction and changes to the DRG and dorsal horn, there may be changes at subcortical and cortical levels. The mechanisms are complex but are thought to be related to a number of factors. One mechanism found in a number of animal studies is that of a switch from descending inhibitory pathways to descending facilitatory pathway, which acts to enhance the nociceptive information entering the dorsal horn (Finnerup et al., 2021). One method of assessing alterations in the descending pathways is through conditioned pain modulation. The premise is that normally one painful stimulus applied at one site becomes less painful when another painful stimulus is applied at a site distant from the original test site (Yarnitsky et al., 2010). It has been postulated that some people have a stronger CPM response than others and that those with a reduced response may be more susceptible to developing persistent pain. However, in a study investigating CPM in people with and without neuropathic pain after spinal cord injury (Gagné et al., 2020), those with neuropathic pain initially had enhanced CPM compared to those without neuropathic pain. However, subsequently, those whose neuropathic pain symptoms increased showed a decrease in CPM, suggesting that neuropathic pain could lead to diminished CPM. Whilst CPM has been demonstrated to be diminished in those with CTS for more than 2 months compared to healthy controls (Soon et al., 2017), it is unknown if the condition has led to the reduced CPM or if an inefficient CPM led to worse neuropathic pain.

Cortical reorganization and structural changes to grey and white matter have been found in people with nerve-related MSK disorders such as CTS (Maeda et al., 2014) and lumbosacral radiculopathy (Luchtmann et al., 2014), potentially contributing to alterations in endogenous pain responses, emotions associated with the experience of pain, as well as alterations in fine motor control and sensory discrimination. Since clinical findings can change rapidly after successful treatment such as injection or surgery, it may suggest that these cortical changes require a peripheral driver to maintain them (Schmid et al., 2020).

Connective Tissue Injury

The repair process of the connective tissue around nerves is similar to that of other viscoelastic tissues within the body, such as ligament. Following a nerve injury, there is an increase in the collagen tissue within the perineurium and endoneurium, indicative of scar formation (Starkweather et al., 1978; Salonen et al., 1985). Additionally, it has been demonstrated in rat sciatic nerves that, 3 weeks after a nerve injury, there is a 28% reduction in nerve length (Clark et al., 1992). Such alterations in nerve motion have been debated to occur in vivo in common nerve-related MSK disorders such as CTS and spinally referred leg pain (Erel et al., 2003; Ridehalgh et al., 2015). However, a recent systematic review (Ellis et al., 2017) concluded that there was likely a reduction in median nerve excursion in people with CTS, with 7 out of 10 studies revealing reduced median nerve excursion compared to controls. In addition, studies utilizing shear wave elastography have found greater stiffness in the peripheral nerves of people with nerve-related MSK pain than control participants (Kantarci et al., 2014; Neto et al., 2020; Paluch et al., 2018).

Common musculoskeletal injuries may also have an element of nerve dysfunction to them. Ankle sprains commonly affect not only the ligamentous structures but also either the common peroneal nerve or the sural nerve (Nitz et al., 1985; Johnston & Howell, 1999). This could be either due to the direct inversion sprain causing a sudden increase in the length of the nerve or secondary to healing and scar tissue formation of structures close to the nerve. Sunderland (1978) termed these conditions friction fibrosis. In such conditions, it may be that the nerve loses its ability to slide and glide through the interfacing tissues (Butler, 2000). Another example of restricted interface movement is the adhesion formation between lumbar nerve roots and the intervertebral foramina that can reduce the ability of the nerve to move (Goddard & Reid, 1965; Kobayashi et al., 2003). This can be caused by local pathological changes or may occur as a result of normal age-related changes (Goddard & Reid, 1965).

A summary of central and local changes can be found in Fig. 6.29.

Nerve Regeneration and Repair

The pathophysiological mechanism explained above tend to follow from a more minor nerve injury where the structural integrity, at least in the first instance, is not affected. Following a more substantial nerve injury, the distal portion of the nerve undergoes Wallerian degeneration. Distal to the site of injury, the Schwann cells proliferate, and the myelin and axoplasm disintegrate and are reabsorbed by macrophagic activity. Proximal to the site of injury, axons grow a large number of sprouts, which grow at approximately 1 mm/day towards the distal segment. If the Schwann cell columns remain intact, the sprouting axons will be guided to reinnervate the target organ. If the Schwann cell columns have been destroyed by the injury, then sprouting axons may grow and innervate inappropriate areas, giving a poorer clinical result.

The reinnervation and sensory restoration following a myocutaneous skin flap have been investigated and highlight the clinical outcome of nerve regeneration. Some axons were found to sprout into Schwann cell columns, whereas a number of axons were found to be unmyelinated and associated with blood vessels (Turkof et al., 1993; Terenghi, 1995). The degree of sensory restoration varied widely between individuals; some flaps were totally numb while others had moderate sensation (Turkof et al., 1993). In patients with CTS, following the resolution of severe compression, recovery is variable and may depend upon an individual's potential for axonal regeneration. Maximal recovery after the removal of compression may take some months and may indeed be incomplete (Chammas et al., 2014).

From this research, it seems that there is a wide variation in the functional regeneration of sensory nerves, from very poor to moderately good.

Centrally, the regeneration of nerve axons occurs at the dorsal horn within 2 weeks of a nerve injury (Doubell & Woolf, 1997). C fibres, which synapse in lamina II of the dorsal horn, atrophy and leave vacant synaptic spaces (Fig. 6.30). Large, myelinated A fibres sprout into these spaces, altering the processing of mechanoreceptor input from A fibres (Woolf et al., 1992; Doubell & Woolf, 1997).

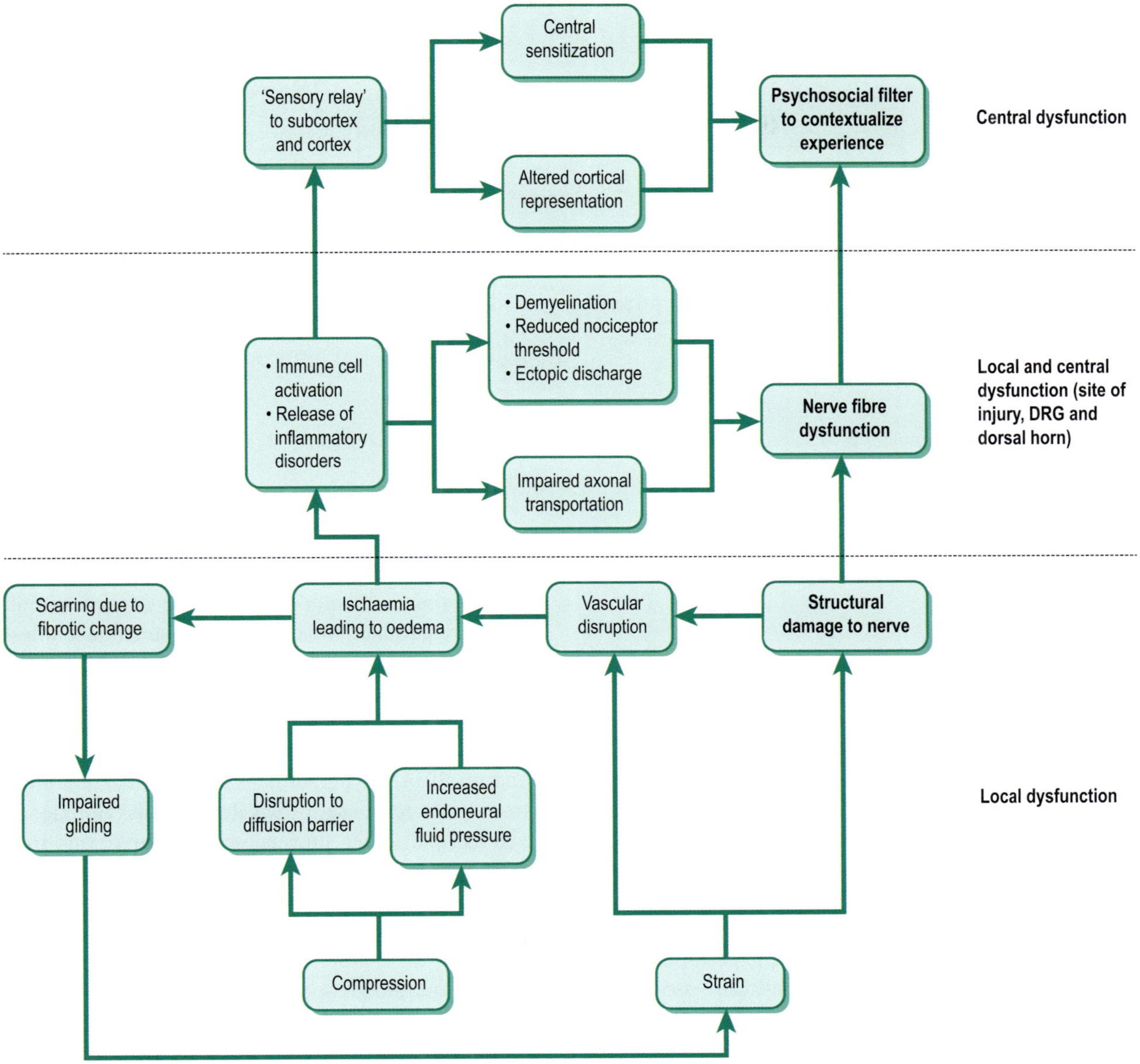

Fig. 6.29 Summary of mechanisms of local and central nerve dysfunction. *DRG*, Dorsal root ganglion.

Pain Mechanisms of Nerve-Related Musculoskeletal Pain

Patients with nerve-related MSK pain might present with different underlying pain mechanisms with characteristics of either somatic or nociceptive pain (caused by activation of nociceptors in cutaneous and deep musculoskeletal tissue such as skin, muscle, and connective tissue), neuropathic pain or a combination of both. Both nociceptive and neuropathic pain can be localized to the site of nociception or can spread (refer) from its source (Freynhagen & Bennett, 2009).

Patients may also present with heightened nerve mechanosensitivity (Yilmaz et al., 2018), with or without alteration in nerve function (e.g. loss of sensation, reflex or muscle weakness) and vice versa (Rainville et al., 2017). These varying pain mechanisms and characteristics result in heterogeneity within and

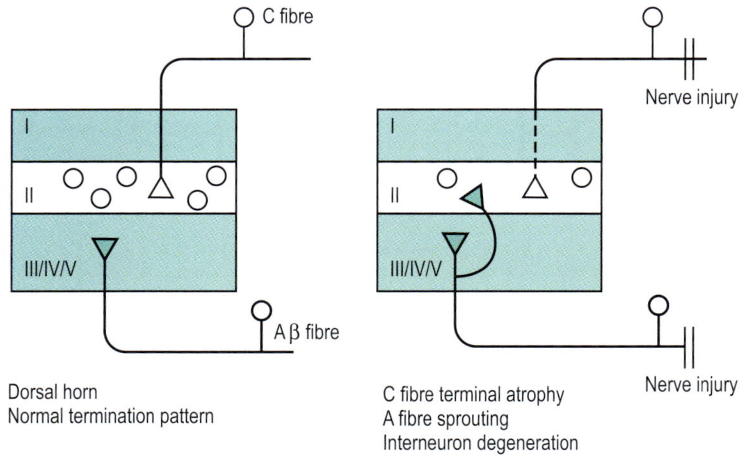

Fig. 6.30 Sprouting of A fibres into lamina II of the dorsal horn to replace atrophied C fibres. (*From Doubell et al. 1999, with permission.*)

between different musculoskeletal aetiologies and will be explored below.

Neuropathic Pain

It is important for the clinician to distinguish neuropathic pain from other pain mechanisms as the presence of neuropathic pain will often influence a patient's treatment and prognosis (see Chapter 7). Mixed pain presentations with features of both nociceptive and neuropathic pain are also common in nerve-related musculoskeletal conditions and require identification to tailor treatment to address both underlying pain processes.

Neuropathic pain can be divided into peripheral and central neuropathic pain. The International Association for the Study of Pain (IASP, 2017) defines peripheral neuropathic pain as pain 'caused by a lesion or disease of the peripheral somatosensory nervous system'. Painful radiculopathy, peripheral nerve injury and painful polyneuropathies (e.g. diabetic neuropathy) are the most common neuropathic pain conditions seen in musculoskeletal practices.

Signs and Symptoms of Neuropathic Pain

Neuropathic pain is characterized by specific painful symptoms. Pain can be persistent and on-going, or there can be spontaneous pain where pain suddenly emerges, sometimes without a precipitating cause. Pain can also be evoked by specific stimuli such as light touch, cool air or heat applied to the area or surrounding tissues. Painful responses to evoked stimuli can be termed allodynia or hyperalgesia. Allodynia is a painful response to a normally nonpainful stimulus (e.g. touch), whereas hyperalgesia is an overtly painful response to a normally painful stimulus (e.g. heightened pain to being stung or pricked with a pin) (Jensen & Finnerup, 2014). Hyperpathia is an abnormal and often extreme pain response to repeated stimuli (Hopkins & Rudge, 1973). Other unusual sensory sensations may also be present, which may be unpleasant (dysaesthesia) and not unpleasant (paraesthesia) (Finnerup et al., 2001). Combinations of these different symptoms can often occur; for example, a patient might have ongoing pain with additional spontaneous shoots of pain and paraesthesia. The symptoms of evoked pain and spontaneous pain are often intermittent in nature, and therefore quantitative sensory testing (QST) (where loss or gain of function is objectively assessed) does not always match with patients' reported symptoms as they may not be present during the time period of testing (Finnerup et al., 2021).

Certain pain descriptors have been considered to be specifically associated with neuropathic pain, including burning, tingling, pins and needles, shooting and numbness (Freynhagen & Bennett, 2009). These descriptors have been utilized in a number of neuropathic pain questionnaires (see screening tools below) although there is little evidence to support the validity of such descriptors. One systematic review on sensory descriptors to identify neuropathic low back pain (Heraughty & Ridehalgh, 2020) found that only self-reported allodynia and numbness could differentiate between somatic and neuropathic low back pain, while dysaesthesia may raise its suspicion. Only 8 studies were included in the review, however, reflecting the lack of high-quality literature to support the diagnostic accuracy of pain descriptors in patients with low back pain. In addition, no data were reported on the sensitivity or specificity of sensory descriptors in identifying neuropathic LBP, and it was concluded that there is not currently enough evidence to support or refute the use of these descriptors in clinical practice.

KNOWLEDGE CHECK

1. Describe the features of neuropathic pain and how these differ from somatic pain.
2. Describe the difference between allodynia, hyperalgesia, and hyperpathia.

Classification Systems of Neuropathic Pain

There is currently no 'gold standard' for diagnosing neuropathic pain in any aetiology or musculoskeletal condition. The Neuropathic Pain Special Interest Group (NeuPSIG) (a sub-group of IASP) developed a global grading system to identify the level of confidence that a patient has possible, probable and definite neuropathic pain (Treede et al., 2008), and this was revised to reflect clinical practice in 2016 (Fig. 6.31) (Finnerup et al., 2016). Possible neuropathic pain is identified with pain descriptors typical of neuropathic pain such as burning sensations, electric shocks and paraesthesia, pain on light touch or heat and cold. The history should suggest a relevant neurological disease, and the pain distribution should fit with the expected neuroanatomical pattern. Probable neuropathic pain is identified with objective sensory examination including light touch and vibration (to assess large fibre function) and pinprick, cold, or warm sensation (to assess small fibre function). Definite neuropathic pain is confirmed through diagnostic tests (such as imaging) which confirm a lesion or disease of the nervous system.

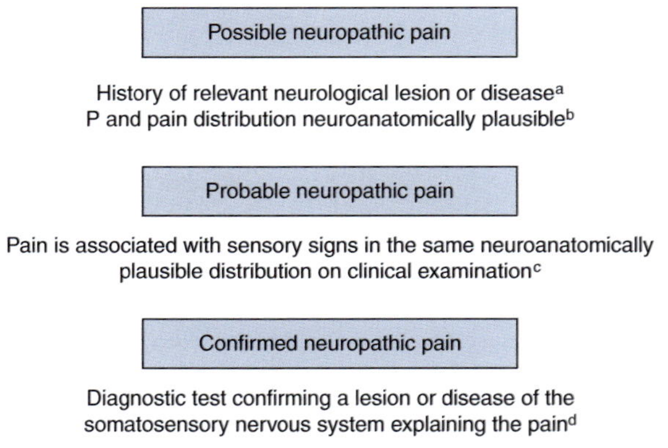

Fig. 6.31 Neuropathic pain grading system. (*From Finnerup et al. 2016 with permission.*)

There are, however, limitations to the use of the NeuPSIG grading system when used in musculoskeletal conditions. The requirement for 'neuroanatomically plausible' patterns of pain or sensory change is an ambiguous concept, as it is well known that patterns of symptoms referral, typical of specific nerve fibres or dermatomes, are often imprecise and based on old data from small case-controlled studies (Murphy et al., 2009). Recent research into the symptom distributions of nerve-related MSK conditions such as CTS has also refuted the traditional referral patterns in favour of often more widespread diffuse symptoms (Schmid et al., 2018).

The requirement within the grading system to confirm 'definite' neuropathic pain through diagnostic tests is also fraught with complexity, as in many musculoskeletal conditions, for example, low back–related leg pain, it is well recognized that MRI results do not always correlate with symptom presentation (Boden, 1990). Diagnostic tests to confirm the presence of neuropathic pain in musculoskeletal conditions should therefore be used with caution.

Physiotherapists will often examine muscle strength to assess the motor nerve conduction or reflexes as part of the neurological assessment. This assessment is not represented in the NeuPSIG grading criteria, as these changes can occur in the absence of neuropathic pain and vice versa. In clinical practice, however, positive neurological signs such as reduced muscle strength and reflex changes are considered significant finding by clinicians that can increase the index of suspicion of neuropathic pain (Mistry et al., 2020a),

In the absence of a 'gold standard' to diagnose neuropathic pain in musculoskeletal conditions, clinicians will often rely on a combination of patient history, physical examination and screening tools (Mistry et al., 2020b) to make a pragmatic decision about the presence of neuropathic pain. Physical examination following the subjective examination can include, for example, mapping pain or sensory change referral and distribution, muscle strength changes and pain/symptom provocation with tests for heightened nerve mechanosensitivity such as SLR and nerve palpation. Many of these tests, however, have been shown to have a high risk of bias in their diagnostic accuracy as they are based on a reference standard of either clinician's opinions or MRI results, both of which have low validity in diagnosing neuropathic pain (Mistry et al., 2020b).

Signs and symptoms of nerve-related musculoskeletal pain will often present as an evolving picture over time. An example of this can be seen in CTS, where intermittent paraesthesia and alteration in sensation, particularly at night, are often some of the first symptoms; this may be due to changes in the intraneural circulation, with some oedema accumulating at night and disappearing during the day (Lundborg et al., 1983; Chammas et al., 2014). Later in the progression of nerve compression, there is increased numbness and paraesthesia, impaired dexterity and muscle weakness. These symptoms may be present during the day as well as at night and may be related to altered circulation and the presence of epineural and intrafascicular oedema (Fuchs et al., 1991; Chammas et al., 2014). Compression and the resulting oedematous change may disrupt the diffusion barrier, impair axonal transportation and cause demyelination, leading to disruption of conductivity and ectopic discharge (Schmid et al., 2013). Minor mechanical irritation can lead to radiating pain (Smyth & Wright, 1958; MacNab, 1972; Howe et al., 1977; Rydevik et al., 1984). Finally, atrophy of the thenar muscles and permanent sensory changes may be due to demyelination and axonal degeneration of the motor and sensory nerve fibres (Lundborg & Dahlin, 1996).

Classification Algorithm

Establishing the most pertinent pain mechanisms can be challenging for nerve-related musculoskeletal pain, and often most confusing for clinicians is establishing the contribution of pain mechanisms in people with spinally referred leg pain. An algorithm has been developed by Schmid and Tampin (2018) (Fig. 6.32) to assist clinicians to navigate through the complexity of different mechanisms responsible for the patient's leg pain, ranging from a nociceptive presentation (somatic referred pain) to a more severe presentation with loss of nerve function (radiculopathy). The algorithm demonstrates the importance of considering pain distribution, pain descriptors and neurological integrity changes and how each of these factors can co-exist.

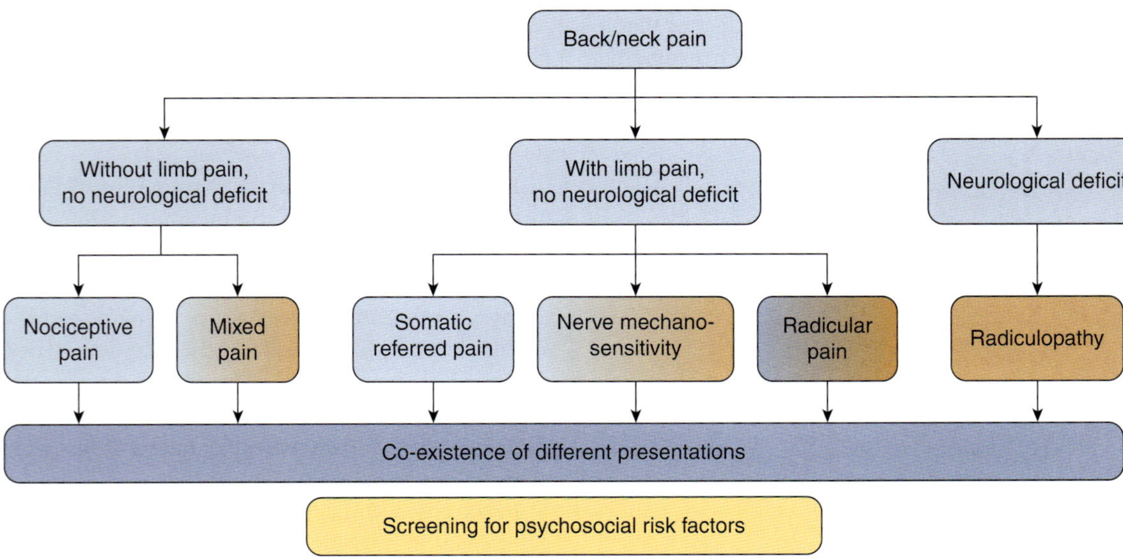

Fig. 6.32 Classification of spinally referred leg pain. (*From Schmid and Tampin 2018 with permission.*)

TABLE 6.3 Summary of Neuropathic Pain Screening Tools

	Pain Detect	LANSS	S-LANSS	DN4	NPQ	ID Pain	StEP
Descriptor							
Pain constancy	x						x
Burning	x	x	x	x	x	x	x
Tingling, pins and needles	x	x	x	x	x	x	x
Pain evoked by light touch	x	x	x		x	x	
Electric shocks or shooting	x	x		x			
Pain evoked by heat/cold	x						x
Painful cold or freezing pain				x	x		x
Numbness	x			x	x	x	x
Pain evoked by pressure	x						x
Itching				x			
Autonomic changes		x	x				x
Radiation of pain	x						
Temporal pain pattern	x						
Body chart	x		x				
Clinical examination							
Brush allodynia		x		x			x
Decreased response to brush movement							x
Touch hyperesthesia				x			
Pin prick hypoesthesia		x					x
Pin prick hyperesthesia		x					x
Decreased response to blunt pressure							x
Decreased response to cold temperature							x
Cold-evoked pain							x
Temporal summation							x
Pain on straight leg raise testing							x

DN4, Douleur Neuropathique en 4 questions; *LANSS,* Leeds Assessment of Neuropathic Symptoms and Signs; *NPQ,* Neuropathic Pain Questionnaire; *StEP,* Standardized Evaluation of Pain; *S-LANSS,* Self-administered Leeds Assessment of Neuropathic Symptoms and Signs.

Source: Schmid and Tampin, 2018 Lumbar Spine Textbook » Section 10: Non-operative Spine Care » Section 10, Chapter 10: Spinally Referred Back and Leg Pain https://www.wheelessonline.com/issls/section-10-chapter-10-spinally-referred-back-and-leg-pain/

KNOWLEDGE CHECK

1. Describe the difference between radicular pain and radiculopathy in patients with low back–related leg pain.

Screening Tools

In the absence of a gold standard to diagnose neuropathic pain, certain screening tools have been developed to aid in the identification of neuropathic pain. Most screening tools are based on verbal pain descriptors whilst some include an objective examination component (Table 6.3).

The sensitivity and specificity of these screening tools vary widely, and the risk of bias in diagnostic accuracy remains high. Many of the screening tools have been developed for use with nonmusculoskeletal neuropathic pain conditions such as generalized chronic pain (Bennett, 2001) or nervous system or somatic lesions (Bouhassira et al., 2005). The pain DETECT questionnaire is the only screening tool developed specifically for patients with chronic LBP (Freynhagen et al., 2006), and on original testing it demonstrated high sensitivity and specificity (85%, 80%, respectively). However, when using the tool in people with radiculopathy in the Netherlands, it was found to have moderate sensitivity of 75% (95% CI: 61.6–85.0) and poor specificity of 51% (95% CI: 42.0–60.4) (Epping et al., 2017), indicating the inherent issues with using descriptors translated from one language to another. Since the questionnaire was originally validated in German and has not been validated in English, caution should be made when using the English version. Similarly, the French DN4 (Bouhassira et al., 2005) has also not been validated in English.

The StEP tool has been tested for use in musculoskeletal conditions such as lumbar or radicular pain, as well as more systemic neuropathic pain conditions such as diabetic polyneuropathy and postherpetic neuralgia (Scholz et al., 2009). In a systematic review (Mistry et al., 2020b), this tool was found to have a low risk of bias. However, the reference standard for determining the presence of neuropathic pain was clinician judgement, which is not considered a 'gold standard' of assessment. This undermines the validity of this tool.

Bedside Clinical Examination

Clinical examination of the neurological system can aid in diagnosing nerve-related musculoskeletal pain and can help to differentiate clinical presentations such as radicular pain, radiculopathy, nociceptive or neuropathic pain presentations and is therefore an essential component of the patient assessment.

Assessment of sensation relevant to the distribution of symptoms can be helpful in assessing the integrity of the sensory nerve fibres. Sensory information from the skin to the central nervous system is conveyed via different sensory nerve fibres, including large myelinated Aβ fibres which convey nonpainful mechanical information (such as light touch and vibration), and smaller thinly myelinated (Aδ) and unmyelinated (C) nerve fibres, which convey painful mechanical stimulation (pin prick) as well as thermal changes (Aδ fibres: cold sensation, heat pain, C-fibres: warm sensation, cold pain) (Millan, 1999; Baron et al., 2012; Von Hehn et al., 2012).

Traditionally, sensory testing in patients with nerve-related musculoskeletal pain has focused on large fibre function (Ridehalgh et al., 2018). This can be broadly assessed with bedside examination of light touch sensibility, although in a research environment, the most sensitive physical tests of large-diameter nerve impairment are vibration sensibility (Gelberman et al., 1983; Szabo et al., 1983) using a 256-cycles-per-second tuning fork (Dellon, 1980, 1981) or vibrameter (Goldberg & Lindblom, 1979; Martina et al., 1998) and mechanical threshold testing (Gelberman et al., 1983; Szabo et al., 1983) using von Frey monofilaments (Levin et al., 1978).

Assessment of sensory loss based solely on large-diameter nerve fibre function must be considered with caution, as large fibre tests may be negative despite the report of subjective sensory symptoms. An example of this is seen in CTS, where during nerve conduction studies, up to 25% of patients had false negative results for distal sensory latency (Demino & Fowler, 2021).

Small fibre nerve function has also been shown to deteriorate in nerve-related musculoskeletal conditions, and this may occur prior to large fibre degeneration and to a greater extent (Schmid et al., 2014; Tamburin et al., 2011). Tests for small fibre function include pin prick sensation, warm detection thresholds and cold detection thresholds. The validity of pin prick and cold/warm detection to assess small fibre nerve function was explored by Ridehalgh et al. (2018) in 85 patients with CTS, compared to 22 healthy controls. Skin biopsy was used as a gold standard to objectively determine intraepidermal nerve fibre density (a measure of the density of the small fibres within the epidermis), and this was compared to the outcomes of pin prick and cold-warm detection threshold using QST. The results demonstrated reduced pin prick was highly specific (0.88: 95% CI: 0.72, 0.95) and therefore able to rule in small fibre degeneration, whereas normal warm AND cold sensation was highly sensitive to rule out small fibre degeneration (0.98: 95% CI 0.85: 0.99). A cluster of tests was therefore recommended, first using pin prick, followed by cold and warm sensation testing if pin prick is normal.

Small and large nerve fibre function can be assessed formally using QST, which involves a selection of psychophysical tests to evaluate an individual's response to graded stimulus, such as static mechanical (calibrated pins), static thermal, dynamic mechanical (standardized brush), and vibration sensations. The patient is required to participate by either pressing a button (i.e. when determining a thermal threshold) or verbally to judge whether or not a stimulus can be felt or is painful. The different tests broadly assess loss or gain of sensory nerve function (Backonja et al., 2009). QST is often used in research settings; however it requires specialist equipment, training and is time-consuming to perform. Therefore more simple bedside examinations might be used in a clinical setting to assess somatosensory function (Zhu et al., 2019). Bedside examination techniques can include static and dynamic light touch using cotton wool, vibration using a tuning fork, pin prick and cold and warm sensation, using for example cold and warm coins. The patient may report sensory loss, or there may be positive symptoms including hyperalgesia (increased sensitivity to pain), paraesthesia (nonpainful abnormal sensation), allodynia (pain to normally nonpainful stimuli) and changed sensations to heat and cold. A summary of bedside sensory assessment is provided in Table 6.4.

KNOWLEDGE CHECK

1. Describe bedside clinical examination tests used to assess small and large nerve fibre function.
2. Why is small nerve fibre testing an important part of your clinical examination?

The validity of bedside sensory testing has been compared with the gold standard QST by Zhu et al. (2019) to explore rates of agreement between the two modalities. Three patient cohorts were recruited with CTS, nonspecific neck and arm pain and lumbar radicular pain/radiculopathy. Thirteen bedside examination tests were then performed, including thermal sensation (with coins, ice cubes and hot test tubes), mechanical sensation (with tuning forks, toothpicks, cotton wool, von Frey hairs, thumb and eraser pressure) and pain detection thresholds. Several bedside tests, including cold, warm and mechanical detection threshold, as well as cold and pressure pain thresholds, were significantly correlated with QST, with most showing greater than 60% agreements rates, varying according to aetiology (Zhu et al., 2019).

Mapping of sensory changes can be done using body charts to document small and large fibre loss or gain of function, and the reported percentage of change can be recorded as an outcome measure. Sensory loss correlated with dermatome distribution might suggest involvement of the nerve root (radiculopathy), although traditional dermatome maps are known to have areas of inconsistency and overlap between the different sensory projections (Foerster, 1933; Keegan, 1947). Sensory changes should therefore be considered within the context of a full clinical examination, including myotomes and reflexes, which if altered, might also raise suspicion of radiculopathy or peripheral neuropathy.

Clinicians must also consider the potential bias of these clinical examination tests. Sensory testing can be impacted by patient's motivation, attention, and cognitive impairment. In studies of diagnostic accuracy, physical examination findings are often subject to a high risk of bias caused by poor reference standards (often based on clinician opinion or MRI findings), limited patient selection and poor blinding, patient flow and timing of tests, all of which limits the clinical utility of these tests (Mistry et al., 2020b).

Prevalence of Neuropathic Pain

Bearing in mind the challenges of accurately identifying neuropathic pain, assessing the prevalence in a musculoskeletal population is equally as complex. In a review of the prevalence, characteristic and prognosis of neuropathic pain in primary care by Harrisson et al. (2020), the diagnostic accuracy of different methods to diagnose neuropathic pain (within the same cohort) was examined. Diagnosis based on symptom descriptions alone showed the highest prevalence of 74%, diagnosis on symptoms and positive MRI findings showed a 46% prevalence, and diagnosis using a screening tool (sLANSS) showed a 49% prevalence. Interestingly, patients classified as having neuropathic pain from sLANSS appeared to have distinctly different profiles, including lower pain self-efficacy and higher use of medication, when compared with clinical diagnosis alone, suggesting there may be subgroups of patients with distinct neuropathic pain profiles (Harrisson et al., 2020).

TABLE 6.4 **Bedside Sensory Examination**					
Type of Stimulus	**Axon Type**	**Tool**		**Sensory**	**Loss Gain**
Static light touch	Aβ	Q-tip, cotton wool	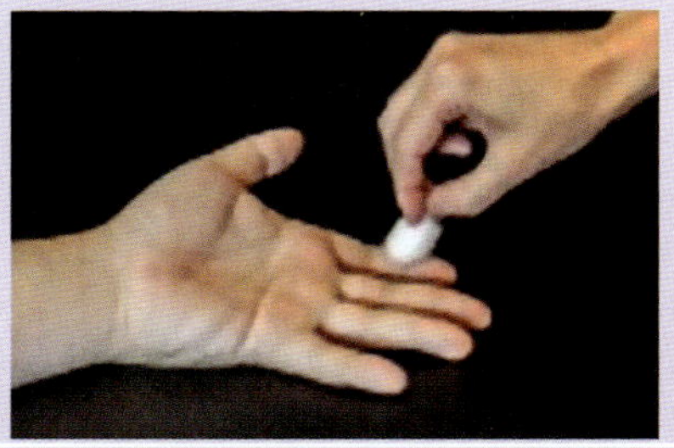	✓	✓
Vibration	Aβ	Tuning fork	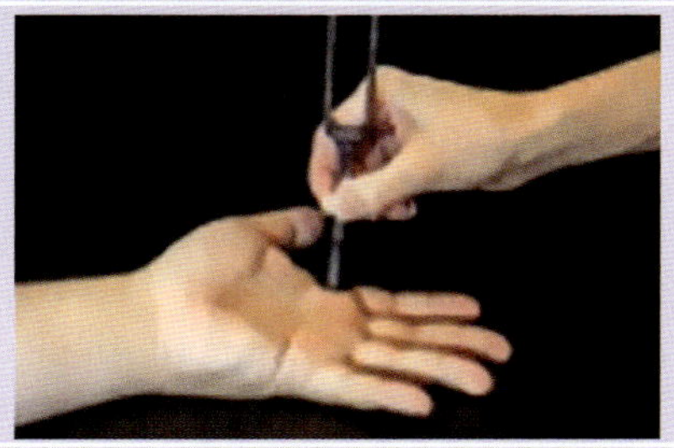	✓	
Dynamic mechanical	Aβ	Brush, cotton wool, Q-tip	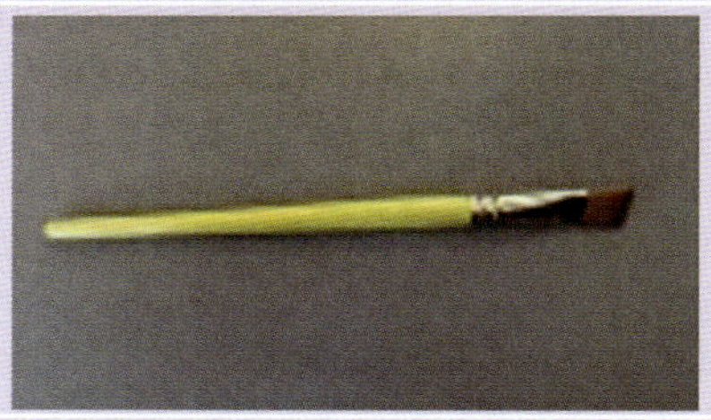	✓	✓
Pin prick	Aδ and C	Toothpick	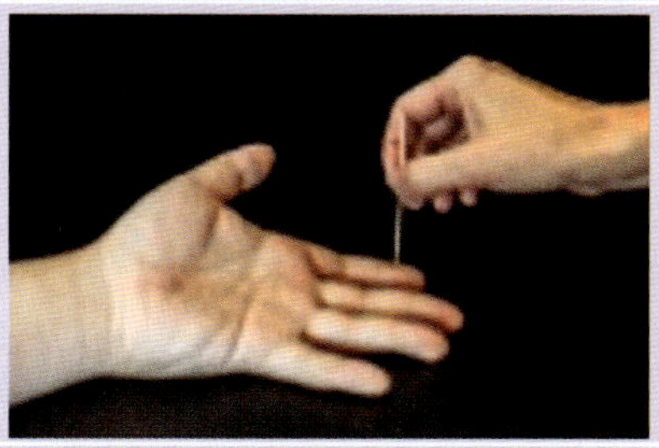	✓	✓
Cold/warm detection	Aδ and C	A5 Cold and warm and C coins/ thermo-rollers, tiptherm	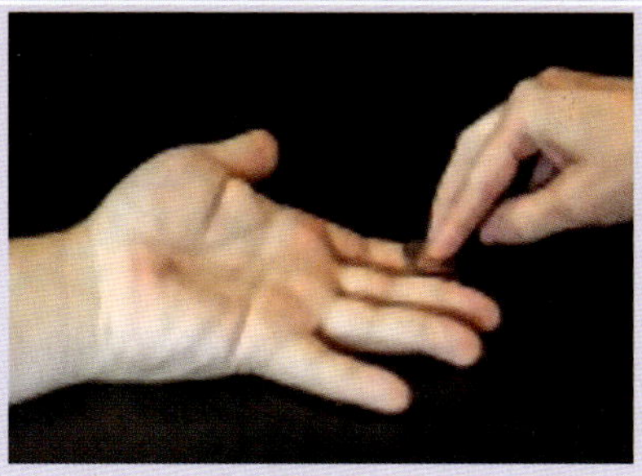	✓	

From: Schmid, A.B., Fundaun, J., Tampin, B., 2020. Entrapment neuropathies: a contemporary approach to pathophysiology, clinical assessment, and management. Pain Rep. 5 (4), e829.

Patients with conditions traditionally considered to be nociceptive in nature may also have symptoms of neuropathic pain. In a recent systematic review and meta-analysis of patients with knee or hip osteoarthritis, 23% of patients were found to have neuropathic pain characteristics (French et al., 2017). However, the review was based mainly on observational studies where a diagnosis of OA was often made on symptom descriptions or x-ray findings rather than physical examination. In most studies, the neuropathic pain screening tools used were not validated for use in measuring peripheral pain conditions. There was also significant heterogeneity between studies ($I2 = 97.9\%$, $P < .001$), because of inadequate sample sizes and lack of controlling of other potential causes of neuropathic pain which limits the interpretation of the results.

The prevalence of neuropathic pain in patients with musculoskeletal conditions is not necessarily dependent upon the existing diagnosis or aetiology. In a recent systematic review with meta-analysis, it was suggested that the prevalence of neuropathic pain in chronic low back pain was up to 54.4%, and in soft tissue syndromes such as fibromyalgia, tendinopathy, chronic widespread pain and myofascial pain syndrome was up to 43.3%. However, the methods used to diagnose neuropathic pain in the included studies were again highly variable, contributing to significant differences in prevalence rates between studies (Fishbain et al., 2014).

Risk Factors for Developing Neuropathic Pain

Risk factors for neuropathic pain in non-musculoskeletal conditions have been extensively explored and, although not necessarily specific to conditions seen in physiotherapy clinics, it is likely that some of these risk factors might be relevant to all patients:

- Clinical factors such as diabetes, peripheral artery disease, HDL cholesterol and preexisting pain (Van Acker et al., 2009; Ziegler et al., 2009).
- Psychosocial factors such as depression, anxiety (Calvo et al., 2019), sleep disturbance (Stocks et al., 2018), low physical activity, pain catastrophizing, alcohol, smoking and high BMI (Bouhassira et al., 2013).
- Genetic factors which might influence neurotransmission, ion channels, iron metabolism and immune response (Momi et al., 2015).
- Demographic factors including older age (Van Acker et al., 2009), female gender, deprivation and manual occupation (Smith & Torrance, 2012).
- Environmental factors may also play a role in the development of neuropathic pain. In carpal tunnel, for example, the increasing use of computer keyboards has been postulated for a rise in CTS (Keir et al., 1999). However, more recently, this has been refuted with one systematic review finding insufficient epidemiological evidence to postulate that computer use caused CTS (Thomsen et al., 2008) and another large cohort study of 1551 workers finding no association between new cases of CTS and computer use. Indeed, it was found more commonly in those with non-computer-related employment (Mediouni et al., 2015). There is, however, strong evidence that tasks requiring 'repetition and forceful exertion', and moderate evidence that exposure to vibration tools may increase the risk of developing CTS (Kozak et al., 2015). Individuals with CTS who are regularly exposed to hand-held vibration tools have been found to have demyelination and incomplete regeneration of the dorsal interosseous nerve at the wrist (Stromberg et al., 1997).

Each of these factors might contribute to the development and persistence of neuropathic pain in conditions such as radiculopathy, CTS and cubital tunnel syndrome, and this reinforces the need for a holistic person-centred approach to treatment and management of nerve-related musculoskeletal pain.

> **KNOWLEDGE CHECK**
> 1. List five potential risk factors for developing neuropathic pain.

CLINICAL EXAMPLE OF NERVE-RELATED MUSCULOSKELETAL PAIN

Lady With Low Back and Leg Pain

A 45-year-old care assistant presented with a 6-month history of pain in the right side of her lumbar spine and down the right lateral thigh and calf. There was an area of maximal pain, which she described as a burning pain in her lateral foot and associated tingling in the same area. There was no pain or sensory changes in the left leg. The pain had started after lifting an oven into the boot of the car. She felt a sudden pop in her back and immediate pain. The pain was aggravated by sitting or driving for more than 15 minutes and bending over while standing. She was able to continue driving once the pain started but often chose to get out of the car and walk around for a few minutes to ease the pain; otherwise, the pain would increase to an 8 or 9 out of 10 on the VAS. Systemically, she was fit and well, although she did have a history of anxiety and depression, which she relates to the challenges of caring for her son, who has autism and suffers from night terrors. She was also waking at night time with pain. She had tried taking over-the-counter paracetamol and ibuprofen but did not find this helpful and was not currently taking any medication. She had previously enjoyed attending gym classes, but had stopped at the onset of back and leg pain. There were no changes in bladder or bowel function, saddle sensation changes or gait disturbance.

Based on the history, her pain was not considered irritable but had the potential to be severe if aggravated. Therefore examinations were performed only at the initial onset of symptoms, positions were not held for long periods of time and a recovery time was provided between each assessment technique.

On examination, she had normal reflexes and muscle strength, but there was some reduced sensation to light touch and pin prick in the lateral foot. Her pain in the back and leg was reproduced on lumbar spine flexion, and after testing this movement, there was a slight delayed onset of P&N in her foot. Slump testing was as follows:

Neutral sitting √/ Lumbo-thoracic flexion √/ cervical flexion√/ right foot PF √/right foot inversion√/knee extension – immediate pain/P&N in lateral foot at −45 degrees from neutral + pain/P&N reduced with cervical extension

Pain in the foot was also reproduced on unilateral PA of the L5/S1 level in prone.

Based on the subjective and physical examination, the patient was classified as having a right-sided S1 radiculopathy (sensory loss on light touch and pin prick sensation) with components of neuropathic pain (burning pain with P&N) and heightened nerve mechano-sensitivity (positive slump).

MRI Findings

It is well known that MRI findings do not necessarily correlate with clinical symptoms. In asymptomatic subjects, a high prevalence of disc abnormalities has been found on MRI, including disc bulges and protrusions (Jensen et al., 1994; Boden, 1990). In patients with LBP, MRI findings do not appear to correlate with the incidence of pain and do not help to predict the patient's prognosis (McNee et al., 2011). There does, however, appear to be some evidence of the role of MRI investigations in patients with leg pain or radiculopathy, which suggests better prognosis in the presence of small disc herniations in a large spinal canal (Carragee & Kim, 1997), annular rupture, nerve root compression (Vroomen et al., 2002) and disc extrusion (Takada et al., 2001), and worse prognosis in exit foramina compression (Vroomen et al., 2002) (Fig. 6.33). MRI finding, should, therefore, be considered only in the context of patient symptoms and more often to explore potential serious pathology or in light of failed conservative management.

This patient had an MRI of the lumbar spine, based on poor response to previous treatment which showed:

> *At the L5/S1 level a combination of circumferential bulging of the disc and ligamentum flavum and facet hypertrophy is resulting in impingement of the right S1 nerve root as it courses through the lateral recess*

Canal, Lateral Recess and Foraminal Narrowing

Narrowing of the lateral recess is a common presentation in patients presenting with a posterolateral disc bulge or protrusion (see Fig. 6.33C). The descending nerve root may be compressed in isolation or in combination with the exiting nerve root at that level. For example, at the level of L5–S1, the L5 nerve root is located in the intervertebral foramen, and the S1 nerve root is located in the lateral recess on its journey caudally to leave the spinal canal at the level of S1. For this reason, patients with L5–S1 lateral recess stenosis may experience signs and symptoms emanating from either the L5 and S1 levels or both. A more lateral disc protrusion, however, produces narrowing to the

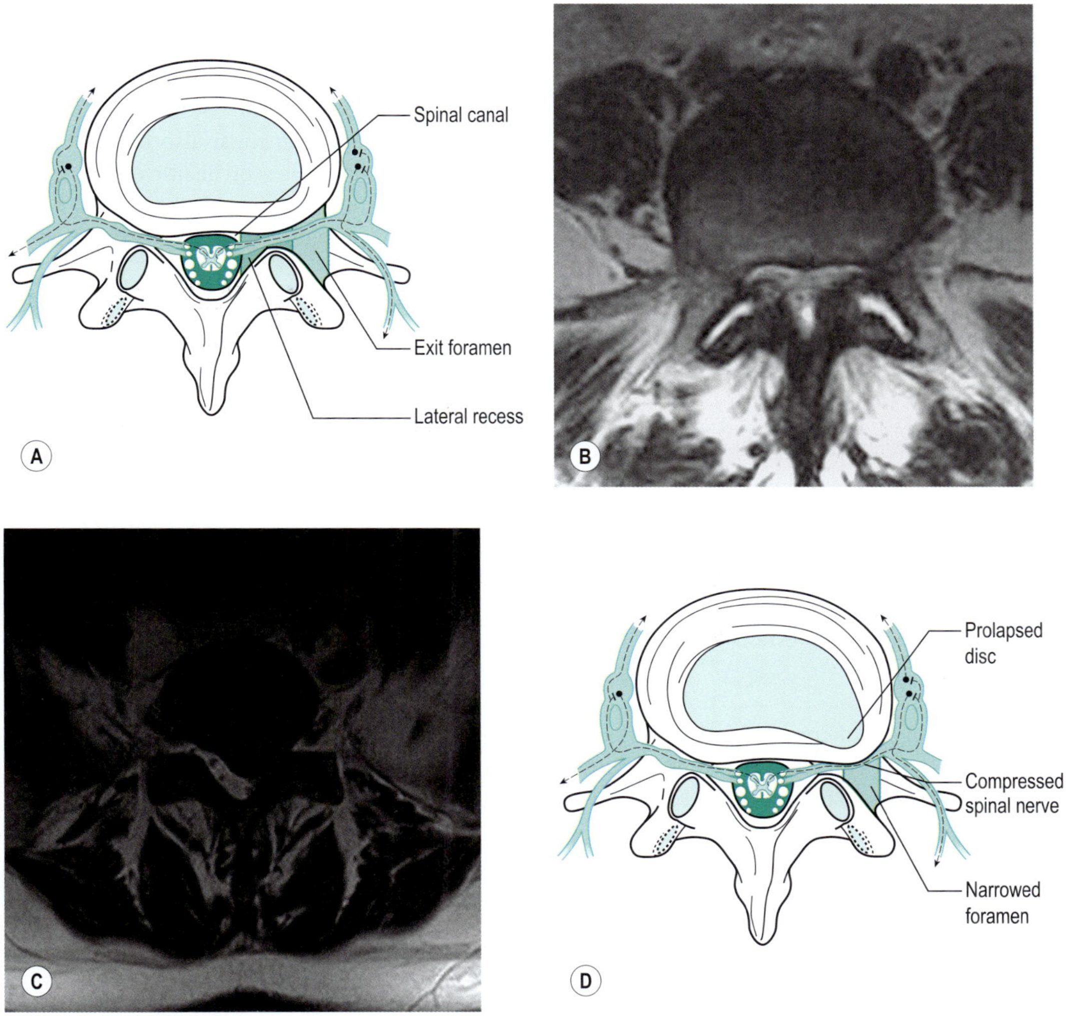

Fig. 6.33 Types of disc prolapse in the lumbar spine. (A) Cross-sectional anatomy of the spinal canal. *DRG*, dorsal root ganglion. (B) Spinal canal stenosis. (C) Lateral recess stenosis. (D) Exit foramen stenosis. (*A and D adapted from Palastanga & Soames 2012, B from Resnick & Kransdorf 2005, C from McNair & Breakwell 2010, reproduced with permission.*)

intervertebral exit foramen, where the nerve has already exited the spinal canal (see Fig. 6.33D). At the level of L5–S1, these patients may experience only L5 signs and symptoms as only the L5 root is located in the exit foramen and can be mechanically affected.

The management of this lady can be followed in Chapter 7.

Summary of Nerve-Related Musculoskeletal Pain

This chapter demonstrates the complexity of nerve-related musculoskeletal pain, where patients can present with varied and differing signs and symptoms as well as a plethora of different pathophysiological mechanisms. Identifying nerve-related MSK pain and distinguishing the pain mechanisms responsible is vital in order to plan patient management, but challenges remain in the accuracy of tools used to categorize the conditions. A thorough examination including detailed subjective questioning, bedside neurological examination and tests for heightened nerve mechanosensitivity are required to distinguish different pain mechanisms responsible. Screening tools and diagnostic testing are also important to determine the main mechanism responsible, but the clinician must use clinical judgement to make a pragmatic decision about the role of nerve-related and neuropathic pain in each individual patient. Consideration of risk factors for nerve-related and neuropathic pain must also be discussed with the patient, and principles of health coaching and shared decision-making can support the patient to implement behavioural change to reduce their modifiable risk factors.

REVIEW AND REVISE QUESTIONS

1. The perineurial barrier means that immune cells cannot freely enter the axons to counter an attack from pathogens. How does the nervous system counter this?
2. Explain how the connective tissue of a nerve can be a direct source of pain.
3. The three main mechanical events occurring with joint movement are ...., ... and ....
4. List three consequences of compression to the nerve.
5. Why might symptoms outside of an anatomical territory (e.g. a dermatome) still be considered a neuropathic pain condition?
6. Which of these terms describes allodynia?
   a. Overtly painful response to a normally painful stimulus.
   b. Painful response to a normally nonpainful stimulus.
   c. An abnormal and often extreme pain response to repeated stimulus.
   d. An unusual unpleasant sensory sensation.
7. Aβ fibres convey ...., Aδ fibres convey .... sensation and ....pain and unmyelinated (C) nerve fibres convey .... sensation and .... pain.

REFERENCES

Adams, M.A., Burton, K., Dolan, P., et al., 2006. The Biomechanics of Back Pain, second ed. Churchill Livingstone, Edinburgh.

Andrade, R.J., Nordez, A., Hug, F., Ates, F., Coppieters, M.W., Pezarat-Correia, P., et al., 2016. Non-invasive assessment of sciatic nerve stiffness during human ankle motion using ultrasound shear wave elastography. J. Biomech. 49 (3), 326–331.

Backonja, M.M., Walk, D., Edwards, R.R., Sehgal, N., Moeller-Bertram, T., et al., 2009. Quantitative sensory testing in measurement of neuropathic pain phenomena and other sensory abnormalities. Clin. J. Pain 25 (7), 641–647.

Bahns, E., Ernsberger, U., Janig, W., et al., 1986. Discharge properties of mechanosensitive afferents supplying the retroperitoneal space. Pflügers Arch. 407, 519–525.

Baron, R., Förster, M., Binder, A., 2012. Subgrouping of patients with neuropathic pain according to pain-related sensory abnormalities: a first step to a stratified treatment approach. Lancet Neurol. 11 (11), 999–1005.

Baron, E.M., Tunstall, R., Standring, S., 2015. Gray's Anatomy: The Anatomical Basis of Clinical Practice. Elsevier Health Sciences, Edinburgh.

Bennett, M., 2001. The LANSS Pain Scale: the Leeds assessment of neuropathic symptoms and signs. Pain 92 (1–2), 147–157.

Bisby, M.A., 1982. Functions of retrograde axonal transport. Fed. Proc. 41, 2307–2311.

Boden, S.D., 1990. The incidence of abnormal lumbar spine: MRI scans in asymptomatic patients: A prospective and blinded investigation. Orthop. Trans. 14, 66.

Bouhassira, D., Attal, N., Alchaar, H., Boureau, F., Brochet, B., Bruxelle, J., et al., 2005. Comparison of pain syndromes associated with nervous or somatic lesions and development of a new neuropathic pain diagnostic questionnaire (DN4). Pain 114 (1–2), 29–36.

Bouhassira, D., Letanoux, M., Hartemann, A., 2013. Chronic pain with neuropathic characteristics in diabetic patients: a French cross-sectional study. PLoS One 8 (9), e74195.

Bove, G.M., Light, A.R., 1995. Unmyelinated nociceptors of rat paraspinal tissues. J. Neurophysiol. 73, 1752–1762.

Boyd, B.S., Puttlitz, C., Jerylin, G., et al., 2005. Strain and excursion in the rat sciatic nerve during a modified straight leg raise are altered after traumatic nerve injury. J. Orthop. Res. 23, 764–770.

Boyd, B.S., Topp, K.S., Coppieters, M.W., 2013. Impact of movement sequencing on sciatic and tibial nerve strain and excursion during the straight leg raise test in embalmed cadavers. J. Orthop. Sports Phys. Ther. 43, 398–403.

Breig, A., 1960. Biomechanics of the Central Nervous System: Some Basic Normal and Pathologic Phenomena. Almqvist & Wiksell, Stockholm.

Breig, A., Marions, O., 1963. Biomechanics of the lumbosacral nerve roots. Acta Radiol. 1, 1141–1160.

Brochwicz, P., von Piekartz, H., Zalpour, C., 2013. Sonography assessment of the median nerve during cervical lateral glide and lateral flexion. Is there a difference in neurodynamics of asymptomatic people? Man. Ther. 18 (3), 216–219. https://doi.org/10.1016/j.math.2012.10.001.

Butler, D.S., 2000. The Sensitive Nervous System. Noigroup, Adelaide.

Calvo, M., Davies, A.J., Hébert, H.L., Weir, G.A., Chesler, E.J., Finnerup, N.B., et al., 2019. The genetics of neuropathic pain from model organisms to clinical application. Neuron. 104 (4), 637–653.

Caridi, J.M., Pumberger, M., Hughes, A.P., 2011. Cervical radiculopathy: a review. HSS J. 7 (3), 265–272.

Carragee, E.J., Kim, D.H., 1997. A prospective analysis of magnetic resonance imaging findings in patients with sciatica and lumbar disc herniation: correlation of outcomes with disc fragment and canal morphology. Spine 22 (14), 1650–1660.

Chammas, M., Boretto, J., Burmann, L.M., et al., 2014. Carpal tunnel syndrome – part I (anatomy, physiology, etiology and diagnosis). Rev. Bras. Ortop. 49, 429–436.

Clark, W.L., Trumble, T.E., Swiontkowski, M.F., et al., 1992. Nerve tension and blood flow in a rat model of immediate and delayed repairs. J. Hand Surg. Am. 17A, 677–687.

Coppieters, M.W., Alshami, A.M., Babri, A.S., et al., 2006. Strain and excursion of the sciatic, tibial, and plantar nerves during a modified straight leg raising test. J. Orthop. Res. 24, 1883–1889.

Coppieters, M.W., Butler, D.S., 2008. Do 'sliders' slide and 'tensioners' tension? An analysis of neurodynamic techniques and considerations regarding their application. Man. Ther. 13 (3), 213–221. https://doi.org/10.1016/j.math.2006.12.008.

Coppieters, M.W., Hough, A.D., Dilley, A., 2009. Different nerve-gliding exercises induce different magnitudes of median nerve longitudinal excursion: an in vivo study using dynamic ultrasound imaging. J. Orthop. Sports Phys. Ther. 39, 164–171.

Coppieters, M.W., Crooke, J.L., Lawrenson, P.R., et al., 2015. A modified straight leg raise test to differentiate between sural nerve pathology and Achilles tendinopathy. A cross-sectional cadaver study. Man. Ther. 20, 587–591.

Cox, J.J., Reimann, F., Nicholas, A.K., et al., 2006. An SCN9A channelopathy causes congenital inability to experience pain. Nature 444, 894–898. https://doi.org/10.1038/nature05413.

Crossman, A., Neary, D., 2015. Neuroanatomy: An Illustrated Colour Text, fifth ed. Elsevier Health Sciences, London.

Dahlin, L.B., Lundborg, G., 1990. The neurone and its response to peripheral nerve compression. J. Hand Surg. Am. 15B, 5–10.

Dahlin, L.B., McLean, W.G., 1986. Effects of graded experimental compression on slow and fast axonal transport in rabbit vagus nerve. J. Neurol. Sci. 72, 19–30.

Dellon, A.L., 1980. Clinical use of vibratory stimuli to evaluate peripheral nerve injury and compression neuropathy. Plast. Reconstr. Surg. 65, 466–476.

Dellon, A.L., 1981. Evaluation of Sensibility and Re-Education of Sensation in the Hand. Williams and Wilkins, Baltimore.

Demino, C., Fowler, J.R., 2021. The sensitivity and specificity of nerve conduction studies for diagnosis of carpal tunnel syndrome: a systematic review. Hand 16 (2), 174–178.

Dilley, A., Greening, J., Lynn, B., et al., 2001. The use of cross-correlation analysis between high-frequency ultrasound images to measure longitudinal median nerve movement. Ultrasound Med. Biol. 27, 1211–1218.

Dilley, A., Lynn, B., Pang, S.J., 2005. Pressure and stretch mechanosensitivity of peripheral nerve fibres following local inflammation of the nerve trunk. Pain 117, 462–472.

Dilley, A., Bove, G.M., 2008. Disruption of axoplasmic transport induces mechanical sensitivity in intact rat C-fibre nociceptor axons. J. Physiol. 586 (2), 593–604. https://doi.org/10.1113/jphysiol.2007.144105.

Doubell, T.P., Woolf, C.J., 1997. Growth-associated protein 43 immunoreactivity in the superficial dorsal horn of the rat spinal cord is localized in atrophic C-fiber, and not in sprouted A-fiber, central terminals after peripheral nerve injury. J. Comp. Neurol. 386, 111–118.

Doubell, T.P., Mannion, R.J., Woolf, C.J., 1999. The dorsal horn: state-dependent sensory processing, plasticity and the generation of pain. In: Wall, P.D., Melzack, R. (Eds.), Textbook of Pain, fourth ed. Churchill Livingstone, Edinburgh, pp. 165–181.

Dubin, A.E., Patapoutian, A., 2010. Nociceptors: the sensors of the pain pathway. J. Clin. Invest. 120 (11), 3760–3772.

Dyck, P.J., Lais, A.C., Giannini, C., et al., 1990. Structural alterations of nerve during cuff compression. Proc. Natl. Acad. Sci. USA 87, 9828–9832.

Ellis, R.F., Hing, W.A., McNair, P.J., 2012. Comparison of longitudinal sciatic nerve movement with different mobilization exercises: an in vivo study utilizing ultrasound imaging. J. Orthop. Sports Phys. Ther. 42, 667–675.

Ellis, R., Blyth, R., Arnold, N., Miner-Williams, W., 2017. Is there a relationship between impaired median nerve excursion and carpal tunnel syndrome? A systematic review. J. Hand Ther. 30 (1), 3–12. https://doi.org/10.1016/j.jht.2016.09.002.

Epping, R., Verhagen, A.P., Hoebink, E.A., Rooker, S., Scholten-Peeters, G.G.M., 2017. The diagnostic accuracy and test-retest reliability of the Dutch PainDETECT and the DN4 screening tools for neuropathic pain in patients with suspected cervical or lumbar radiculopathy. Musculoskelet. Sci. Pract. 30, 72–79. https://doi.org/10.1016/j.msksp.2017.05.010.

Erel, E., Dilley, A., Greening, J., et al., 2003. Longitudinal sliding of the median nerve in patients with carpal tunnel syndrome. J. Hand Surg. Br. 28, 439–443.

Finnerup, N.B., Johannesen, I.L., Sindrup, S.H., Bach, F.W., Jensen, T.S., 2001. Pain and dysesthesia in patients with spinal cord injury: a postal survey. Spinal Cord 39 (5), 256–262.

Finnerup, N.B., Haroutounian, S., Kamerman, P., Baron, R., Bennett, D.L., Bouhassira, D., et al., 2016. Neuropathic pain: an updated grading system for research and clinical practice. Pain 157 (8), 1599.

Finnerup, N.B., Kuner, R., Jensen, T.S., 2021. Neuropathic pain: from mechanisms to treatment. Physiol. Rev. 101 (1), 259–301. https://doi.org/10.1152/physrev.00045.2019.

Fishbain, D.A., Cole, B., Lewis, J.E., Gao, J., 2014. What is the evidence that neuropathic pain is present in chronic low back pain and soft tissue syndromes? An evidence-based structured review. Pain Med. 15 (1), 4–15. https://doi.org/10.1111/pme.12229.

Foerster, O., 1933. The dermatomes in man. Brain 56 (1), 1–39.

French, H.P., Smart, K.M., Doyle, F., 2017. Prevalence of neuropathic pain in knee or hip osteoarthritis: a systematic review and meta-analysis. Semin. Arthritis Rheum. 47 (1), 1–8. https://doi.org/10.1016/j.semarthrit.2017.02.008.

Freynhagen, R., Baron, R., Gockel, U., Tölle, T.R., 2006. painDETECT: a new screening questionnaire to identify neuropathic components in patients with back pain. Curr. Med. Res. Opin. 22 (10), 1911–1920. https://doi.org/10.1185/030079906X132488.

Freynhagen, R., Bennett, M.I., 2009. Diagnosis and management of neuropathic pain. BMJ 339, b3002.

Fuchs, P.C., Nathan, P.A., Myers, L.D., 1991. Synovial histology in carpal tunnel syndrome. J. Hand Surg. Am. 16A, 753–758.

Gagné, M., Côté, I., Boulet, M., Jutzeler, C.R., Kramer, J.L.K., Mercier, C., 2020. Conditioned pain modulation decreases over time in patients with neuropathic pain following a spinal cord injury. Neurorehabil. Neural. Repair 34 (11), 997–1008. https://doi.org/10.1177/1545968320962497.

Gelberman, R.H., Hergenroeder, P.T., Hargens, A.R., et al., 1981. The carpal tunnel syndrome. A study of carpal canal pressures. J. Bone Joint Surg. Am. 63, 380–383.

Gelberman, R.H., Szabo, R.M., Williamson, R.V., et al., 1983. Sensibility testing in peripheral-nerve compression syndromes, an experimental study in humans. J. Bone Joint Surg. Am. 65A, 632–638.

Giardini, A.C., Dos Santos, F.M., da Silva, J.T., de Oliveira, M. E., Martins, D.O., Chacur, M., 2017. Neural mobilization treatment decreases glial cells and brain-derived neurotrophic factor expression in the central nervous system in rats with neuropathic pain induced by CCI in rats. Pain Res. Manag. 2017, 7429761. https://doi.org/10.1155/2017/7429761.

Gilbert, K.K., Brismée, J.M., Collins, D.L., et al., 2007. 2006 Young Investigator Award winner: lumbosacral nerve root displacement and strain: part 2. A comparison of 2 straight leg raise conditions in unembalmed cadavers. Spine 32, 1521–1525.

Goddard, M.D., Reid, J.D., 1965. Movements induced by straight leg raising in the lumbo-sacral roots, nerves and plexus, and in the intrapelvic section of the sciatic nerve. J. Neurol. Neurosurg. Psychiatry 28, 12–18.

Goldberg, J.M., Lindblom, U., 1979. Standardised method of determining vibratory perception thresholds for diagnosis and screening in neurological investigation. J. Neurol. Neurosurg. Psychiatry 42, 793–803.

Greening, J., Lynn, B., Leary, R., et al., 2001. The use of ultrasound imaging to demonstrate reduced movement of the median nerve during wrist flexion in patients with non-specific arm pain. J. Hand Surg. Am. 26B, 401–406.

Greening, J., Dilley, A., 2017. Posture-induced changes in peripheral nerve stiffness measured by ultrasound shear-wave elastography. Muscle Nerve 55 (2), 213–222. https://doi.org/10.1002/mus.25245.

Grossmann, L., Gorodetskaya, N., Baron, R., et al., 2009. Enhancement of ectopic discharge in regenerating A-and C-fibers by inflammatory mediators. J. Neurophysiol. 101, 2762–2774.

Harrisson, S.A., Ogollah, R., Dunn, K.M., Foster, N.E., Konstantinou, K., 2020. Prevalence, characteristics, and clinical course of neuropathic pain in primary care patients consulting with low back-related leg pain. Clin. J. Pain 36 (11), 813–824.

Hatashita, S., Sekiguchi, M., Kobayashi, H., Konno, S., Kikuchi, S.-I., 2008. Contralateral neuropathic pain and neuropathology in dorsal root ganglion and spinal cord following hemilateral nerve injury in rats. Spine 33 (12), 1344–1351. https://doi.org/10.1097/BRS.0b013e3181733188.

Heraughty, M., Ridehalgh, C., 2020. Sensory descriptors which identify neuropathic pain mechanisms in low back pain: a systematic review. Curr. Med. Res. Opin. 36 (10), 1695–1706.

Hopkins, A., Rudge, P., 1973. Hyperpathia in the central cervical cord syndrome. J. Neurol. Neurosurg. Psychiatry 36 (4), 637–642.

Hough, A.D., Moore, A.P., Jones, M.P., 2000. Peripheral nerve motion measurement with spectral Doppler sonography: a reliability study. J. Hand Surg. Am. 25B, 585–589.

Howe, J.F., Loeser, J.D., Calvin, W.H., 1977. Mechanosensitivity of dorsal root ganglia and chronically injured axons: a physiological basis for the radicular pain of nerve root compression. Pain 3, 25–41.

Hromada, J., 1963. On the nerve supply of the connective tissue of some peripheral nervous system components. Acta Anat. (Basel) 55, 343–351.

International Association for the Study of Pain. IASP Taxonomy. Pain terms. Neuropathic pain. Updated 2017 Dec 14. www.iasp-pain.org/Taxonomy#Neuropathicpain.

International Association for the Study of Pain 2014 IASP taxonomy. Available online at: http://www.iasp-pain.org/Taxonomy#Peripheralneuropathicpain. (Accessed 4 December 2016).

Jensen, M.C., Brant-Zawadzki, M.N., Obuchowski, N., Modic, M.T., Malkasian, D., Ross, J.S., 1994. Magnetic resonance imaging of the lumbar spine in people without back pain. N. Engl. J. Med. 331 (2), 69–73.

Jensen, T.S., Finnerup, N.B., 2014. Allodynia and hyperalgesia in neuropathic pain: clinical manifestations and mechanisms. Lancet Neurol. 13 (9), 924–935.

Johnston, E.C., Howell, S.J., 1999. Tension neuropathy of the superficial peroneal nerve: associated conditions and results of release. Foot Ankle Int. 20, 576–582.

Kandel, E.R., Schwarz, J.H., Jessel, T.M., 2000. Principles of Neural Science, fourth ed. McGraw-Hill, New York.

Kantarci, F., Ustabasioglu, F.E., Delil, S., Olgun, D.C., Korkmazer, B., Dikici, A.S., et al., 2014. Median nerve stiffness measurement by shear wave elastography: a potential sonographic method in the diagnosis of carpal tunnel syndrome. Eur. Radiol. 24 (2), 434–440.

Keir, P.J., Bach, J.M., Rempel, D., 1999. Effects of computer mouse design and task on carpal tunnel pressure. Ergonomics 42, 1350–1360.

Keegan, J.J., 1947. Relations of nerve roots to abnormalities of lumbar and cervical portions of the spine. Arch. Surg. 55 (3), 246–270.

Kiguchi, N., Kobayashi, Y., Kishioka, S., 2012. Chemokines and cytokines in neuroinflammation leading to neuropathic pain. Curr. Opin. Pharmacol. 12, 55–61.

Kingwell, K., 2019. Nav1.7 withholds its pain potential. Nat. Rev. Drug Discov. 18, 321–323.

Kobayashi, S., Shizu, N., Suzuki, Y., et al., 2003. Changes in nerve root motion and intraradicular blood flow during an intraoperative straight leg raise test. Spine 28, 1427–1434.

Kozak, A., Schedlbauer, G., Wirth, T., et al., 2015. Association between work-related biomechanical risk factors and the occurrence of carpal tunnel syndrome: an overview of systematic reviews and a meta-analysis of current research. BMC Musculoskelet. Disord. 16, 231.

Lee, E.Y., Lim, A.Y., 2019. Nerve compression in the upper limb. Clin. Plastic Surg. 46 (3), 285–293.

Levin, S., Pearsell, G., Ruderman, R.J., 1978. Von Frey's method of measuring pressure sensibility in the hand: an engineering analysis of the Weinstein–Semmes pressure aesthesiometer. J. Hand Surg. Am. 3, 211–216.

Luchtmann, M., Steinecke, Y., Baecke, S., Lützkendorf, R., Bernarding, J., Kohl, J., et al., 2014. Structural brain alterations in patients with lumbar disc herniation: a preliminary study. PLoS ONE 9 (3), e90816. https://doi.org/10.1371/journal.pone.0090816.

Lundborg, G., 1975. Structure and function of the intraneural microvessels as related to trauma, edema formation, and nerve function. J. Bone Joint Surg. Am. 57A, 938–948.

Lundborg, G., 2004. Nerve injury and repair. In: Regeneration, Reconstruction and Cortical Remodelling, second ed. Churchill Livingstone, Edinburgh.

Lundborg, G., Dahlin, L.B., 1992. The pathophysiology of nerve compression. Hand Clin. 8, 215–227.

Lundborg, G., Dahlin, L.B., 1996. Anatomy, function, and pathophysiology of peripheral nerves and nerve compression. Hand Clin. 12, 185–193.

Lundborg, G., Gelbermann, R.H., Minteer-Convery, M., et al., 1982. Median nerve compression in the carpal tunnel: functional response to experimentally induced controlled pressure. J. Hand Surg. Am. 7, 252–259.

Lundborg, G., Myers, R., Powell, H., 1983. Nerve compression injury and increased endoneurial fluid pressure: a miniature compartment syndrome. J. Neurol. Neurosurg. Psychiatry 46, 1119–1124.

Lundborg, G., Rydevik, B., Manthorpe, M., et al., 1987. Peripheral nerve: the physiology of injury and repair. In: Woo, S.L.-Y., Buckwalter, J.A. (Eds.), Injury and Repair of the Musculoskeletal Soft Tissues. American Academy of Orthopaedic Surgeons, Park Ridge, IL, pp. 295–352.

MacNab, I., 1972. The mechanism of spondylogenic pain. In: Hirsch, C., Zotterman, Y. (Eds.), Cervical Pain. Pergamon Press, Oxford, pp. 89–95.

Maeda, Y., Kettner, N., Holden, J., et al., 2014. Functional deficits in carpal tunnel syndrome reflect reorganization of primary somatosensory cortex. Brain 137, 1741–1752.
Manvell, J.J., Manvell, N., Snodgrass, S.J., Reid, S.A., 2015a. Improving the radial nerve neurodynamic test: an observation of tension of the radial, median and ulnar nerves during upper limb positioning. Man. Ther. 20 (6), 790–796. https://doi.org/10.1016/j.math.2015.03.007.
Manvell, N., Manvell, J.J., Snodgrass, S.J., Reid, S.A., 2015b. Tension of the ulnar, median, and radial nerves during ulnar nerve neurodynamic testing: observational cadaveric study. Phys. Ther. 95 (6), 891–900. https://doi.org/10.2522/ptj.20130536.
Marieb, E.N., 1995. Human Anatomy and Physiology, third ed. Benjamin/Cummings, San Francisco, CA.
Martina, I.S.J., van Koningsveld, R., Schmitz, P.I.M., et al., 1998. Measuring vibration threshold with a graduated tuning fork in normal aging and in patients with polyneuropathy. J. Neurol. Neurosurg. Psychiatry 65, 743–747.
McNair, C., Breakwell, L.M., 2010. Disc degeneration and prolapse. Orthop. Trauma 24, 430–434.
McNee, P., Shambrook, J., Harris, E.C., Kim, M., Sampson, M., Palmer, K.T., Coggon, D., 2011. Predictors of long-term pain and disability in patients with low back pain investigated by magnetic resonance imaging: a longitudinal study. BMC Musculoskelet. Disord. 12 (1), 1–12.
Mediouni, Z., Bodin, J., Dale, A.M., et al., 2015. Carpal tunnel syndrome and computer exposure at work in two large complementary cohorts. BMJ Open 5, e008156. https://doi.org/10.1136/bmjopen-2015-008156.
Michaelis, M., Häbler, H.J., Jäenig, W., 1996. Silent afferents: a separate class of primary afferents? Clin. Exp. Pharmacol. Physiol. 23 (2), 99–105. https://doi.org/10.1111/j.1440-1681.1996.
Middleditch, A., Oliver, J., 2005. Functional Anatomy of the Spine, second ed. Butterworth Heinemann, Edinburgh.
Millan, M.J., 1999. The induction of pain: an integrative review. Prog. Neurobiol. 57 (1), IASP1–164.
Mistry, J., Falla, D., Noblet, T., Heneghan, N.R., Rushton, A.B., 2020a. Clinical indicators to identify neuropathic pain in low back-related leg pain: protocol for a modified Delphi study. BMJ Open 10 (2), e033547.
Mistry, J., Heneghan, N.R., Noblet, T., Falla, D., Rushton, A., 2020b. Diagnostic utility of patient history, clinical examination and screening tool data to identify neuropathic pain in low back related leg pain: a systematic review and narrative synthesis. BMC Musculoskelet. Disord. 21 (1), 1–18.
Momi, S.K., Fabiane, S.M., Lachance, G., Livshits, G., Williams, F.M., 2015. Neuropathic pain as part of chronic widespread pain: environmental and genetic influences. Pain 156 (10), 2100.
Mtui, E., Gruener, G., Dockery, P., et al., 2015. Fitzgerald's Clinical Neuroanatomy and Neuroscience. Elsevier Health Sciences, Philadelphia.
Murphy, D.R., Hurwitz, E.L., Gerrard, J.K., Clary, R., 2009. Pain patterns and descriptions in patients with radicular pain: Does the pain necessarily follow a specific dermatome? Chiropr. Osteopat. 17 (1), 1–9.
Neto, T., Freitas, S.R., Andrade, R.J., Vaz, J.R., Mendes, B., Firmino, T., et al., 2020. Shear wave elastographic investigation of the immediate effects of slump neurodynamics in people with sciatica. J. Ultrasound Med. 39, 675–681. https://doi.org/10.1002/jum.15144.
Nitz, A.J., Dobner, J.J., Kersey, D., 1985. Nerve injury and grades II and III ankle sprains. Am. J. Sports Med. 13, 177–182.
Nora, D.B., Becker, J., Ehlers, J.A., et al., 2005. What symptoms are truly caused by median nerve compression in carpal tunnel syndrome? Clin. Neurophysiol. 116, 275–283.
Nitta, H., Tajima, T., Sugiyama, H., Moriyama, A., 1993. Study on dermatomes by means of selective lumbar spinal nerve block. Spine (Phila Pa 1976) 18 (13), 1782–1786. https://doi.org/10.1097/00007632-199310000-00011. PMID: 8235861.
Palastanga, N., Soames, R., 2012. Anatomy and Human Movement, Structure and Function, sixth ed. Churchill Livingstone, Edinburgh.
Palastanga, N., Field, D., Soames, R., 2002. Anatomy and Human Movement: Structure and Function, fourth ed. Butterworth-Heinemann, Oxford.
Paluch, L., Noszczyk, B.H., Walecki, J., Osiak, K., Kiciński, M., Pietruski, P., 2018. Shear-wave elastography in the diagnosis of ulnar tunnel syndrome. J. Plast. Reconstr. Aesthet. Surg. 71 (11), 1593–1599. https://doi.org/10.1016/j.bjps.2018.08.018. ISSN 1748-6815.
Panjabi, M.M., White, A.A., 2001. Biomechanics in the Musculoskeletal System. Churchill Livingstone, New York.
Peltonen, S., Alanne, M., Peltonen, J., 2013. Barriers of the peripheral nerve. Tissue Barriers 1, e24956.
Powell, H.C., Myers, R.R., 1986. Pathology of experimental nerve compression. Lab. Invest. 55, 91–100.
Rainville, J., Joyce, A.A., Laxer, E., Pena, E., Kim, D., Milam, R.A., et al., 2017. Comparison of symptoms from C6 and C7 radiculopathy. Spine 42 (20), 1545–1551.
Reid, J.D., 1960. Effects of flexion-extension movements of the head and spine upon the spinal cord and nerve roots. J. Neurol. Neurosurg. Psychiatry 23 (3), 214–221. https://doi.org/10.1136/jnnp.23.3.214.
Rempel, D., Dahlin, L., Lundborg, G., 1999. Pathophysiology of nerve compression syndromes: response of peripheral nerves to loading. J. Bone Joint Surg. Am. 81A, 1600–1610.

Resnick, D., Kransdorf, M.J., 2005. Degenerative disease of the spine. In: Bone and Joint Imaging. Elsevier, Richmond, VA (Chapter 30).

Ridehalgh, C., Moore, A., Hough, A., 2012. Repeatability of measuring sciatic nerve excursion during a modified passive straight leg raise test with ultrasound imaging. Man. Ther. 17, 572–576.

Ridehalgh, C., Moore, A., Hough, A., 2014. Normative sciatic nerve excursion during a modified straight leg raise test. Man. Ther. 19, 59–64.

Ridehalgh, C., Moore, A., Hough, A., 2015. Sciatic nerve excursion during a modified passive straight leg raise test in asymptomatic participants and participants with spinally referred leg pain. Man. Ther. 20, 564–569.

Ridehalgh, C., Sandy-Hindmarch, O.P., Schmid, A.B., 2018. Validity of clinical small-fiber sensory testing to detect small-nerve fiber degeneration. J. Orthop. Sports Phys. Ther. 48 (10), 767–774.

Rydevik, B., Lundborg, G., 1977. Permeability of intraneural microvessels and perineurium following acute, graded experimental nerve compression. Scand. J. Plast. Reconstr. Surg. 11, 179–187.

Rydevik, B., Lundborg, G., Bagge, U., 1981. Effects of graded compression on intraneural blood flow. An in vivo study on rabbit tibial nerve. J. Hand Surg. Am. 6, 3–12.

Rydevik, B., Brown, M.D., Lundborg, G., 1984. Pathoanatomy and pathophysiology of nerve root compression. Spine 9, 7–15.

Rydevik, B., Lundborg, G., Skalak, R., 1989. Biomechanics of peripheral nerves. In: Nordin, M., Frankel, V.H. (Eds.), Basic Biomechanics of the Musculoskeletal System, second ed. Lea & Febiger, Philadelphia, pp. 75–87.

Salonen, V., Lehto, M., Vaheri, A., et al., 1985. Endoneurial fibrosis following nerve transection. Acta Neuropathol. (Berlin) 67, 315–321.

Schmid, A.B., Bland, J.D., Bhat, M.A., Bennett, D.L., 2014. The relationship of nerve fibre pathology to sensory function in entrapment neuropathy. Brain 137 (12), 3186–3199.

Schmid, A.B., Fundaun, J., Tampin, B., 2020. Entrapment neuropathies: a contemporary approach to pathophysiology, clinical assessment, and management. Pain Rep. 5 (4), e829. https://doi.org/10.1097/PR9.0000000000000829. Published 2020 Jul 22.

Schmid, A.B., Tampin, B., 2018. Spinally referred back and leg pain. In: Lumbar Spine Online Textbook. ISftSotL Spine. Available at: http://www.wheelessonline.com/ISSLS/section-10-chapter-10-spinally-referredback-and-leg-pain/.

Schmid, A., 2015. The peripheral nervous system and its compromise in entrapment neuropathies. In: Jull, G., Moore, A.P., Falla, D., et al. (Eds.), Grieve's Modern Musculoskeletal Physiotherapy. Churchill Livingstone, Edinburgh.

Schmid, A.B., Nee, R.J., Coppieters, M.W., 2013. Reappraising entrapment neuropathies – mechanisms, diagnosis and management. Man. Ther. 18, 449–457.

Schmid, A.B., Hailey, L., Tampin, B., 2018. Entrapment neuropathies: challenging common beliefs with novel evidence. J. Orthop. Sports Phys. Ther. 48 (2), 58–62.

Scholz, J., Mannion, R.J., Hord, D.E., Griffin, R.S., Rawal, B., Zheng, H., et al., 2009. A novel tool for the assessment of pain: validation in low back pain. PLoS Med. 6 (4), e1000047.

Scholz, J., Finnerup, N.B., Attal, N., Aziz, Q., Baron, R., Bennett, M.I., et al., 2019. Classification Committee of the Neuropathic Pain Special Interest Group (NeuPSIG). The IASP classification of chronic pain for ICD-11: chronic neuropathic pain. Pain 160 (1), 53–59. https://doi.org/10.1097/j.pain.0000000000001365.

Schwartz, J.H., 1991. Synthesis and trafficking of neuronal proteins. In: Kandel, E.R., Schwartz, J.H., Jessell, T.M. (Eds.), Principles of Neural Science, third ed . Elsevier, New York, pp. 49–65.

Smith, B.H., Torrance, N., 2012. Epidemiology of neuropathic pain and its impact on quality of life. Curr. Pain Headache Reports 16 (3), 191–198.

Smyth, M.J., Wright, V., 1958. Sciatica and the intervertebral disc, an experimental study. J. Bone Joint Surg. Am. 40A, 1401–1418.

Sommer, C., Leinders, M., Üçeyler, N., 2018. Inflammation in the pathophysiology of neuropathic pain. Pain 159 (3), 595–602. https://doi.org/10.1097/j.pain.0000000000001122.

Soon, B., Vicenzino, B., Schmid, A.B., Coppieters, M.W., 2017. Facilitatory and inhibitory pain mechanisms are altered in patients with carpal tunnel syndrome. PLoS ONE 12 (8), e0183252. https://doi.org/10.1371/journal.pone.0183252.

Starkweather, R.J., Neviaser, R.J., Adams, J.P., et al., 1978. The effect of devascularization on the regeneration of lacerated peripheral nerves: an experimental study. J. Hand Surg. Am. 3, 163–167.

Stocks, J., Tang, N.K., Walsh, D.A., Warner, S.C., Harvey, H.L., Jenkins, W., et al., 2018. Bidirectional association between disturbed sleep and neuropathic pain symptoms: a prospective cohort study in post-total joint replacement participants. J. Pain Res. 11, 1087.

Stromberg, T., Dahlin, L.B., Brun, A., et al., 1997. Structural nerve changes at wrist level in workers exposed to vibration. Occup. Environ. Med. 54, 307–311.

Sunderland, S., 1978. Nerves and Nerve Injuries, second ed. Churchill Livingstone, Edinburgh, pp. 39–680.

Sunderland, S., 1990. The anatomy and physiology of nerve injury. Muscle Nerve 13, 771–784.

Szabo, R.M., Gelberman, R.H., Williamson, R.V., et al., 1983. Effects of increased systemic blood pressure on the tissue fluid pressure threshold of peripheral nerve. J. Orthop. Res. 1, 172–178.

Takada, E., Takahashi, M., Shimada, K., 2001. Natural history of lumbar disc hernia with radicular leg pain: spontaneous MRI changes of the herniated mass and correlation with clinical outcome. J. Orthop. Surg. 9 (1), 1–7.

Takahata, S., Takebayashi, T., Terasima, Y., Tanimoto, K., Wada, T., Yamashita, T., Sohma, H., Kokai, Y., 2011. Activation of glial cells in the spinal cord of a model of lumbar radiculopathy. J. Orthop. Sci. 16 (3), 313–320. https://doi.org/10.1007/s00776-011-0052-4. ISSN 0949-2658.

Tamburin, S., Cacciatori, C., Praitano, M.L., et al., 2011. Median nerve small- and large-fiber damage in carpal tunnel syndrome: a quantitative sensory testing study. J. Pain 12, 205–212.

Takahashi, K., Shima, I., Porter, R., 1999. Nerve root pressure in lumbar disc herniation. Spine 24 (19), 2003.

Tencer, A.F., Allen, B.L., Ferguson, R.L., 1985. A biomechanical study of thoracolumbar spine fractures with bone in the canal, part III, mechanical properties of the dura and its tethering ligaments. Spine 10, 741–747.

Terenghi, G., 1995. Peripheral nerve injury and regeneration. Histol. Histopathol. 10, 709–718.

Thacker, M.A., Clark, A.K., Marchand, F., et al., 2007. Pathophysiology of peripheral neuropathic pain: immune cells and molecules. Anesth. Analg. 105, 838–847.

Thaxton, C., Bhat, M.A., 2009. Myelination and regional domain differentiation of the axon. Results Probl Cell Differ 48, 1–28. https://doi.org/10.1007/400_2009_3.

Thomsen, J.F., Gerr, F., Atroshi, I., 2008. Carpal tunnel syndrome and the use of computer mouse and keyboard: a systematic review. BMC Musculoskelet. Disord. 9, 134.

Todd, A.J., Koerber, R., 2006. Neuroanatomical substrates of spinal nociception. Wall and Melzack's Textbook of Pain, fifth ed. Churchill Livingstone, Edinburgh.

Topp, K.S., Boyd, B.S., 2006. Structure and biomechanics of peripheral nerves: nerve responses to physical stresses and implications for physical therapist practice. Phys. Ther. 86, 92–109.

Turkof, E., Jurecka, W., Sikos, G., et al., 1993. Sensory recovery in myocutaneous, noninnervated free flaps: a morphologic, immunohistochemical, and electron microscopic study. Plast. Reconstr. Surg. 92, 238–247.

Treede, R.D., Jensen, T.S., Campbell, J.N., Cruccu, G., Dostrovsky, J.O., Griffin, J.W., et al., 2008. Neuropathic pain: redefinition and a grading system for clinical and research purposes. Neurology 70 (18), 1630–1635.

Van Acker, K., Bouhassira, D., De Bacquer, D., Weiss, S., Matthys, K., Raemen, H., et al., 2009. Prevalence and impact on quality of life of peripheral neuropathy with or without neuropathic pain in type 1 and type 2 diabetic patients attending hospital outpatients clinics. Diabetes Metab. 35 (3), 206–213.

Vicuna, L., Strochlic, D.E., Latremoliere, A., Bali, K.K., Simonetti, M., Husainie, D., et al., 2015. The serine protease inhibitor SerpinA3N attenuates neuropathic pain by inhibiting T cell-derived leukocyte elastase. Nat. Med. 21, 518–523. https://doi.org/10.1038/nm.3852.

Von Hehn, C.A., Baron, R., Woolf, C.J., 2012. Deconstructing the neuropathic pain phenotype to reveal neural mechanisms. Neuron. 73 (4), 638–652.

Vroomen, P.C.A.J., Wilmink, J., de Krom, M.C.T.F., 2002. Prognostic value of MRI findings in sciatica. Neuroradiology 44 (1), 59–63.

Williams, P.L., Warwick, R., 1980. Gray's Anatomy, thirty-sixth ed. Churchill Livingstone, Edinburgh.

Williams, P.L., Bannister, L.H., Berry, M.M., et al., 1995. Gray's Anatomy, thirty-eighth ed. Churchill Livingstone, New York.

Woolf, C.J., Shortland, P., Coggeshall, R.E., 1992. Peripheral nerve injury triggers central sprouting of myelinated afferents. Nature 355, 75–77.

Yarnitsky, D., 2010. Conditioned pain modulation (the diffuse noxious inhibitory control-like effect): its relevance for acute and chronic pain states. Curr. Opin. Anaesthesiol. 23 (5), 611–615. https://doi.org/10.1097/ACO.0b013e32833c348b.

Yılmaz, S., Taş, S., Yılmaz, Ö.T., 2018. Comparison of median nerve mechanosensitivity and pressure pain threshold in patients with nonspecific neck pain and asymptomatic individuals. J. Manipulative Physiol. Ther. 41 (3), 227–233.

Zhu, G.C., Böttger, K., Slater, H., Cook, C., Farrell, S.F., Hailey, L., et al., 2019. Concurrent validity of a low-cost and time-efficient clinical sensory test battery to evaluate somatosensory dysfunction. Eur. J. Pain 23 (10), 1826–1838.

Ziegler, D., Rathmann, W., Dickhaus, T., Meisinger, C., Mielck, A., 2009. Neuropathic pain in diabetes, prediabetes and normal glucose tolerance: the MONICA/KORA Augsburg Surveys S2 and S3. Pain Med. 10 (2), 393–400.

Zoech, G., Reihsner, R., Beer, R., et al., 1991. Stress and strain in peripheral nerves. Neuro-orthopaedics 10, 73–82.

7

Management of Nerve Related Musculoskeletal Pain

Colette Ridehalgh and Jennifer Ward

LEARNING OUTCOMES

After studying this chapter, you should be able to:

- Understand and explain how nerve management strategies can influence a number of neurophysiological mechanisms including oedema, immune cells, descending inhibitory pain mechanisms, blood flow and axonal transport mechanisms.
- Explain how injury can lead to changes in biomechanical properties of nervous tissue.
- Understand the concept and underlying literature on sliders and tensioners.
- Understand the current literature base to support or refute nerve gliding techniques in the management of persons with nerve-related MSK pain.
- Describe the use and efficacy of exercise in the management of persons with nerve-related MSK pain.
- Have an understanding of what medications may be useful in the management of persons with nerve-related MSK pain.
- Understand the limitations of studies in this field of practice.
- Debate the benefits of sub-profiling persons with nerve-related pain.

CHAPTER CONTENTS

Management of persons with nerve-related musculoskeletal pain consists of a multimodal approach, utilizing a variety of techniques designed to enhance function, reduce pain and optimize health and well-being. No one technique can result in such changes; rather, it is the careful detailed examination of the patient, meticulous clinical reasoning processes and shared management planning and goal setting that produce a detailed, comprehensive and, most importantly, individualized management plan. The focus of this chapter is on the

TABLE 7.1 **Aims of Treatment for Nerve Related Musculoskeletal Pain**

Nerve Treatment Technique	Aim of Treatment	Examples of Treatment
Direct slider or tensioner	• Restore normal movement • Improve circulation • Improve axonal transport • Reduce oedema • Reduce pain • Reduce fear of movement • Reduce activation of immune cells	• Straight-leg raise • Slump • Femoral nerve mobilization (side-lying slump) • ULNT1 median nerve • ULNT2a median nerve or 2b radial nerve • ULNT3 ulnar nerve
Indirect interface	• Reduce pain • Improve circulation • Restore normal biomechanics of the nerve—nerve interface • Reduce oedema	• Fibular head mobilizations for common peroneal nerve • Supinator soft-tissue mobilizations for posterior interosseous nerve • Piriformis hold/relax for sciatic nerve • Carpal bone mobilizations for median nerve
Exercise	• Reduce pain • Improve circulation • Improve axonal transport • Reduce oedema • Reduce fear of movement • Reduce activation of immune cells	• Swimming • Walking • Running

ULNT, Upper-limb neurodynamic test.

principles underlying the management of people with nerve-related musculoskeletal pain and specific techniques available to the clinician but in the context of an overall management strategy ensuring person-centred care to deliver the best outcomes.

The main focus of management is to normalize nerve function (both in terms of reducing heightened nerve mechanosensitivity as well as restoring nerve conduction where possible and feasible), enhancing normal range of motion and restoring a normal healthy nerve environment (reducing oedema and inflammatory mediators). A summary of the aims and types of nerve techniques can be found in Table 7.1, and some specific techniques are illustrated in Figs 7.1–7.5. The reader is referred to the accompanying examination book for a full description of the neurodynamic tests (Ryder & Barnard, 2024).

OVERVIEW OF TYPES OF NERVE TREATMENT

There are many ways to manage a person with nerve-related musculoskeletal pain, but primarily the focus should always be on person-centred care. Person-centred care is aimed at the person's 'preferences, needs and values to guide clinical decisions, and provide care that is respectful of and responsive to them' (NHS Health Education England). As such, management strategies will encapsulate shared decision making about the use of specific techniques considered suitable for the underlying condition, as well as ensuring that these align with the person's understanding and beliefs.

Advice is often the most important part of any management strategy. A person with tingling in their hand after an hour of typing for example may need to consider reducing the amount of typing before breaking. This may enhance circulation and prevent the build of oedema within the carpal tunnel. Appropriate explanations of why this is helpful, ensuring understanding and appropriate time to answer questions, will be essential to support any behaviour change.

There are several specific nerve treatment techniques. Two commonly used techniques involve either influencing the nerve directly (moving the nerve through the tissues, most commonly referred to as sliders or tensioners) or influencing the structures

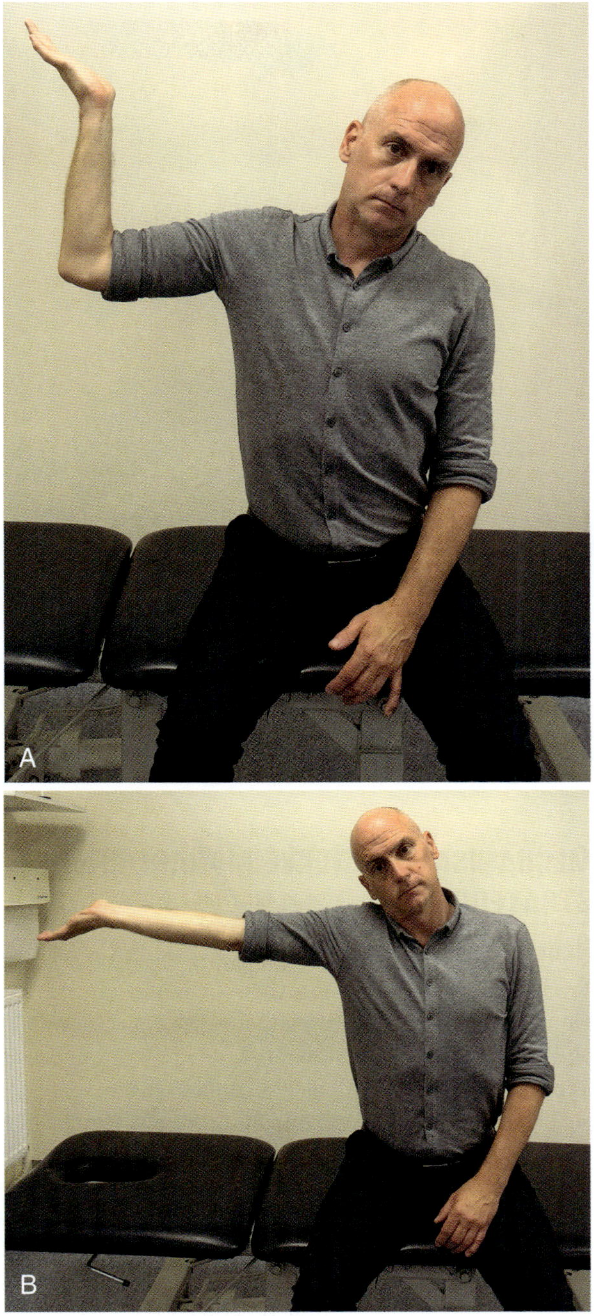

Fig. 7.1 Upper-limb neurodynamic test 1 (ULNT1) slider technique.

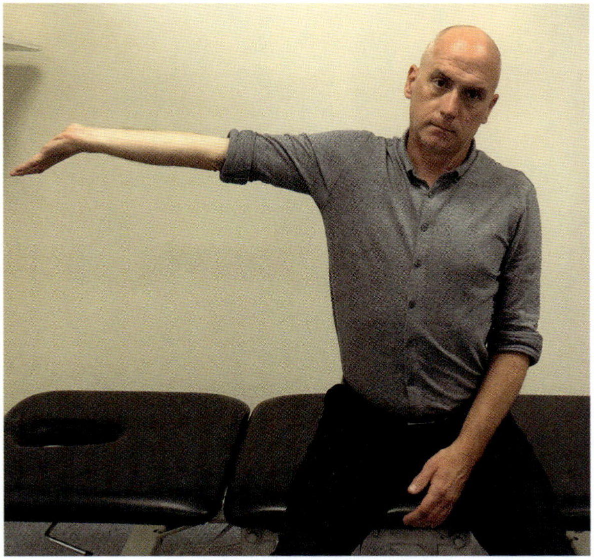

Fig. 7.2 Upper-limb neurodynamic test 1 (ULNT1) tensioner technique.

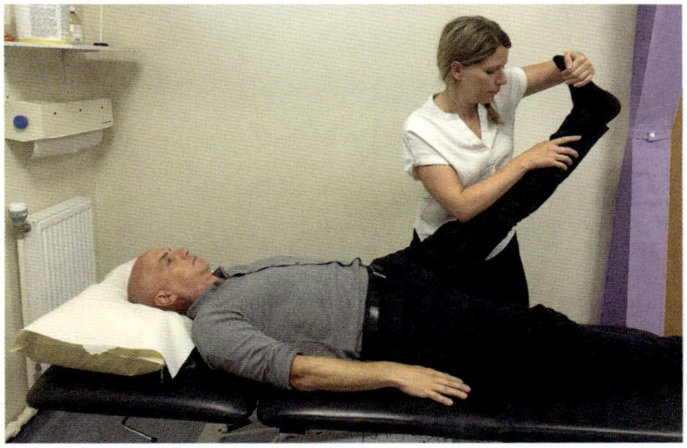

Fig. 7.3 Straight-leg raise tensioner technique.

which the nerve passes through or close to (interface techniques). As detailed in Chapter 6, combining joint movements which lengthen the path that the nerves travel can be used to test heightened nerve mechanosensitivity and are termed neurodynamic tests (see Figs 7.1–7.4). These movements can be converted into treatment techniques by repeatedly oscillating one joint to produce an overall nerve mobilization.

The choice of technique will relate to the severity, irritability and nature of the condition as well as the potential source of symptoms and contributing factors (see Chapter 3 in the companion text, Ryder & Barnard, 2024). In a situation where the person's symptoms are severe and irritable, care must be taken not to reproduce their symptoms. Where an obvious interface is suspected, it may be useful to consider treatment of this

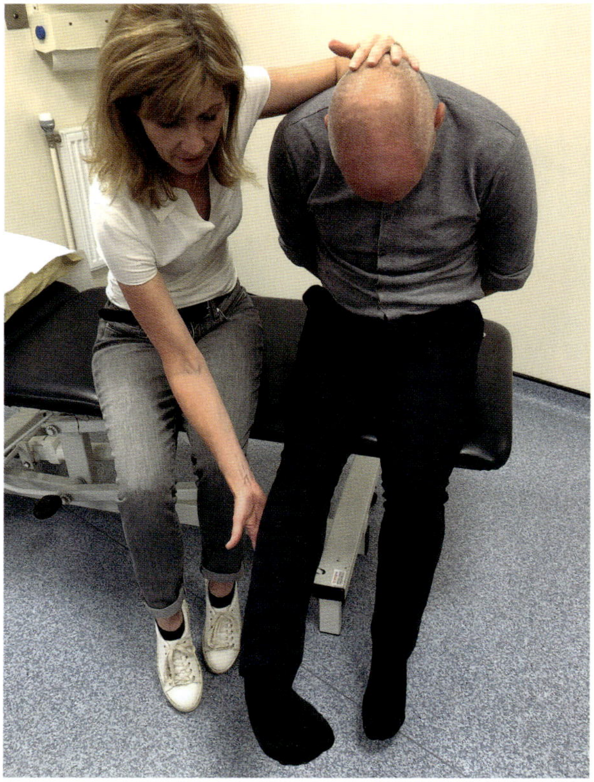

Fig. 7.4 Slump tensioner technique.

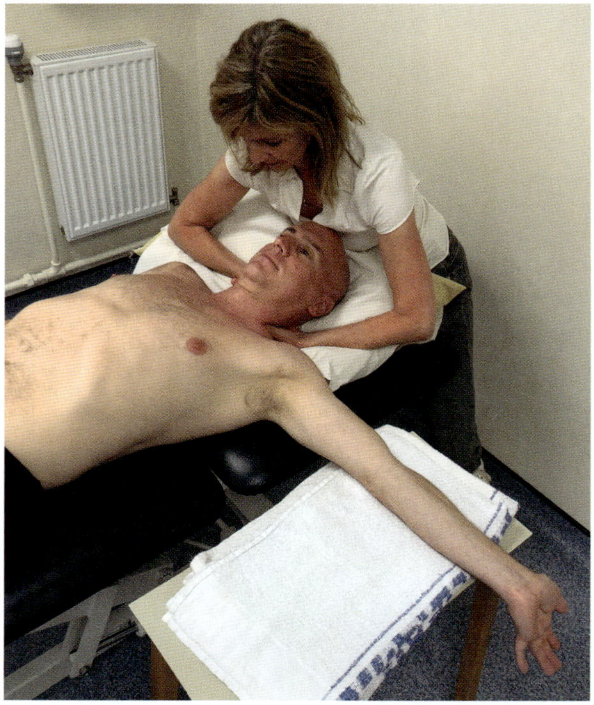

Fig. 7.5 Lateral glide technique in upper-limb neurodynamic test 1 (ULNT1) position.

structure first to restore a normal relationship between the nerve and the interfacing tissue. The postulated effects of such treatments will be discussed later in this chapter. An example of such a technique may be mobilization of the fibular head to influence the common peroneal nerve or a soft-tissue technique to supinator muscle to influence the radial nerve. A combination of both an interface treatment with a direct nerve mobilizing technique may also be considered to target the affected tissue, for example, mobilizing the fibular head whilst the leg is in a straight-leg raise (SLR) position.

Alternatively, more generic exercise may be a beneficial management strategy to either directly influence the nerve due to mechanical loading, and potential improvements in macro- and micro-circulation (Dobson et al., 2014) but also to enhance neurophysiological mechanisms. Simply advising the person to stay active may be important within 6–8 weeks of injury (Ostelo, 2020).

MECHANISMS OF NERVE MANAGEMENT STRATEGIES

Neurophysiological Mechanisms

Traditionally, nerve gliding techniques focused on the biomechanical effects (Butler, 1991), but a growing body of evidence has demonstrated a number of important neurophysiological changes which occur after these treatments. Arguably, these effects may have a greater influence on restoring the healthy nerve environment than the biomechanical effects.

Many studies assessing the mechanisms associated with nerve gliding techniques have utilized animal models, although some cadaveric and human studies have also demonstrated some potential desirable effects. Animal models have also been used to assess the mechanisms associated with exercise, and these will also be reviewed in the following sections.

Oedema

One way in which the nerve adapts to injury or disease is with an inflammatory response, and the resultant oedema can cause further compressive load and provide an acidic environment enhancing peripheral nerve sensitivity (Steen et al., 1996). Reducing oedema would therefore be particularly beneficial to patients with peripheral neuropathic pain.

It has been postulated that both slider and tensioner techniques could disperse oedema due to a milking or pumping effect caused by oscillatory techniques (Coppieters & Butler, 2008). Intraneurally injected dye has been demonstrated to disperse along the nerve after nerve mobilization techniques in both the peripheral nerve (Brown et al., 2011; Boudier-Reveret et al., 2017) and the nerve root (Gilbert et al., 2007) in cadavers. Whilst the limitations of cadaveric research reduce to an extent the extrapolation to clinical practice, an in vivo study (Schmid et al., 2012) demonstrated a reduction in signal intensity on T2 weighted MRI images, suggesting a reduction in oedema proximal to the carpal tunnel in participants with carpal tunnel syndrome (CTS). Whilst this was not significantly different to a group of participants who only wore resting night splints, this suggests the use of both may be favourable to ensure that unintended pressure doesn't escalate in sleeping individuals as well as to utilize movement-based therapy to enhance not only neurophysiological mechanisms but to reduce psychological factors such as kinesiophobia or fear avoidance.

Immune Cell Changes

Inflammation is a feature in some nerve-related musculoskeletal disorders (Kobayashi et al., 2004; Rothman & Winkelstein, 2007; Hubbard & Winkelstein, 2008; Schmid et al., 2013). Inflammatory mediators can lower the threshold for firing and may therefore result in spontaneous pain. Such lowered firing of afferent nerves would warrant caution when applying movement-based treatment approaches, especially techniques such as tensioners where elongation of the nerve may provoke further discharge (Dilley et al., 2005). Glial cells become activated in neuropathic pain conditions, and these cells synthesize proinflammatory cytokines, glutamate and nitrous oxide (DeLeo & Yezierski, 2001) as well as increase the production of nerve growth factor. Hence an elevation of glial cells may result in heightened nerve sensitivity (Herzberg et al., 1997; DeLeo & Yezierski, 2001).

Normalization of both glial cells and nerve growth factor have been demonstrated in rats with experimentally induced neuritis after neural mobilizations (Martins et al., 2011; Santos et al., 2012) and in animals exposed to exercise regimes such as swimming (Almeida et al., 2015) and treadmill walking (Sumizono et al., 2018). These changes suggest that both neural mobilization and cardiovascular exercise may lead to a downplay in the immune response after peripheral nerve injury. These changes were associated with a decrease in mechanical hyperalgesia after neural mobilizations (Martins et al., 2011; Santos et al., 2012) and exercise (Shen et al., 2013; Tian et al., 2018) as well as thermal hyperalgesia (Santos et al., 2012 neural mobilization, Shen et al., 2013 exercise).

Descending Inhibitory Pain Pathways

Supraspinal pain-inhibitory mechanisms have been suggested as one way in which neurodynamic mobilization may be beneficial. Animal studies have demonstrated improvements in pain-related behaviour after nerve mobilizations in rats with nerve injury (Bertolini et al., 2009; Martins et al., 2011; Santos et al., 2012).

More compelling evidence of descending inhibitory pain mechanisms have been demonstrated after neurodynamic mobilizations and exercise. After chronic constriction injury (CCI) of the sciatic nerve in rats, a decrease in opioid receptor levels in the periaqueductal grey matter was shown which normalized after 10 sessions of neurodynamic tensioner treatment undertaken every other day (Santos et al., 2014). Likewise, after CCI, rats who swam for 3 or 5 days per week for 5 weeks were found to have an increase in the expression of endogenous opioids in the midbrain/periaqueductal grey matter compared to the non-swimming CCI injured rats (Sumizono et al., 2018). Taken together with the pain behaviour changes, this suggests that one of the mechanisms responsible for beneficial changes after nerve mobilizations and exercise is an endogenous pain-inhibitory mechanism.

Blood Flow and Axonal Transport Systems

Improvements in blood flow and axonal transport systems after mobilizations and exercise are one of the theories proposed for many tissues around the body. Improvements in these systems would be of potential benefit to enhance normal healing processes and provide the nerve with essential nutrients and an oxygen supply which may be restricted due to the deleterious effects of compression (Rydevik & Lundborg, 1977;

Rydevik et al., 1981; Ogata & Naito, 1986). Limited research exists which demonstrates changes to these systems, particularly the changes to axonal transport systems due to the complexities of the methodology required to do so. Compression of nerves can cause impairment of axonal transport systems; pressure as low as 20 mmHg (much lower than those demonstrated to occur in patients with compression neuropathies) have been shown to detrimentally affect transport systems in animal studies (Dahlin et al., 1986). In addition, heightened nerve trunk sensitivity has been demonstrated in rats after disruption in axonal transport (Dilley & Bove, 2008), and therefore if such techniques could improve these transport systems, substantial benefits may be associated with such changes.

With respect to blood flow, Driscoll et al. (2002) found that stretching rabbits' sciatic nerves beyond 8% of their resting length for an hour resulted in a decrease in blood flow, but on release, an increase of around 151% of baseline occurred. Whilst the amount of strain may be similar during nerve mobilization techniques (Coppieters et al., 2006; Boyd et al., 2013), the duration of the stretch is clearly well outside those given during those techniques, and therefore it is not known how well this applies to clinical practice. It does suggest, however, that circulation can be affected by applying a technique which lengthens and then releases the nerve and its accompanying circulatory system.

KNOWLEDGE CHECK

1. How might neural mobilization techniques reduce oedema, and why might this be helpful in a patient's recovery?
2. What immune cells have been shown to be reduced in rats after exercise and neural mobilization?
3. What mechanism might reduce pain during neural mobilization?

BIOMECHANICAL EFFECTS OF NERVE TREATMENT

The presence of oedema in neuropathic pain presentations may result in intra- and extraneural fibrosis if not dispersed (Sunderland, 1989; Mackinnon, 2002), resulting in a restriction in the nerve's ability to glide through the interfacing structures as well as gliding of the nerve's connective tissue layers. Such restrictions in nerve gliding may be one situation where the concept of influencing the connective tissue properties of the nerve via creep and hysteresis (see Chapter 2) is an attractive proposition. However, it is not well established if nervous tissue becomes restricted after injury. Some studies demonstrated no differences in nerve excursion between those with and without painful neuropathies (Erel et al., 2003; Dilley et al., 2008; Ridehalgh et al., 2015), although others demonstrated reduced excursion in patient groups (Hough et al., 2007; Korstanje et al., 2012). In a systematic review exploring median nerve excursion measured by ultrasound imaging in people with CTS, 7/10 studies found a reduction in excursion compared to healthy controls (Ellis et al., 2017).

Tensioners and sliders have been proposed as techniques which differently influence the biomechanical effects on the nerve during joint movements. A slider is a combination of a series of joint movements which lengthen one end of the nerve bed whilst simultaneously shortening the other end. An example would be that, during upper-limb neurodynamic test 1 (ULNT1), the cervical spine is contralaterally side flexed whilst the wrist is flexed. A tensioner is described as a technique where the two ends of the system are simultaneously lengthened, e.g. in ULNT1 the cervical spine is contralaterally side flexed whilst the wrist is extended. Coppieters and Butler (2008) examined strain and excursion in both the median and ulnar nerves during tensioning and sliding movements in two embalmed cadavers (Coppieters & Butler, 2008). The median nerve was tensioned by extending the elbow and wrist, whilst the sliding manoeuvre consisted of elbow extension with wrist flexion (Fig. 7.6). The ulnar nerve was tensioned by extending the wrist, flexing the elbow and abducting the shoulder, whilst the sliding manoeuvre consisted of elbow extension with shoulder abduction. Although there was no statistical confirmation of the trends identified, the sliding techniques produced more excursion (12.6 mm at the wrist) than the tensioning techniques (6.1 mm) whilst producing less strain (0.8% slider, 6.8% tensioner at the wrist). Along with the small sample size and lack of statistical confirmation, a major limitation of cadaveric studies is not knowing to what extent these findings could be extrapolated into living humans.

Subsequently, studies using ultrasound imaging further supported the biomechanical events during the

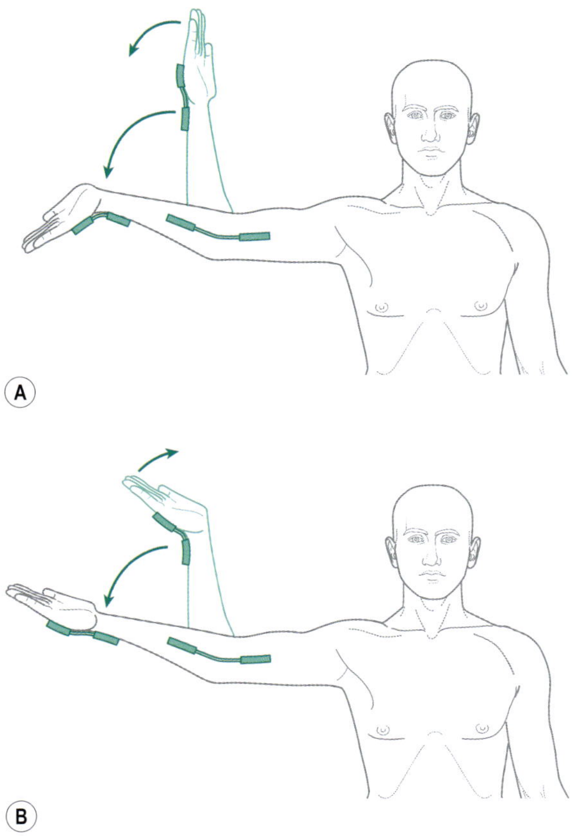

Fig. 7.6 Tensioning (A) and sliding (B) upper-limb neurodynamic test 1 (ULNT1) mobilization techniques. (*From Coppieters & Butler 2008, with permission.*)

two techniques (Coppieters et al., 2009, 2015; Ellis et al., 2012). Whilst this technology has not yet been able to give accurate estimates of strain, measurements of excursion have been shown to be reliable (Ellis et al., 2008; Ridehalgh et al., 2012) and valid (Dilley et al., 2001; Ridehalgh, 2014). Coppieters et al. (2009) found 3.6 mm of median nerve excursion measured proximal to the elbow during the tensioner manoeuvre and 10.2 mm in the slider manoeuvre. During a modified SLR (Coppieters et al., 2015) (Fig. 7.7), sciatic nerve excursion in the posterior thigh during the tensioner manoeuvre was in the region of 3.2 mm, and the slider was 17 mm.

Taken together, the studies suggest that a slider technique produces larger amounts of overall nerve excursion with smaller amounts of nerve strain. This may suggest that, where the patient has severe and irritable symptoms, movements which impose less strain on the nerve may be warranted. However, where symptoms are not severe and irritable and to ensure that nerves are able to tolerate the biomechanical loads during normal everyday activities, tensioners may be indicated. Ultimately it is the close monitoring and reassessment after treatment which will determine the effectiveness of the technique.

In addition to strain and excursion, in vivo measures of stiffness are now possible by utilizing ultrasound imaging with a novel technique called shear wave elastography. When high-intensity acoustic pulses mechanically excite the underlying tissues, this leads to the production of shear waves which are perpendicular to the inputted pulse. The velocity of the returning shear waves are measured and are considered to be an indication of nerve stiffness. Increased shear wave velocity (hence nerve stiffness) has been demonstrated during upper limb neurodynamic test 1 (median nerve bias) and SLR test (Greening & Dilley, 2017).

Changes to nerve stiffness measured via shear wave elastography have also been demonstrated after a statically held neurodynamic technique (SLR, and long sitting slump) but not during a muscle stretching technique in asymptomatic participants (Andrade et al., 2020). Stiffness was also found to be reduced in participants with spinally referred leg pain after slump treatment (effect size = 0.65; P = .019) but not in asymptomatic participants (effect size = 0.05; P = .75) (Neto et al., 2020). However, only eight participants were included in both groups, and further studies are needed to corroborate these results.

KNOWLEDGE CHECK

1. What biomechanical effects occur during neural mobilizations?
2. Describe a slider and tensioner technique for someone with a positive ULNT 2b (radial nerve bias).

Nerve Interface Treatments

Nerve interfaces are specific locations where the nerve passes through or around bone muscle or fascia. Examples of nerve interfaces include the median nerve passing beneath the flexor retinaculum of the wrist, the common peroneal nerve passing around the superior tibiofibular joint and the tibial nerve passing through

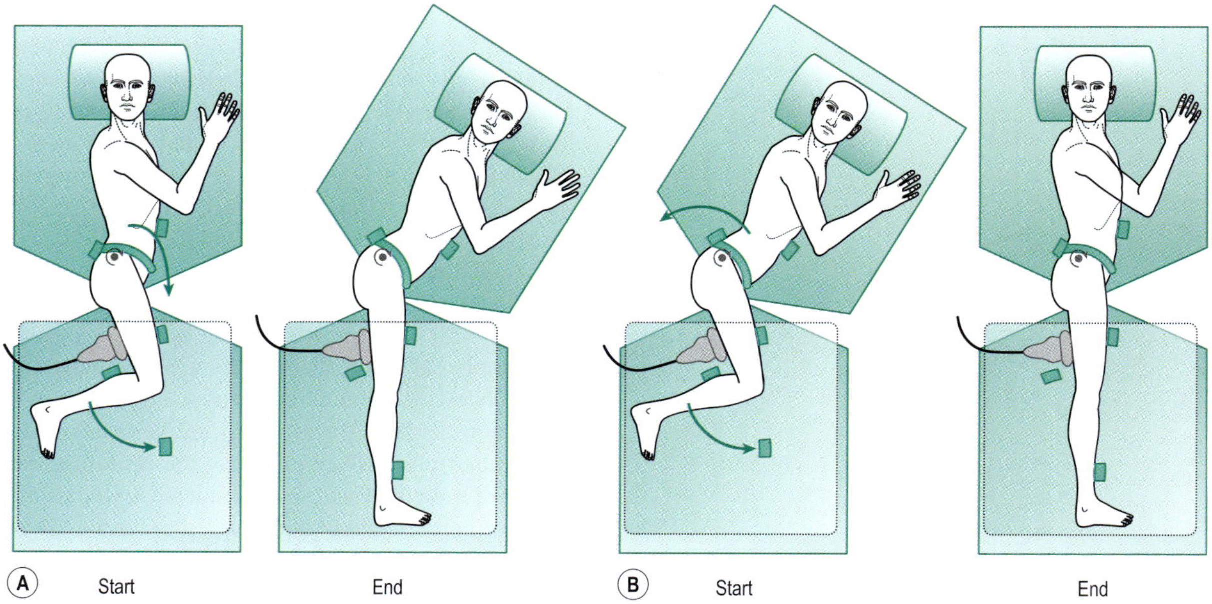

Fig. 7.7 Modified slider and tensioner straight-leg raise mobilization techniques. (A) Tensioner. (B) Slider. (*From Coppieters et al. 2015.*)

the tarsal tunnel into the foot. If an interface is involved in the pathophysiological mechanism, the aim of treatment may be to move the interface relative to the nerve. For example, mobilizations of the zygapophyseal joint or giving contralateral side flexion exercises may influence an affected nerve root. Treating the interface to offload the neural structures may be a priority to improve the nerve root environment (e.g. reduce oedema, improve circulation, reduce compression and improve pain through descending inhibitory pain pathways).

Soft-tissue techniques could also be applied as an appropriate interface technique. Examples of common soft-tissue interfaces include the supinator as it interfaces with the posterior interosseous nerve or the piriformis muscle as it interfaces with the sciatic nerve.

If the condition is non-severe and non-irritable, the clinician may wish to replicate a neurodynamic test position corresponding to an aggravating factor and apply the interface technique in this position. Where the symptoms are severe and/or irritable, the interface technique may be performed away from a position of pain. It has been found that the point of the symptomatic range of SLR coincides with the point of greatest restriction of the nerve root adjacent to lumbosacral disc herniation, which reduces after surgical disc removal (Kobayashi et al., 2003). It is possible therefore that there may be a greater effect on the nerve when positioned in the first onset of pain during the neurodynamic test. Examples of this could be to perform a unilateral posteroanterior to the lumbar spine with the leg in an SLR position if the patient complained of pain on heel strike during gait, or in a slump position if the patient complained of pain in sitting or flexion.

KNOWLEDGE CHECK

1. Name three common nerve interface treatment techniques.

Treatment Dose: Considerations in Relation to Nerve Treatment

Time and Repetition of Nerve Gliding Techniques

There is limited evidence to support specific treatment doses when utilizing neurodynamic techniques. Indeed many studies have used a variety of treatment doses (see Table 7.2 for an example of some of these). Spinal joint mobilizations led to a statistically significant

TABLE 7.2 Examples of Treatment Dose Utilized in Some Studies on Effectiveness of Neurodynamic Treatment

Authors	Neurodynamic Treatment	Dose
Adel (2011)	SLR tensioner	5 sets sustained for 30 s
Bialosky et al. (2009)	ULNT1 tensioner	5 sets of 10 repetitions for sessions 1–3, then 7 sets of 10 repetitions for sessions 4–6
Cleland et al. (2006)	Slump tensioner	5 sets sustained for 30 s
Lewis et al. (2020)	ULNT1 slider	5–10 repetitions of each exercise five times a day
Nagrale et al. (2012)	Slump tensioner	5 sets sustained for 30 s. HER 2 × 30 s hold
Nee et al. (2012)	ULNT1 slider and tensioner	10–15, 3 times daily as HER
Ridehalgh et al. (2016)	SLR tensioner	3 sets of oscillations for 60 s
Schäfer et al. (2011)	Side-lying SLR slider	5 sets of oscillations for 30 s
Schmid et al. (2012)	ULNT1 slider	10 repetitions
Tal-Akabi and Rushton (2000)	ULNT1 mobilization	Dose not specified

Cx, Cervical; *HER*, home exercise regime; *SLR*, straight-leg raise; *ULNT*, upper-limb neurodynamic test.

hypoalgesic effect after four sets, but no difference was found between 30 and 60 seconds (Pentelka et al., 2012). However, participants for this study were asymptomatic, and it is unclear if the same trend would occur in symptomatic participants, nor if the same time frames are relevant to nerve mobilization. More research is needed on symptomatic participants to see if the same trend follows.

The clinician is guided by the patient's symptoms and rigorous evaluation of reassessment asterisks as a guide to the optimal treatment time for the individual patient. Additionally, the choice of time and repetition that has been demonstrated to be beneficial in the treatment room should be maintained for any home exercises prescribed.

EFFICACY OF NERVE MANAGEMENT STRATEGIES

Neurodynamic Treatment

There has been a steady stream of studies examining the effectiveness of nerve treatments over the past 20 years. In general, these studies tend to support nerve treatment (Cleland et al., 2006; Adel, 2011; Nagrale et al., 2012; Nee et al., 2012), whilst others show no difference compared to standard care alone (Scrimshaw & Maher, 2001; Akalin et al., 2002; Heebner & Roddey, 2008; Bardak et al., 2009). Tensioner treatments in addition to standard care have been found to be superior to standard care alone in patients with spinally referred leg pain (Cleland et al., 2006; Adel, 2011; Nagrale et al., 2012), but there are limitations associated with these study designs. Such limitations include the use of multiple T tests (Cleland et al., 2006; Adel, 2011) which could lead to a type 1 error (risk of falsely accepting the alternative hypothesis) and the disparity of time/attention that the participants in the standard care plus nerve treatment group received, which could account in part for the more favourable findings in this group. Schäfer et al. (2011) and Ridehalgh et al. (2016) investigated whether the effectiveness of nerve treatment differed dependent on the subgroup that participants with spinally referred leg pain were allocated to. Schäfer et al. (2011) found that the group with heightened nerve mechanosensitivity (without neurological loss) showed significant improvements in a number of outcomes (including Global Perceived Change Scale and functional disability) over other subgroups; however, the small number of participants in this group ($n = 9$) makes the extrapolation of these results less convincing. Ridehalgh et al. (2016) looked at the immediate changes to pain, vibration threshold and sciatic nerve excursion after a single session of an SLR tensioner and found no significant differences in outcomes between subgroups (somatic referred, radicular and radiculopathy) or indeed after treatment. However, the short treatment duration (3 × 1 minute) may not be sufficient to show changes in pain, and measurement only immediately after treatment may have missed any longer-term effects. Indeed, De-la-Llave-Rincon et al. (2012) found significant changes to pressure pain thresholds 1 week after nerve treatment but no immediate changes.

Studies investigating treatment for CTS have produced some equivocal results. In a systematic review exploring the efficacy of nerve gliding techniques, it was concluded that there was no evidence to support the use of nerve gliding techniques for pain or disability (Basson et al., 2017). Conversely, in a recent systematic review, Núñez de Arenas-Arroyo et al. (2021) found statistically significant short term improvements in pain and function after neural mobilisations, although the qualify of evidence was considered "very low certainty" as measured by GRADE. Combinations of physical therapy, not surprisingly, including nerve gliding techniques, show some promising results. In a randomized controlled trial, one session of education, nerve gliding, tendon gliding and night splints resulted in a statistically significant reduction in surgery compared to a waiting list (Lewis et al., 2020). Comparable improvements in pain and disability were found for conservative management strategies including nerve gliding in a randomized clinical trial of women with CTS compared to surgery at 6 and 12 months (Fernández-de-Las Peñas et al., 2015).

Cervical radicular pain has been investigated with some positive midterm findings (Deepti et al., 2008; Nee et al., 2012; Thoomes et al., 2021). Nee et al. (2012) found that the numbers-needed-to-treat analysis favoured neurodynamic treatment using sliders and tensioners in addition to cervical spine mobilizations compared to a control group on a number of measures including pain, Global Rating of Change Scale and disability. Deepti et al. (2008) found significant improvements in pain and disability in a neurodynamic tensioner group compared to participants who had a cervical lateral glide treatment.

Increases in nerve excursion (median excursion at wrist 0.5 mm baseline to 1.96 mm post treatment and at the elbow 1.21 mm baseline to 2.63 mm post treatment, $P < .01$) were found after 3 months of conservative physiotherapy treatment which included neural sliders and cervical contralateral glide techniques in people with cervical radicular pain (Thoomes et al., 2021). Importantly, the increases in nerve movement at the elbow were significantly correlated with improvements in pain ($P < .001$), scores on global perceived effect ($P < .001$) and patient-specific functional scale ($P < .010$). However, the study was a case-controlled study, and therefore it is not possible to say whether these changes would have occurred by natural recovery alone. Nonetheless, this study demonstrated that changes to nerve excursion may be associated with improvements in pain and function.

Despite some assertions of the potentially harmful effects of neurodynamic tensioner techniques, there is little literature published which supports such a notion. Ridehalgh et al. (2016) found no statistical differences in vibration thresholds after an SLR tensioner in participants with and without identifiable neurological loss of function, suggesting that nerve function is not detrimentally affected even in those with a reduction in function. Nee et al. (2012) found that patients with cervical radicular pain who reported adverse symptoms after neurodynamic treatment recovered quickly and did no worse than those who did not report adverse effects.

Exercise

Like many conditions, the type of exercise prescribed for nerve-related musculoskeletal (MSK) pain is varied within the literature and at times non-specific. Long-term improvements (1 year) in global perceived effect were found in people with acute lumbosacral radicular pain who were given physiotherapy prescribed exercise in comparison to GP advice (Luijsterburg et al., 2008). However, the secondary outcomes which included pain and disability did not reach statistical significance at short, medium or long term, indicating that self-reported improvements in pain do not always correlate with other outcome measures. In addition, the methods did not detail the type of exercise given, nor adherence to the exercises which limits the interpretation of the results.

Both active exercise and motor control exercise have demonstrated beneficial effects compared to sham or control groups but not superiority between interventions. Participants with radicular leg pain were divided into two groups, with one group receiving cardiovascular exercise (sham group) and the other given both McKenzie exercises and lumbosacral stability exercises (Albert & Manniche, 2012). After 8 weeks of treatment, there was a significant improvement in the McKenzie group compared to the sham group on the global outcome at both 8 weeks and 1 year ($P < .008$, ~90% much better McKenzie, ~60% sham group) but no significant difference between the groups for pain or disability. Both intervention groups showed statistical and clinical significant differences compared to baseline at both time points. However, the sham group could choose to do the exercises or not, meaning it is not possible to ascertain overall the efficacy of either intervention. Similarly, Akkan and Gelececk (2018) compared stability exercises to a combination of electrotherapy, stretching and isometric exercises in participants with cervical radicular pain. Both groups showed statistically significant improvements in an array of measures immediately after treatment and 3 months later, including disability, pain and hand grip, but there were no significant differences between the groups. Additionally, the lack of a control group means that improvements could be attributed to natural recovery.

Medications for Neuropathic Pain

Medications which target specific pain mechanisms are considered to be more effective than medications to treat diseases (which are often based on broad diagnostic criteria). An example of this is in inflammatory arthritis, where clear pain mechanisms have been identified and medications are targeted at the specific underlying pathophysiology (Cohen & Mao, 2014). Specific medicines have been developed to treat neuropathic pain, and the NICE pharmacological guidelines for the management of neuropathic pain (2013) suggest a selection of different medicines which can be trialled (see Table 7.3). Table 7.4 summarizes the main mechanisms of action, side effects and precautions of common neuropathic pain medicines.

In clinical practice, however, identifying the pain mechanisms responsible for neuropathic symptoms can be difficult and in addition, patients may present with mixed pain mechanisms including both neuropathic and nociceptive pain. This has translated into pharmacological research which often fails to identify neuropathic pain features or their underlying mechanisms in participants. An example of this is found in a recent systematic review (Enke et al., 2018) which showed moderate to high-quality evidence that anti-convulsant medication was ineffective for the treatment of low back or lumbar radicular pain. There were limited attempts, however, to identify neuropathic pain within the included studies, and in some cases patients with neuropathic symptoms such as paraesthesia (McCleane, 2001) or neurological deficit (Muehlbacher et al., 2006) were excluded from studies. Hence, included participants may have presented with more nociceptive pain features which may respond less favourably to neuropathic pain medication. The poor efficacy found in such studies for neuropathic pain medication has influenced the development of national guidelines, e.g. NICE sciatica guidelines (2020), leading to recommendations that clinicians avoid prescribing certain neuropathic pain medications, such as anticonvulsants.

TABLE 7.3 Neuropathic Pain Medicines
Offer a choice of amitriptyline, duloxetine, gabapentin or pregabalin as initial treatment (except for trigeminal neuralgia).
If the initial treatment is not effective or is not tolerated, offer one of the remaining 3 drugs and consider switching again if the second and third drugs tried are also not effective or not tolerated.
Consider tramadol only if acute rescue therapy is needed.
Consider capsaicin cream for people with localized neuropathic pain who wish to avoid, or who cannot tolerate, oral treatments.

Neuropathic pain—pharmacological management: NICE clinical guideline 173 (November 2013)

KNOWLEDGE CHECK

1. Which medications are suggested as first line treatment in neuropathic pain conditions?

Sub-Profiling of Persons With Nerve Related Pain

Since one major limitation of large RCTs is the heterogeneity of participants included in studies, one solution is to ascertain if there are specific sub-profiles of persons with nerve-related pain. There is evidence emerging that individuals with neuropathic pain may fit within specific clusters based on sensory loss or gain (i.e. hyperalgesia, allodynia etc.) and that these clusters occur regardless of the underlying aetiology (Baron et al., 2017). Importantly, there is emerging evidence that patients lying within a particular cluster might benefit more from specific treatments, compared to those in other clusters.

Quantitative sensory testing (QST) is one method that has been used to identify these clusters in patients with peripheral neuropathic pain (Baron et al., 2017). As explained in Chapter 6, QST is a psychophysical test which evaluates an individual's response to a range of

TABLE 7.4 **Evidence-Based Recommendations for Pharmacotherapy of Neuropathic Pain**

Drug	Main Mechanism of Action	Very Common Side Effects	Precautions for Use	Other Benefits Beyond Neuropathic Pain
Tricyclic antidepressants (i.e. amitriptyline, nortriptyline, imipramine)	Inhibits the reuptake of neurotransmitters norepinephrine and serotonin, thus increasing their bioavailability. It also blocks the action of acetylcholine.	Mostly occur from the blockade of acetylcholine and include somnolence, tremor, dizziness, headache, drowsiness, speech disorder (dysarthria), low BP on standing, mood changes, palpitations, dry mouth constipation, nausea	Cardiac disease, glaucoma, prostatic adenoma, seizure, concurrent use of tramadol	Improvement of depression, (although only when used at higher dosages) and sleep (amitriptyline)
Gabapentinoids (i.e. gabapentin and pregabalin)	Binds to the α2δ-1 subunit of the voltage dependent calcium channels in the CNS and modulates the release of excitatory neurotransmitters and the channel of calcium currents. The α2δ-1 subunit also has a role in the development of new synapse formation by interacting with thrombospondins. Binding to the subunit, gabapentin is therefore able to block formation of new synapses (Eroglu et al., 2009).	Sedation, dizziness, peripheral oedema, weight gain	Reduce dosages in renal insufficiency	Does not interact with other drugs and can cause improvement of generalized anxiety and sleep
Topical lidocaine plasters	Block of sodium channel	Local erythema Itch rash	Itch rash	No systemic side effects
Topical capsaicin	TRPV1 agonist	Pain, erythema, itching. Rare cases of high blood pressure (initial increase in pain)	No overall impairment of sensory evaluation after repeated applications, caution in progressive neuropathy	No systemic side effects

Table adapted from Attal, N., Bouhassira, D., 2015. Pharmacotherapy of neuropathic pain: which drugs, which treatment algorithms? Pain. 156 (Suppl), S104–S114.

applied graded stimuli. In a recent study of a large cohort of patients with peripheral neuropathic pain (including some with radiculopathy), Baron et al. (2017) identified 3 clusters using QST:

- Cluster 1: a sensory loss group, (42%)—deficits in warm/cold and mechanical sensation and thermal and mechanical pain sensitivity.
- Cluster 2: a thermal hyperalgesia group, (33%)—normal sensory function but heat and cold hyperalgesia plus mild dynamic mechanical allodynia.
- Cluster 3: mechanical hyperalgesia, (24%)—gain in mechanical pain perceptions including pinprick hyperalgesia and dynamic mechanical allodynia and diminished temperature sensation and thermal pain sensitivity.

These sensory profiles occurred irrespective of underlying aetiology, suggesting that the value of diagnosing the underlying pathology in neuropathic pain may be less important than identifying the individual's sensory sub-profile.

Similar clusters were found in a more recent trial using the Neuropathic Pain Symptoms Inventory Screening Tool to cluster patients receiving botulinum toxin injections for peripheral neuropathic pain (Bouhassira et al., 2021). Three clusters of sensory profiles were identified:

Cluster 1—pinpointed pain (above average paraesthesia/dysaesthesia and below average evoked pain)
Cluster 2—evoked pain (above average pain on brushing, cold or pressure, but below average deep pain, paraesthesia/dysaesthesia)
Cluster 3—deep pain (above average pressure and squeezing pain and below average paraesthesia/dysaesthesia).

Post hoc analysis found statistically significant improvements from botulinum toxin in clusters 2 and 3 but not in cluster 1. Additional studies on subgrouping are required to further explore responses to medication in patients with neuropathic pain conditions and to confirm if screening tools are useful to allow subgrouping of participants.

An individual's psychological and social factors might also influence their response to pain medication and allow sub-profiling of participants. In a recent large prospective cohort study on 609 patients with low back pain, or sciatica (Konstantinou et al., 2018), negative prognostic factors included the person's belief that the problem would last a long time (odds ratio (OR) 0.70: confidence interval (CI) 0.13—0.57), as well as longer leg pain duration (OR 0.41; CI 0.19—0.90) and a stronger belief that specific symptoms (such as fatigue, insomnia) were related to the underlying condition (known as an identity score) (OR 0.70; CI 0.53—0.93). In a secondary subgroup analysis in this same cohort of patients, Harrisson et al. (2020) found that high neuropathic pain screening tool scores were associated with higher levels of depression, anxiety and use of 2 or more medications. Retrospective reviews of other studies on patients with neuropathic MSK pain have suggested pain catastrophizing is one of the most important pretreatment variables predicting the effectiveness of topical analgesics (Mankovsky et al., 2012), cortisone (Makarawung et al., 2013), and oral acetaminophen and tramadol combination (Schiphorst Preuper et al., 2014).

KNOWLEDGE CHECK

1. Why might sub-profiling be useful to establish optimal treatment effects in persons with neuropathic pain conditions?

Case Study

Mrs X

Mrs. X, a 45-year-old care assistant with 6-month history of low back and leg pain (see Chapter 6 for examination findings).

Treatment 1

Symptoms were severe, and the description of symptoms (with associated paraesthesia) suggested a neuropathic pain component. The commencement of a course of neuropathic pain medication was therefore discussed (see Table 7.3), and the patient under her doctor's guidance opted to start a course of low-dose amitriptyline, taken at night.

The impact of her anxiety and depression was also explored, and the patient was aware of a link between her low mood and worsening symptoms. Strategies were discussed for managing her mood, and the patient made a plan to restart meditation, which in the past she had found helpful for managing her depression.

Follow-Up 1

After starting her course of amitriptyline, Mrs. X was tolerating the medication well and had noticed a significant improvement in her symptoms, with the maximum pain score reduced to 4/10. She was able to tolerate sitting for up to 30 min and only had to walk for a few minutes to relieve the pain after sitting. She also expressed an interest in trialling some manual therapy, as past treatment had provided some temporary relief of symptoms.

Objective markers were reassessed with pain in the back and leg again reproduced on lumbar flexion. Slump testing was still positive, but the knee extension had improved by 10 degrees. Neurological integrity remained the same with reduced sensation to light touch and pinprick in the right lateral foot.

As the condition was no longer deemed severe and there was no irritability, a slump position was chosen to start manual therapy treatment. In this position, with the knee extended just short of the onset of pain a right unilateral PA mobilization (grade III) to the L5 transverse process was performed for 4 × 1 min of treatment. On reassessment, lumbar flexion was pain free, but adding left side flexion brought on P&N in her foot. Knee extension on slump was nearly full, and sensation to light touch and pinprick remained the same. As the response to treatment was favourable, the patient was asked if they could replicate the manual therapy technique by sitting on a hard backed chair, in a slump position (with her foot up on a small stool), place a tennis ball into the same area of her spine and bounce gently into the tennis ball to apply the same oscillating pressure as the manual therapy for 4 × 1 min. Given her other commitments to caring for her son, the patient felt she could manage to do this home exercise at this dose once or twice a day.

The session also included a discussion about how she was managing to find time for meditation, how effective this was and a general discussion about what support networks she had to help care for her son.

Follow-Up 2

Mrs. X's subjective markers had improved; reporting that she could drive for up to 45 min, watch TV in the evening without pain and able to bend and put her shoes on more comfortably. She was also waking less at night mainly with P&N in the foot. Physical examination revealed the improved lumbar flexion had been maintained and leg pain (but no P&N) was only reproduced on combined flexion with left side flexion. Slump testing was unchanged, and there was still reduced sensation to light touch and pinprick in the lateral foot.

Treatment was progressed by positioning the patient in a slump with knee extension into full pain reproduction and applying the same grade III PA mobilization to the right L5 transverse process for 4 × 1 min. On reassessment, lumbar flexion combined with side flexion was now pain free; however, the slump and sensation markers remained the same, and therefore the clinician applied an additional treatment to address the nerve mechanosensitivity. Mrs. X was again positioned in a slump position, knees flexed at 90 degrees, right ankle plantar flexed and inverted and then asked to perform a slump slider, by slowly extending their knee while simultaneously extending their cervical spine for 4 × 30 s. On reassessment, Mrs. X was able to achieve a full and pain-free slump position, and there was improved sensation to light touch and pinprick on sensation testing. Mrs. X felt she could include this slump slider in her home exercise programme once or twice a day.

Follow-Up Session 3

Mrs. X's subjective markers had improved; she had no limitations to how long she could sit and was sleeping through the night without pain or P&N. She only occasionally felt pain driving more than 30 min and had begun to wean off her amitriptyline by taking it every other day. Physical examination revealed full and pain free lumbar spine range of movement, including combined positions, normal sensation to light touch and pinprick and only some mild discomfort in her foot when her knee was nearly fully extended on slump testing.

Given the significant improvement, a tensioner slump technique was performed by maintaining cervical flexion during knee extension for 3 × 30 s (Fig. 7.8). On reassessment slump testing was full and pain free, and the bilateral slump was also unremarkable. The patient was advised to continue under her GPs advice weaning off the amitriptyline, given an open appointment and advised to continue her home exercise programme until her symptoms had completely resolved.

To conclude, this case study demonstrates how personalized prescribing of pain medication can be used

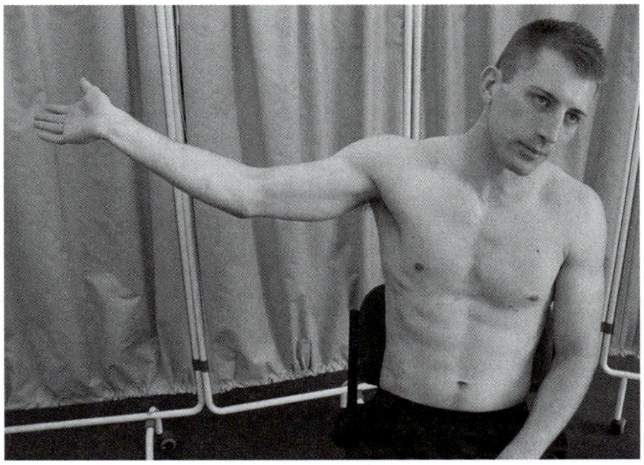

Fig. 7.8 Upper-limb neurodynamic test 1 (ULNT1) tensioner in sitting.

as an adjunct to treatment, particularly in a patient with severe or irritable symptoms, which might otherwise be a barrier to effective treatment and self-management techniques. The use of nerve interface and gliding techniques can be used alone or in combination with each other, but patient symptoms must be monitored throughout the treatment to decide how and when to progress treatment techniques and ensure the symptoms are not unduly aggravated. A demonstration of how these treatments can then be translated to a tailored home exercise programme which fits with lifestyle commitments is also provided to support the patient in implementing a self-management plan.

REVIEW AND REVISE QUESTIONS

1. Nerve gliding techniques have been found to have the following effects (please tick all that apply):
   - **a.** Increased nerve length
   - **b.** Dispersal of oedema
   - **c.** Increased pain
   - **d.** Reduced activation of immune cells
2. A slider is (tick all that are correct):
   - **a.** A nerve gliding procedure
   - **b.** Causes greatest strain to the nerve
   - **c.** May be useful in more irritable situations
   - **d.** Only possible with combinations of joint movements
3. How might exercise be beneficial to people with nerve-related MSK pain?
4. What is one of the challenges of RCTs in people with spinally referred leg pain?
5. Which of the following medications may be useful for people with neuropathic pain?
   - **a.** Opioids
   - **b.** Paracetamol
   - **c.** Anticonvulsants (e.g. gabapentin)
   - **d.** Tricyclic antidepressants (e.g. amitriptyline)

REFERENCES

Adel, S.M., 2011. Efficacy of neural mobilization in treatment of low back pain dysfunctions. J. Am. Sci. 7, 566–573.

Akalin, E., El, O., Peker, O., et al., 2002. Treatment of carpal tunnel syndrome with nerve and tendon gliding exercises. Am. J. Phys. Med. Rehabil. 81, 108–113.

Akkan, H., Gelecek, N., 2018. The effect of stabilization exercise training on pain and functional status in patients with cervical radiculopathy. J. Back Musculoskelet. Rehabil. 31, 247–252.

Albert, H.B., Manniche, C., 2012. The efficacy of systematic active conservative treatment for patients with severe sciatica: a single-blind, randomized, clinical, controlled trial. Spine 37, 531–542.

Almeida, C., DeMaman, A., Kusuda, R., et al., 2015. Exercise therapy normalizes BDNF upregulation and glial hyperactivity in a mouse model of neuropathic pain. Pain 156 (3), 504–513. https://doi.org/10.1097/01.j.pain.0000460339.23976.12.

Andrade, R.J., Freitas, S.R., Hug, F., et al., 2020. Chronic effects of muscle and nerve-directed stretching on tissue mechanics. J. Appl. Physiol. 129 (5), 1011–1023.

Bardak, A.N., Alp, M., Erhan, B., et al., 2009. Evaluation of the clinical efficacy of conservative treatment in the management of carpal tunnel syndrome. Adv. Ther. 26, 107–116.

Baron, R., Maier, C., Attal, N., et al., 2017. German Neuropathic Pain Research Network (DFNS), and the EUROPAIN, and NEUROPAIN consortia. Peripheral neuropathic pain: a mechanism-related organizing principle based on sensory profiles. Pain 158 (2), 261–272. https://doi.org/10.1097/j.pain.0000000000000753.

Basson, A., Olivier, B., Ellis, R., et al., 2017. The effectiveness of neural mobilization for neuromusculoskeletal conditions: a systematic review and meta-analysis. J. Orthop. Sports Phys. Ther. 47 (9), 593–615. https://doi.org/10.2519/jospt.2017.7117.

Bertolini, G.T.F., Silva, T.S., Trindade, D.L., et al., 2009. Neural mobilization and static stretching in an experimental sciatica model – an experimental study. Braz. J. Phys. Ther. 13, 493–498.

Bialosky, J.E., Bishop, M.D., Price, D.D., et al., 2009. A randomised sham-controlled trial of a neurodynamic technique in the treatment of carpal tunnel syndrome. J. Orthop. Sports Phys. Ther. 39, 709–723.

Boudier-Revéret, M., Gilbert, K.K., Allégue, D.R., et al., 2017. Effect of neurodynamic mobilization on fluid dispersion in median nerve at the level of the carpal tunnel: a cadaveric study. Musculoskelet. Sci. Pract. 31, 45–51. https://doi.org/10.1016/j.msksp.2017.07.004.

Bouhassira, D., Branders, S., Attal, N., et al., 2021. Stratification of patients based on the Neuropathic Pain Symptom Inventory: development and validation of a new algorithm. Pain 162 (4), 1038–1046. https://doi.org/10.1097/j.pain.0000000000002130.

Boyd, B.S., Topp, K.S., Coppieters, M.W., 2013. Impact of movement sequencing on sciatic and tibial nerve strain and excursion during the straight leg raise test in embalmed cadavers. J. Orthop. Sports Phys. Ther. 43, 398–403.

Brown, C.L., Gilbert, K.K., Brismee, J.-M., et al., 2011. The effects of neurodynamic mobilization on fluid dispersion within the tibial nerve at the ankle: an unembalmed cadaveric study. J. Man. Manip. Ther. 19, 26–34.

Butler, D.S., 1991. Mobilisation of the nervous system. Churchill Livingstone, Melbourne.

Cleland, J.A., Childs, J.D., Palmer, J.A., et al., 2006. Slump stretching in the management of non-radicular low back pain: a pilot clinical trial. Man. Ther. 11, 279–286.

Cohen, S.P., Mao, J., 2014. Neuropathic pain: mechanisms and their clinical implications. BMJ 5, 348.

Coppieters, M.W., Alshami, A.M., Babri, A.S., et al., 2006. Strain and excursion of the sciatic, tibial, and plantar nerves during a modified straight leg raising test. J. Orthop. Res. 24, 1883–1889.

Coppieters, M.W., Andersen, L.S., Johansen, R., et al., 2015. Excursion of the sciatic nerve during nerve mobilization exercises: an in vivo cross-sectional study using dynamic ultrasound imaging. J. Orthop. Sports Phys. Ther. 45, 731–737.

Coppieters, M.W., Butler, D.S., 2008. Do 'sliders' slide and 'tensioners' tension? An analysis of neurodynamic techniques and considerations regarding their application. Man. Ther. 13, 213–221.

Coppieters, M.W., Hough, A.D., Dilley, A., 2009. Different nerve gliding exercises induce different magnitudes of median nerve longitudinal excursion: an in vivo study using dynamic ultrasound imaging. J. Orthop. Sports Phys. Ther. 39, 164–171.

Dahlin, L., Danielsen, N., Ehira, T., et al., 1986. Mechanical effects of compression of peripheral nerves. J. Biomech. Eng. 108, 120–122.

Deepti, C., Kavitha, R., Ganesh, B., et al., 2008. Effectiveness of neural tissue mobilization over cervical lateral glide in cervico-brachial pain syndrome – a randomized clinical trial. Indian J. Physiother. Occup. Ther. 2, 47–52.

De-La-Llave-Rincon, A.I., Ortega-Santiago, R., Ambite-Quesada, S., et al., 2012. Response of pain intensity to soft tissue mobilization and neurodynamic technique: a series of 18 patients with chronic carpal tunnel syndrome. J. Manipulative Physiol. Ther. 35, 420–427.

DeLeo, J.A., Yezierski, R.P., 2001. The role of neuroinflammation and neuroimmune activation in persistent pain. Pain 90, 1–6.

Dilley, A., Bove, G.M., 2008. Disruption of axoplasmic transport induces mechanical sensitivity in intact rat C-fibre nociceptor axons. J. Physiol. 586 (2), 593–604. https://doi.org/10.1113/jphysiol.2007.144105.

Dilley, A., Greening, J., Lynn, B., et al., 2001. The use of cross-correlation analysis between high-frequency ultrasound images to measure longitudinal median nerve movement. Ultrasound Med. Biol. 27, 1211–1218.

Dilley, A., Lynn, B., Pang, S., 2005. Pressure and stretch mechanosensitivity of peripheral nerve fibres following local inflammation of the nerve trunk. Pain 117, 462–472.

Dilley, A., Odeyinde, S., Greening, J., et al., 2008. Longitudinal sliding of the median nerve in patients with non-specific arm pain. Man. Ther. 13, 536–543.

Dobson, J.L., McMillan, J., Li, L., 2014. Benefits of exercise intervention in reducing neuropathic pain. Front. Cell. Neurosci. 8, 102. https://doi.org/10.3389/fncel.2014.00102.

Driscoll, P.J., Glasby, M.A., Lawson, G.M., 2002. An in vivo study of peripheral nerves in continuity: biomechanical and physiological responses to elongation. J. Orthop. Res. 20, 370–375.

Ellis, R., Blyth, R., Arnold, N., et al., 2017. Is there a relationship between impaired median nerve excursion and carpal tunnel syndrome? A systematic review. J. Hand Ther. 30 (1), 3–12. https://doi.org/10.1016/j.jht.2016.09.002.

Ellis, R., Hing, W., Dilley, A., et al., 2008. Reliability of measuring sciatic and tibial nerve movement with diagnostic ultrasound during a neural mobilisation technique. Ultrasound Med. Biol. 34, 1209–1216.

Ellis, R., Hing, W., McNair, P., 2012. Comparison of longitudinal sciatic nerve movement with different mobilization exercises: an in vivo study utilizing ultrasound imaging. J. Orthop. Sports Phys. Ther. 42, 667–675.

Enke, O., New, H.A., New, C.H., et al., 2018. Anticonvulsants in the treatment of low back pain and lumbar radicular pain: a systematic review and meta-analysis. CMAJ 190 (26), E786–E793.

Erel, E., Dilley, A., Greening, J., et al., 2003. Longitudinal sliding of the median nerve in patients with carpal tunnel syndrome. J. Hand Surg. Br. 28B, 439–443.

Eroglu, C., Allen, N.J., Susman, M.W., et al., 2009. Gabapentin receptor α2δ-1 is a neuronal thrombospondin receptor responsible for excitatory CNS synaptogenesis. Cell 139 (2), 380–392. https://doi.org/10.1016/j.cell.2009.09.025.

Fernández-de-Las Peñas, C., Ortega-Santiago, R., de la Llave-Rincón, A.I., et al., 2015. Manual physical therapy versus surgery for carpal tunnel syndrome: a randomized parallel-group trial. J. Pain 16 (11), 1087−1094. https://doi.org/10.1016/j.jpain.2015.07.012.

Gilbert, K.K., Brismee, J.-M., Collins, D.L., et al., 2007. Lumbosacral nerve root displacement and strain: part 2: straight leg raise conditions in unembalmed cadavers. Spine 32, 1521−1525.

Greening, J., Dilley, A., 2017. Posture-induced changes in peripheral nerve stiffness measured by ultrasound shear-wave elastography. Muscle Nerve 55 (2), 213−222. https://doi.org/10.1002/mus.25245.

Harrisson, S.A., Ogollah, R., Dunn, K.M., et al., 2020. Prevalence, characteristics, and clinical course of neuropathic pain in primary care patients consulting with low back-related leg pain. Clin. J. Pain 36 (11), 813−824.

Heebner, M.L., Roddey, T.S., 2008. The effects of neural mobilization in addition to standard care in persons with carpal tunnel syndrome from a community hospital. J. Hand Ther. 21, 229−241.

Herzberg, U., Eliav, E., Dorsey, J.M., et al., 1997. NGF involvement in pain induced by chronic constriction injury of the rat sciatic nerve. Neuroreport 8, 1613−1618.

Hough, A.D., Moore, A.P., Jones, M.P., 2007. Reduced longitudinal excursion of the median nerve in carpal tunnel syndrome. Arch. Phys. Med. Rehabil. 88, 569−576.

Hubbard, R.D., Winkelstein, B.A., 2008. Dorsal root compression produces myelinated axonal degeneration near the biomechanical thresholds for mechanical behavioural hypersensitivity. Exp. Neurol. 212, 482−489.

Kobayashi, S., Shizu, N., Suzuki, Y., et al., 2003. Changes in nerve root motion and intraradicular blood flow during an intraoperative straight leg raise test. Spine 28, 1427−1434.

Kobayashi, S., Yoshino, N., Yamada, S., 2004. Pathology of lumbar nerve root compression. Part 1: intraradicular inflammatory changes induced by mechanical compression. J. Orthop. Res. 22, 170−179.

Konstantinou, K., Dunn, K.M., Ogollah, R., et al., 2018. Prognosis of sciatica and back-related leg pain in primary care: the ATLAS cohort. Spine J. 18 (6), 1030−1040.

Korstanje, J.-W.H., Scheltens-de boer, M., Blok, J.H., et al., 2012. Ultrasonographic assessment of longitudinal median nerve and hand flexor tendon dynamics in carpal tunnel syndrome. Muscle Nerve 45, 721−729.

Lewis, K.J., Coppieters, M.W., Ross, L., et al., 2020. Group education, night splinting and home exercises reduce conversion to surgery for carpal tunnel syndrome: a multicentre randomised trial. J. Physiother. 66 (2), 97−104. https://doi.org/10.1016/j.jphys.2020.03.007.

Luijsterburg, P.A., Verhagen, A.P., Ostelo, R.W., et al., 2008. Physical therapy plus general practitioners' care versus general practitioners' care alone for sciatica: a randomised clinical trial with a 12-month follow-up. Eur. Spine J. 17 (4), 509−517. https://doi.org/10.1007/s00586-007-0569-6.

McCleane, G.J., 2001. Does gabapentin have an analgesic effect on background, movement and referred pain? A randomised, double-blind, placebo controlled study. Pain Clin. 13 (2), 103−107.

Mackinnon, S.E., 2002. Pathophysiology of nerve compression. Hand Clin. 18, 231−241.

Makarawung, D.J., Becker, S.J., Bekkers, S., et al., 2013. Disability and pain after cortisone versus placebo injection for trapeziometacarpal arthrosis and de Quervain syndrome. Hand (N Y) 8, 375−381.

Mankovsky, T., Lynch, M., Clark, A., et al., 2012. Pain catastrophizing predicts poor response to topical analgesics in patients with neuropathic pain. Pain Res. Manag. 17, 10−14.

Martins, D.F., Mazzardo-Martins, L., Gadotti, V.M., et al., 2011. Ankle joint mobilization reduces axonotmesis-induced neuropathic pain and glial activation in the spinal cord and enhances nerve regeneration in rats. Pain 152, 2653−2661.

Muehlbacher, M., Nickel, M.K., Kettler, C., et al., 2006. Topiramate in treatment of patients with chronic low back pain: a randomized, double-blind, placebo-controlled study. Clin. J. Pain 22 (6), 526−531.

Nagrale, A.V., Patil, S.P., Ghandi, R.A., et al., 2012. Effect of slump stretching versus lumbar mobilization with exercises in subjects with non-radicular low back pain: a randomized clinical trial. J. Man. Manip. Ther. 20, 35−42.

National Institute for Health and Clinical Excellence, 2013. Neuropathic pain: the pharmacological management of neuropathic pain in adults in non-specialist settings. Clinical guideline 173. www.nice.org.uk/CG173.

National Institute for Health and Clinical Excellence, 2020. Overview | Low back pain and sciatica in over 16s: assessment and management | Guidance | NICE.

Nee, R.J., Vincenzino, B., Jull, G.A., et al., 2012. Neural tissue management provides immediate clinically relevant benefits without harmful effects for patients with nerve-related neck and arm pain: a randomised trial. J. Physiother. 58, 23−31.

Neto, T., Freitas, S.R., Andrade, R.J., et al., 2020. Shear wave elastographic investigation of the immediate effects of slump neurodynamics in people with sciatica. J. Ultrasound Med. 39, 675−681. https://doi.org/10.1002/jum.15144.

NHS Health Education England. https://www.hee.nhs.uk/our-work/person-centred-care. Accessed 23/7/21.

Núñez de Arenas-Arroyo, S., Cavero-Redondo, I., Torres-Costoso, A., et al., 2021. Short-term effects of neurodynamic techniques for treating carpal tunnel syndrome: A systematic review with meta-analysis. J. Orthop. Sports Phys. Ther. 51(12), 566−580.

Ogata, K., Naito, M., 1986. Blood flow of peripheral nerves effects of dissection, stretching and compression. J. Hand Surg. Am. 11B, 10–14.
Ostelo, R.W.J.G., 2020. Physiotherapy management of sciatica. J. Physiother. 66 (2), 83–88.
Pentelka, L., Hebron, C., Shapleski, R., et al., 2012. The effect of increasing sets (within one treatment session) and different set durations (between treatment sessions) of lumbar spine posteroanterior mobilisations on pressure pain thresholds. Man. Ther. 17, 526–530.
Ryder, D., Barnard, K., 2024. Petty's musculoskeletal examination and assessment: a handbook for therapists, sixth ed. Elsevier, Oxford.
Ridehalgh, C., 2014. Straight leg raise treatment for individuals with spinally referred leg pain: exploring characteristics that influence outcome. Doctoral thesis. University of Brighton. Available online at: http://eprints.brighton.ac.uk/12511/.
Ridehalgh, C., Moore, A., Hough, A., 2012. Repeatability of measuring sciatic nerve excursion during a modified passive straight leg raise test with ultrasound imaging. Man. Ther. 17, 572–576.
Ridehalgh, C., Moore, A., Hough, A., 2015. Sciatic nerve excursion during a modified passive straight leg raise test in asymptomatic participants and participants with spinally referred leg pain. Man. Ther. 20, 564–569.
Ridehalgh, C., Moore, A., Hough, A., 2016. The short term effects of straight leg raise neurodynamic treatment on pressure pain and vibration thresholds in individuals with spinally referred leg pain. Man. Ther. 23, 40–47.
Rothman, S.M., Winkelstein, B.A., 2007. Chemical and mechanical nerve root insults induce differential behavioural sensitivity and glial activation that are enhanced in combination. Brain Res. 1181, 30–43.
Rydevik, B., Lundborg, G., 1977. Permeability of intraneural microvessels and perineurium following acute graded experimental nerve compression. Scand. J. Plast. Reconstr. Surg. 11, 179–187.
Rydevik, B., Lundborg, G., Bagge, U., 1981. Effects of graded compression on intraneural blood flow: an in vivo study on rabbit tibial nerve. J. Hand Surg. Am. 6, 3–12.
Santos, F.M., Grecco, L.H., Pereira, M.G., 2014. The neural mobilization technique modulates the expression of endogenous opioids in the periaqueductal gray and improves muscle strength and mobility in rats with neuropathic pain. Behav. Brain Funct. 10, 19.
Santos, F.M., Silva, J.T., Giardini, A.C., et al., 2012. Neural mobilization reverses behavioral and cellular changes that characterize neuropathic pain in rats. Mol. Pain 8, 57.
Schäfer, A., Hall, T., Müller, G., et al., 2011. Outcomes differ between subgroups of patients with low back and leg pain following neural manual therapy: a prospective cohort study. Eur. Spine J. 20, 482–490.
Schiphorst Preuper, H.R., Geertzen, J.H., van Wijhe, M., et al., 2014. Do analgesics improve functioning in patients with chronic low back pain? An explorative tripleblinded RCT. Eur. Spine J. 23, 800–806.
Schmid, A., Coppieters, M.W., Ruitenberg, M.J., et al., 2013. Local and remote imuune-mediated inflammation after mild peripheral nerve compression in rats. J. Neuropathol. Exp. Neurol. 72, 662–680.
Schmid, A., Elliott, J.M., Strudwick, M.W., et al., 2012. Effect of splinting and exercise on intraneural edema of the median nerve in carpal tunnel syndrome – an MRI study to reveal therapeutic mechanisms. J. Orthop. Res. 1343–1350.
Scrimshaw, S.V., Maher, C.G., 2001. Randomized controlled trial of neural mobilization after spinal surgery. Spine 26, 2647–2652.
Shen, J., Fox, L.E., Cheng, J., 2013. Swim therapy reduces mechanical allodynia and thermal hyperalgesia induced by chronic constriction nerve injury in rats. Pain Med. 14 (4), 516–525. https://doi.org/10.1111/pme.12057.
Steen, K.H., Steen, A.E., Kreysel, H.W., et al., 1996. Inflammatory mediators potentiate pain induced by experimental tissue acidosis. Pain 66, 163–170.
Sumizono, M., Sakakima, H., Otsuka, S., et al., 2018. The effect of exercise frequency on neuropathic pain and pain-related cellular reactions in the spinal cord and midbrain in a rat sciatic nerve injury model. J. Pain Res. 11, 281–291. https://doi.org/10.2147/JPR.S156326.
Sunderland, S., 1989. Features of nerves that protect them during normal daily activities. In: Paper presented at: Manipulative Therapy Association Australia (Adelaide).
Tal-Akabi, A., Rushton, A., 2000. An investigation to compare the effectiveness of carpal bone mobilisation and neurodynamic mobilisation as methods of treatment for carpal tunnel syndrome. Man. Ther. 5, 214–222.
Tian, J., Yu, T., Xu, Y., et al., 2018. Swimming training reduces neuroma pain by regulating neurotrophins. Med. Sci. Sports Exer. 50 (1), 54–61. https://doi.org/10.1249/MSS.0000000000001411.
Thoomes, E., Ellis, R., Dilley, A., et al., 2021. Excursion of the median nerve during a contra-lateral cervical lateral glide movement in people with and without cervical radiculopathy. Musculoskelet. Sci. Pract. 52, 102349. https://doi.org/10.1016/j.msksp.2021.102349.

8

Vascular Flow Limitations: A Source of Pain and Dysfunction

Alan Taylor and Nathan Hutting

LEARNING OUTCOMES

After studying this chapter, you should be able to:

- Understand how vascular dysfunction may present in physiotherapy clinics.
- Recognize a range of mechanisms of vascular flow limitations.
- Identify appropriate and timely management for patients of all ages.

CHAPTER CONTENTS

INTRODUCTION

The vascular system has been of interest to physiotherapists since the 1800s, from the early days of the profession's origin in Sweden at the Royal Central Institute of Gymnastics for Manipulation and Exercise in 1813, and the 'Society of Trained Masseuses' (UK in 1894). However, physiotherapists became ever more sophisticated and branched out into electrotherapies and developed manual therapies; vascular knowledge and principles were gradually side-lined as the profession branched further into complex specialisms such as 'pain science'. With the current worldwide impact of COVID-19, which has been described as a vascular disease (Siddiqi et al., 2021), there has never been a more appropriate time for physiotherapists to review and enhance their vascular knowledge.

It is well accepted that the vascular system plays a crucial role in bringing oxygen to every organ and tissue in the body (including the brain) and removing waste products via a series of interconnected blood vessels. Bodily function therefore relies on sound haemodynamic function, a combination of healthy blood contained within responsive and fully functioning blood vessels. This chapter will consider how vascular dysfunction, with a particular emphasis on some of the lesser known (arterial) vascular flow limitations, may manifest and present in clinical situations. It will offer a practical guide to the recognition and management of a broad range of regional anatomical presentations.

Why Is Considering the Vascular System Important?

Whilst atherosclerosis is a leading cause of vascular disease in older adults worldwide (Barquera et al., 2015), there are a number of peripheral vascular syndromes that are rare, and because of that rarity, and because they affect younger adults, they are commonly overlooked. They classically present as pain syndromes which mimic or masquerade as more common musculoskeletal (MSK) presentations. As a result, many patients pass through physiotherapy clinics and are offered a range of inappropriate interventions and referral pathways prior to the origin of their presentation being discovered. Often his process leads to long delays in the appropriate management of the condition and considerable distress to the patient in the process. A case study by Taylor and Kerry (2017) described a 35-year history of delayed diagnosis of low back and leg pain in a 53-year-old cyclist who had been subjected to a range of inappropriate interventions and management strategies. The arterial source of his 'chronic pain' was finally (35 years after onset) revealed via simple clinic-based exercise testing; he then went on to have further vascular tests and eventually underwent surgery on an extensive stenosis of his common and external iliac arteries. He made a complete recovery from his symptoms and returned to leisure cycling. The case is illustrative of how faulty clinical reasoning can lead to a 'best fit' approach, and how key elements of this patient's presentation (exercise induced leg pain) were overlooked by a range of clinicians and medics. This chapter will attempt to provide guidance on how to recognize a range of mechanisms of vascular flow limitations and offer appropriate and timely management for patients of all ages.

PERIPHERAL VASCULAR CONDITIONS THAT CAN MASQUERADE AS MUSCULOSKELETAL PRESENTATIONS

Non-Atherosclerotic Lower Limb Arterial Flow Limitations

External Iliac Artery Endofibrosis

External iliac artery endofibrosis (EIAE) is a fibrous arterial lesion (distinct pathologically from atherosclerosis) which leads to asymmetrical stenosis or narrowing of the external iliac artery.

Presentation. EIAE commonly affects young, fit, high-mileage cyclists or triathletes leading to reduced flow to the affected limb at times of maximal effort. There are reports in the literature of marathon runners, fell runners, speed skaters and weightlifters who have been diagnosed with the condition (Gähwiler et al., 2021). Affected athletes will commonly complain of lower limb pain and dysfunction and poor performance. Thigh pain is commonly reported, calf pain is rare and this generally differentiates the condition clinically from distal lesions. There is usually no pain at rest, except in advanced cases. Numbness in the affected limb is often described. Symptoms occur commonly at times of maximal effort. Athletes will often describe a 'loss of force' in the affected leg. The symptoms rapidly diminish if the exercise level is reduced marginally.

The condition is thought to be related to abnormal haemodynamic stress combined with kinking and tethering of the artery, leading to vessel wall injury (Fig. 8.1). The symptoms commonly masquerade as pain of musculoskeletal or neural origin and long delays to diagnosis have been documented (Abraham et al., 1997).

Assessment. Resting vascular tests such as pulse palpation are usually normal. A bruit (the sound of turbulence) may be detected on auscultation over the external iliac artery. Ankle to brachial pressure (ABPI) at rest usually falls within normal limits. In the clinic, pulse palpation after exercise may be diminished. If this is the case, the patient should be referred on for a maximal exercise test to reproduce the symptoms. Post exercise systolic blood pressure may be lowered on the affected side resulting in an abnormal ABPI (<0.66) (Peach et al., 2012). This test will reveal the presence of a blood flow problem in 85% of cases. Duplex

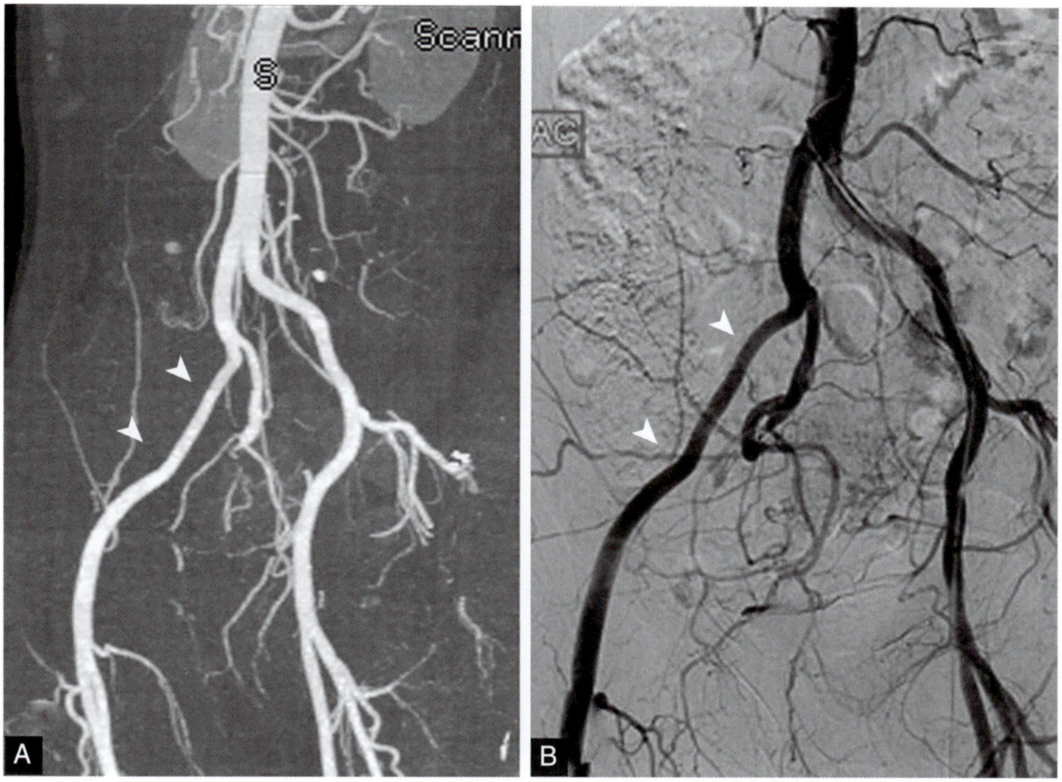

Fig. 8.1 External iliac artery endofibrosis. (A) On maximum intensity projection of CT images, the endofibrosis lesion appears as a mild stenosis of the right external iliac artery involving more than two-thirds of the arterial length (arrowheads). (B) Intra-arterial digital subtraction angiography shows similar findings (arrowheads). Surgical findings and histology confirmed the diagnosis of arterial endofibrosis of the right external iliac artery. (Source: Perrier, L., Feugier, P., Goutain-Majorel, C., et al., July–August 2020. Arterial endofibrosis in endurance athletes: prospective comparison of the diagnostic accuracy of intra-arterial digital subtraction angiography and computed tomography angiography. Diagn. Interv. Imaging 101 [7–8], 463–471.)

ultrasound flow studies after exercise, magnetic resonance angiogram (MRA) or standard arteriogram will usually reveal the exact site of the lesion.

Management. Management is dependent on the competitive level of the affected athlete and the extent of the lesion. Professional or Olympic standard athletes will often demand remedial surgery. Surgery involves endofibrosectomy (removal and shortening of the damaged section of vessel) with saphenous vein patching or grafting. A number of professional cyclists have returned to world-class competition following this type of surgery. Sports participants at lower levels are advised against surgery due to the lack of long-term follow-up and relative risk/benefit of the procedure.

Note: Some cases of endofibrosis in athletes have been reported to affect the common iliac artery.

KNOWLEDGE CHECK

1. What is EIAE?
2. How does it present?

Adductor Canal Syndrome

Adductor canal syndrome is a rare condition defined by mechanical stenosis or occlusion of the femoral artery in the aponeurotic tunnel (Hunter's canal) in the middle third of the thigh (Fig. 8.2). The mechanism is

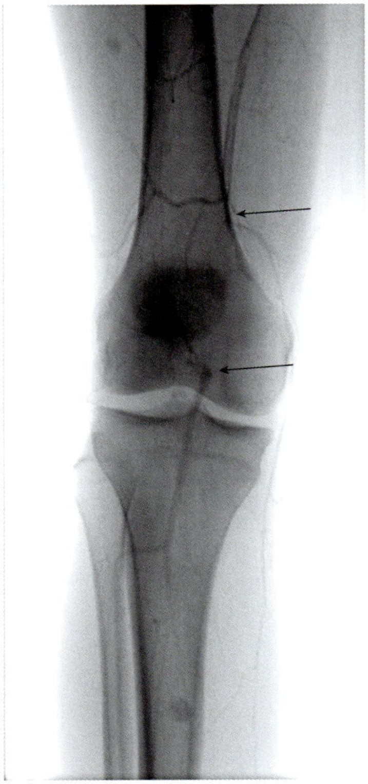

Fig. 8.2 Adductor canal syndrome. (Source: Menon, D., Onida, S., & Davies, A.H., August 2019. Overview of arterial pathology related to repetitive trauma in athletes. J. Vasc. Surg. 70 [2], 641–650.)

thought to be due to the scissor-like action of adductor magnus and vastus medialis. Anatomical abnormalities may be combined with muscle or tendon hypertrophy. Of note, the condition may present as acute occlusion with or without thrombosis.

Presentation. This rare condition has been reported in young fit athletes such as skiers and runners (Menon et al., 2019). Symptoms depend on the extent of the flow limitation, with mild cases experiencing intermittent muscle pains or cramps distal to the lesion (calf) and specifically related to activity or effort. Commonly the complaint is of calf pain or numbness in the toes. For this reason, mild cases may be mistaken for nerve entrapment. The condition may progress rapidly if a thrombus forms at the occluded vessel. At this stage, the diagnosis becomes more straightforward as the patient presents with typical claudication symptoms such as pain/numbness/weakness in the medial knee region and distal lower limb.

Assessment. The condition may present with similar symptoms as popliteal artery entrapment syndrome (PAES). Indeed, it may be difficult to differentiate between the two clinically. As the lesion exists on the aorto-femoro-popliteal axis, the condition may be revealed by chance during exercise testing for EIAE or PAES. In the presence of an arterial lesion, results may reveal lowered post exercise systolic pressure and ABPI results on the affected leg (compared to the normal side). In advanced cases, there may be pain during normal daily activity (i.e. walking), pulses may be reduced or absent at the foot. The foot may be cold or blanch white with minimal repetitive dorsiflexion/plantarflexion exercise at the ankle. ABPI at rest may be significantly lowered (<0.9; see Table 8.1).

Management. Acute cases should be referred urgently for a full vascular diagnostic workup. Irreversible damage to the limb may occur if the condition progresses rapidly (usually in association with thrombus). Arteriogram or MRA will confirm diagnosis and differentiate it from PAES. Emergency surgery is performed to explore and repair the affected portion of the artery (endarterectomy with a saphenous vein patch or via saphenous vein bypass).

KNOWLEDGE CHECK

1. Where and how is the femoral artery stenosed/occluded?
2. How should you manage such a case, if discovered?

Popliteal Artery Entrapment Syndrome

PAES is a condition which leads to vascular flow limitation affecting the distal lower limb (calf/foot). It is associated with a gradual progressive stenosis of the popliteal artery. The condition has been linked to mechanical trauma from a range of abnormal anatomical variants in the popliteal fossa. Various anatomical anomalies are reported relating to the medial head of gastrocnemius, popliteus or localized fibrous bands (Fig. 8.3).

Presentation. The condition is commonly associated with pain, weakness and paraesthesia in the calf or foot at times of effort during sport. Discomfort is usually elicited by specific levels of exercise, for example, runners may report symptoms only when sprinting or

TABLE 8.1 Ankle to Brachial Pressure

Right ABI	**Left ABI**
$\frac{\text{Higher right ankle pressure}}{\text{Higher arm pressure}} = \frac{\text{mm Hg}}{\text{mm Hg}}$ ________	$= \frac{\text{Higher left ankle pressure}}{\text{Higher arm pressure}} = \frac{\text{mm Hg}}{\text{mm Hg}}$ ________

EXAMPLE

$\frac{\text{Higher ankle pressure}}{\text{Higher arm pressure}} = \frac{\text{92 mm Hg}}{\text{164 mm Hg}} = 0.56$ See ABI Interpretation Chart

How to Perform and Calculate the ABI

Partners Program ABI Interpretation

Above 0.90 – Normal
0.71–0.90 – Mild Obstruction
0.41–0.70 – Moderate Obstruction
0.00–0.40 – Severe Obstruction

Source: Goldman L, Schafer AI: Goldman's Cecil medicine, ed 24, Philadelphia, 2012, WB Saunders.

running on slopes/hills. Symptoms are commonly relieved by reducing the intensity of the activity. Rarely, in advanced cases, the athlete may need to stop exercising to gain relief.

Assessment. Vascular examination, such as pulse palpation, at rest is usually normal. Pulse palpation after exercise is classically diminished at the posterior tibial and dorsalis pedis sites. If the condition has progressed to an aneurysm, a pulsatile mass may be palpable in the popliteal fossa, although this is a rare presentation (Hameed et al., 2018).

In the clinic, a simple clinical test is to ask the patient to hop on the spot until symptoms are reproduced. A loss or reduction of pulses is an indication for non-invasive vascular studies such as ABPI before and after provocative exercise. This may reveal the abnormality. Loss of pulses, reduced systolic pressure on the affected leg or a significantly lowered ABPI post-exercise compared to the normal limb raises the suspicion of an arterial cause for the pain (Hameed et al., 2018).

If the index of suspicion for arterial impingement is high, referral to a vascular specialist is required. Continuous-wave Doppler ultrasonography may reveal a change in flow or pulse loss. Duplex flow studies (ultrasound) allow visualization of the artery with simultaneous monitoring of arterial flow. This may reveal the lesion with the use of provocative manoeuvres such as during passive dorsiflexion or active plantarflexion (Hameed et al., 2018). However, the sensitivity of the testing is likely to be higher after exercise at a time of high blood flow. An MRA or standard arteriogram will usually confirm the site of the lesion and differentiate it from adductor canal syndrome (Hameed et al., 2018).

Management. Surgical intervention involves exploration and decompression of the underlying cause. This may require simple release of fascial or musculotendinous slips through to thrombectomy or endarterectomy and saphenous vein grafting.

KNOWLEDGE CHECK

1. What is PAES?
2. Which movements of the ankle will provoke symptoms?

Atherosclerotic Lesions

Atherosclerosis of the lower limbs or lower extremity arterial disease (LEAD) is known to result in either stenosis (Fig. 8.4) or aneurysm at a range of locations in the lower, most commonly, femoral or popliteal arteries. Both stenotic and aneurysmal lesions may mimic MSK presentations and be mistaken for referred pain from somatic or neural structures (Kasapis & Gurm, 2010). It is therefore essential that the astute clinician has a high index of suspicion for the presence of potential vascular lesions and is able to perform an

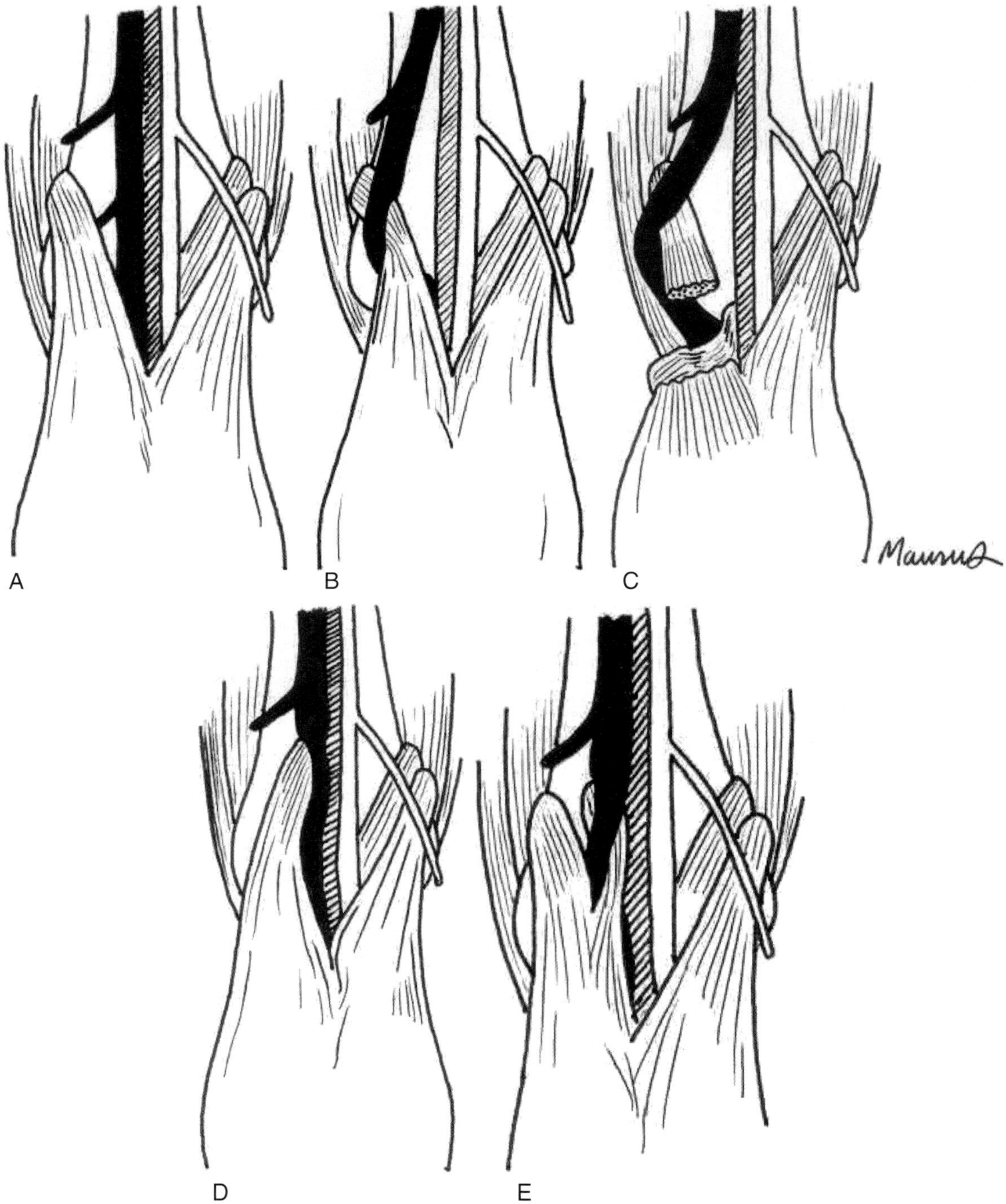

Fig. 8.3 Popliteal artery entrapment syndrome. (A) Normal anatomy. (B) The artery runs medial to the medial head of gastrocnemius. (C) Accessory muscle slip affects the arterial course. (D) The artery is compressed by lateralized gastrocnemius insertion. (E) An accessory slip of the medial head of the gastrocnemius muscle inserts into the inter-condylar region and compresses the artery. (Source: Modified from Rich N.M., et al. Arch Surg. 1979;114:1377.)

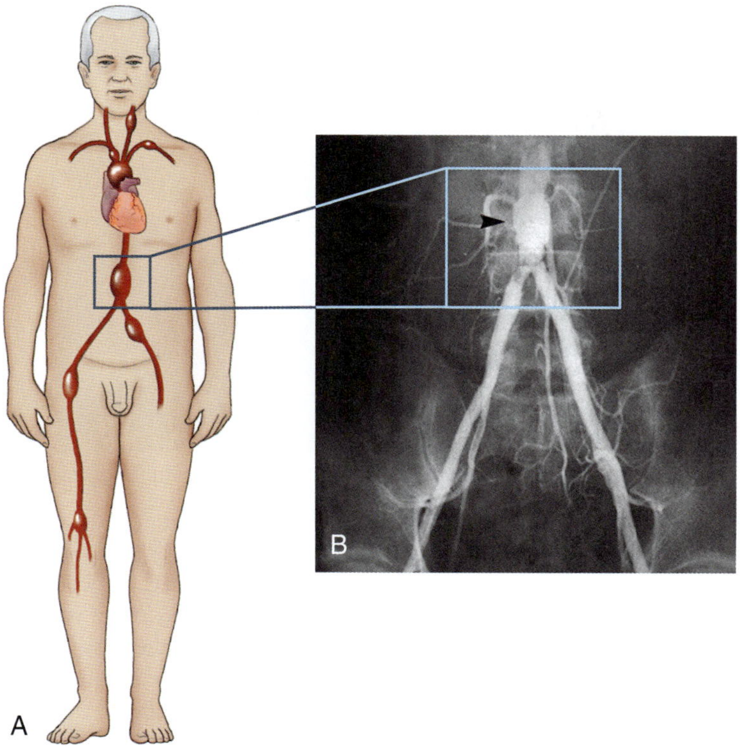

Fig. 8.4 (A) Common anatomic sites of arterial aneurysms. (B) Arteriogram of an abnormal aortic aneurysm. (Source: Quick & Easy Medical Terminology, ninth ed. Elsevier.)

appropriate examination which fit with the presenting symptoms and the general health of the patient (Box 8.1). The key elements of clinical reasoning and physical examination remain the same, for both atherosclerotic and non-atherosclerotic entities. The bottom line is that arterial stenosis leads to flow limitation, leading to claudication pain/symptoms, and that the pattern is most commonly exercise induced.

BOX 8.1 Key Questions for the Clinician

1. Is there an exercise/movement induced component to the presentation?
2. Does this present as a claudication pattern?
3. Could this patient have a vascular flow limitation?
4. Does the limb have normal colour at rest?
5. Does the limb have normal pulses at rest?
6. Is the blood pressure of the limb normal at rest?
7. Is it appropriate to consider an exercise test?
8. Are the pulses normal after exercise (if appropriate)?
9. Is the blood pressure normal after exercise (if appropriate)?
10. Is the patient stable or critical?
11. Is this a routine or urgent referral?
12. Either way, how should I communicate my findings?

UPPER LIMB ARTERIAL CONDITIONS

Upper Limb Arterial Flow Limitations Within the Thoracic Outlet

The Subclavian-Axillary Artery

The aetiology of arterial flow limitation in the subclavian-axillary region may occur due to external or internal factors. External occlusion can occur due to compression of the artery lumen by surrounding anatomical structures, leading to transient flow limitations. Muscular structures which can cause arterial compression include the anterior scalene, subclavius and pectoralis minor. Muscular hypertrophy may result in the occlusion of distal blood flow and create local and peripheral altered hemodynamics (Gannon, 2018). Bony structures within the costoclavicular space include the presence of a cervical rib (Fig. 8.5) or an anomalous

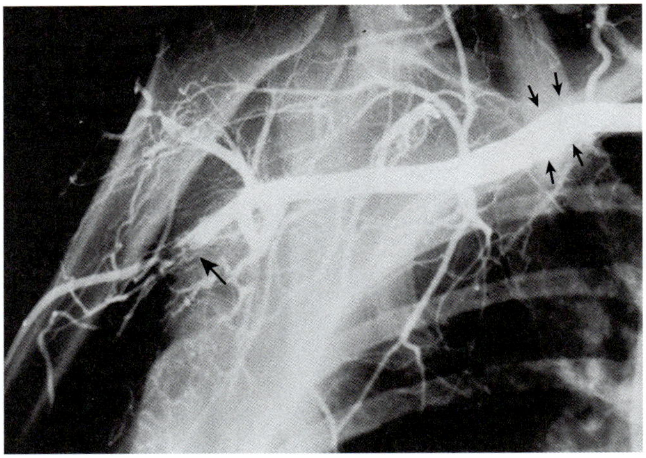

Fig. 8.5 Cervical rib. (Source: Vascular Surgery, sixth ed. Elsevier.)

first rib (Gannon, 2018). Symptoms may occur during repetitive upper limb activity or direct trauma. Internal occlusion is related to atherosclerotic disease. Of note, case series regarding distal thrombosis from subclavian-axillary inducible occlusion (i.e. transient and as a result of the throwing action and concomitant glenohumeral instability) have been reported (Gannon, 2018).

Presentation. The condition may present as pain in the region of the affected supra-clavicular fossa and arm. The vascular origin of the symptoms may be overlooked, especially in the younger population. Other MSK conditions that may be mistaken for arterial thoracic outlet syndrome (TOS) include glenohumeral pathology and instability, ulna nerve injury, cervical spine referred pain, lateral epicondylalgia and non-vascular TOS (Brantigan & Roos, 2004). A description of distal symptoms including weakness, fatigue, coldness, and dysesthesia related to activity are common. A Raynaud's-type intolerance to cold should also raise the clinician's index of suspicion to an arterial cause.

Assessment. Vascular examination is usually normal at rest. Clinical examination must reproduce comparable positions and effort. Pulse palpation may reveal reduced or absent distal pulses during positional change; therefore classic 'thoracic outlet' tests, such as Adson's, Allen's, Halstead's manoeuvre and Roos's EAST test, may or may not be positive (Brantigan & Roos, 2004). Negative positional tests do not exclude an arterial cause. The exertional component must be explored fully.

Management. The primary aim of treatment would be to prevent further repetitive external trauma to the vessel, as this may result in pathology developing on the intimal layer of the vessel. Activity cessation or modifications of aggravating activities is important (Ohman & Thompson, 2020). Antiplatelet therapy may be required (Kargiotis et al., 2016) in persistent cases that have failed to respond to previous intervention. Surgical removal of the anomalous anatomical structures may be the only option. Surgical intervention may be avoided by physical therapies designed to address the underlying MSK dysfunction, together with a carefully planned rehabilitation of muscle training and reloading.

KNOWLEDGE CHECK

1. What causes thoracic outlet syndrome?
2. Do negative clinical tests exclude an arterial cause?

Arterial Conditions Outside the Thoracic Outlet

Quadrilateral Space Syndrome

The posterior circumflex humeral artery (PCHA) is a branch artery, coming off the distal third of the axillary artery. In some individuals, upper limb activity can cause repetitive tension and mechanical stress to the PCHA as it stretches around the surgical neck of the humerus. Injury to this site includes external compression, leading to potential thrombus formation and aneurysm (Hangge et al., 2018). Compression of the PCHA falls outside the anatomical region of the

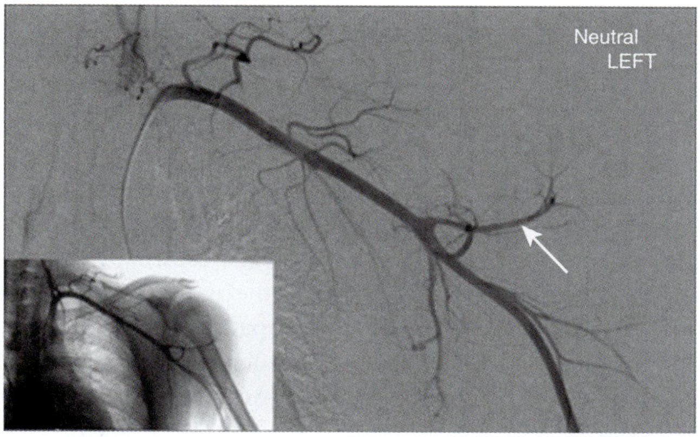

Fig. 8.6 Quadrilateral space syndrome. (Source: Atlas of Uncommon Pain Syndromes, 4th ed. Elsevier)

'thoracic outlet' and is usually associated with compression from the humeral head during upper limb activity (Fig. 8.6). Commonly the throwing action involving abduction and external rotation is implicated. The condition is commonly associated with cases of glenohumeral instability. Clinicians should consider the presence of PCHA involvement when assessing glenohumeral instability in people who report unusual recalcitrant distal upper limb symptoms.

Presentation. True MSK dysfunction, e.g. glenohumeral instability, is a common confounder, and the clinical presentation may include localized glenohumeral pain, 'clunking' of joint etc. Concomitantly there will be distal symptoms such as transient weakness of the hand/arm during overhead activities such as swimming strokes, throwing and baseball pitching. Clinicians need to differentiate between a neural or vascular cause for these symptoms.

Assessment. If the patient's symptoms can be reproduced, transient pulse obliteration may be revealed during pulse palpation. The use of arm-to-arm blood pressure measurements may provide objective measures of the degree of arterial compromise. However, clinicians should note that these may need to be taken in the positions of dysfunction, e.g. arm overhead. Blanching of the hand may also suggest an arterial cause.

Management. Management will largely be dependent on the time line of the condition. The aim will be to reduce further repetitive external trauma to a vessel (i.e. repeated compression from the humeral head), which may lead to pathological atherosclerotic changes on the intimal lining of the vessel (Hangge et al., 2018). Rehabilitation and muscle training to address any underlying glenohumeral instability (i.e. the underlying cause of the injury or flow limitation) should be initiated and may be successful. However, if arterial signs remain, or worsen, during the rehabilitation period as other measures are improving, then possible intimal pathology may have developed and surgical exploration/intervention may be the only solution.

KNOWLEDGE CHECK

1. What actions of the upper limb might produce symptoms of a vascular nature?
2. What are the early management options for quadrilateral space syndrome?

Subclavian Steal Syndrome

Subclavian steal syndrome (SSS) is also known as subclavian-vertebral artery (VA) steal syndrome, as it commonly causes retrograde flow in the VA of the same side (Fig. 8.7). This occurs due to narrowing of the subclavian artery, proximal to the origin of the VA. It manifests with symptoms of vertebral artery insufficiency (VBI) and/or the upper extremity ischaemia, classically associated with overhead movements or effort of the upper limb.

It is more common on the left side, perhaps due to the more acute origin of the left subclavian artery. This may lead to increased turbulence, causing accelerated atherosclerosis and stenosis of the vessel subclavian stenosis and leading to the phenomenon of flow

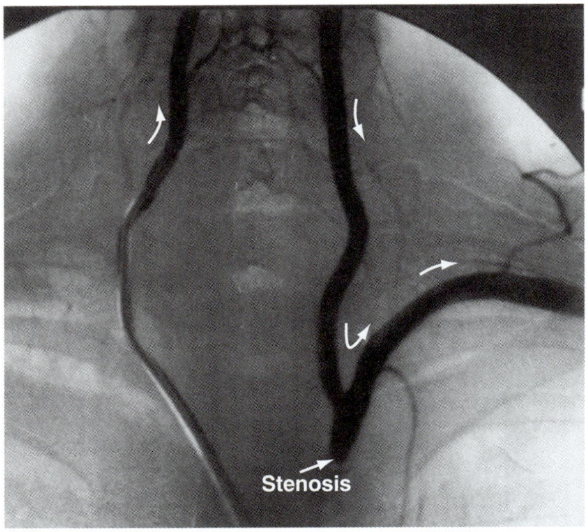

Fig. 8.7 Subclavian steal syndrome. (Source: Youmans & Winn Neurological Surgery, eighth ed. Elsevier)

reversal in the VA, resulting in posterior circulation ischemia of the brain. This occurs when the demand increases for blood flow to the upper limb but is impaired by the significantly narrowed subclavian or innominate artery and so steals from the vertebrobasilar system (Kargiotis et al., 2016; Potter & Pinto, 2014). The presence of congenital anatomical anomalies such as a cervical rib or right aortic arch may also be a source of flow limitation (Kargiotis et al., 2016).

Presentation. The most common complaint is of transient dizziness/disequilibrium or associated symptoms of vertebra-basilar insufficiency such as drop attacks or double vision during overhead movements or efforts of the upper limb. Patients may also complain of transient ischaemic symptoms in the upper limb such as numbness, tingling or fatigue/weakness (Boettinger et al., 2009).

Assessment. The patient's subjective history (interview) as described above may raise the index of suspicion for SSS. If patients are not suffering serious symptoms (e.g. drop attacks), then careful physical examination may include pulse palpation (radial) and/or arm-to-arm blood pressures taken in neutral and or provocative positions as described by the patient. Cases of underlying atherosclerotic stenosis may have reduced pulses and BP (affected arm) at rest, which is exacerbated by functional demonstrations, e.g. overhead activity. In healthy subjects with no underlying vascular pathology, aggravating positions or activities will be required to reveal the mechanical flow limitation.

Management. Subclavian stenosis is most often a marker of cardiovascular risk, and patients will benefit from aggressive secondary prevention. Medical therapy includes aspirin, β-blockade, angiotensin-converting enzyme inhibition, and statins (Aboyans et al., 2010). For patients with mild symptoms, medical therapy and observation may be appropriate, as symptomatic improvement without intervention has been described.

In persistent and troublesome cases, subclavian artery occlusion can be successfully treated either surgically or percutaneously (Babic et al., 2012). Balloon angioplasty and stenting may be performed when stenting is unlikely to compromise the vertebral circulation. However, longer, or more distal occlusions may require surgical intervention. Post-surgical rehabilitation is commonly required.

KNOWLEDGE CHECK

1. What symptoms does subclavian steal syndrome cause?
2. What actions/movements may reproduce those symptoms?

TRUNK

Aortic Coarctation

Aortic coarctation is a rare congenital abnormality of the aorta which may present in young otherwise fit athletes. This commonly overlooked stenosis results in reduced blood flow to the lower limbs during times of effort.

Presentation. The condition may manifest in early childhood and commonly be dismissed as 'growing pains'. Otherwise, it may present around the late teenage years and may present as pain and fatigue during effort related activities in sport. This non-arteriosclerotic aetiology is rare, and this commonly leads to delayed diagnosis resulting in incapacity and diminished athletic ability. It has been reported in a range of sports activities. Sufferers may describe chronic (bilateral) leg fatigue and complain of difficulty 'keeping up' during training. Symptoms became apparent as the demands of the sport increase. The athlete may describe 'heaviness' in the legs, intermittent pain or cramping in the thighs or calves (nondermatomal) and poor performance (Rossi et al., 2020). Classically, sufferers may present for sports medicine assessment complaining of sports-related fatigue.

Assessment. The condition is very rare and as such is usually revealed after exclusion of other causes. Auscultation of the aorta reveals a loud bruit. The condition may be confirmed by ultrasound examination. Doppler flow studies will usually reveal the stenosis and alteration of blood velocity at the site of the lesion. Further confirmation may be sought via arteriogram, MRA or computerized tomographic angiogram (CTA).

Management. Depends largely on the exact site and nature of the abnormality and if there is systemic hypertension. Surgery interventions may result in a return to sport together with a marked improvement in overall fitness and ability to run.

> **KNOWLEDGE CHECK**
> 1. How does aortic coarctation manifest?
> 2. What clinical tests may be helpful to diagnose it?

Aortic Stenosis

Presentation. Aortic stenosis (narrowing of the vessel) is known to produce bilateral leg symptoms (pain, tingling, reduced walking tolerance) usually in patients over the age of 60 years, which may or may not be associated with low back pain (LBP) (Anagnostakos & Lal, 2021). The symptoms occur due to reduced blood flow to the lower limbs during times of effort, e.g. walking or stair climbing (claudication). The presenting symptoms diminish as the effort is stopped or reduced in intensity. It is essential to ask patients if their symptoms are affected by activity, exercise or effort to aid differentiation. It is wise to consider that comorbidities such as obesity and diabetes commonly co-exist and can cloud the clinical picture.

Laslett (2000) described a classic case of bilateral buttock and leg symptoms in a 51-year-old woman who had co-existing LBP. The patient had presented with a deterioration of her ability to walk due to the developing symptoms and a primary outcome of wanting to return to her previous level of walking—three to four times per week. The source of this patient's symptoms was revealed by a simple bicycle test of van Gelderen (Dyck & Doyle, 1977), and the patient was referred on with a suspected vascular cause of her symptoms. Eventually, after some delay (related to her co-existing LBP) she was referred to the vascular team, where further testing revealed significant aortic stenosis, and she underwent balloon angioplasty which provided complete resolution of her buttock and leg symptoms, and she was able to achieve her primary objective of returning to walking without pain.

Assessment. Whenever distal lower limb symptoms are associated (specifically increased) with exercise, clinicians should perform a vascular examination. Resting pulse palpation may be entirely normal. Distal pulses, however, may be diminished after exercise. Bicycle testing as described by van Gelderen will commonly reproduce the lower limb symptoms (Dyck & Doyle, 1977). Resting lower limb blood pressures may be reduced at rest (in advanced cases) or post exercise (Table 8.1).

Management. Suspected cases should be referred on to a vascular team for a full diagnostic work up (Joseph et al., 2017) without delay. Confirmed cases may go on to balloon angioplasty or surgical stenting.

> **KNOWLEDGE CHECK**
> 1. How does aortic stenosis manifest?
> 2. What are the management options?

Abdominal Aortic Aneurysm

Abdominal aortic aneurysms (AAAs) are a ballooning of the arterial wall associated with atherosclerotic pathology (Fig. 8.4). They affect older adults usually over the age of 60 years and can cause significant morbidity and mortality if not identified and managed in a timely fashion. The aetiology of the condition is topic of continued debate. There are a range of known causes, including trauma, infection and inflammatory disorders. Risk factors include cigarette smoking, advanced age, dyslipidaemia, hypertension and coronary artery disease.

Presentation. Many AAAs are asymptomatic and may be picked up during routine screening. However, some are known to present with concomitant LBP, loin pain and abdominal pain (Anagnostakos & Lal, 2021). In some cases distal embolization may occur, giving rise to limb ischaemia.

Assessment. Pulse palpation may reveal a pulsatile abdominal mass. Auscultation may reveal a bruit. Observation may reveal signs of retro-peritoneal haemorrhage, though this is rare. If the aorta has ruptured, the patient may present with acute pain (abdominal, lower back or loin) and may go on to syncope, i.e. faint.

Management. Suspected acute cases should be urgently referred to an emergency department for further diagnostic workup. Stable cases will require referral for assessment of the size of the aneurysm. Surgical repair or stenting may be required depending on presenting symptoms and the size of the aneurysm.

> **KNOWLEDGE CHECK**
> 1. What risk factors are associated with AAA?
> 2. What clinical tests may help with the diagnosis of AAA?

CRANIO-CERVICAL FLOW LIMITATIONS

There are a wide range of potential pathological and nonpathological mechanisms of vascular flow limitations relating to the arterial system which supplies blood to the brain (Golomb et al., 2020; Rushton et al., 2020). As such this section uses tables to assist the reader. Within the cervical spine, events and presentations of vascular flow limitation are rare (Kranenburg et al., 2017) but are an important consideration as part of the patient assessment (Rushton et al., 2020). If pathological and nonpathological mechanisms of vascular flow limitations are not recognized by clinicians, the pathological process may continue or be potentially aggravated by therapeutic encounters, either assessment or management.

It is challenging to distinguish the different pathological and nonpathological mechanisms of vascular flow limitations. Therefore, with regard to pattern recognition, developing an index of suspicion is important, rather than trying to make a clinical diagnosis. Therefore, this section will focus on the more general presentation of pathological and nonpathological mechanisms of vascular flow limitations. It is important that all clinicians managing people with neck pain, headache and/or orofacial symptoms develop an index of suspicion of vasculogenic sources of clinical presentations and familiarize themselves with the underlying mechanisms that may lead to vessel pathology, injury or mechanical flow limitations (Hutting et al., 2021).

Presentation. There are a wide range of haemodynamic mechanisms which have the potential to present as musculoskeletal pain and dysfunction, with patients presenting to the physical therapist with an underlying vascular flow limitation which may present as neck pain, headache or orofacial pain (Rushton et al., 2020).

Potential vascular flow limitations, including their symptoms/presentation which may affect brain perfusion, are presented in Table 8.2. It is important to emphasize that many of the presentations include headache and/or neck pain. These complaints are often reported to have an acute onset of pain and are described as 'unlike any other' (Kerry & Taylor, 2009). However, although this is the case in the majority of the cases (e.g. in craniocervical artery dissections), these characteristics can differ between people, meaning that not all people will not report an acute onset or worst pain ever (Matsumoto et al., 2019).

It is vitally important that clinicians be aware that vascular flow limitation can occur due to mechanical reasons, in healthy vessels and in the absence of frank vascular pathology (e.g. Eagle syndrome, Bow Hunters syndrome and the previously mentioned subclavian steal syndrome) (Westbrook et al., 2020; Hutting et al., 2021). Therefore, it is important to consider the wider implications of mechanical flow limitations (in the absence of vessel pathology) which may contribute to brain ischaemia (Hutting et al., 2021).

Tables 8.3 and 8.4 present symptoms for dissection and nondissection vascular events in the neck region. The percentage figures refer to the proportion of all observed patients with the specified condition (e.g. 'Dissection vascular event') who exhibit the specific symptoms stated in the first column. These data are not intended to inform any judgement on relative risk but rather contribute to the clinician's reasoning regarding the developing clinical pattern (Rushton et al., 2020).

More specifically, signs of vertebrobasilar artery dissection and internal carotid artery are presented in Tables 8.5 and 8.6.

The pain distribution of vertebrobasilar artery dissection and internal carotid artery dissection is presented in Fig. 8.8A and B. Often, the pain is 'unlike any other' (Kerry & Taylor, 2009). However, although less

TABLE 8.2 **Range of Vascular Pathologies of the Neck**

Anatomical Region	Mechanism of Flow Limitation	Symptoms/Presentation
Carotid artery	Atherosclerotic, stenotic, thrombotic, aneurysmal	Carotidynia, neck pain, facial pain, headache, cranial nerve dysfunction, Horner's syndrome, transient ischaemic attack (TIA), stroke
	Hypoplasia (congenital variation)	Commonly silent, rare cerebral ischaemia
	Dissection (vessel wall injury)	Neck pain, facial pain, headache, TIA, stroke, cranial nerve palsies, Horner's syndrome
	Eagle syndrome. Mechanical compression with or without vascular pathology	Neck pain, facial pain, headache, cranial nerve dysfunction, TIA, stroke
	Carotid sinus hypersensitivity (CSH). Vessel may be normal or atherosclerotic	Syncope
Vertebral artery	Atherosclerotic, stenotic, thrombotic, aneurysmal	Neck pain, occipital headache, drop attacks, possible TIA, stroke, cranial nerve palsies
	Hypoplasia (congenital variation)	Commonly silent, rare cerebral ischaemia
	Dissection (vessel wall injury)	Neck pain, occipital headache, TIA, cranial nerve palsy
	Bow Hunters syndrome. Mechanical compression with or without vascular pathology	Neck pain, occipital headache, drop attacks, possible TIA, stroke
	Vertebral artery compression syndrome (VACS). Vascular compression of the medulla or spinal cord	Dizziness, vertigo, inalante, ataxia, limb weakness
Temporal/vertebral/occipital/carotid arteries	Giant cell arteritis (inflammation)	Temporal pain (headache), scalp tenderness, jaw and tongue claudication, visual symptoms, (diplopia or vision loss–may be permanent)
Cerebral vessel	Reversible cerebral vasoconstriction syndrome (RCVS). Vasoconstriction of normal (nonpathological) vessels.	Severe 'thunderclap' headache
	Aneurysm	Sudden severe headache, stiff neck, visual disturbance, photophobia, slurred speech, sickness, unilateral weakness
	Subarachnoid haemorrhage	Sudden severe headache, stiff neck, visual disturbance, photophobia, slurred speech, sickness, unilateral weakness
Jugular vein	Thrombosis	Neck pain, headache, fever, swelling around neck/angle of jaw
Any other cervicocranial or aortic vessel	Vascular anomaly, i.e. intracranial aneurysm	Possible headache/neck pain
Any other vessel	Subclavian steal syndrome. Stenosis of the subclavian vessels	Drop attacks and VBI symptoms as above

Reprinted with permission from Rushton, A., Carlesso, L.C., Flynn, T., Hing, W.A., Rubinstein, S.M., Vogel, S., Kerry, R., Position Statement: International Framework for Examination of the Cervical Region for potential of vascular pathologies of the neck prior to Musculoskeletal Intervention: International IFOMPT Cervical Framework. J Orthop Sports Phys Ther. 2022 Sep 13:1-62. doi: 10.2519/jospt.2022.11147. Epub ahead of print. PMID: 36099171.

TABLE 8.3 Reported Symptoms for Dissection Events (In Order of Most-to-Least Common)

Symptoms	Dissection Vascular Event %
Headache	81
Neck pain	57–80
Visual disturbance	34
Paraesthesia (upper limb)	34
Dizziness	32
Paraesthesia (face)	30
Paraesthesia (lower limb)	19

Reprinted with permission from Rushton, A., Carlesso, L.C., Flynn, T., Hing, W.A., Kerry, R., Rubinstein, S.M., Vogel, S., International Framework for Examination of the Cervical Region for potential of vascular pathologies of the neck prior to Orthopaedic Manual Therapy (OMT) Intervention. J Orthop Sports Phys Ther. 2020.

TABLE 8.4 Reported Symptoms for Nondissection Events (In Order of Most-to-Least Common)

Symptoms	Nondissection Vascular Event %
Headache	51
Paraesthesia (upper limb)	47
Paraesthesia (lower limb)	33
Visual disturbance	28
Paraesthesia (face)	19
Neck pain	14
Dizziness	7

Reprinted with permission from Rushton, A., Carlesso, L.C., Flynn, T., Hing, W.A., Kerry, R., Rubinstein, S.M., Vogel, S., International Framework for Examination of the Cervical Region for potential of vascular pathologies of the neck prior to Orthopaedic Manual Therapy (OMT) Intervention. J Orthop Sports Phys Ther. 2020.

frequently, gradual onset and pain may occur in people with a cervical artery dissection (Matsumoto et al., 2019; Hutting et al., 2021).

Figure 8.8A: Typical pain distribution relating to extracranial VA dissection—ipsilateral posterior upper cervical pain and occipital headache (Kerry & Taylor, 2010).

TABLE 8.5 Signs of Vertebrobasilar Artery Dissection (In Order of Most-to-Least Common)

Signs	VBA Dissection %
Unsteadiness/ataxia	67
Dysphasia/dysarthria/aphasia	44
Weakness (lower limb)	41
Weakness (upper limb)	33
Dysphagia	26
Nausea/vomiting	26
Facial palsy	22
Dizziness/disequilibrium	20
Ptosis	19
Loss of consciousness	15
Confusion	7
Drowsiness	4

Reprinted with permission from Rushton, A., Carlesso, L.C., Flynn, T., Hing, W.A., Kerry, R., Rubinstein, S.M., Vogel, S., International Framework for Examination of the Cervical Region for potential of vascular pathologies of the neck prior to Orthopaedic Manual Therapy (OMT) Intervention. J Orthop Sports Phys Ther. 2020.

TABLE 8.6 Signs of Internal Carotid Artery Dissection (In Order of Most-to-Least Common)

Signs	Nondissection Vascular Event %
Weakness (upper limb)	74
Dysphasia/dysarthria/aphasia	70
Weakness (lower limb)	60
Ptosis	5–50
Facial palsy	47
Unsteadiness/ataxia	35
Confusion	14
Nausea/vomiting	14
Dysphagia	5
Loss of consciousness	5
Drowsiness	2

Reprinted with permission from Rushton, A., Carlesso, L.C., Flynn, T., Hing, W.A., Kerry, R., Rubinstein, S.M., Vogel, S., International Framework for Examination of the Cervical Region for potential of vascular pathologies of the neck prior to Orthopaedic Manual Therapy (OMT) Intervention. J Orthop Sports Phys Ther. 2020.

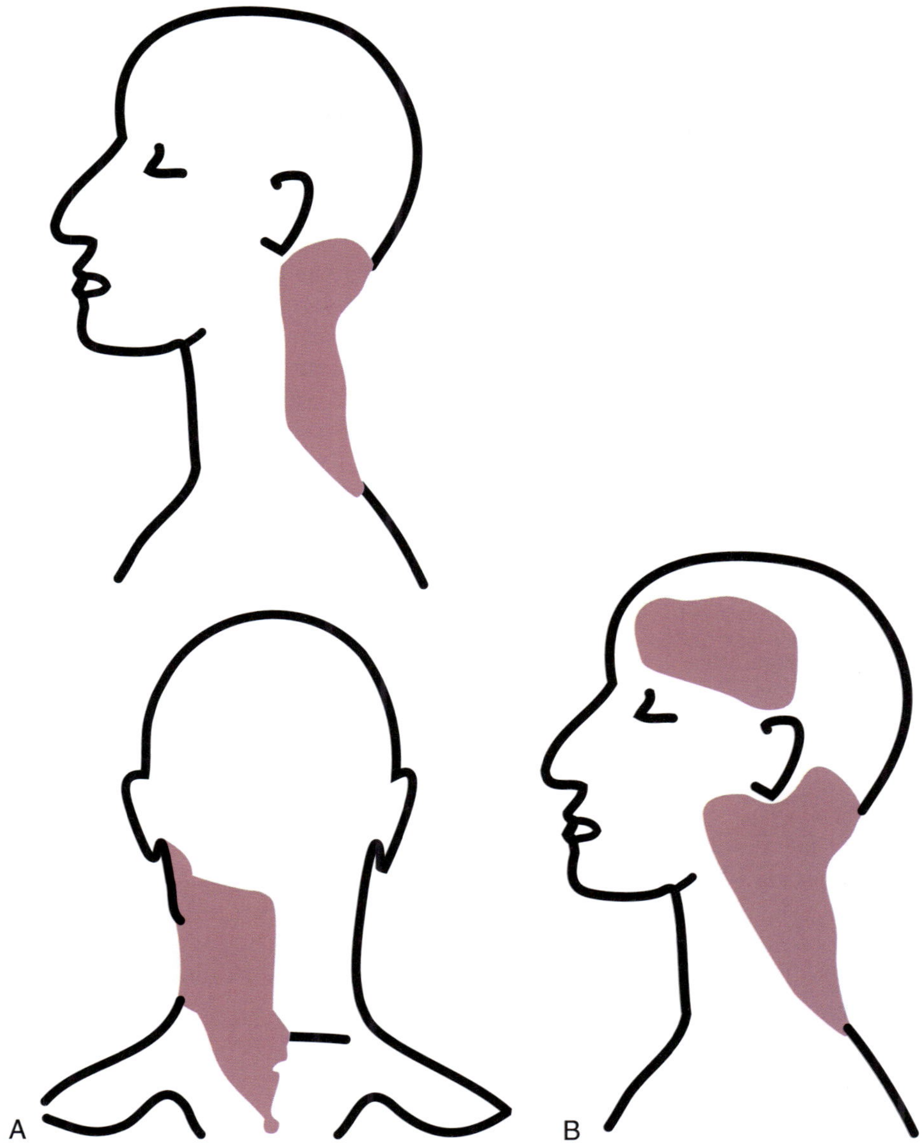

Fig. 8.8 (A) Pain distribution vertebral artery. (B) Pain distribution internal carotid artery. (Source: Kenneth A. Olson. Manual Physical Therapy of the Spine, third ed. Elsevier.)

Figure 8.8B: Typical pain distribution relating to dissection of the internal carotid artery—ipsilateral frontotemporal headache, and upper/mid cervical pain (Kerry & Taylor, 2010).

Table 8.7 presents signs of nondissection events, related to the VA or internal carotid artery.

KNOWLEDGE CHECK

1. Name at least three mechanisms of flow limitations in the head/neck region.
2. Describe the differences between reported symptoms for dissection events and nondissection events.

TABLE 8.7 **Signs of Nondissection Event (Vertebral Artery or Internal Carotid Artery - In Order of Most-to-Least Common)**

Signs	Nondissection vascular event %
Weakness (upper limb)	74
Dysphasia/dysarthria/aphasia	70
Weakness (lower limb)	60
Ptosis	5–50
Facial palsy	47
Unsteadiness/ataxia	35
Confusion	14
Nausea/vomiting	14
Dysphagia	5
Loss of consciousness	5
Drowsiness	2

Reprinted with permission from Rushton, A., Carlesso, L.C., Flynn, T., Hing, W.A., Kerry, R., Rubinstein, S.M., Vogel, S., International Framework for Examination of the Cervical Region for potential of vascular pathologies of the neck prior to Orthopaedic Manual Therapy (OMT) Intervention. J Orthop Sports Phys Ther. 2020.

Assessment

Patient history. In the clinical reasoning process, data obtained from the patient history and the physical examination are used to make the best decision regarding management of the patients' complaints, in shared decision making with the patient (Rushton et al., 2020). An important initial aim in the clinical reasoning process in this context is to assess if there is a vasculogenic hypothesis for the patient presenting with headache and neck pain (Hutting et al., 2018; Rushton et al., 2020). The patient history and the physical examination are used to establish and test hypotheses related to either the predisposition of vascular pathologies of the neck, the presence of frank vascular pathologies of the neck (Rushton et al., 2020), or potential mechanical flow limitations.

It has been suggested that underlying vascular pathologies may be recognizable if appropriate questions are asked during the patient history. Furthermore, if interpretation of elicited data enables recognition of this potential, then physical examination can be adapted to explore any potential vasculogenic hypothesis further (Rushton et al., 2020).

Of primary importance is the fact that vascular pathologies or flow limitations of the head and neck region have the potential to mimic musculoskeletal dysfunction, i.e. head/neck/orofacial pain in the early stages of their presentation (Rushton et al., 2020). Subtle signs and symptoms of the suspected pathologies or blood flow limitations should be recognized in the patient history. Therefore, questions aimed at identifying signs and symptoms are important to ask.

It is important to recognize risk factors indicating the potential for neuro-vascular pathology (Rushton et al., 2020). Cardiovascular risk factors are not strongly associated with dissection-related vascular events in younger people (<38 years) (Thomas et al., 2011; Hutting et al., 2018; Rushton et al., 2020). For example, high total cholesterol and hypertension were only found to be present in 23% and 19%, respectively, of people with an arterial dissection (Rushton et al., 2020). More important risk factors for dissection-related vascular events are recent trauma, vascular anomalies and smoking, which are present in 40%–64%, 39%, and 30% respectively, of people with a dissection-related vascular event (Rushton et al., 2020). See Table 8.8 for an overview of risk factors for dissection vascular events.

Conversely, cardiovascular risk factors are strongly associated with nondissection-related vascular events, e.g. embolization. Atherosclerosis-related risk factors

TABLE 8.8 **Risk Factors for Dissection Vascular Events (In Order of Most-to-Least Common)**

Risk Factor	Dissection Event (%)
Recent trauma	40–64
Vascular anomaly	39
Current or past smoker	30
Migraine	23
High total cholesterol	23
Recent infection	22
Hypertension	19
Oral contraception	11
Family history of stroke	9

Reprinted with permission from Rushton, A., Carlesso, L.C., Flynn, T., Hing, W.A., Rubinstein, S.M., Vogel, S., Kerry, R. Position Statement: International Framework for Examination of the Cervical Region for potential of vascular pathologies of the neck prior to Musculoskeletal Intervention: International IFOMPT Cervical Framework. J Orthop Sports Phys Ther. 2022 Sep 13:1-62. doi: 10.2519/jospt.2022.11147. Epub ahead of print. PMID: 36099171.

are often present in older age groups (>50 years). Therefore, in the over 50s, it is logical to address atherosclerosis-related factors in the patient interview, as their presence is a risk factor for vascular pathology (Hutting et al., 2018). An overview of risk factors for nondissection vascular events is presented in Table 8.9.

Spontaneous dissection events are not associated with the historical risk factors detailed in Table 8.9. Therefore, clinical reasoning must recognize that an absence of risk factors does not necessarily rule out the risk of serious neurovascular events (Rushton et al., 2020).

Clear communication is considered very important and can potentially contribute to the identification of underlying vasculogenic problems and risk factors. A language barrier or low (health) literacy can be a barrier to the communication between healthcare providers and patients. Therefore, it is important to verify that the patient properly understands the questions asked during the patient interview and physical examination (Hutting et al., 2021).

Asking specific questions is important to optimize communication between the physiotherapist and the patient (e.g. instead of asking about overall health, ask specifically about current or previous vascular pathologies, risk factors and contraindications) (Hutting et al., 2021). Moreover, asking about specific signs and symptoms of dissecting as well as nondissecting stroke is important. Clinicians should not assume that patients will always relate these specific symptoms to their complaint (i.e. headache or neck pain) (Hutting et al., 2021).

TABLE 8.9 Risk Factors for Nondissection Vascular Events (In Order of Most-to-Least Common)

Risk Factor	Nondissection Event (%)
Current or past smoker	65–74
Hypertension	53–74
High total cholesterol	53
Migraine	19
Vascular anomaly	16
Family history of stroke	14
Oral contraception	9
Recent infection	9
Recent trauma	7

Reprinted with permission from Rushton, A., Carlesso, L.C., Flynn, T., Hing, W.A., Kerry, R., Rubinstein, S.M., Vogel, S., International Framework for Examination of the Cervical Region for potential of vascular pathologies of the neck prior to Orthopaedic Manual Therapy (OMT) Intervention. J Orthop Sports Phys Ther. 2020.

Physical examination. The purpose of the physical examination is to continue to test the vascular hypothesis generated during the history. The results of the history and physical examination serve to determine whether or not a medical referral for further investigation is warranted. Following the evaluation of the history and physical examination, a specific diagnosis is not rendered, rather the decision to refer for further vascular workup or proceed with physical therapy management is made (Rushton et al., 2020).

Differentiation of a patient's symptoms originating from a vasculogenic cause with complete certainty is not currently possible from the physical examination (Rushton et al., 2020). Thus, it is important for the physical therapist to understand that headache/neck pain/orofacial symptoms may be the early presentation of an underlying vascular pathology, albeit on rare occasions. The task of the physiotherapist is to differentiate the symptoms by (1) having a high index of suspicion and (2) testing the vascular hypothesis (Rushton et al., 2020).

Positional testing. Historically, positional testing for vertebrobasilar insufficiency (VBI) was often used in the physical examination. However, the diagnostic accuracy, rationale and value of the VBI tests have been questioned. The totality of the existing data evaluating functional positional tests for the identification of VA pathology does not support the continued recommendation of these tests (Hutting et al., 2013, 2018, 2020; Rushton et al., 2020). However, in some countries positional testing is still recommended and used clinically, despite its limitations (Thomas et al., 2017; Thomas & Treleavan, 2019).

Blood pressure measurement. Although the diagnostic validity and reliability of blood pressure measurement (in addition to the patient history) with regard to assessing vascular risk factors are unknown (Hutting et al., 2018), in the IFOMPT Cervical Framework (Rushton et al., 2020) examination of blood pressure is an important physical measurement to inform clinical reasoning to assess for risk of stroke, particularly from the carotid origin and to assess for acute arterial trauma in situ (as an increase in blood pressure may be related to acute carotid/vertebral arterial trauma). Information about blood pressure measurement can be found in the NICE guideline 'hypertension in adults' (NICE, 2019).

Neurological examination. Examination of the peripheral nerves, cranial nerves and upper motor neuron testing will assist in evaluating the potential for neurovascular conditions (Rushton et al., 2020). Knowledge of a wide range of testing procedures is required owing to the diversity of possible clinical presentations associated with vascular pathologies of the neck (Rushton et al., 2020). Musculoskeletal clinicians are generally well trained in the examination of the peripheral nerves. However, evidence suggests that clinicians are not always sufficiently trained in the examination of the cranial nerves (Mourad et al., 2021).

Cranial nerve examination is particularly important when examining for the potential of arterial pathology within the cervical region (Rushton et al., 2020), as both vertebral and carotid artery dissection can lead to cranial nerve dysfunction (Taylor et al., 2021). Subtle cranial nerve palsy is known to be a preischemic feature of carotid artery dissection due to the anatomical proximity of the lower cranial nerves (IX, X and XII) to the carotid sheath. Lower CN lesions should be considered in cases of neck pain/headache, neuralgic pain, disturbed speech, swallowing, coughing, deglutition (swallowing), sensory dysfunctions, taste, or autonomic dysfunction, dysphagia, pharyngeal pain, cardiac or gastrointestinal compromise, or weakness of the trapezius, sternocleidomastoid, or the tongue muscles (Finsterer & Grisold, 2015; Taylor et al., 2021). An overview of the cranial nerves, their functions and examination is presented in Table 8.10.

Note that musculoskeletal clinicians are well used to testing function, and for that reason, the order and grouping of the tests have been changed into a more logical function-based order (Taylor et al., 2021). Table 8.11 presents subjective cranial nerve questions.

For more detailed information with regard to the cranial nerves and the cranial nerve examination we refer to Taylor et al. (2021). There are no specific data to support the reliability and validity of examination of a complete cranial nerve examination, and the absence of clinical findings in these examinations does not rule out an underlying pathology or impending dissection (Rushton et al., 2020).

Examination of the carotid artery. Palpation and auscultation of the common and internal carotid arteries are possible due to the size of these vessels and their relatively superficial anatomy (Kerry & Taylor, 2010; Pickett et al., 2011) (Fig. 8.9). Pulses are found in the mid-cervical region with gentle pressure applied medial to the sternocleidomastoid muscle against the vertebral transverse process. The internal carotid pulse can be felt from the mid-cervical region upwards, whilst the more obvious carotid bifurcation is felt more distally towards the angle of the mandible (Kerry & Taylor, 2010). These are common sites for aneurysm formation (Kerry & Taylor, 2010). There is some evidence to support that an alteration of pulse has been identified as a feature of internal carotid disease (Rushton et al., 2020). It is unlikely that transient changes in flow rate or velocity can be perceived in the cervical vessels by palpation (Kerry & Taylor, 2010). However, palpating for gross pathologies—specifically aneurysms—is feasible (Kerry & Taylor, 2010). An extra-cranial aneurysmal pulse will classically feel like a localized mass which is more pulsatile (more noticeable) and more expandable (greater tissue excursion) than a nonpathological pulse (Kerry & Taylor, 2010). A bruit on auscultation (controlling for normal turbulence) is indicative of a significant finding and should be considered in the context of other clinical findings (Rushton et al., 2020). In isolation, pulse palpation is neither sensitive nor specific, but it can offer important data leading to specific diagnoses and treatment (Kerry & Taylor, 2010; Rushton et al., 2020).

Gait/proprioception. Assessment of gait and proprioception is essential for testing cerebellar dysfunction and to differentiate from vestibular problems and sensory loss. Including standard gait assessment, heel-to-toe gait, Romberg's test, assessment of resting tremor (hands), upper limb tone, and co-ordination tests (dysdiadochokinesis, finger-to-nose, heel-to-shin) is appropriate.

Management. If a suspicion of vasculogenic contribution to the patient's complaints is raised, the patient should be referred for further medical investigation. In case a serious event is suspected (e.g. craniocervical artery dissection), immediate referral to an emergency department is warranted.

KNOWLEDGE CHECK

1. Describe the differences between dissection vascular events and nondissection vascular events.
2. Explain why optimizing communication between the physiotherapist and the patient is important.

Name the components of the physical examination.

TABLE 8.10 Cranial Nerves, Their Functions and Examination (Diagonal Lines – Sensory Function – Smell/Hearing; Horizontal Lines – Motor and Sensory Function of the Eyes; Vertical Lines – Motor and Sensory Function of the Face/Jaw/Throat/Tongue; Crossed Lines – Motor Function of the Head/Neck/Shoulders)

Number/Name	Function	Examination	
I Olfactory	Smell (olfaction)	Identify a familiar smell (soap/perfume)	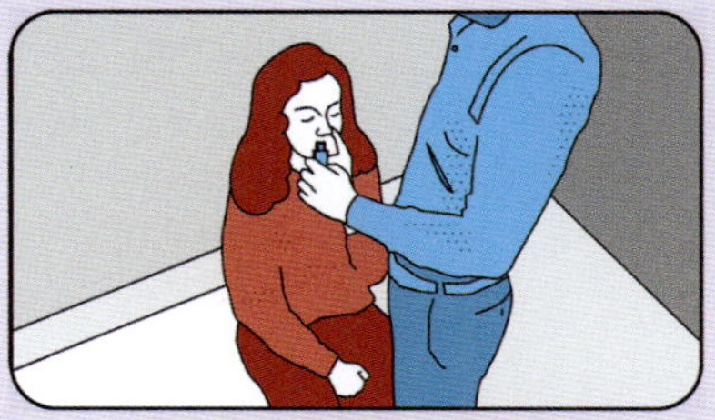
VIII Vestibulocochlear (auditory)	Hearing, balance/ equilibrium	Ask patient if they can hear fingers rubbing (close to ear) or whispered number sequence	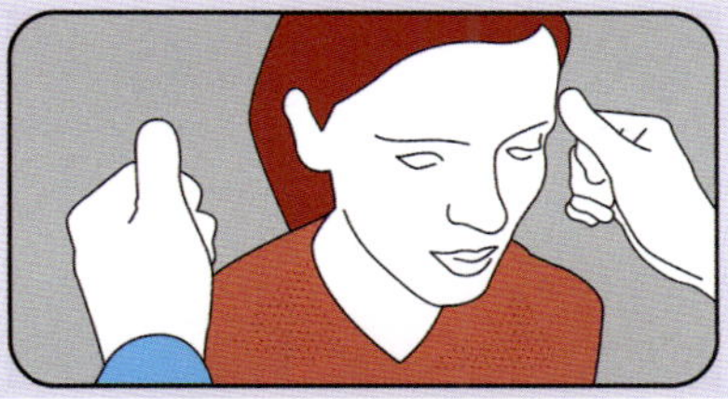
II Optic	Vision (acuity and field)	Test each eye with Snellen chart or newspaper Test visual fields in four quadrants	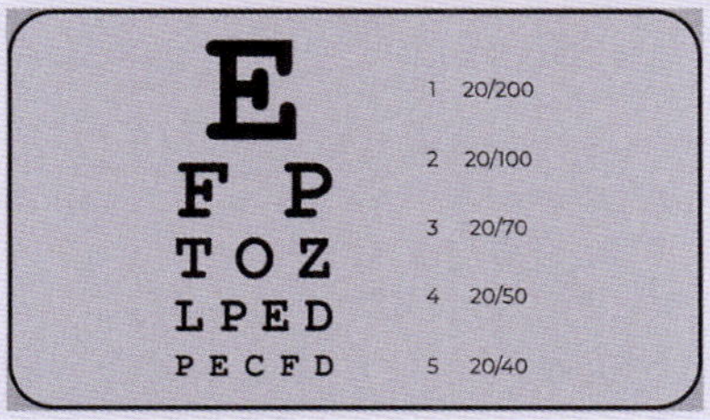
III Oculomotor	Eye movements, elevation of eyelid Pupil size and reactivity to light	Check pupil reaction to light (both should constrict). Check all EOMS (H-test). Check accommodation (finger to nose)	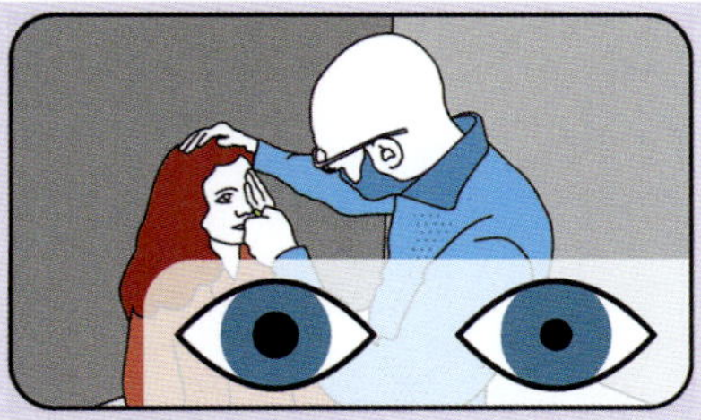
IV Trochlear	Eye movement (vertical and adduction)	H-Test–observe down and in	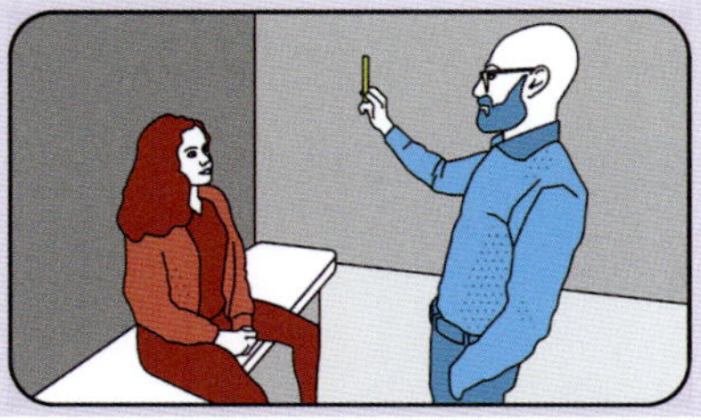
VI Abducens	Eye movements–abduction	H-Test–observe side to side	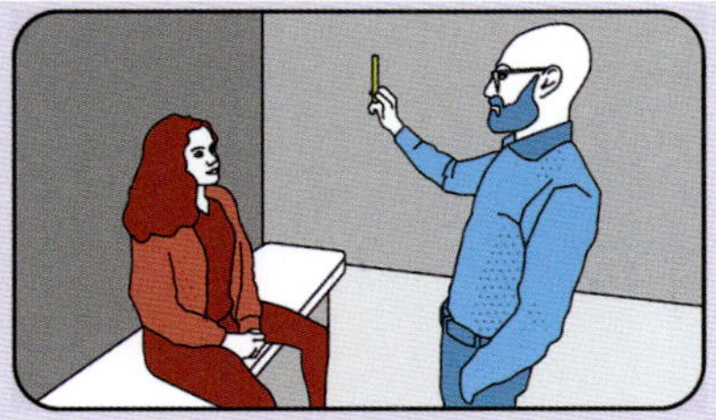

Continued

TABLE 8.10 Cranial Nerves, Their Functions and Examination (Diagonal Lines – Sensory Function – Smell/Hearing; Horizontal Lines – Motor and Sensory Function of the Eyes; Vertical Lines – Motor and Sensory Function of the Face/Jaw/Throat/Tongue; Crossed Lines – Motor Function of the Head/Neck/Shoulders)—cont'd

Number/Name	Function	Examination	
V Trigeminal	Chewing, face/mouth sensation Corneal reflex (sensory)	Test jaw strength (open mouth)–try to close/move laterally Check facial sensation–sharp/blunt	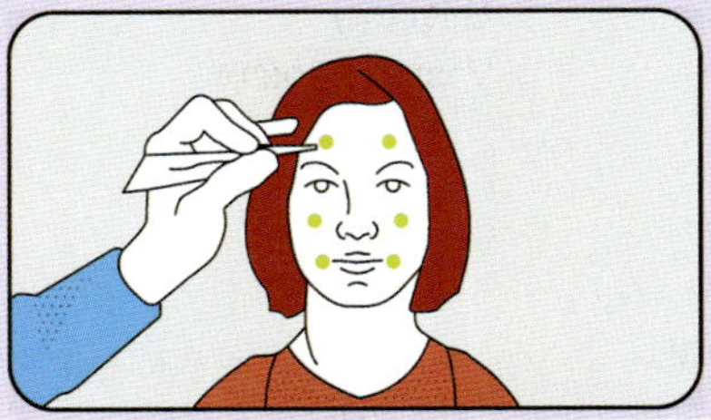
VII Facial	Facial expression, eyelid and lip closure, taste. Corneal reflex (motor)	Ask patient to smile, raise eyebrows, puff out cheeks. Check for symmetry. Ask about taste	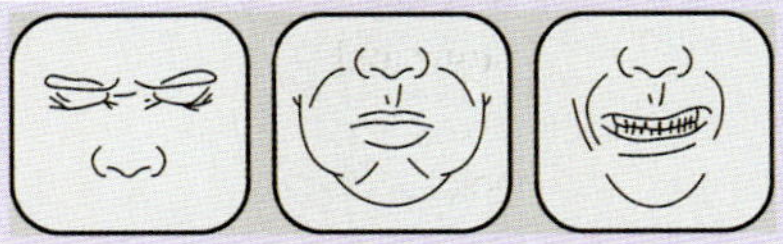
IX Glossopharyngeal	Gagging, swallowing (sensory), taste	Assess gag reflex with tongue depressor Ask patient to swallow	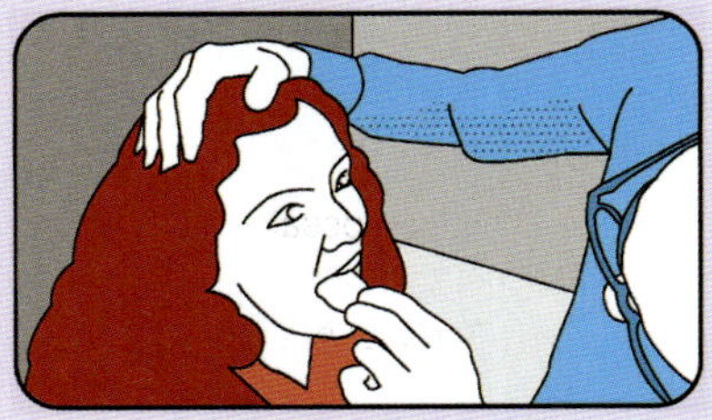
X Vagus	Gagging, swallowing (motor), speech (sound)	Ask patient to say 'Aaaaaaaaah', observe for symmetrical elevation of palate [a] and uvula [b]	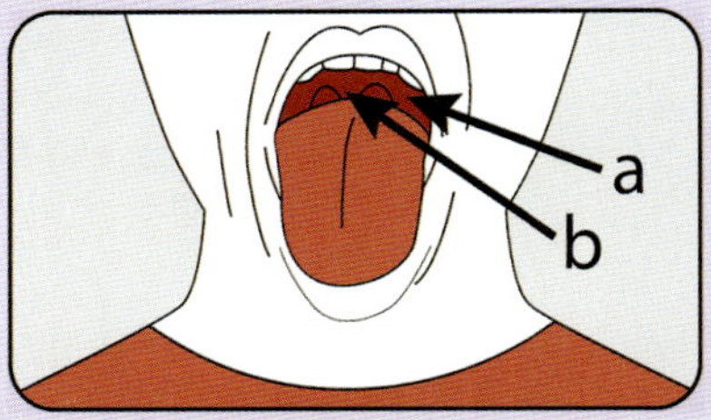
XII Hypoglossal	Tongue movement, speech (articulation)	Patient protrudes tongue, check for deviation, look for fasciculations Patient pushes out cheek with tongue, check power by pushing cheek	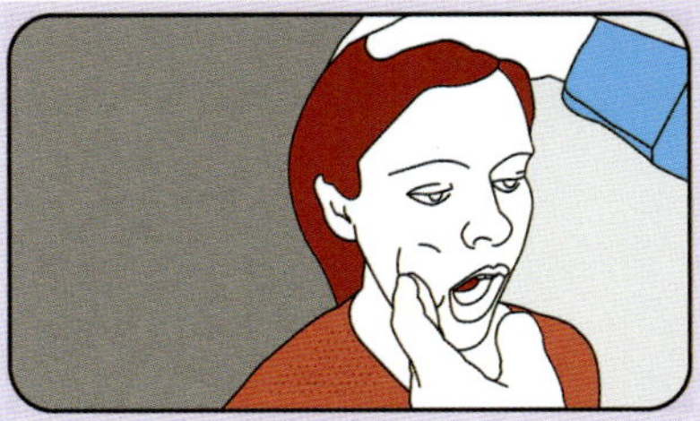
XI Accessory	Head/neck/shoulder movement	Check resisted head rotation (sternocleidomastoid) and shoulder elevation (trapezius—upper fibres)	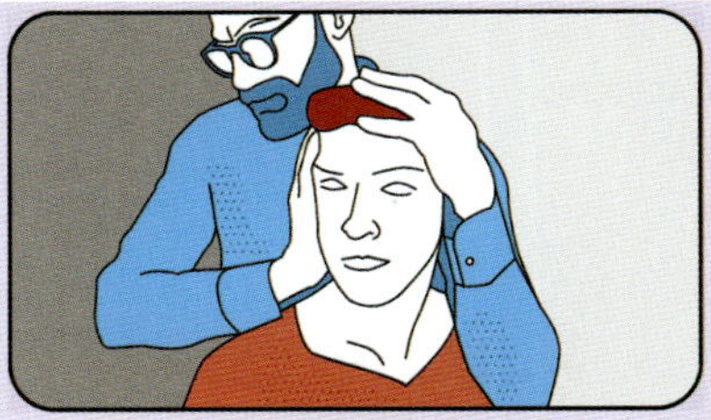

Source: Taylor et al. (2021).

TABLE 8.11 **Cranial Nerve Subjective Questions (Diagonal Lines – Sensory Function – Smell/Hearing; Horizontal Lines – Motor and Sensory Function of the Eyes; Vertical Lines – Motor and Sensory Function of the Face/Jaw/Throat/Tongue; Crossed Lines – Motor Function of the Head/Neck/Shoulders)**

Number	Name	Subjective Examination Questions
I	Olfactory	Have you noticed any recent changes of the ability to smell?
VIII	Vestibulocochlear	Have you noticed any recent alteration to your hearing? Any balance issues, motion sickness or tinnitus linked to eye movements?
II	Optic	Have you noticed any recent difficult reading or alteration to your vision? Have your extremes/fields of vision altered?
III and VI	Oculomotor and abducens	Have you noticed any recent alteration to your vision?
IV	Trochlear	Have you noticed any recent alteration to your vision or unsteadiness?
V	Trigeminal	Have you noticed any recent alteration to your ability to eat or chew? Have you noticed any recent alteration to your facial sensation?
VII	Facial	Have you noticed any recent alteration to your facial features, e.g. smile? Any recent alteration to taste?
IX and X	Glossopharyngeal and vagus	Have you noticed any recent alteration to eating, taste or ability to swallow? Does your cough sound the same as usual? Any change in the sound of your voice or hoarseness?
XII	Hypoglossal	Have you noticed any recent alteration to eating, swallowing, speech (articulation) or tongue function?
XI	Accessory	Have you noticed any recent alteration to your head, neck or shoulder function?

Taylor et al. (2021).

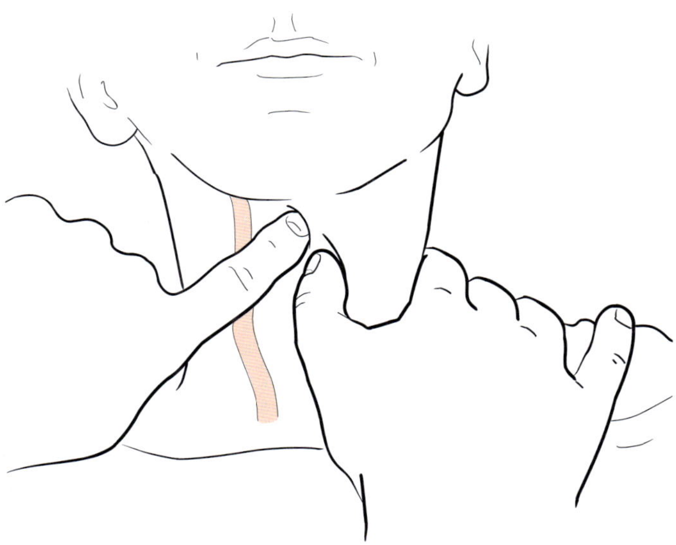

Fig. 8.9 Palpation C/ICA. (Source: Leon Chaitow, Judith DeLany. Clinical Application of Neuromuscular Techniques: Volume 1 – The Upper Body, second ed. Elsevier)

CONCLUSION AND DIRECTIONS FOR THE FUTURE

This chapter provides an overview of the topic and the key considerations for clinicians who may encounter such presentations. Awareness of haemodynamics and mechanisms of vascular flow limitations has progressed enormously in the last two decades and allowed for a greater understanding of how such flow limitations may occur. This has allowed translation of knowledge from the lower and upper limbs to inform how we think about and risk-assess craniocervical flow limitations.

The chapter illustrates the wide range of potential mechanism and presentations which clinicians should be aware of. Despite the rarity of the described conditions, the potential sequelae of misdiagnosis mean that a consideration of a vascular cause should be an initial priority before moving on to other potential causes for a patient's presentation. Recalcitrant, worsening presentations or those with unusual patterns should alert the clinician to a series of targeted questions and an appropriate vascular physical examination.

The astute clinician will be aware that such presentations are very rare but may be a significant finding for both the clinician and the patient. As physiotherapists increasingly adopt the role of first contact practitioners (FCPs), there is an increasing need for clinicians to have an index of suspicion for vascular presentations in all anatomical locations.

REVIEW AND REVISE QUESTIONS

1. What assessment tools can be utilized to investigate endofibrosis (EIAE)?
2. What symptom and signs might alert you to a case of adductor canal syndrome?
3. Which pulses should be palpated if PAES is suspected?
4. How does thoracic outlet syndrome present?
5. Are any conditions associated with quadrilateral space syndrome?
6. How should subclavian steal syndrome be managed?
7. What are the management options for aortic coarctation?
8. What clinical tests may be helpful to diagnose aortic stenosis?
9. How should an AAA be managed?
10. Describe the typical pain distribution relating to extracranial vertebral artery dissection

REFERENCES

Aboyans, V., Kamineni, A., Allison, M.A., et al., 2010. The epidemiology of subclavian stenosis and its association with markers of subclinical atherosclerosis: the Multi-Ethnic Study of Atherosclerosis (MESA). Atherosclerosis 211 (1), 266–270.

Abraham, P., Chevalier, J.M., Saumet, J.L., 1997. External iliac artery endofibrosis: a 40-year course. J. Sports Med. Phys. Fitness 37, 297–300.

Anagnostakos, J., Lal, B.K., 2021. Abdominal aortic aneurysms. Prog. Cardiovasc. Dis. 65, 34–43.

Babic, S., Sagic, D., Radak, D., et al., 2012. Initial and long-term results of endovascular therapy for chronic total occlusion of the subclavian artery. Cardiovasc. Intervent. Radiol. 35 (2), 255–262.

Barquera, S., Pedroza-Tobías, A., Medina, C., et al., 2015. Global overview of the epidemiology of atherosclerotic cardiovascular disease. Arch. Med. Res. 46 (5), 328–338.

Boettinger, M., Busl, K., Schmidt-Wilcke, T., et al., 2009. Neuroimaging in subclavian steal syndrome. BMJ Case Rep. 2009, bcr11.2008.1198.

Brantigan, C.O., Roos, D.B., 2004. Diagnosing thoracic outlet syndrome. Hand Clin. 20 (1), 27–36.

Dyck, P., Doyle, J.B., 1977. 'Bicycle test' of van Gelderen in diagnosis of intermittent cauda equina compression syndrome. Case report. J. Neurosurg. 46, 667–670.

Finsterer, J., Grisold, W., 2015. Disorders of the lower cranial nerves. J. Neurosci. Rural Pract. 6, 377–391.

Gähwiler, R., Hirschmüller, A., Grumann, T., et al., 2021. Exercise induced leg pain due to endofibrosis of external iliac artery. Vasa – Eur. J. Vasc. Med. 50 (2), 92–100.

Gannon, M.X., 2018. Thoracic outlet syndrome. In: Tips and Tricks in Thoracic Surgery. Springer, London.

Golomb, M.R., Ducis, K.A., Martinez, M.L., 2020. Bow hunter's syndrome in children: a review of the literature and presentation of a new case in a 12-year-old girl. J. Child Neurol. 35, 767–772.

Hameed, M., Coupland, A., Davies, A.H., 2018. Popliteal artery entrapment syndrome: an approach to diagnosis and management. Br. J. Sports Med. 52 (16), 1073–1074.

Hangge, P., Breen, I., Albadawi, H., et al., 2018. Quadrilateral space syndrome: diagnosis and clinical management. J. Clin. Med. 7 (4), 86.

Hutting, N., Kerry, R., Coppieters, M.W., et al., 2018. Considerations to improve the safety of cervical spine manual therapy. Musculoskelet. Sci. Pract. 33, 41–45.

Hutting, N., Kranenburg, H.A., 'Rik', Kerry, R., 2020. Yes, we should abandon pre-treatment positional testing of the cervical spine. Musculoskelet. Sci. Pract. 49, 102181.

Hutting, N., Verhagen, A.P.A.P., Vijverman, V., et al., 2013. Diagnostic accuracy of premanipulative vertebrobasilar insufficiency tests: a systematic review. Man. Ther. 18, 177–182.

Hutting, N., Wilbrink, W., Taylor, A., et al., 2021. Identifying vascular pathologies or flow limitations: Important aspects in the clinical reasoning process. Musculoskelet. Sci. Pract. 53, 102343.

Joseph, J., Naqvi, S.Y., Giri, J., et al., 2017. Aortic stenosis: pathophysiology, diagnosis, and therapy. Am. J. Med. 130 (3), 253–263.

Kargiotis, O., Siahos, S., Safouris, A., et al., 2016a. Subclavian steal syndrome with or without arterial stenosis: a review. J. Neuroimaging. 26 (5), 473–480.

Kasapis, C., Gurm, H.S., 2010. Current approach to the diagnosis and treatment of femoral-popliteal arterial disease. A systematic review. Curr. Cardiol. Rev. 5, 296–311.

Kerry, R., Taylor, A., 2010. Haemodynamics. In: McCarthy, C. (Ed.), Combined Movement Theory – Rational Mobilization and Manipulation of the Vertebral Column. Churchill Livingstone, London.

Kerry, R., Taylor, A.J., 2009. Cervical arterial dysfunction: knowledge and reasoning for manual physical therapists. J. Orthop. Sports Phys. Ther. 39, 378–387.

Kranenburg, H.A., Schmitt, M.A., Puentedura, E.J., et al., 2017. Adverse events associated with the use of cervical spine manipulation or mobilization and patient characteristics: a systematic review. Musculoskelet. Sci. Pract. 28, 32–38.

Laslett, M., 2000. Bilateral buttock pain caused by aortic stenosis: a case report of claudication. Man Ther. 5 (4), 227-33.

Matsumoto, H., Hanayama, H., Sakurai, Y., et al., 2019. Investigation of the characteristics of headache due to unruptured intracranial vertebral artery dissection. Cephalalgia 39, 504–514.

Menon, D., Onida, S., Davies, A.H., 2019. Overview of arterial pathology related to repetitive trauma in athletes. J. Vasc. Surg. 70 (2), 641–650.

Mourad, F., Lopez, G., Cataldi, F., et al., 2021. Assessing cranial nerves in physical therapy practice: findings from a cross-sectional survey and implication for clinical practice. Healthcare (Switzerland) 9, 1262.

NICE, 2019. Hypertension in adults: diagnosis and management [WWW Document]. URL. https://www.nice.org.uk/guidance/ng136.

Ohman, J.W., Thompson, R.W., 2020. Thoracic outlet syndrome in the overhead athlete: diagnosis and treatment recommendations. Curr. Rev. Musculoskelet. Med. 13 (4), 457–471.

Peach, G., Schep, G., Palfreeman, R., et al., 2012. Endofibrosis and kinking of the iliac arteries in athletes: a systematic review. Eur. J. Vasc. Endovasc. Surg. 43 (2), 208–217.

Pickett, C.A., Jackson, J.L., Hemann, B.A., et al., 2011. Carotid artery examination, an important tool in patient evaluation. Southern Med. J. 104, 526–532.

Potter, B.J., Pinto, D.S., 2014. Subclavian steal syndrome. Circulation 129 (22), 2320–2323.

Rossi, U.G., Ierardi, A.M., Carrafiello, G., et al., 2020. Aortic coarctation. AORTA 8, 46–47.

Rushton, A., Carlesso, L.C., Flynn, T., et al., 2020. International Framework for Examination of the Cervical Region for potential of vascular pathologies of the neck prior to Orthopaedic Manual Therapy (OMT) Intervention: International IFOMPT Cervical Framework. IFOMPT, Auckland.

Siddiqi, H.K., Libby, P., Ridker, P.M., 2021. COVID-19 – a vascular disease. Trends Cardiovasc. Med. 31 (1), 1–5.

Taylor, A., Mourad, F., Kerry, R., et al., 2021. A guide to cranial nerve testing for musculoskeletal clinicians. J. Man. Manip. Ther. 29, 376–389.

Taylor, A.J., Kerry, R., 2017. When chronic pain is not 'chronic pain': lessons from 3 decades of pain. J. Orthop. Sports Phys. Ther. 47 (8), 515–517.

Thomas, L., Shirley, D., Rivett, D., 2017. Clinical guide to safe manual therapy practice in the cervical spine (Part 1). Australian Physiotherapy Association.

Thomas, L., Treleavan, J., 2019. Should we abandon positional testing for vertebrobasilar insufficiency? Musculoskelet. Sci. Pract. 46, 102095.

Thomas, L.C., Rivett, D.A., Attia, J.R., et al., 2011. Risk factors and clinical features of craniocervical arterial dissection. Man. Ther. 16, 351–356.

Westbrook, A.M., Kabbaz, V.J., Showalter, C.R., 2020. Eagle's syndrome, elongated styloid process and new evidence for pre-manipulative precautions for potential cervical arterial dysfunction. Musculoskelet. Sci. Pract. 50, 102219.

9

Understanding and Managing Persistent Pain

Hubert van Griensven

LEARNING OUTCOMES

After studying this chapter, you should be able to:

- Explain the definition of pain.
- Discuss ways of categorizing pain.
- Explain what nociceptive pain is.
- Understand that the central nervous system can reduce or enhance pain.
- Explain how the brain may alter pain processing.
- List behavioural changes in response to pain.
- Explain the boom or bust cycle.
- Discuss when behaviour changes may be adaptive or maladaptive.
- Discuss social aspects of persistent pain.
- Explain how these aspects may affect clinical encounters.
- Explain what catastrophizing is.
- Explain what fear-avoidance is.
- Discuss aspects of psychologically informed physiotherapy.
- Discuss why the assessment of a patient with persistent pain may differ from a routine musculoskeletal assessment.
- Explain differences between these two types of assessment.
- Understand the importance of communicating findings with your patient.
- Discuss the role of pain education.
- Explain how to approach active pain rehabilitation.
- Explain why relaxation and mindfulness can be important for patients with pain.

CHAPTER CONTENTS

INTRODUCTION

The assessment, examination and management of specific musculoskeletal conditions are discussed in this book and by Ryder and Barnard, 2024. Clinicians ask patients specific questions about their pain and carefully apply tests to hypothesize about the pain. Once a physical source of pain has been identified, a treatment and management programme can be devised. Addressing the tissue pathology or dysfunction is assumed to lead to resolution of the pain. This way of thinking may be referred to as the *tissue-pathology model of pain*.

When pain has persisted beyond the normal healing time or is not clearly associated with an injury or disease, the tissue-pathology model may no longer be meaningful. The level and duration of pain may be out of proportion with the original injury. The pain may not correlate well with a specific pathology, making it difficult for the patient and clinician to devise an effective treatment. Pain-related disability and distress can form a greater obstacle to the patient's recovery than the physical problem. A tissue-focused approach may therefore no longer be feasible or even be counterproductive.

This chapter provides an understanding of the physiological, behavioural, psychological and social aspects associated with persistent pain. These are discussed in separate sections for didactic purposes, but a few or all of these can be relevant in an individual patient. The theoretical concepts will be applied in a general approach to the assessment and management of patients with persistent pain, complementing the information provided in Ryder and Barnard, 2024 and other chapters in this book.

TERMINOLOGY

The recently updated definition of pain is an unpleasant sensory and emotional experience associated with, or resembling that associated with, actual or potential tissue damage (www.iasp-pain.org).

The definition makes it clear that:

- Pain is a conscious, unpleasant experience.
- It combines sensory and emotional aspects. A sensation without emotion cannot be called pain.
- The experience may be associated with:
  - Actual tissue damage—pain tells us that something is wrong with the body.
  - Potential tissue damage—pain signals the threat of tissue damage.
  - A subjective experience as if there is actual or potential tissue damage. Someone's pain must therefore be accepted as real, even if there is no demonstrable damage or threat to the tissues.

Pain is sometimes classified according to the length of time that it has been present. Pain associated with injury or recovery from injury is classed as acute or subacute, respectively (Loeser & Melzack, 1999). Once pain has been present for more than 3–6 months, it may be called chronic or persistent (ibid.). Some authors call pain persistent once the time for the body to restore its normal homeostasis has passed (ibid.), or when it is clear that the body fails to respond to curative treatment or pain control (Merskey et al., 1994).

Chronic pain was recently added to the International Classification of Diseases (ICD-11), which classes pain as chronic if it persists or recurs for more than 3 months (Treede et al., 2019). Chronic pain as a consequence of an injury or disease is called *secondary*. It is called *primary chronic pain* if:

- It is also associated with significant emotional distress and/or significant functional disability.
- And the symptoms are not better accounted for by another diagnosis (ibid.).

Another classification of pain is based on its neurophysiological mechanisms. *Nociceptive pain* tends to be associated with tissue pathology, such as injury and inflammation. *Neuropathic pain* originates from injury or disease of the nervous system, be it peripheral or central. Finally, pain may be referred to as *centrally mediated* or *nociplastic* if an altered function of the central nervous system contributes to the pain. These categories will be used in the next section of this chapter.

> **KNOWLEDGE CHECK**
> 1. List three criteria for classifying pain as chronic.
> 2. List three pain categories based on neurophysiological mechanisms.

UNDERSTANDING PERSISTENT PAIN

Nociceptive Pain

Pain is the body's warning system in the tissue-pathology model. As such, it can be referred to as *adaptive*: it drives us to modify our behaviour in order to deal with injury. Pain makes us avoid certain things while making us take actions that may be helpful. We avoid circumstances, postures and activities that are likely to aggravate or maintain our injury. Actions may include applying compression, taking medication or seeking help. As the injury resolves, the pain settles down, and our protective behaviour reduces. We gradually return to normal function, although some local pain and functional limitation may remain if healing was incomplete or inadequate.

The pain described in this scenario is *nociceptive pain* (www.iasp-pain.org), pain as a result of the stimulation of nociceptive neurones, types C and Aδ. Their receptors (nociceptors) have a high stimulation threshold and are therefore normally activated only when a stimulus has a high intensity (i.e. when there is actual or potential tissue damage). The stimulation threshold of nociceptors may be lowered by sensitizing chemicals such as bradykinin or prostaglandin, which are released as part of the inflammatory process and tissue injury. When this happens, stimuli which are normally too weak to reach the stimulation threshold may now activate nociceptive neurones. For example, a fresh bruise may have concentrations of inflammatory mediators, lowering the nociceptive stimulation threshold. Even gentle pressure can make it sore because the local nociceptors are sensitized. This is called *mechanical allodynia* (i.e. pain in response to mechanical stimulation which is not normally painful (www.iasp-pain.org)).

Although nociception and pain often go together, the two are different. Nociception is sensation as a consequence of stimulation of, or activity in, nociceptive neurones. Pain, on the other hand, is a subjective experience. It is possible to create nociception without pain, for instance by electrically stimulating Aδ or C fibres. It is also possible to experience pain in the absence of nociceptive stimulation (Fisher et al., 1995). It is tempting to always interpret pain as a consequence of a specific pathology, but this is not always true and may lead to inappropriate and unhelpful treatment.

If pain persists beyond the natural healing time despite our best efforts, it becomes an unreliable indicator of what is happening in the body. It no longer fulfils its protective function and can therefore be called *maladaptive*. Reasons for this can be found in changes in neurophysiology, psychology, behaviour and social circumstances. Physiologically, the patient's sensory nervous system may become hyperresponsive and create an inaccurate and exaggerated experience of physical sensations. Persistent pain is likely to influence a patient's emotions, behaviour, thoughts and beliefs, especially if it is unpredictable. Socially, ongoing pain may affect relationships, work and leisure activities. Conversely, psychological and social aspects can influence pain.

Sensory Transmission in the Dorsal Horn

Fig. 9.1 shows how primary nociceptive neurones, type C and Aδ, terminate in the dorsal horn of the spinal cord and synapse with secondary neurones (Galea, in press). Aβ neurones carrying mechanoreceptor signals continue up the dorsal column without synapsing but have collateral fibres which influence nociceptive processing in the dorsal horn. Secondary neurones in the dorsal horn which receive input from nociceptive fibres only are called *nociceptive specific*, but *wide dynamic range (WDR)* neurones receive stimulation from both nociceptive and Aβ fibres (Gardner, 2021; Fig. 9.2). A complex of local inhibitory interneurones keeps transmission of nociceptive information under control under normal circumstances (Sandkühler, 2013; Todd & Koerber, 2013).

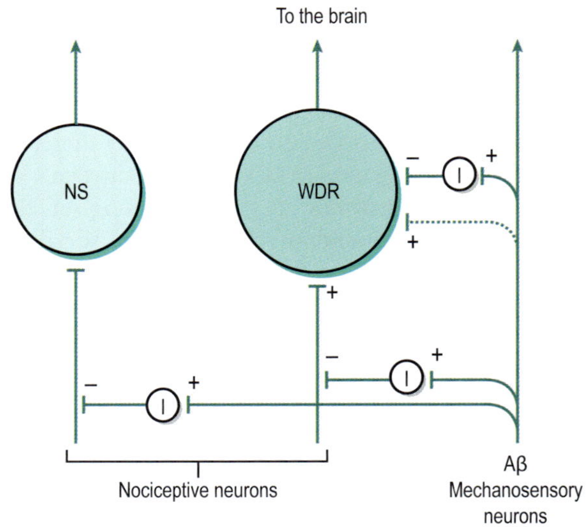

Fig. 9.1 Simplified diagram of sensory transmission in the dorsal horn. Nociceptive neurones terminate at the dorsal horn and synapse either with nociceptive specific neurones NS or wide dynamic range neurones WDR. Aβ neurones do not terminate at dorsal horn level but stimulate local inhibitory interneurones I. They also have a low-level excitatory influence on the WDR (faint line). The interneurones play a role in controlling nociceptive transmission, either pre-synaptically or post-synaptically. Neurones can exert either an excitatory + or inhibitory – influence.

Nociplastic Changes

The central sensory nervous system plays an active role in filtering and modifying sensory information, including pain. Patients with persistent pain may have alterations in central processing that cause heightened responsiveness to sensory input, despite a lack of evidence of a nociceptive or neuropathic cause. This is called *nociplastic pain* (www.iasp-pain.org). It may manifest as *hyperalgesia* (increased response to a normally painful stimulus), *allodynia* (pain in response to signals which are normally not painful, such as light touch) and spreading pain and sensitivity (Woolf, 2011). Signs and symptoms inconsistent with a purely

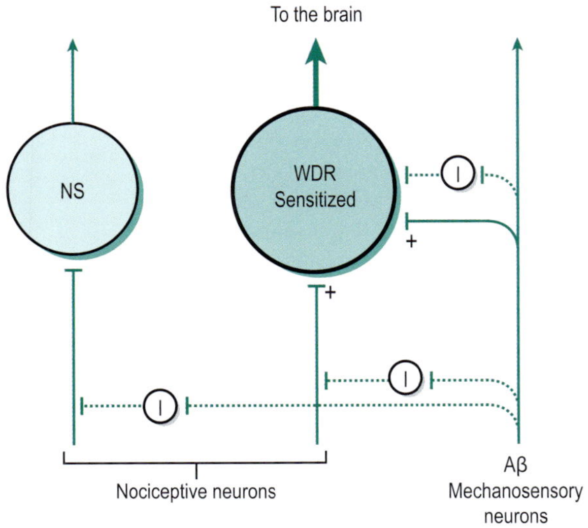

Fig. 9.2 Simplified diagram of central sensitization in the dorsal horn. When wide dynamic range neurones WDR become sensitized, input from nociceptive neurones and Aβ neurones is amplified. This leads to hyperalgesia and tactile allodynia, respectively. Part of the central sensitization process is a reduction in inhibitory influence (faint lines). As a consequence, control of nociceptive input is reduced, and the WDR is more easily excited. Neurones can exert either an excitatory + or inhibitory – influence.

TABLE 9.1 Findings Suggestive of Nociplastic Pain

- Normal, non-noxious stimuli may cause, or contribute to, pain.
- Painful stimuli may be felt more intensely than before (allodynia, hyperalgesia).
- It can take a long time for pain to settle once it has been evoked.
- Pain may be widespread and nonanatomical.
- Inconsistent responses to tests.
- Poor response to analgesic medication.
- Poor or unpredictable response to passive treatment.

Other causes of these findings must be investigated and addressed.

musculoskeletal diagnosis may therefore suggest changes in central sensory processing, but other causes must be considered (Table 9.1).

Nociplastic changes are likely to take place throughout the sensory central nervous system. One of the neurophysiological mechanisms that may contribute to nociplastic pain is *central sensitization* in the dorsal horn, the increased responsiveness of secondary nociceptive neurones. These neurones may develop a lower stimulation threshold, a responsiveness to input that is normally below their stimulation threshold and possibly spontaneous activity (Woolf, 2011). Central sensitization can only be established by measuring the input and output of neurones in vitro, so it is more appropriate to use the term nociplastic pain in clinic (van Griensven et al., 2020).

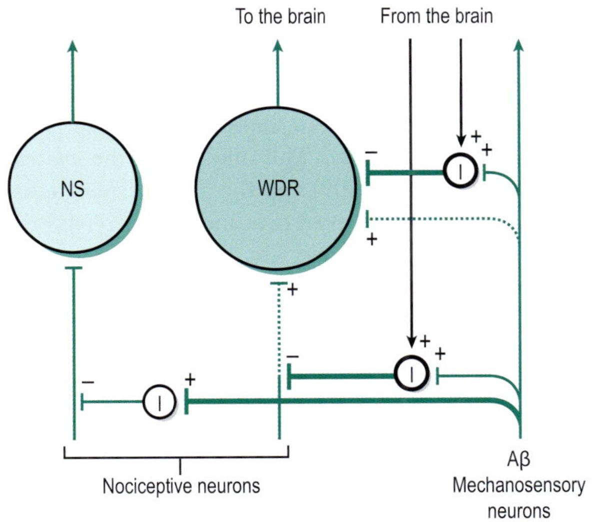

Fig. 9.3 Simplified diagram of descending inhibition. Inhibitory neurones descending from the brain (wide arrows) stimulate inhibitory interneurones I at the level of the dorsal horn. This enhances presynaptic inhibition of primary nociceptive input and postsynaptic inhibition of the WDR, thus controlling both the input and transmission of nociceptive signals. Neurones can exert either an excitatory + or inhibitory – influence.

Descending Inhibition and Facilitation

Sensory processing is controlled by neurones from the brain that suppress nociception in the dorsal horn by activating inhibitory interneurones (Fig. 9.3). They originate from the periaqueductal grey (PAG), the rostro-ventromedial medulla (RVM) and the locus coeruleus (Basbaum, 2021; Heinricher & Fields, 2013). These neurones terminate in the dorsal horn, releasing noradrenaline (norepinephrine) or serotonin (5-HT) which stimulate the local inhibitory systems. This system, referred to as *descending inhibition*, *Diffuse*

Noxious Inhibitory Control System (DNIC) or *endogenous analgesia*, provides the brain with a way to control nociception (Ramaswamy & Wodehouse, 2021).

Under normal circumstances, the central nervous system responds to painful stimuli by activating the DNIC (Villanueva & Fields, 2004). This can be demonstrated by *conditioned pain modulation*: the response to a painful stimulus can be reduced by applying another painful stimulus. The DNIC can be activated from anywhere in the body and may underpin *counter-irritation treatment* (i.e. inhibition of pain by applying a strong stimulus elsewhere). Clinical examples include strong stimulation with transcutaneous electrical nerve stimulation (TENS), acupuncture or pressure. It is important to note that there are similar pathways for *descending facilitation*, enabling the brain to enhance nociception.

Pain inhibitory systems can be activated in life-threatening situations in which pain may prevent one from escaping to safety. This is known as *stress-induced analgesia* (Butler & Finn, 2009). They can also be activated when there is an expectation of pain relief (Benedetti et al., 1999). This underpins the *placebo response* (Benedetti, 2009) and the pain-relieving effect of focusing away from pain (Bushnell et al., 2004; Price & Bushnell, 2004). Conversely, expectation of worsening of pain can lead to the activation of pain facilitatory systems (*nocebo response*) (ibid.). It is likely that a patient's concerns and uncertainties about the origin and nature of their pain reduce descending inhibition and drive descending facilitation, so realistic reassurance, patient empowerment and good communication are important.

KNOWLEDGE CHECK

1. What is the difference between nociception and pain?
2. When can pain be called maladaptive?
3. How can mental processes influence pain perception?

Behavioural Aspects of Persistent Pain

In acute and subacute pain, changing one's behaviour is an adaptive response that reduces the risk of further harm and enhances recovery. In the early stages of an injury, a patient may avoid activities associated with harm and suspend personal autonomy while undertaking activities which are likely to promote healing (Table 9.2). These pain behaviours may alleviate the pain temporarily but may have a detrimental impact on the overall person and become maladaptive if they persist. It is therefore important to interpret an individual's coping strategies in the context of their overall function and wellbeing. Decisions about what is adaptive or maladaptive should be made in collaboration with the patient.

TABLE 9.2 Acute and Subacute Pain Behaviours

Adaptive avoidance behaviour may consist of:
- Reducing or avoiding painful activities.
- Not loading an affected limb.
- Taking time off work and sports.
- Suspending social activities.

Adaptive actions may include:
- Asking others for help.
- Taking medication.
- Seeking information and advice.
- Using aids such as walking aids or supportive bandages.
- Applying ice, compression or getting a massage.
- Seeking treatment.

Using the examples in Table 9.2, potential downsides of long-term pain behaviour include the following:

1. Actions avoided:
   - Reducing or avoiding painful activities can reduce one's fitness, flexibility and strength over time. Not only does this increase the chance of ongoing pain and further injury, it can also interfere with one's ability to work or take part in social activities and relationships.
   - Not bearing weight on an affected leg may create problems for the other leg and spine.
   - Not working reduces distractions from pain and motivations to overcome pain and injury. A lack of financial independence and social interaction can also have a negative effect on the individual.
   - Suspending activities can lead to social isolation.
2. Actions taken:
   - Long-term intake of analgesic medication can lead to drowsiness, lack of concentration and gastro-intestinal disturbance (Waller & Sampson, 2015). Analgesics may be regarded as maladaptive if the side effects interfere with overall function.

- Patients may seek advice from multiple practitioners if the pain continues, and they receive conflicting information. Even when referring to similar problems, different practitioners may use different terms (e.g. zygapophyseal joint dysfunction, facet joint arthritis or spondylitis).
- Persistent searching for answers can be a way of avoiding current situation and finding ways to manage the pain.
- Reliance on aids may be necessary but carries the risk of maintaining disability.
- Targeted treatment can be appropriate for a specific injury or dysfunction. In the longer term, pain treatment may need to be either supplemented or replaced by pain management.

An example of an unhelpful combination of avoidance and action is the *overactivity-underactivity (boom and bust) cycle*: long periods of rest to allow the pain to subside, followed by a rush of activity to catch up (Harding & Watson, 2000). The excessive periods of rest are likely to lead to deconditioning, which in turn increases the risk of further pain and injury. Over time, function and pain are likely to deteriorate.

KNOWLEDGE CHECK

1. Explain when avoidance of activities is helpful and when it may not be.
2. Explain why overactivity-underactivity cycles may cause problems.

Social Aspects of Persistent Pain

The social environment has an influence on various aspects of persistent pain (Craig & Fashler, in press). For example, the patient's experience of, and response to, their pain is influenced by the opinions and behaviour of relatives, carers, friends and colleagues. Conversely, social aspects affect the way a patient expresses their pain to those around them. There is a complex interaction between the social environment and the patient which influences pain-related behaviour. Engaging with carers and relatives can therefore be important for the rehabilitation process. For example, if the patient is asked to tolerate some pain in order to make functional gains, the relatives have to understand that they should not step in whenever the patient expresses pain. They may also need to be included when educating the patient about their pain, for instance when explaining that pain does not equal harm.

Clinicians' own behaviour also influences the patient's behaviour in relation to their pain. When clinicians have a biomedical orientation and think that painful activities are harmful, their patients are more likely to avoid painful activities because they fear negative consequences (Darlow et al., 2013). These patients are also more likely to receive sick certification, increasing the risk of long-term disability (ibid.). Clinicians are advised to assess their own pain beliefs by completing relevant questionnaires (Bishop et al., 2007). The results can be used for reflection on practice and training.

Interaction between patient and clinician is complex. Patients may modify the way they present their pain depending on their impression of the clinician (Froud et al., 2014; Toye et al., 2013; van Griensven, 2016). For example, they may present their symptoms more forcefully if they sense that they are not believed (van Griensven, 2016). Patients with persistent pain tend to value an open and collaborative attitude from their clinician, a willingness to listen, a clear explanation of tests and outcomes, clarity, realistic reassurance and a clear plan of action (Cooper et al., 2008; Slade et al., 2009; Kidd et al., 2011; Holopainen et al., 2018). They appreciate supported autonomy (Holopainen et al., 2018).

KNOWLEDGE CHECK

1. Why is it important to involve the patient's relatives?
2. What do patients expect from their therapist?

Psychological Aspects of Persistent Pain

Psychological aspects of pain can be divided into cognitive and affective components, which are interrelated. *Cognitive* or *evaluative* aspects include thoughts, interpretations, beliefs, attitudes and expectations. *Affective* or *emotional* aspects may include joy, anxiety or anger. A patient's psychology is part of their pain experience. It influences the impact of the pain and the way the patient responds to or deals with it (Linton & Shaw, 2011). Physiotherapists who are sensitive to these issues are more likely to help the patient recover and reduce disability. This has been referred to as *psychologically informed* practice (Main & George, 2011).

TABLE 9.3 Psychological Factors Which May Predict the Development of Persistent Musculoskeletal Pain

- Anxiety and/or depression.
- Higher somatic perceptions.
- Higher psychological distress.
- Having poor coping strategies.
- Somatization, or the unconscious expression of psychological distress as physical symptoms.
- Pain cognitions such as catastrophizing.
- Fear-avoidance beliefs.

Linton (2000), Artus et al. (2017) Pincus et al. (2002).

Numerous psychological factors of pain have been, and continue to be, identified (see Table 9.3). Two well-researched factors associated with the development and maintenance of persistent pain are catastrophizing and fear-avoidance. *Catastrophizing* is a set of exaggerated cognitions in relation to current or anticipated pain (Sullivan et al., 2001). In includes *rumination* (an inability to divert attention away from pain), *magnification* (persistent focus on pain and its potential impact), *helplessness* and *beliefs about worst-case scenarios* (Amtmann et al., 2018). There is a strong link between catastrophizing and poor function in patients with persistent pain (ibid). It may be assessed using the Pain Catastrophizing Scale (Sullivan et al., 1995) or the more recent free Concerns About Pain Scale (Amtmann et al., 2020).

Fear-avoidance is the tendency not to undertake activities associated with pain because the pain is experienced as threatening (Vlaeyen & Linton, 2000). High threat value of the pain is thought to be associated with catastrophizing, leading to pain-related fear (Haythornthwaite, 2013). The fear-avoidance model suggests that patients who are willing and able to confront and/or accept their pain have a better chance of actively engaging with their recovery and reducing their chance of pain-related disability (Vlaeyen & Linton, 2000). The shortened Tampa Scale for Kinesiophobia is a simple assessment tool (Woby et al., 2005). A tool more reflective of the complexities of painful activities and disability is the Fear-Avoidance Components Scale (Neblett et al., 2015, 2017).

Physiotherapists can deal with unhelpful cognitions and behaviours by giving the patient a realistic explanation of their pain, addressing concerns and providing structured self-management strategies. They can also help their patient to engage with their rehabilitation programme, allowing them to set their own pace and helping them to set personally meaningful goals. Physiotherapists should seek appropriate training and get support from more experienced colleagues (Holopainen et al., 2020).

It is important for physiotherapists to remain aware of their professional boundaries when dealing with the psychological aspects of persistent pain. As a rule of thumb, they can deal with psychological issues that are a consequence of the patient's pain and physical problems, e.g. worries about loss of income or fears about the pain. They can offer a practical problem-solving approach. On the other hand, extreme distress and underlying psychological conditions may be beyond the scope of physiotherapy practice. Physiotherapists are not expected to diagnose or manage psychological states or traits and should suggest professional help for psychological and psychiatric conditions as appropriate. In line with this, it is advisable to use layman's terms in notes and letters, for example 'low mood' or 'feeling anxious' rather than psychological diagnostic terms 'depression' or 'anxiety disorder'.

KNOWLEDGE CHECK

1. What is the relevance of catastrophizing for pain?
2. How can you assess fear-avoidance?
3. What kind of psychological issues are within a physiotherapist's remit?

ASSESSING PERSISTENT PAIN—GENERAL APPROACH

Musculoskeletal assessment is detailed in Ryder and Barnard, 2024, so this section provides a brief overview of the assessment of a patient with persistent pain. It will be clear from the preceding sections that persistent pain presents the clinician with diagnostic challenges because

- It does not correlate well with a lesion or injury.
- It may involve multiple body regions.
- It may not respond to tests in a predictable fashion.
- It may be associated with general dysfunction, as well as psychological and social difficulties.

These issues can have the following consequences for the assessment:

- Musculoskeletal findings may be misleading.
- Musculoskeletal problems may be less relevant for the patient's overall progress than, for example, overall function, work status and social life.
- The clinician needs to decide what to prioritize in the assessment.

By the end of the subjective examination, the physiotherapist should consider whether the patient's history of the present complaint, symptom behaviour and other factors point to a *specific* musculoskeletal problem. One of the issues to look out for is consistency: a musculoskeletal problem may be multifactorial, but history and presentation tend to suggest specific mechanisms and tissues.

Examples of issues that may *not* fit a musculoskeletal model well are:

- A patient feels that using a crutch helps his pain, but is using it on the wrong side, i.e. it does not take pressure off the affected area and may even load it more.
- A patient diagnosed with fibromyalgia syndrome experiences pain in varying places in the body at different times.
- A patient has pain and hyperaesthesia in the whole of the right leg, which developed over years following a back injury years ago.
- A patient has given up work, is finding it increasingly difficult to leave the house, and has become stiff, weak and unfit. The patient has become socially isolated and finds it difficult to go out because of the pain.

For patients with a persistent pain presentation, the assessment has to be adapted to accommodate aspects beyond the strictly musculoskeletal. The traditional physiotherapy examination consists of *ruling in* conditions which are involved. For example, if a patient has back pain radiating to the hip area, the clinician will test various structures of the lumbar region, pelvis and hips. All the tissues which yield a positive test tend to be ruled in, and the clinician will clinically reason how the findings can be combined to form a consistent diagnostic hypothesis.

This examination approach is not appropriate when symptoms are widespread, nonspecific or to a large extent of a nonmusculoskeletal nature. In this case, focusing on local structures carries a risk of missing the barriers to the patient's recovery and therapeutic targets. The clinician is therefore advised to direct attention to more general issues such as overall posture and movement, behavioural response to pain and general sensitivity to gentle stimuli. Where a specific musculoskeletal condition is tested, the clinician adopts an approach whereby tissues are *ruled out*: the examination is used to decide whether there is consistent evidence of a *specific* condition. This is similar to the examination of a patient with a stroke: the overall physical and mental function forms the main target of the examination, but within that approach, the clinician may check whether a frozen shoulder can be ruled out as a contributor to the patient's overall presentation.

The use of objective examination markers to provide an evaluation of the patient's progress that is not pain contingent is recommended; see Ryder & van Griensven (in press). These can take the form of functional outcome measures, pain scores and questionnaires.

At the end of the examination, the patient should be given an explanation of the findings. This ought to include what has been identified and what has been ruled out and address all concerns voiced by the patient. If the patient has been given conflicting information by others, the clinician must try to explain what this information may mean in the light of the examination findings. The clinician should explain what they can and can't do for the patient, and agree with the patient on how to proceed (Main et al., 2010).

KNOWLEDGE CHECK

1. What findings can suggest that a routine musculoskeletal assessment is not appropriate?
2. Why should you try to rule out specific musculoskeletal problems in patients with pain, rather than ruling them in?
3. Name three things that must be discussed with the patient at the end of the assessment.

Managing Persistent Pain

Overview

Physiotherapists need to have an understanding of strategies to deal with wider aspects of persistent pain. By necessity, physiotherapy training tends to have a biomedical focus, but communication skills and an understanding of psychological and social aspects are important for the management of persistent pain (Synnott et al., 2015). Elements of a physiotherapy approach to persistent pain are listed in Table 9.4.

TABLE 9.4 Elements of Physiotherapy for Persistent Pain

Depending on the issues that the patient presents with, physiotherapy for persistent pain may include the following:
• Providing the patient with a helpful understanding of their pain. This can also help to reduce pain-related fear.
• Maximizing factors that are likely to enhance the patient's pain inhibitory systems, such as:
  • Education about pain
  • Empowering the patient
  • Suggesting exercises and changes that are within the patient's control
  • Giving positive and realistic feedback.
• Helping the patient to identify what is important to them as an individual, setting goals accordingly, and developing an approach to rehabilitation that works towards those goals.
• Adopting an active approach to rehabilitation in a way that demonstrates to the patient that activity can be improved without making the pain worse. This can also help to reduce fear.
• Relaxation techniques and sleep management.
• Mindfulness-based approaches.

Pain Education

Pain education is important because patients who understand their condition are more likely to manage their pain appropriately and adapt to changes. It is also likely to reduce the patient's uncertainty and vigilance and potentially enhance descending inhibition (Moseley & Butler, 2015). For education and reassurance to be effective, it is essential that it addresses all of the patient's concerns; a blanket explanation is unlikely to reassure and may be counterproductive (Dowrick et al., 2004). The therapist should therefore elicit the patient's concerns and insight. This can be done by asking questions such as "What do you think is causing (or maintaining) your pain?" or "What is the best explanation you have had for your pain?" It is best to be open and listen to the patient's own answers, resisting the temptation to prompt (Laerum et al., 2006). Chapter 2 in Ryder and Barnard, 2024 provides more information.

If the patient's interpretation of their pain is maladaptive and/or if there are nociplastic changes, it may be advisable to educate the patient regarding pain physiology. Patients are capable of understanding pain physiology better than clinicians may anticipate (Moseley, 2003b). The patient's new understanding of pain and central sensitization can be used to develop self-management strategies that are likely to enhance descending inhibition.

Active Pain Rehabilitation

Patients with persistent pain may lose function, with consequences for their work, leisure activities and other aspects of their life. Patients are more likely to engage in rehabilitation if they can see how it will contribute to their overall recovery. It is therefore advisable to help patients to set personal goals that are meaningful to them. These goals can be used to formulate a rehabilitation strategy, which may include stretches, strengthening exercises and increases in fitness and general activity (Harding & Williams, 1995). A structured programme with clearly identified outcomes can provide the patient with a view of how and when they are likely to achieve their goals. This aids motivation but also helps to shift their focus from pain (and pain reduction) to activities and life goals.

One of the strategies used to increase activity levels while avoiding lasting aggravation of pain is called *activity pacing* (Gil et al., 1988; Harding & Williams, 1995). The patient starts with exercises and functional activities at a level that feels safe to them and is unlikely to exacerbate the pain. The activity is then increased over time by very small amounts. Patients are asked to apply these activities in their daily life. For example, if a patient has increased their walking time to 5 minutes but wishes to be able to walk for 15 minutes to meet friends, they could divide their walk into three sections and have a short rest in between.

Patients are usually asked to apply objective markers to their activity pacing, such as the time that they stand, sit or walk, walking distance, or the number of steps when using the stairs. Alternatively, patients can be taught to recognize when they are approaching their safe activity limit. This may be a more appropriate way for patients to learn to manage their activities long-term, but it is essential that they recognize their limit before the pain forces them to stop.

Before embarking on a pain rehabilitation programme, patients need to be clear that the focus is on their function and valued goals. The pain may or may not reduce. The initial aim is to overcome deconditioning and to restore function, to help the patient to return to (or maintain) activities that are important to them.

Some patients become so fearful of activities associated with pain that they end up doing very little (Vlaeyen & Linton, 2000). For these patients, a programme of graded exposure may be more appropriate (Meeus et al., 2016). Fear of movement can be further reduced by breaking the movements down into smaller, less threatening components or by asking the patient to imagine performing the movement in a pain-free manner (Moseley, 2003a).

Apart from pain management approaches, patients may be helped by advice on healthy posture and movement, ergonomics such as the setup of a workstation or other equipment, and manual handling. If necessary, a graded approach can help the patient to increase their tolerance to postures and activities required for work (Main et al., 2008). Success may rely on the involvement of family members and liaison with the employer and general practitioner, as mentioned above.

Relaxation and Mindfulness

Our discussion so far has focused on active approaches to pain rehabilitation, but it is equally important for patients to be able to relax. Relaxation techniques can help the patient learn to relax both their body and mind. It can also help in the treatment of negative pain-related emotions such as fear, distress or low moods (Linton & Shaw, 2011). There are many books and CDs with relaxation techniques on the market. The CD/mp4 by pain psychologist Neil Berry (www.paincd.org.uk) has relaxation tracks, as well as tracks about pain, its impact and approaches to management. Another resource is the relaxation CD in the self-help book The Pain Management Plan (www.pain-management-plan.co.uk) (Lewin & Bryson, 2010). A note of caution: while many patients benefit from relaxation techniques, some find a quiet environment without activity extremely uncomfortable.

Finally, pain management approaches based on *mindfulness* have come into prominence in recent years. It is not possible to provide a full introduction to the field in this context, so the clinician is advised to access the resources below or others. At its core, mindfulness trains patients to pay attention to what can be perceived in the present moment, without judgement and with curiosity. Thoughts and feelings associated with the past and future, including regrets, hopes and fears, are acknowledged but not adhered to or acted on. With practice, negative thoughts, emotions, blame and attempts to escape from pain can reduce. An important aspect of mindfulness is *acceptance*, which is not a passive 'giving up' but an acknowledgement of where one is at the present moment without judgement.

There is a growing body of literature about the efficacy of mindfulness in the management of persistent pain (Theadom et al., 2015; Hilton et al., 2017). A pioneer in the application of mindfulness in the treatment of stress and pain is John Kabat-Zinn, whose book *Full Catastrophe Living* continues to be one of the most thorough and accessible introductions to the approach (Kabat-Zinn, 1990). Patients may also benefit from a self-help book with CD such as Burch and Penman (2013). One of the most progressive yet traditionally rooted approaches in the UK has been developed by Breathworks (www.breathworks-mindfulness.org.uk), which provides training and resources for patients and professionals. It must, however, be stressed that the only way to fully appreciate mindfulness and learn how to help others with it is to practise it.

KNOWLEDGE CHECK

1. What is activity pacing?
2. Name 5 objective outcome measures for a pain rehabilitation programme.
3. What is the aim of mindfulness?

CONCLUSION

This chapter has described how persistent pain may vary from acute and subacute pain in terms of neurophysiology, psychology, behaviour and social circumstances. It has provided a general strategy for assessing a patient with persistent pain and discussed psychologically informed physiotherapy techniques that can be used to manage or treat them. When applied appropriately, physiotherapy can play an important role in the management and treatment of persistent pain.

REVIEW AND REVISE QUESTIONS

1. What is primary chronic pain?
2. Nociceptors are normally inactive. Please discuss when they may be activated.
3. Name three ways of activating the body's pain inhibiting systems.
4. How can behaviour influence pain?
5. What are the three aspects of catastrophizing (or being concerned about pain) called? What does each mean for the patient?
6. How is the assessment of persistent widespread pain different from assessment of a specific musculoskeletal problem?
7. Please name three approaches to the treatment or management of a patient with persistent pain.

REFERENCES

Amtmann, D., Bamer, A., Liljenquist, K., et al., 2020. The concerns about pain (CAP) scale: a patient-reported outcome measure of pain catastrophizing. J. Pain. 21, 1198–1211.

Amtmann, D., Liljenquist, K., Bamer, A., et al., 2018. Measuring pain catastrophizing and pain-related self-efficacy: expert panels, focus groups, and cognitive interviews. Patient 11, 107–117.

Artus, M., Campbell, P., Mallen, C., et al., 2017. Generic prognostic factors for musculoskeletal pain in primary care: a systematic review. BMJ Open 7 (1), e012901.

Basbaum, A., 2021. Pain. In: Kandel, E., Koester, J., Mack, S., Siegelbaum, S. (Eds.), Principles of Neural Science, sixth ed. McGraw Hill, New York.

Benedetti, F., 2009. Placebo Effects. Understanding the Mechanisms in Health and Disease. Oxford University Press, Oxford.

Benedetti, F., Arduino, C., Amanzio, M., 1999. Somatotopic activation of opioid systems by target-directed expectations of analgesia. J. Neurosci. 19, 3639–3648.

Bishop, A., Thomas, E., Foster, N., 2007. Health care practitioners' attitudes and beliefs about low back pain: a systematic search and critical review of available measurement tools. Pain 132, 91–101.

Burch, V., Penman, D., 2013. Mindfulness for health. A practical guide to relieving pain, reducing stress and restoring wellbeing. Piatkus, London.

Bushnell, M., Villemure, C., Duncan, G., 2004. Psychophysical and neurophysiological studies of pain modulation by attention. In: Price, D., Bushnell, M. (Eds.), Psychological Methods of Pain Control: Basic Science and Clinical Perspectives. IASP Press, Seattle.

Butler, R., Finn, D., 2009. Stress-induced analgesia. Prog. Neurobiol. 88, 184–202.

Cooper, K., Smith, B., Hancock, E., 2008. Patient-centredness in physiotherapy from the perspective of the chronic low back pain patient. Physiotherapy 94, 244–252.

Craig, K., Fashler, S., (in press). Social determinants of pain. In: van Griensven, H., Strong, J., (Eds.), Pain. A Textbook for Health Professionals, third ed. Churchill Livingstone, Edinburgh.

Darlow, B., Dowell, A., Baxter, G., et al., 2013. The enduring impact of what clinicians say to people with low back pain. Ann. Fam. Med. 11, 527–534.

Dowrick, C., Ring, A., Humphris, G., et al., 2004. Normalisation of unexplained symptoms by general practitioners: a functional typology. Br. J. Gen. Prac. 54, 165–170.

Fisher, J., Hassan, D., O'Connor, N., 1995. Minerva. Br. Med. J. 310, 70.

Froud, R., Patterson, S., Eldridge, S., et al., 2014. A systematic review and meta-synthesis of the impact of low back pain on people's lives. BMC Musculoskeletal Dis 15.

Galea, M (in press). Neuroanatomy of the nociceptive system. In: van Griensven, H, Strong, J (Eds). Pain – a Textbook for Health Professionals, third ed. Churchill Livingstone, Edinburgh.

Gardner, E., 2021. Receptors of the somatosensory system. In: Kandel, E., Koester, J., Mack, S., Siegelbaum, S. (Eds.), Principles of Neural Science. Mc Graw Hill, New York.

Gil, K., Ross, S., Keefe, F., 1988. Behavioural treatment of chronic pain: four pain management protocols. Chronic Pain. American Psychiatric Press, Washington.

Harding, V., Watson, P., 2000. Increasing acitivity and improving function in chronic pain management. Physiotherapy 86, 619–630.

Harding, V., Williams, A.C.D.C., 1995. Extending physiotherapy skills using a psychological approach: cognitive-behavioural management of chronic pain. Physiotherapy 81, 681–688.

Haythornthwaite, J., 2013. Assessment of pain beliefs, coping, and function. In: McMahon, S., Koltzenburg, M., Tracey, I., Turk, D. (Eds.), Wall & Melzack's Textbook of Pain, sixth ed. Saunders, Philadelphia.

Heinricher, M., Fields, H., 2013. Central nervous system mechanisms of pain modulation. In: McMahon, S., Koltzenburg, M., Tracey, I., Turk, D. (Eds.), Wall & Melzack's Textbook of Pain, sixth ed. Saunders, Philadelphia.

Hilton, L., Hempel, S., Ewing, B., et al., 2017. Mindfulness meditation for chronic pain: systematic review and meta-analysis. Ann Behav. Med. 51, 199–213.

Holopainen, R., Piirainen, A., Heinonen, A., et al., 2018. From "non-encounters" to autonomic agency. Conceptions of patients with low back pain about their encounters in the health care system. Musculoskeletal Care 16, 269–277.

Holopainen, R., Simpson, P., Piirainen, A., et al., 2020. Physiotherapists' perceptions of learning and implementing a biopsychosocial intervention to treat musculoskeletal pain conditions: a systematic review and metasynthesis of qualitative studies. Pain 161, 1150–1168.

Kabat-Zinn, J., 1990. Full catastrophe living. How to cope with stress, pain and illness using mindfulness meditation. Piatkus, London.

Kidd, M., Bond, C., Bell, M., 2011. Patients' perspectives of patient-centredness as important musculoskeletal physiotherapy interactions: a qualitative study. Physiotherapy 97, 154–162.

Laerum, E., Indahl, A., Skouen, J., 2006. What is 'the good back-consultation'? A combined qualitative and quantitative study of chronic low back pain patients' interaction with and perceptions of consultations with specialists. J. Rehabil. Med. 38, 255–262.

Lewin, R., Bryson, M., 2010. The Pain Management Plan: How People Living With Pain Found a Better Life. Npowered, New York.

Linton, S., 2000. A review of psychological risk factors in back and neck pain. Spine 25, 1148–1156.

Linton, S., Shaw, W., 2011. Impact of psychological factors in the experience of pain. Phy. Ther. 91, 700–711.

Loeser, J., Melzack, R., 1999. Pain: an overview. Lancet 353, 1607–1609.

Main, C., Buchbinder, R., Porcheret, M., et al., 2010. Addressing patient beliefs and expectation in the consultation. Best Pract. Res.: Clin. Rheumatol. 24, 219–225.

Main, C., George, S., 2011. Psychologically informed practice for management of low back pain: future directions in practice and research. Phy. Ther. 91, 820–824.

Main, C., Sullivan, M., Watson, P., 2008. Pain Management. Practical applications of the biopsychosocial perspective in clinical and occupational settings. Churchill Livingstone, Edinburgh.

Meeus, M., Nijs, J., Van Wilgen, C., et al., 2016. Moving on to movement in patients with chronic joint pain. Pain XXIV, 1–8.

Merskey, H., Lindblom, U., Mumford, J., et al., 1994. Pain terms, a current list with definitions and notes on usage. In: Merskey, H., Bogduk, N. (Eds.), Classification of Chronic Pain. IASP Press, Seattle.

Moseley, G., 2003a. A pain neuromatrix approach to patients with chronic pain. Man. Ther. 8, 130–140.

Moseley, G., 2003b. Unraveling the barriers to reconceptualization of the problem in chronic pain: the actual and perceived ability of patients and health professionals to understand the neurophysiology. J. Pain. 4, 184–189.

Moseley, G., Butler, D., 2015. Fifteen years of explaining pain: the past, present, and future. J. Pain 16, 807–813.

Neblett, R., Mayer, T., Hartzell, M., et al., 2015. The Fear-avoidance Components Scale (FACS): development and psychometric evaluation of a new measure of pain-related fear avoidance. Pain Pract 16, 435–450.

Neblett, R., Mayer, T., Williams, M., et al., 2017. The Fear-Avoidance Components Scale (FACS). Responsiveness to functional restoration treatment in a chronic musculoskeletal pain disorder (CMPD) population. Clin. J. Pain. 33, 1088–1099.

Pincus, T., Burton, A., Vogel, S., et al., 2002. A systematic review of psychological factors as predictors of chronicity/disability in prospective cohorts of low back pain. Spine 27, E109–E120.

Price, D., Bushnell, M., 2004. Psychological Methods of Pain Control: Basic Science and Clinical Perspectives. IASP Press, Seattle.

Ramaswamy, S., Wodehouse, T., 2021. Conditioned pain modulation – a comprehensive review. Clin. Neurophysiol. 51, 197–208.

Ryder, D., Barnard, K., 2024. Musculoskeletal Examination and Assessment: A Handbook for Therapists, sixth ed. Elsevier, Oxford.

Sandkühler, J., 2013. Spinal cord plasticity and pain. In: McMahon, S., Koltzenburg, M., Tracey, I., Turk, D. (Eds.), Wall & Melzack's Textbook of Pain, sixth ed. Saunders, Philadelphia.

Slade, S., Molloy, E., Keating, J., 2009. 'Listen to me, tell me': a qualitative study of partnership in care for people with non-specific chronic low back pain. Clin. Rehabil. 23, 270–280.

Sullivan, M., Bishop, S., Pivik, J., 1995. The pain catastrophizing scale: development and validation. Psychol. Assess. 7, 524–532.

Sullivan, M., Thorn, B., Haythornthwaite, J., et al., 2001. Theoretical perspectives on the relation between catastrophizing and pain. Clin. J. Pain 17, 52–64.

Synnott, A., O'keeffe, M., Bunzli, S., et al., 2015. Physiotherapists may stigmatise or feel unprepared to treat people with low back pain and psychosocial factors that influence recovery: a systematic review. J. Physiother. 61, 68–76.

Theadom, A., Cropley, M., Smith, H., et al., 2015. Mind and body therapy for fibromyalgia. Cochrane Database of Syst. Rev. 2015 (4), CD001980.

Todd, A., Koerber, H., 2013. Neuroanatomical substrates of spinal nociception. In: McMahon, S., Koltzenburg, M., Tracey, I., Turk, D. (Eds.), Wall & Melzack's Textbook of Pain, sixth ed. Saunders, Philadelphia.

Toye, F., Seers, K., Allcock, N., et al., 2013. Patients experiences of chronic non-malignant musculoskeletal pain: a qualitative systematic review. Br. J. Gen. Pract. e829–e841.

Treede, R., Rief, W., Barke, A., et al., 2019. Chronic pain as a symptom or a disease: the IASP Classification of Chronic Pain for the International Classification of Diseases (ICD-11). Pain 160, 19–27.

van Griensven, H., 2016. Patients' experiences of living with persistent back pain. Int. J. Osteopath. Med. 19, 44–49.

van Griensven, H., Schmid, A., Trendafilova, T., et al., 2020. Central sensitization in musculoskeletal pain: lost in translation? J. Orthop. Sports Phys. Ther. 50, 592–596.

Villanueva, L., Fields, H., 2004. Endogenous central mechanisms of pain modulation. In: Villanueva, L., Dickenson, A., Ollat, H. (Eds.), The Pain System in Normal and Pathological States: A Primer for Clinicians. IASP Press, Seattle.

Vlaeyen, J., Linton, S., 2000. Fear-avoidance and its consequences in chronic musculoskeletal pain: a state of the art. Pain 85, 317–332.

Waller, D., Sampson, A., 2015. Medical Pharmacology & Therapeutics. Saunders, Edinburgh.

Woby, S., Roach, N., Urmston, M., et al., 2005. Psychometric properties of the TSK-11: a shortened version of the Tampa Scale for Kinesiophobia. Pain 117, 137–144.

Woolf, C., 2011. Central sensitisation: implications for the diagnosis and treatment of pain. Pain 152, S2–S15.

10

Principles of Exercise Rehabilitation

Lee Herrington and Simon Spencer

LEARNING OUTCOMES

After studying this chapter, you should be able to:

- Understand the concepts of tissue homeostasis and mechanotherapy and how they apply to load application in exercise rehabilitation.
- Understand how skill and motor control are developed.
- Identify means for assessing and impacting on proprioceptive deficits.
- Outline the progression from closed skill to open skill random movement tasks in rehabilitation.
- Identify the differences in exercise prescription for force development and work capacity.
- Understand how to tailor exercise programmes for individual specific performance needs.
- Identify means for monitoring the exercise programme for signs of tissue overload and inflammatory stress.
- Understand the importance of building chronic load.

CHAPTER CONTENTS

INTRODUCTION

The goal when treating musculoskeletal injuries is the restoration of function, to the greatest degree, in the shortest possible time. For all clinicians, the overarching aim when rehabilitating a patient is to achieve a safe return of the individual to, or as close as possible to, preinjury levels of function. It becomes clear that with this as the primary goal of the therapeutic intervention, to relieve the patient of symptoms solely, though significant, does not necessarily mean this primary goal has been attained. The tissues of the body are designed to function under and adapt to the loads applied to them; consequently, the absence of load has a negative impact on these tissues. The simplest means to relieve the primary symptom patients present with, that is pain, is to offload the irritated tissue. This takes away the cause of the pain, and symptoms can be resolved. This situation then presents the clinician with a dilemma: resting/offloading the tissues relieves pain and irritation, but it also weakens the tissue, making it more likely to reinjure and moving the patient further away from the goal of restoring full function. The primary aim of this chapter is to introduce concepts which will aid the clinician in the decision-making process regarding when, how and by how much to reload the tissues, in order to rebuild the patient's level of function through the use of targeted exercise intervention.

RELOADING IN REHABILITATION: A PHYSIOLOGICAL CONSTRUCT

This section will present the concept of tissue homeostasis and how this relates to the development of both acute and overuse injury and their rehabilitation. The section will also look at how loading of the tissues impacts tissue homeostasis through the process of mechanotherapy.

Mechanotherapy and Tissue Homeostasis

Injuries occur when a tissue is stressed beyond its ability to cope with the load applied to it. In a biomechanics laboratory, this is easy to visualize: the two ends of a muscle, tendon or ligament are pulled apart and eventually the forces applied are great enough that the structure tears. This is shown graphically in the load deformation curve (Fig. 10.1). Initially as a biological structure is loaded, the tissue deforms slowly (toe

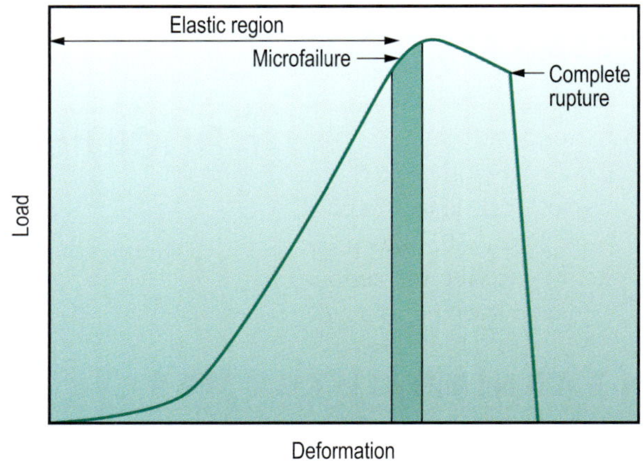

Fig. 10.1 Load deformation curve.

region), then more rapidly, until it reaches a point of microfailure. Prior to this point if the load is removed the tissue returns to its previous form. Once the tissue has been loaded beyond the elastic region it is permanently changed. This model applies equally to all musculoskeletal tissues when loaded; the shape of the curve varies slightly, and the loads required to bring about change might be different, but the overall processes are the same.

The model of loading presented above has significant implications for those working in the field of injury rehabilitation. If we wish to bring about changes in a tissue and make it more tolerant to load, for example, that is, shifting the microfailure zone to the right in Fig. 10.1, then we must create some tissue damage in a controlled manner. This brings about a sequence of physiological events which create an anabolic environment causing positive adaptive changes in the tissues loaded. Mueller and Maluf (2002) describe this process within the Physical Stress Theory (PST).

The basic premise of the PST (Mueller & Maluf, 2002) is that changes in the relative level of load cause a predictable adaptive response in all biological tissue. Tissues accommodate to physical stress by altering their structure and composition to meet the mechanical demands of routine loading best. Deviations from routine or steady-state loading provide a stimulus for tissue adaptation that allows tissues to meet the mechanical demands of the new loading environment. Response to loading is believed to occur along a continuum of threshold levels, defining the highest and lowest loads required to produce a specific tissue response. These thresholds can be viewed as boundaries for the effective dose-response to physical loading. There are five qualitative responses to physical stress depending on the level of load applied: decreased stress tolerance (e.g. atrophy); maintenance (tissue homeostasis); increased stress tolerance (e.g. hypertrophy); injury; and permanent damage.

Scott Dye (2005) has presented a tissue homeostasis model to describe the aetiology of patellofemoral pain. This model can be expanded potentially to describe what happens to any tissue and fits nicely with the PST model. The model of tissue homeostasis is shown in Fig. 10.2. Most uninjured biological structures can accept a broad range of loading (from less than one to nearly eight times body weight) and still maintain tissue homeostasis, a balance between cellular breakdown and growth. This range of load acceptance is called the zone of homeostatic loading, the outer limits of which are defined by the envelope of function. If an increased load is placed on a tissue, for example, repetitive low loading involved in distance running or the single high load of a rugby tackle, loss of soft- or hard-tissue homeostasis can result, characterized by low-level (cellular) damage to the tissue. This application of increased loading, insufficient to cause immediate overt structural damage, is termed to be within the zone of supraphysiological overload. At this point the tissue is weakened (losing its current homeostatic envelope) and, if subjected to repeated loads, is likely to deteriorate further (be less tolerant of load—its envelope of function shifting further to the left), eventually resulting in tissue failure. If sufficient recovery is allowed prior to application of repeated loading, the tissues develop a tolerance to that load; they adapt and become stronger through reinforcement and orientation of tissue in direct response to the stress loading.

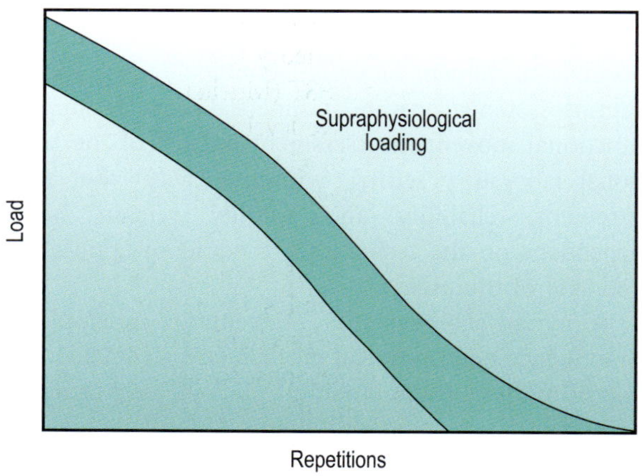

Fig. 10.2 Tissue homeostasis model.

The PST model (Mueller & Maluf, 2002) also describes the process, whereby persistent loading levels below the maintenance level (homeostatic envelope of function) lead to tissue atrophy and decreased tolerance to load (in Fig. 10.1 the microfailure zone moves to the left, and in Fig. 10.2 the envelope of function moves to the left). If loading occurs within the maintenance range, there is no net change in load tolerance, and homeostasis is maintained. Loading beyond this level results in tissue overload and increased load tolerance (the zones moving to the right in Figs. 10.1 and 10.2), or, conversely, tissue breakdown, injury, and cell death. A major consideration in determining which of these situations occurs is dependent on the nature of the applied load—a composite value, relating to magnitude, time, direction, and recovery (repetition rate), with tissue breakdown typically resulting from high-magnitude, short-duration or low-magnitude, long-duration loading.

Wolff's law of soft tissue states that tissue remodelling and the response to load (and so any exercise) are determined by the specific adaptation of the tissue to the imposed level of demand. Khan and Scott (2009) have described the overarching process as 'mechanotransduction', which is the process whereby cells convert physiological mechanical stimuli into biochemical responses. They break down mechanotransduction into three steps: (1) mechanocoupling, (2) cell-cell communication, and (3) the effector response. The mechanocoupling refers to physical load (often shear, tensile or compression) causing a physical perturbation to cells that make up a tissue. These forces elicit a deformation of the cell that can trigger a wide array of responses depending on the nature of loading. The forces need to perturb the cell directly or indirectly, which then acts as a trigger to a variety of chemical responses both within and between cells, the extent of which is dependent on the magnitude and duration of the load. The effector response following the transmission of chemical triggers from cell to cell is increased protein synthesis and, therefore, the addition of tissue in response to the stress loading. These physiological explanations lead logically to the development of 'mechanotherapy', where mechanotransduction is utilized therapeutically for the stimulation of tissue repair and remodelling.

It can be seen from the discussion above that movement and load appear to be critical in not only maintaining normal musculoskeletal tissue function but in improving load tolerance (strengthening/hypertrophy of the tissue) to enhance function, sporting performance or recovery from injury. The tissue response to loading is likely to be a dynamic one, with a myriad of factors influencing how the tissue responds to loading, especially repetitive loading. A significant factor is likely to be the direction force that is applied. This is likely to be more specifically reflected in the alignment of the limb as it is loaded, as malalignment has the potential to cause the application of asymmetrical loads and concentration of those loads on specific tissues or even areas of tissues. An obvious example here is an increased Q angle increasing the load on the lateral facet of the patellofemoral joint. The components of movement and alignment which are very significant to maintaining optimal movement patterns are muscle performance (force development and capacity), motor control, posture and alignment, and physical activity, all of which will be discussed later.

A major emphasis within this chapter will be placed on the assessment and application of targeted progressive loading within the rehabilitation process.

FUNDAMENTALS OF MOBILITY AND MOTOR CONTROL TRAINING

Here the basic principles of motor control and skill learning will be covered, how they practically apply to injury rehabilitation and how rehabilitation exercise programmes can be progressed to reflect the chaotic environments individuals have to function in, to prepare patients best for return to their chosen activities.

Mobility and Stability Paradox

Mobility is defined as freedom of movement at articular segments, where a joint or series of joints demonstrates the ease of motion through an appropriate anatomical range. In that sense, mobility forms the basis of motor control, where the performance of a skilled motor task is governed by an appropriate balance of mobility, passive stability (form closure), active stability and neuromuscular control (force closure). Vleeming et al. (2008) define functional stability as the effective accommodation of the joints to each specific load demand through an adequately tailored joint compression, as a function of gravity, coordinated muscle and ligament forces, to produce effective joint reaction forces under changing conditions. Maintenance of joint integrity during skilled movement tasks is therefore dependent not only on muscular capacity, but also on the ability to process sensory input, interpret the status of stability and motion, and establish strategies to overcome predictable and unexpected movement challenges (Hodges & Moseley, 2003).

Considerations When Rehabilitating to Regain Mobility

Deficits in movement are frequently identified in patients with a history of pain and pathology, where changes in mobility are a product of the interaction between soft tissue and articular dysfunction. Whilst aberrant connective tissue remodelling following injury may influence joint mobility, it is also plausible that abnormal movement patterns or repetitive directional loading could result in the consistent absence of mechanical tension, associated with connective tissue remodelling and eventual loss of muscle fibre length (Sahrmann, 2002; Langevin & Sherman, 2007). Loss of mobility could also represent an adaptive or maladaptive mechanism by which the body attempts to achieve active stability and maintain a level of function in the presence of pain, physical stress or failed motor control. Clinical assessment of a joint range of motion (ROM) typically involves the use of goniometry or inclinometry as an accurate means of measuring and comparing joint displacement against normative reference angles in appropriate planes of motion and directions permitted at a specific joint. The development of affordable and portable movement analysis technologies (e.g. motion capture systems/software and inertial sensors) supports functional movement assessment outside of the traditional laboratory setting, with the caveat that measurement reliability and validity remain highly dependent on the technology, method of application, and skill of the user.

A myriad of therapeutic interventions are employed to influence neurophysical mechanisms associated with loss of mobility (hypomobility), such as focal articular/tissue restriction, pain and altered muscular tone. Mechanical loading strategies attempt to influence the biomechanical properties of soft tissue and facilitate collagen reorganization, neural function and restoration of optimal movement kinematics. The nature of exercise prescription required to bring about an intended adaptation is highly individualized, as are the expectations of an intervention outcome. For example, consider a healthy, active individual presenting with an adaptive loss of mobility following an acute episode of low-back pain versus a sedentary patient presenting with a chronic loss of mobility 24 months post ankle surgery. Practitioners must therefore carefully consider how, in context, mechanical loading variables (e.g. direction, intensity, duration) could facilitate the desired physical effect. Increases in ROM following mobility (stretching) exercises are a product of the passive extensibility of the muscle-tendon unit (MTU), where joint ROM is unrestricted by bony or other nonmuscular limitations (Gajdosik, 2001). Following the application of sustained longitudinal loading (typically >30 seconds; Behm & Chaouachi, 2011), the MTU has been shown to exhibit a significant viscoelastic stress relaxation response (Magnusson et al., 2000). This viscoelastic behaviour appears to be the result of both mechanical and neural adaptations (Guissard & Duchateau, 2004). The adaptations manifest themselves as hysteresis and creep (Linke & Leake, 2004), where the reduction in MTU stiffness may explain immediate (elastic) changes in passive joint ROM (Magnusson et al., 1997).

Alongside decreased MTU stiffness, the mechanisms responsible for chronic (plastic) increases in ROM are also attributed to increases in stretch tolerance (Magnusson et al., 1996). Strategies to influence soft-tissue mobility through exercise prescription are not just limited to passive stretching. 'Stretching' variations such as proprioceptive neuromuscular facilitation and active/dynamic exercises are all effective methods of increasing flexibility and muscle extensibility (Page, 2012). In addition, resistance training (with evidence specifically supporting the use of eccentric strength training) is an effective method of influencing the length-tension relationship in soft tissue (O'Sullivan et al., 2012).

Motor Control and Pain

The presence of musculoskeletal pain often creates deficits in motor control (ability to coordinate movement and posture); this will not only affect tissue loading but could also contribute to deficits in general features of motor output such as poor strength and endurance; the patient essentially becomes less efficient. The impact of pain on motor coordination could be at a local (peripheral) level with the failure of activation or delay in activation of specific muscles. For example, quadriceps function is significantly disrupted with any knee injury or pathology, with the presence of this arthrogenic inhibition creating issues with activation and overall force development/muscular capacity. Similar relationships have been found in the deep muscles of the spine in the presence of low-back pain, and in the rotator cuff with shoulder joint pain or structural damage.

Equally the failure in motor coordination could be at a global (central) level and result in, for example, an antalgic gait. Antalgic or pain-avoiding gait patterns initially develop as an adaptive strategy to avoid placing a load on the injured structure to minimize any pain. Often these gait patterns become counterproductive and actually create more load and stress within tissues, both perpetuating the injury and potentially increasing the risk of developing further injuries. Consider an individual walking on a plantar flexed foot following an injury to the lateral ankle ligaments. If this gait is maintained it rapidly creates a situation where the patient has lost ankle dorsiflexion ROM, leading to increased compensatory foot pronation or knee valgus in midstance to maintain gait; there is inappropriate quadriceps control of knee extension (the knee is held in flexion by overactive hamstring muscles); and the patient fails to hip extend fully, which creates reduced activity in the gluteal muscles (further impacted upon by increased hamstring activity), resulting in suboptimal control of frontal and transverse plane loads. All this could happen simply because the patient does not maintain a simple heel-toe gait pattern, which does not load the lateral ankle complex in the first place!

In the presence of pain, suboptimal motor control is driven by simplification—the cortex typically switches to simple stability mechanisms, where maladaptive movement patterns can result in considerable secondary consequences both locally and remotely to the original injury. When assessing the patient following injury the clinician needs to consider how the sensorimotor system is impacting on the patient's presentation. The strategy of the movement/muscle activation can create conditions which lead to excessive loading of the tissues. Examples could include compromised activation leading to muscle atrophy so the muscle can no longer meet the demands of the task; inaccurate sensory information leading to inaccurate control; movement which now involves too much (excessive movement and instability) or too little variability (excessive stiffness and rigidity). This can often lead to a situation where the original reason for the patient developing injury and pain may be different from the reason it is maintained. To complicate this situation further, though the initial traumatic load or the suboptimal mechanics from a less-than-ideal sensorimotor strategy may be the initial stimulus for tissue damage and pain, other mechanisms could become involved in the creation of persistent pain and altered sensorimotor control. Central sensitization, cognitive and psychological factors can significantly impact sensorimotor control. The abhorrent processing of nociceptive input through the processes of peripheral and central sensitization can have a direct effect on motor output; likewise, kinesiophobia (fear of movement) and catastrophizing (exaggeration of the impact of an action) will also change the way the individual moves and so how tissues are loaded. In improving the patient's movement, the focus should therefore be on rehabilitating not only the biomechanical and physiological issues but also the psychological ones.

The Role of Proprioception in Motor Control

The term proprioception is best used when referring to the detection of one or all the following sensations:

- position and movement of joints (joint position sense)
- sensation of force and contraction
- sensation of orientation of body segments as well as of the body as a whole.

Most experts believe that the muscle mechanoreceptors are the primary source of this proprioceptive information, especially in the middle ranges of motion, with ligamentous receptors only contributing toward the extremes of motion. This has implications for rehabilitation, where joint inflammation and loss of ROM could change the nature, accuracy and reliability of information from the ligamentous receptors, whilst muscle atrophy could likewise change information from the muscle receptors. It is unclear though whether proprioception can be trained in the strictest sense, that is, altering the physiological function of the mechanoreceptors themselves. What can be achieved, however, is an improvement in the efficiency of signal processing, an increase in the use of convergent feedback from other receptors and the development of triggered (automatic subconscious) reactions, all of which could lead to improved proprioceptive acuity.

The nervous system uses three sources of sensory information in order to maintain postural stability (hold the body's centre of mass within or close to its base of support):

- somatosensory (or proprioceptive) feedback
- vestibular feedback
- visual feedback.

When developing a rehabilitation programme, consideration should be given to fully and progressively challenging all these systems, in order to prepare the patient fully for return to unrestricted activity. In order to understand the level of challenge required, it is critical to understand the levels of deficit the individual may have; therefore valid and reliable means of testing are needed.

Clinical Testing for Proprioceptive Deficits

Testing for Postural Stability

When testing for postural stability the two most common tests which can easily be replicated clinically are the balance error scoring system (BESS) and the star excursion balance test (SEBT). These assess slightly different aspects of static balance, with BESS probably being more a test of static balance stability and SEBT dynamic balance dissociation.

Balance error scoring system. This test assesses the number of errors occurring during a 20-second static hold in a variety of positions (stances). The BESS test has three stances: double-leg stance (hands on pelvis and feet together), single-leg stance (standing on one leg with hands on pelvis) and tandem stance (non-dominant (or noninjured limb) foot behind the dominant foot) in a heel-to-toe fashion. The stances are performed on both a firm and foam surface with eyes closed. The errors are counted during the 20-second trials. Typical errors to be scored are opening eyes, lifting forefoot or heel, abducting the hip by more than 30 degrees or failing to return to the test position in more than 5 seconds. Bell et al. (2011) produced a systematic review of the test's reliability, validity and sensitivity, concluding overall that the test was good to excellent in all of these areas. In Iverson and Koehle's (2013) paper, they provide normative data for this test across a range of ages and both genders.

Star excursion balance test. Participants perform the test by standing in the middle of a testing grid of eight lines, placed at 45 degrees to each other; they then reach with one foot as far as possible along the different grid lines and then return to the starting position. The measure of dynamic postural control movement dissociation is inferred from how far a participant has reached whilst maintaining balance. When undertaking the test there appears to be a significant learning effect, with Munro and Herrington (2010) establishing that SEBT scores are reliable after the fourth trial. The test has been shown to be a reliable measure, has validity to identify balance deficits in patients with a variety of lower-limb injuries and is sensitive to changes generated with training (Gribble et al., 2012).

Testing for Joint Position Sense

This test involves assessing joints' accuracy at identifying and replicating joint positions. Knee and shoulder (tested in 90 degrees abducted position) joint position sense (repositioning accuracy) should improve as the knee moves towards full extension and the shoulder towards full lateral rotation in the abducted position, so it is important to test joint position sense in both a mid and relatively (though not fully) end-range position (Herrington et al., 2009; Relph & Herrington, 2016). The tests can be undertaken either using photography and then analyzing the angles (via angle-measuring software) or using goniometry (ideally from a smartphone app). The process is essentially the same: the subject, with eyes closed or blindfolded, has the joint moved passively to a target angle (this angle is measured); the position is held for 5 seconds, and then the limb is returned to the start position. The individual is then asked to try to reproduce the joint angle actively, this attempt is measured, and the difference between target and actual is the patient's joint position sense, with smaller being better and typical errors being less than 5 degrees.

Considerations When Rehabilitating to Regain Proprioceptive Acuity

Progressively Challenging Static Balance

On the surface static balance exercises to minimize postural sway seem relatively simple to train, in that the patient just needs to practise standing on two then one leg, thus reducing the base of support. The question is: how is this activity to be progressed in a way which challenges but does not overload the system, resulting in excessive muscle co-contraction and rigidity? If we first consider the starting position, standing flat-footed with an extended knee, we can simply add more challenge to the system here by standing up on to the toes or standing with the knees flexed, for example; both will increase postural sway and so increase the challenge on the sensorimotor control mechanisms. Which progression is chosen will be dictated by the goal (i.e. focusing a challenge on the ankle or the hip–knee). The surface the individual stands on potentially provides further challenge, where standing on a yielding soft surface presents a greater challenge than a hard floor so is a logical progression. Challenging the visual or vestibular systems adds further challenge (e.g. rotating the head slowly from side to side whilst trying to maintain a static limb position or closing the eyes whilst undertaking a balance task).

Movement Dissociation Training

Movement dissociation is the ability to move one part of the body whilst keeping another part still. For example, kicking a ball requires good movement dissociation skill, where the stance leg needs to stay still during the performance of the motor task. Training movement dissociation is a progression from static balance training; Riemann and Schmitz (2012) found an only limited association between static balance and movement dissociation tests. It would appear necessary that, once the patient has progressed through static balance and can balance on soft surfaces at a variety of joint angles whilst having a visual or vestibular challenge applied, the next progression would be to start to undertake movement dissociation activities. These tasks could include standing on one leg and catching or throwing a ball or kicking it or undertaking movements of the trunk or other leg whilst maintaining limb position.

Movement Control in Motor Skill Learning

Skill acquisition is the process which is followed to acquire new skills. The skill is considered to be acquired when a particular criterion can be fulfilled. The skills should be able to be demonstrated consistently, alongside appropriate mobility and movement efficiency in the task undertaken. It is no use if the individual can only perform a single strategy in an isolated circumstance. For example, the recruitment of the transversus abdominis muscle is often cited as critical in the motor control of the spine, but the act of recruiting this muscle in isolation is only a small part of the bigger picture of integrating its action into functional tasks (Spencer et al., 2016). Motor learning is measured by assessing an individual's performance with the consideration of three distinct factors:

1. acquisition: the initial performance of a new skill
2. retention: the ability to replicate the movement after a time delay in which the skill is not practised
3. transfer: the ability to perform a similar, although different, movement to the original task demonstrated in the acquisition phase.

The motor skill which is being undertaken is then defined in terms of the size of the movement involved (which may vary from gross to fine) and the stability of the environment in which it is performed (which may be very closed with considerable internal control or very open with considerable external influences and variability). In addition, the skill may be very discrete, with clear start and end points, or may be continuous.

How practice is undertaken has a significant impact on the ability to acquire, retain and transfer any particular skill, so practice needs to be optimized to improve requisition and retention. Practice could involve undertaking the whole or only part of the skill task. Whole practice relates to practising the entire movement from the start to the end point while part practice refers to segmenting the movement into specific areas to focus upon. To identify the optimal approach the movement must be analyzed based on the number of segments involved in the task and the extent that the segments influence subsequent actions. For instance, continuous tasks are reliant upon the previous movement and thus should be practised as a whole (e.g. running), where breaking down the movement into segmented activities (initial contact, midstance and propulsion phases) is unlikely to be as successful as practising the skill as a whole. Skills consisting of several coupled movements may be best broken down into separate components—for example, the power clean Olympic lift is often taught in segments before sequencing the whole movement.

Extrinsic Versus Intrinsic Training Feedback Cues

Feedback can be provided both internally and externally. Internal feedback is often referred to as the knowledge of performance and is a major component in motor skill learning; however, an excessive focus on internal feedback can have limitations, as will be discussed later. External feedback (augmented feedback) can come from various sources, for example, visual demonstrations or using a mirror, verbal instruction or physical elements such as manual guidance. Augmented feedback can greatly improve an individual's ability to learn a skill; however, consideration of the content, timing and frequency of the feedback is important. Verbal augmented feedback aims to provide supplementary information regarding knowledge of performance and results of the movement, both of which are critical to skill learning. Knowledge of performance is related to the execution of the movement, typically the quality of the movement. Conversely, knowledge of results pertains to the actual outcome of the movement—whether it is successful or not.

Often feedback is very descriptive in style. It is often better to engage with individuals via questioning to understand the style of feedback which works best for them. Presenting feedback through open questions which encourage individuals actively to problem solve deficiencies related to their movement is likely to be most effective. Additional considerations relate to the specificity of the information—are you focusing on the movement as a whole or individual segments that need focusing on? Is the information intended to result in an internal focus of attention or an external focus of attention? For a more detailed review of these principles see Kal et al. (2021) and Sherman et al. (2020).

Feedback can be provided at different times either during or after the movement and at different intervals. Concurrent feedback has previously been thought to be beneficial in immediately preventing a problem; however, research suggests that concurrent augmented feedback ('in action') can actually impede motor skill learning (retention and transfer) because the individual becomes reliant on such information. Equally, post-practice feedback can hinder learning if the frequency of feedback causes the recipient to become passive in problem-solving movement errors. Feedback should question individuals' beliefs about the performance, not just give them information overload about the performance. Thus as the skill is developed, augmented feedback should be reduced.

Guidance for Providing Feedback

- Provide feedback only when the magnitude of the error is very large (or very small).
- Use a reducing feedback schedule as training progresses.
- Allow the individual athlete/patient to have control over the areas receiving feedback.
- Use summary feedback after a number of attempts rather than after individual attempts.

Modelling is when actions are reproduced based on observing another. Demonstrations are a very effective method of providing an individual with information about the general movement pattern, especially when related to movement sequences and velocities that would be challenging to verbalize accurately. However, care must be taken to demonstrate the movement correctly, as evidence suggests that observed movements are readily adopted, whether they are the correct form or not. This demonstration can also be provided through a video of the task. Even when the demonstration is less than perfect, when carefully thought through, modelling using a less than perfect model can prove beneficial in promoting the client to problem solve and identify how the movement pattern can be improved.

When performing a movement, the individual can focus either internally or externally. Internal focus of attention relates to the movement and positioning of the body; this could include focusing on contracting the bicep while lifting a barbell. Conversely, an external focus of attention relates to focusing on the effect of the movement, so in the same example, this would be the movement of the barbell. A range of research has identified that in skill learning and execution adopting an external focus of attention is beneficial. Examples have included greater movement efficiency, reduced muscle activity, greater accuracy of movement and increased force when using an external focus; however, a recent review has questioned the evidence base (Herrington & Comfort, 2013). Language must be carefully considered to use instructions which promote an external focus of attention (Sherman et al., 2020).

In the context of injury, Benjaminse et al. (2015) provide an excellent review of the use of feedback in relation to anterior cruciate ligament injury prevention programmes, while Agresta and Brown (2015) provide another on running gait retraining. These provide great examples of how using the appropriate feedback has positive outcomes.

Adding Complexity to Movement Skill Training

The learning process that individuals utilize to acquire movement skill has been proposed to have three stages: cognitive, associative, and autonomous. The cognitive stage is characterized by a conscious attempt to determine what exactly needs to be done, step by step, involving considerable repetition of the same task. The associative phase starts when the basic movement pattern has been acquired. The movement outcome is now more reliable, consistent, automatic and economical. Once this is accomplished, more attention can be directed to other aspects of performance. After extensive practice, the performer reaches the autonomous phase, which is characterized by fluent and seemingly effortless motions. Movements are accurate, very consistent and efficiently produced. The skill is performed largely automatically at this stage, and movement execution requires little or no attention. It is commonly believed that directing the athlete's attention to step-by-step components of a skill is necessary during the early stages of acquisition. Gaining cognitive control (explicit knowledge) of the task is a necessary phase that athletes must go through. It is in this stage that the athlete practises a new skill over and over to reach the autonomous stage, so-called automatic movement control. However, repetition of the same movement patterns may be a suboptimal method compared to utilizing pattern variations, which can stimulate the brain to find optimal solutions to unanticipated events more effectively. What follows is a discussion of how to incorporate these greater levels of complexity into training.

The fundamental aim of any motor skill learning programme is to achieve transference of the skill into sport (or activity of daily living) performance (dynamic correspondence). A lot of training programmes undertake work at or on the conscious (cognitive) level, relying on closed skill activities carried out in a block order. Typically, this involves repeated practising of the closed skill, that is, the same movement tasks, undertaken in stable predictable environments, most often carried out at a pace determined by the participant. To reflect the motor skill requirements of sports and even life more appropriately, motor skill training programmes need to have progressively increasing complexity where more open skill (nonplanned skills/tasks) elements become incorporated in a more and more random fashion once the closed skill tasks have been mastered (Gokeler et al., 2020). This leads to practices that are initially controlled and self-paced, allowing participants to understand and learn the specifics of the appropriate movement patterns in environments that are predictable and static to allow them to plan their movements in advance (closed skill practice). The practices then need to progress to incorporate more random elements, where the environment becomes unpredictable, and performers need to adapt their movements in response (open skill practice). During the whole of the practice practitioners need to consider the appropriate feedback and cues which they use to maximize the skill development, as discussed above. An example of developing skill through this process is reported in the paper of Herrington and Comfort (2013), illustrated in Figs. 10.5 and 10.6 (see below).

Considerations When Rehabilitating to Regain Motor Control Skill

Research indicates that the level of load placed on the musculoskeletal system is different despite doing the same task when a sport-specific context is applied. For example, Dempsey et al. (2012) found knee loads were significantly increased during a landing task when the participants had to catch a ball during the task. This simple more 'functional' addition shows how much greater loading stress could occur in the random chaotic environments presented by sports participation or even a patient walking around the shops on a busy Saturday afternoon. The final stages of rehabilitation, if we are truly going to have full neuromuscular control of the task at hand, must therefore train them to cope with these random chaotic environments. This is as relevant for an 80-year-old with an arthritic knee as an elite sportsperson; both will be exposed to the risk of further, recurrent or other injury if not able to cope with these environmental demands.

Certain fundamentals are required to engage in motor control rehabilitation. Patients must have adequate strength, work capacity (WC), proprioceptive acuity and ranges of movement for the task to be undertaken; otherwise, these become the rate limiters to their progression. As detailed above, motor skill control begins with practice in a closed skill block manner with both internal and external feedback cues, so for instance, this might involve doing repetitive single-leg squats in front of a mirror, attempting to maintain good limb alignment. Once the task is mastered in that context, then it can be challenged by increasing complexity (task demand) by performing a step landing, for example, still as a closed skill, but requiring far greater control because of the increased forces involved. This might further be challenged by stepping onto different surfaces or from different heights. Once each of these tasks has been mastered individually, then they could be undertaken together, which adds variability to the global task of step landing; patients have to land from a variety of heights on to a variety of surfaces, so they cannot preplan to the same extent, hence the task becomes more open. Then further complexity could be added by including perturbation, which makes the situation even more random. So, at the end of this little training progression patients would be able to demonstrate good motor control skill for the task of step landing off a variety of heights of step, onto a variety of surfaces whilst potentially being pushed off balance (perturbed)—that should teach them how to cope with the shops on a Saturday afternoon! The progressions through closed and open skill training are illustrated in Figs. 10.5 and 10.6 (see below).

KNOWLEDGE CHECK

1. Identify some of the best ways to give feedback on movement performance.
2. List the ways increasing complexity could be added to a movement task.

FUNDAMENTALS OF STRENGTH TRAINING AND ADAPTATION

This section identifies the underpinning knowledge required to understand the fundamentals of strength and WC training and then discusses how these concepts could and should be applied when rehabilitating the injured patient. The development of exercise prescriptions tailored to specific outcomes is discussed.

Exercise Prescription by Intention, Adaptation and Physical Outcome

The comprehensive restoration of physical abilities during rehabilitation is fundamental in the attainment of athletic performance and mitigation of injury risk on return to sporting activity, but equally, this construct could be applied to maximizing functional capacity in activities of daily living. In order to achieve this, those rehabilitating the patient need to identify both the current capabilities of the patient and the injured tissue and the patient's 'end goals' (i.e. the nature and level of stress the tissue (and individual) will have to cope with in order to perform). Critically, different exercises produce different effects on neuromuscular performance and effective rehabilitation is underpinned by a clear understanding of exercise specificity and targeted adaptation, where the intended physical outcome (e.g. mobility, motor control, strength/force development) dictates the nature of exercise prescription. The practitioner needs to carefully balance the requirement to re-establish physical qualities and address modifiable (hypothesized) factors contributing to injury causation (described by Wainner et al. (2007) as regional interdependence), alongside the loading capacity of the healing tissue and the inherent physical attributes of each individual patient. The entry point or baseline for loading in rehabilitation will be discussed later in the chapter.

Defining Work Capacity and Strength

Discrepancies between load tolerance and requirements for performance are critical determinants in rehabilitation efficacy. Progressive tissue overload through targeted resistance training and appropriate manipulation of training variables (i.e. exercise selection, tempo, intensity, volume, rest and frequency of performance) enables the practitioner to facilitate optimized improvements in strength and capacity whilst avoiding deleterious loading, which could result in tissue failure and/or reinjury.

Work Capacity

WC is synonymous with local muscular endurance (ACSM, 2009) and can be defined as the ability to produce or tolerate variable intensities and durations of work (Siff, 2003). WC is a training outcome where the accumulation of training over many weeks and months results in chronic local adaptation to muscle, tendon and metabolic biogenesis. This chronic local adaptation increases the ability of the system to produce more work during repeated efforts and allows the local musculature to tolerate (or demonstrate resilience to) a larger training volume of work. By comparison, strength endurance (high-intensity endurance) has been described as a performance outcome test completed in isolation, whereby the goal is to achieve a specific amount of work at a given intensity, such as maximum number of repetitions at 50% of one repetition maximum (1RM) or at a specific submaximal load, with less emphasis placed on the physiological adaptation required for WC development. As a result, strength endurance can be used as a proxy measure of WC or as a training variable within WC. Through specific WC training, the patient is able to produce, transfer, absorb or dissipate (and recover from) repeated or sustained submaximal forces, providing a platform of 'general physical preparedness' for the development and performance of specific strength qualities. The American College of Sports Medicine resistance training guidelines suggest that light to moderate loads (40% to 60% of 1RM) be performed for high repetitions (>15) using short rest periods (<90 seconds) two to three times per week to develop local muscular endurance.

Muscular Strength

Muscular strength can be defined as the ability to produce force, with maximal strength being the largest force the musculature can produce (Stone et al., 2004).

Rate of Force Development

Rate of force development (RFD) has been defined as the rate of rise of contractile force at the beginning of a muscle action and is time dependent (Aagaard et al., 2002). Functionally, globally coordinated RFD augments external power production during maximal velocity movements (e.g. sprinting, kicking, jumping or throwing) or creates segmental 'stiffening' against yielding forces (e.g. bracing against an external impact). The production of force/torque and stiffness depends on morphological and neurological factors from the neuromuscular system. Morphological and neurological factors influencing RFD include muscle cross-sectional area, pennation angle, fascial length, and fibre, motor unit recruitment, firing frequency, motor unit synchronization and intermuscular coordination (Cormie et al., 2009). Strength development in highly trained individuals typically utilizes higher loads corresponding to a repetition range of a 1 to 6 RM using 3- to 5-minute rest periods between sets, as much as 4 to 5 days/week. The loads required in untrained individuals are comparatively low, where a repetition range of an 8 to 12 RM or higher, 2 to 3 days/week, is sufficient to create an increase in maximal strength. Lighter loads (0% to 60% 1RM) performed at a fast contraction velocity with a multi-joint emphasis are appropriate for enhancing RFD/external power production (ACSM, 2009).

EXERCISE PROGRESSION WITHIN RELOADING REHABILITATION

This section explains how to develop a needs analysis for patients, breaking this down into appropriate stages, setting appropriate goals to demarcate the ability to progress to the next stage and monitoring the effect of load on both the injured tissue and the individual. This section will also consider how to regain 'fitness', that is, chronic capacity in the injured tissue and the individual to reduce the risk of recurrence. Finally, it will look at the decision-making around the return to performance.

A concise, comprehensive format detailing the progression of exercise rehabilitation for musculoskeletal injuries is lacking within the research and professional literature. Of the limited examples, it is worth considering the papers of Ralston (2003) on the RAMP principle and Herrington et al. (2013) on anterior cruciate ligament reconstruction rehabilitation, which offer insight into a comprehensive process which could be applied generically to all injuries. This section outlines a structure from which an exercise rehabilitation framework for musculoskeletal injury can be built. A previous section (Reloading in rehabilitation) outlined the underpinning theory as to why progressive appropriate loading is essential in the development of tissue tolerance to load and how this knowledge underpins exercise rehabilitation.

Performance Needs Analysis

A successful outcome of rehabilitation is when the individual is able to return fully to whatever tasks she wishes to participate in without limitation and at no greater risk of further injury to the previously damaged tissues. In reality, however, this is highly unlikely, with previously injured tissues often constraining performance. Part of the reason this happens might be that the individual has not been adequately prepared to return to full activity. When planning any rehabilitation programme it is critical to understand what the 'end goal' is. That is, what is the nature of the activities the individual wishes to return to? Once the performance needs are established, it is important to define the physical abilities underpinning the performance of each activity (Box 10.1). Detailed consideration of mobility and motor control qualities has been described in an earlier section, and readers should also consider the maintenance, restoration and development of cardiovascular qualities within the rehabilitation process. What follows is a conceptual model of how to load the tissues progressively, that is, how to deliver a progressive loading programme to bring about appropriate adaptations within the tissue and re-establish loading tolerance underpinning the mechanical demands of the target activity. The language used within this section will often refer to the athlete and sport, but the concepts and underpinning philosophy could equally be applied to any individual wishing to return to any activity of daily living or work task. Box 10.1 identifies typical information required to assess the activity-specific needs of an individual.

BOX 10.1 Components of an Activity-Specific Needs Analysis

- Sport, role and position
  - What is the person's role/position within the activity/sport?
- Performance duration
  - What is the total duration of the person's whole performance?
  - What is the duration and frequency of training sessions?
- Activity duration
  - Is the activity continuous or does it involve bursts of varying intensity and duration?
- Activities
  - What is involved? Jumping, landing, sprinting, change of direction, kicking, throwing, lifting, carrying?
- Involvement of impact/contact/collisions
- Distances covered and directions moved in
- Predominant muscle groups
- Predominant muscle actions
- Flexibility and range of movement demands
- Motor skill requirements

Progressing Load and Function (Entry Criteria for Progression)

When designing a rehabilitation programme the first stage is to assess the problem; this involves two elements. One is to establish a clear definitive diagnosis of the problem; the establishing of a clinical diagnosis is covered elsewhere within this text. Here we will concentrate on the second element, which is defining the 'problems' associated with the injury (Fig. 10.3).

The status of the injured tissue is the primary consideration. How much load can the injured tissue tolerate? With some injuries, this would appear obvious, where it might be assumed that an acute muscle/ligament/tendon injury would have zero tolerance of load when damaged, or would they? Even these injured structures can often generate or tolerate a level of force (albeit low) without creating any further tissue damage or pain. It is essential that the level of load the tissues can tolerate is clearly identified. For example, if a tendon can only tolerate low repetitions of body weight loads, then it is critical that activities such as walking are restricted or the relative load reduced by using walking aids (e.g. crutches) or a walking boot. Equally, if the tendon only becomes irritated and painful after running for 8 km, it would be inappropriate to stop the individual from running entirely as this is likely to cause significant atrophy of the tissue. Likewise, for muscle, if a 5-kg weight, for example, can be lifted without issue, then that would be the starting point for loading. Significant muscle atrophy can occur within 5 to 14 days of inactivity (Wall et al., 2013), so it is imperative that the minimum activity an athlete can perform is established so that atrophy related to underactivity and disuse is reduced to an absolute minimum.

In addition to allowing the application of 'safe' loads, all extraneous loads which could stress the tissue need to be identified. The second element of this stage is therefore to identify and remove negative external (and internal) forces and factors promoting continued trauma. This could involve the use of gait aids, tape and braces or modification/restriction of certain elements of training. Equally, it could involve the modification of movement patterns, which create asymmetrical loads on the tissues, which may represent an ongoing goal throughout the rehabilitation process.

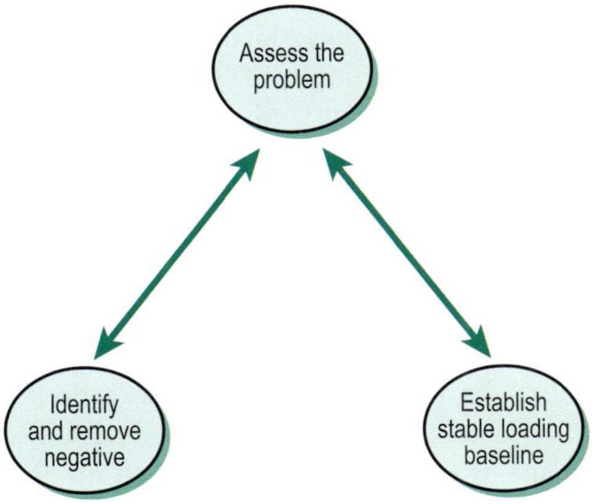

Fig. 10.3 Stage 1 in developing an exercise rehabilitation programme.

Once the starting point for rehabilitation has been established then the exercises themselves can be developed. Whilst undertaking the rehabilitation programme, the athlete needs to be monitored within each session, daily and weekly, for specific markers which may indicate that the tissue is becoming stressed by the level of loading. The athlete's quality of performance and response to loading are monitored continuously throughout the rehabilitation process. This information provides intelligence to ascertain whether the level of exercise is appropriate (to the moving baseline level) and whether the movement patterns are appropriate, which indicates whether external (extra) loading is being controlled with the use of appropriate movement patterns. Methods for monitoring the patient are discussed later in this section.

When introducing the programme it is important to get the initial load right. If the load is too high then there is the potential for further tissue damage, but equally, if the level is too low, it could cause tissue atrophy and set the patient back and prolong the rehabilitation period unnecessarily. Understanding how the tissue responds to the loads applied is a critical element of ongoing exercise rehabilitation programming and prescription. The control of pain is also essential; pain can cause muscle inhibition, alter sensory feedback and alter movement patterns, all of which would limit the effectiveness of the exercise programme. Box 10.2 identifies key elements in setting up and the progression of the exercises chosen.

Tissue Function and Exercise Specificity

When developing specific exercise programmes, the relationship between the role of the injured tissue and the target activity or activities must be carefully considered. Box 10.3 highlights the key issues when reloading the injured tissue.

BOX 10.2 Key Elements to Setting Up Exercises

- Use symptoms to guide the loading programme
- Control pain
- Employ specificity to the nature of the load applied
- Use maximal (tolerated) loads
- Assess and progress the load (regularly)
- Progress towards specific end-goals related to sport-specific tasks

BOX 10.3 Key Issues When Reloading the Injured Tissues

- What is the stable baseline load?
- Has the loading level start point been established?
- What forces stress the injured structure?
- Which forces and loads do not stress the injured structure?
- For ligaments, have the direction and magnitude of injurious force been defined?
- For muscle and tendon, has the nature of contraction load, force velocity and length-tension relationship implications been defined?
- For articular surfaces, define the direction and magnitude of injurious forces and the impact of malalignment.

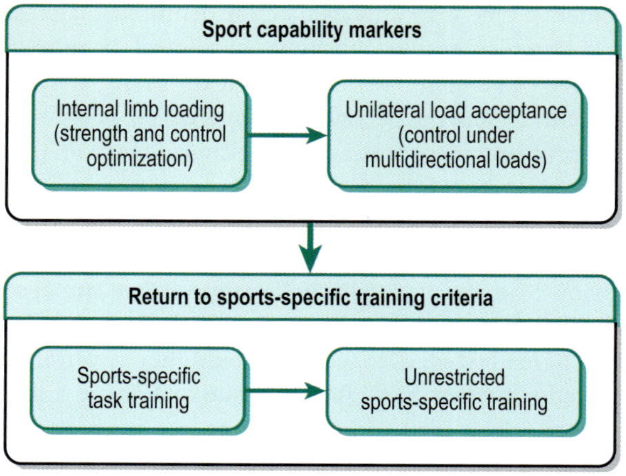

Fig. 10.4 Typical exercise progression.

Tissue Loading

As discussed, when reloading the injured tissue, the first consideration is the level of load it can tolerate. Depending on the tissue injury-specific factors which need to be accounted for in the plan for progressive reloading (highlighted in Fig. 10.4; see below), a starting level of load is established, from which exercises can be progressed. Two critical interrelated concepts need to be considered within the rehabilitation exercise progression plan: Wolf's law and the specific adaptation to imposed demand (SAID) principle. According to Wolf's law, injured tissues are stressed and so stimulated to heal and adapt according to the forces that are applied to them. The SAID principle similarly states that tissue adapts to the specific stress applied to them. The implication of this information is simply that the tissue must be (eventually) exposed to the loads and stresses involved in the sports and activities that the patient wishes to participate in.

It has already been identified that, if tissue is unloaded, it atrophies and its tolerance to load is decreased, so the imperative to prevent reinjury is to make sure the tissue is strong enough to tolerate the loads it will be exposed to during sporting or functional activity. In order to achieve this, a progressive exposure plan must be developed. For muscle that is relatively easy, the load the muscle has to lift and lower can be progressively increased. But even here the situation is not that straightforward. The length-tension and force-velocity relationships must be incorporated into the plan; the muscle must not only generate progressively greater forces but do it at different lengths, during different types of muscular contraction and contraction velocities. Tendon loading would have to follow a similar pattern with the added complication of decisions regarding the impact of tensile versus torsional or compressive loading. Moreover, articular and osseous injuries require gradually increased exposure to axial (compressive) loading, whilst minimizing exposure to torsional and shear loading.

When considering the progression of loading for a ligament, initially the most stressful direction of load would need to be identified and avoided with a focus on controlling the forces (through muscle action) which move the joint in that direction. Gradually, the joint movements would need to be focused towards the stressful direction, to load the ligament and facilitate adaptation in order to restrict movement in that direction, or laxity and unrestrained movement will persist. In addition, mechanical stimulus in the direction of maximum ligamentous tension is needed to generate proprioceptive 'knowledge' of what movement in the stressful position 'feels like'. This increased awareness helps facilitate appropriate reactive muscle action to restrict pathological loading. If the movement is constantly avoided, when it does occur, the body will not know how to react, increasing the risk of reinjury. Furthermore, if the structure is biologically weaker (from limited load exposure) the potential damage may be significantly greater.

Task-Specific Training

In addition to specifically reloading the injured tissue, a holistic approach needs to be taken towards the management of the athlete. There are two main considerations. Firstly, whilst undergoing rehabilitation individuals have the potential to detrain globally with regard to the 'fitness' required to perform their sport. This must be avoided or minimized because of its performance implications; and because an athlete who is poorly conditioned is more likely to get injured. Secondly, progressing the athlete through specific capability markers towards unrestricted sports-specific training will increase the success of a graduated loading programme.

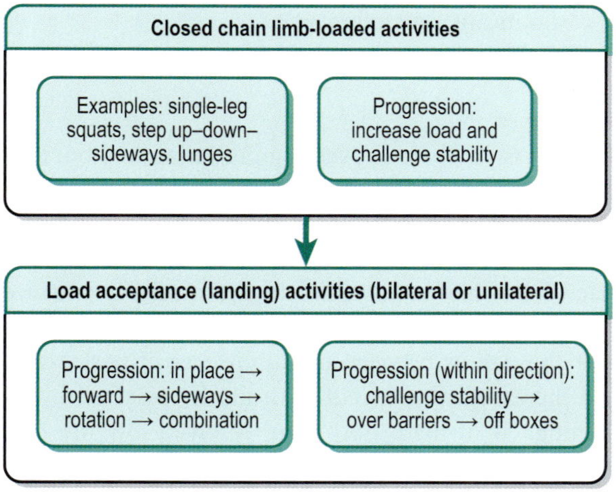

Fig. 10.5 Closed skill exercise progression. (*After Herrington & Comfort 2013.*)

Fig. 10.4 describes a typical progression for rehabilitation, where the athlete initially starts with controlled exercises, often described as closed-chain exercises (though the inclusion of open-chain exercises may be appropriate); some example progressions are outlined in Fig. 10.5. The intent is to develop the fundamental WC and strength qualities underpinning sport-specific progression. When specific capability markers are achieved, the athlete would then progress to load acceptance tasks (landing on the limb and moving towards running). When the athlete is accepting load in multiple directions and running without issues, sport-specific elements can be added based on the sport activity needs analysis. These elements need to consider directions and durations of loading which reflect those in the sport (with the addition of specific technical and tactical elements such as kicking or catching a ball during the task, etc.) and may include open skill and random training when fatigued to reflect end of game situations (Fig. 10.6).

The guiding principle of the sport-specific training element of the rehabilitation programme is to reload athletes in a manner which fully meets the needs of the

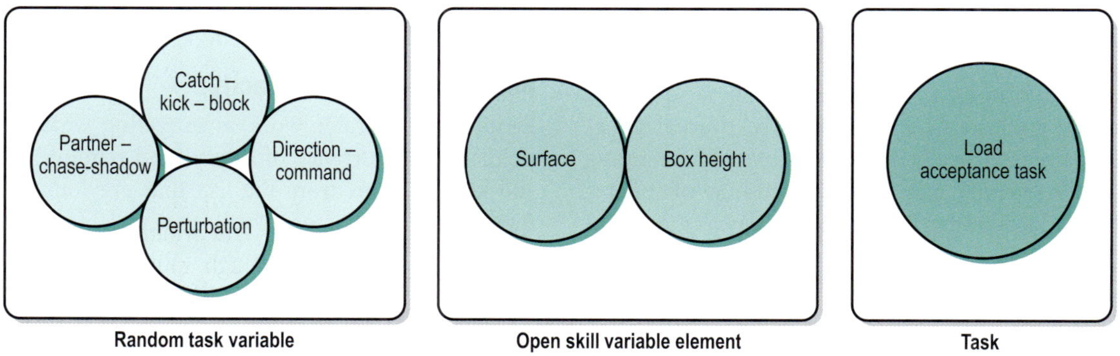

Fig. 10.6 Open skill exercise progression. (*After Herrington & Comfort 2013.*)

sport they wish to return to. This process would work equally well for a return to activities of daily living and work; the example used here just happens to be sport. A key factor is to ensure the athlete's chronic capacity is increased to a sufficient level that any acute increase in load should not significantly overload the system Blanch and Gabbett (2016). It is important to understand fully the demands placed on individuals in order to ensure they are fully prepared for a return to unrestricted activities. The process of regaining and measuring chronic capacity is described below. Once individuals are able to carry out all relevant tasks whilst fatigued (with sport-specific elements incorporated where appropriate), they would then be commenced on unrestricted sport-specific training. Again, comprehensive monitoring is required to assess the tissue reaction during the return to the training phase.

Monitoring the Effect of Rehabilitation Exercise Load

Pain, stiffness and swelling can be used to determine exercise progression as these factors will relate to the loading stresses placed on the tissues and will provide an indirect measure of any tissue inflammation which has been generated as a result of tissue trauma.

Pain

Pain can be monitored using numeric rating scales, for example, on a scale of 0 to 10, with 0 equalling no pain and 10 equating to the worst pain imaginable. This is more useful when placed in a specific context; for example, where 2/10 might be described as the level of discomfort typically experienced following a 'hard' training session (i.e. delayed-onset muscle soreness). Likewise, it is more sensitive to link pain scores to specific events rather than a generic question, for example, rating pain following a rehabilitation session or whilst performing a specific task, such as squatting, walking or going downstairs. Similarly, diurnal variation in pain is typically more sensitive, where rating pain in the evening may identify build-up of inflammatory products in the tissue over the day as a result of repetitive overload. Using numeric rating scales has been shown to be sensitive to changes in pain which affect function (Krebs et al., 2007), with a reduction or increase by 1 point being regarded as the minimal clinically important change (Salaffi et al., 2004). Any change in score from the previous day is noted and significant increases in postrehabilitation scores (>1) which do not resolve by the evening are likely to indicate overload.

Stiffness

Stiffness or resistance to movement of the tissue, especially the next morning, is a strong indicator of an overloaded tissue demonstrating signs of inflammatory stress. A simple scale can be used to monitor stiffness in the morning on rising; again, this works best if linked to a physical task, for example, squatting, sitting, or going downstairs, as appropriate. A typical scale could be:

0 = free movement
1 = some restriction
2 = significant restriction
3 = unable to move as too painfully restricted.

Swelling

Swelling is an obvious overt sign of inflammation. Here the change in swelling is likely to be a more sensitive measure than merely the presence or absence of swelling itself. So assessment of swelling should take place following activity and in the morning and evening. The goal would be that swelling does not vary over the day or between days; however, if postexercise had increased, this would have ideally resolved by the evening. If it had not been resolved by the next morning, then subsequent loading may have to be modified until the situation is resolved. Circumferential measurements are possible in the periphery in joints such as ankles, knees, wrists and fingers and can be used as a monitoring tool for this aspect of response to exposure monitoring.

Regaining Chronic Capacity

Despite considerable work investigating which factors predict the occurrence of injury (and reinjury), little is still known, apart from the fact that previous injury is the greatest predictor of all the variables currently investigated. This poses the question: is it that the tissue is perpetually weak due to 'poor healing' and unable to tolerate the loads it is exposed to, or is it that the tissue has not been exposed to sufficient loading during the rehabilitation process in order to bring about the required adaptation to cope with the return to sport demands? If the latter is the case, then the levels of load applied during rehabilitation need careful consideration. The application of load during rehabilitation has been discussed above; however, an element which was not covered was the frequency with which these loads need to be applied. The occurrence of injury would appear to be related to the application of loads more than what the tissue is capable of withstanding. This indicates that a relative increase in load from these chronic levels could predispose tissue stress; Blanch and Gabbett (2016) called this the acute–chronic load ratio.

The acute–chronic ratio relates to the amount of training the athlete has completed during the rehabilitation period, compared with the amount required when in full training. This ratio is calculated by comparing the acute load (i.e. training performed during the current week) with the chronic load (i.e. the training performed over the last 4 weeks, for example). Training load could be calculated from either external workload, such as kilometres run/amount of weight lifted and/or internal load such as minutes exercised multiplied by a perceived exertion rating. Once calculated, an acute–chronic workload of 0.5 would indicate that an athlete had undertaken only half as much workload in the most recent week as in the previous 4 weeks, whereas a ratio of 2.0 would indicate that the athlete was undertaking twice as much work in the current week as the previous 4 weeks. It has been reported that acute–chronic workload ratios of greater than 1.5 indicate a significant elevation in the injury risk profile (Blanch & Gabbett, 2016). The work in this area indicates that the athlete must have a gradual increase in workload eventually to match the demands required to complete full unrestricted activities. For example, it is easy to see how an athlete recovering from a hamstring strain would be at elevated risk of reinjury on return to gameplay following a period of time off (or very restricted) high-speed running, despite being able to sprint pain-free. Similarly, the patient with osteoarthritis of the knee who has been off her feet with a cold or flu returning to full activity could equally suffer an increased risk of problems with her sudden spike in acute–chronic workload ratio.

Return to Performance: Decision Making and Measuring Effectiveness

Return to performance/play efficacy is measured across three key elements: actually, returning to play (whatever 'play' is—sport, work or walking around the shops on a Saturday); competence (i.e. returning to play at the same competence level or better); and sustained performance over time. Attainment across all three factors presents a significant challenge to the practitioner and provides context to research measuring successful rehabilitation/intervention by 'returning to play' alone. Return to play decision making is often very challenging; clinicians are required to advise when it is 'safe' to resume sports participation, or at the very least, provide information to enable patients to make informed decisions regarding the advantages and disadvantages of returning to sporting activity. The information presented must include a balanced interpretation of the health risks associated with a return to play (i.e. the risk of reinjury or sustaining a new injury) alongside the predicted consequences (which may be minor, significant or even serious/life changing). Whilst a precise calculation of risk/consequence is impossible, the practitioner must provide a reasoned hypothesis based on available knowledge and previous experience. The perceived risk is also amplified or dampened according to the nature of the intended return (e.g. sport, position and role) and the available options to mitigate the threat of further injury (e.g. modified training, the use of padding/strapping). The following section highlights the key considerations for medical practitioners involved in return-to-play decision making. Further reading on this Tripp model (Finch, 2006) is recommended.

As described in detail in this chapter, rehabilitation is not determined by the attainment of a temporal or time-based prognosis. Whilst injury prognostics are inevitably part of the practitioner's role, and often the first question asked by athletes and coaches following injury, rehabilitation must be considered as a progressive, criterion-based journey from injury to return to play/function. It is an interdisciplinary process, where collaboration and collective integration between the support team, coach/parent and athlete are paramount. This optimized approach ensures that the physical qualities underpinning sporting performance (i.e. mobility, motor control, WC and strength/RFD) are fully restored and, where available, mapped against profiling data captured prior to the injury, and the athlete is progressively exposed (and adapts) to the physical and psychological demands of the sport. Quantification of performance parameters in training and competition provides important information during the rehabilitation process. Methods of capturing workload data may be relatively simple or highly complex and can be measured in a variety of different ways. External loads relate to physical work (e.g. distance ran, weight lifted, number and intensity of sprints) and are accompanied by an internal load relating to the physiological or perceptual response (e.g. ratings of perceived exertion and heart rate) (Gabbett, 2016). This information helps practitioners comprehend the biomechanical and physiological stresses during training and competition and provides performance benchmarks to inform functional reintegration and return-to-play criteria based on historical data analysis.

The comprehensive rehabilitation journey ends with a successful and sustained return to unrestricted training, at which stage the athlete is passed ‘fit’ to return to competition. In this sense, the athlete’s response to a traditional field-based ‘fitness test’ becomes redundant. Unfortunately, however, optimized rehabilitation planning often becomes complicated by external factors such as the athlete’s fundamental desire to return, time constraints (i.e. the competition schedule), financial incentives or pressure from parents, coaches and the media. In such cases, the practitioner is faced with a difficult decision regarding the appropriateness of a return to play. The Strategic Assessment of Risk and Risk Tolerance (StARRT) assessment, described by Shrier (2015), introduces a strategic approach underpinning return-to-play decisions in sports. This approach helps practitioners to reason opinions and advice offered to patients in a consistent and transparent way and could be modified to suit any patient’s demands and functional ‘performance’ needs. The model in Fig. 10.7 organizes key information and interactions between factors associated with tissue health (e.g. medical history, symptoms, objective clinical testing) and tissue stress (e.g. type of sport, position

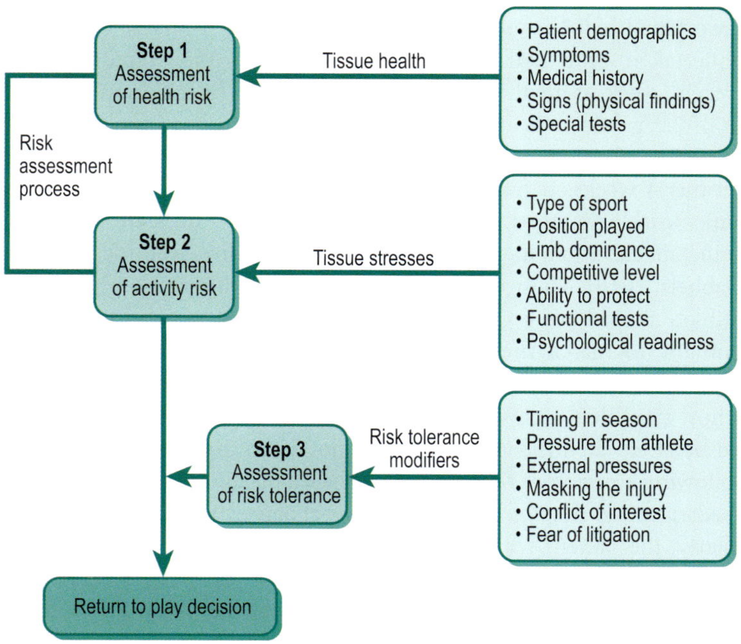

Fig. 10.7 Strategic Assessment of Risk and Risk Tolerance (StARRT) framework.

played, psychological readiness) to determine the risk of participation. Importantly, the risk is then placed in the context of risk tolerance: the clinician's (and athlete's) threshold for acceptable risk. For example, it might be considered that a 20% chance of reinjury to the lateral ankle ligaments is an acceptable risk in order to compete at the Olympic Games, especially if the risk can be mitigated with the use of strapping/bracing. Conversely, however, the potential consequences of allowing an athlete with a suspected concussion to return to play are so severe (regardless of risk tolerance modifiers), that the risk assessment unreservedly exceeds risk tolerance, and the decision should be not to return to play. Whilst the medical team perform an essential role in informing the decision-making process, input from the interdisciplinary team is crucial to determine whether the athlete is ready to return at the level of intensity (and frequency) required to sustain the performance outcomes within the target activity.

KNOWLEDGE CHECK

1. How do Wolff's law and the SAID principle influence exercise selection to meet patients' specific needs?
2. What are the potential ways you can monitor the impacts of your rehabilitation programme (positive and negative)?
3. Consider how the StARRT framework can be applied when assessing the risk of return to performance.

SUMMARY

The primary goals when rehabilitating any musculoskeletal injury are to maximize the patient's potential level of function postinjury whilst minimizing the risk of injury recurrence or secondary injury or other comorbidities. These goals are true whether rehabilitating an Olympic athlete or an octogenarian with a degenerate hip, and the fundamental processes are also the same. A thorough assessment of the presenting problems, the patient's capability (at the injured tissue and global levels) and the patient's end goals is the starting point. From there the injured tissue and the patient globally are exposed to progressively more challenging loads in order to generate adaptation in these systems, so that the capabilities of the tissue and the individual are improved in such a way as to move the person closer to the overarching treatment goals. A comprehensive understanding of the concepts underpinning rehabilitation planning and delivery provides the foundation for a successful return to performance. 'Performance' is not a term reserved for those interested in sporting activity; indeed, meaningful tasks are determined by patients' desire to return to any activity they deem important—this is the outcome measure. The outcome may or may not present a realistic objective, however; the process must always start with a clear and detailed understanding of the physical, physiological and biomechanical demands of the intended target activity. This performance analysis enables the practitioner to consider what physical qualities underpin performance in the context of the clinical assessment/diagnosis, function of the injured tissue and current physical status. The analysis is driven by both the impact of the injury and by factors contributing to injury aetiology. Rehabilitation planning then details the reloading journey and the intervention required to attain progressive, criterion-based goals throughout the process.

Successful rehabilitation requires targeted intervention, defined and measured by the intended outcomes. Pain management is paramount and provides a primary focus, particularly during the initial stages of management, but, wherever possible, the approach should proactively avoid the deleterious effects of offloading. Skilled movement control training provides the basis for optimizing load distribution and mechanical efficiency but can only be achieved on the foundation of adequate tissue mobility and the ability to produce and absorb force—ultimately, the patient must develop tolerance to load through careful exposure and chronic adaptation. The skill of rehabilitation is therefore the prescription of highly individualized exercises/physical activities defined by an intended outcome and physical adaptation (exercises are not defined by name, equipment used or the place where they are performed). As patients are functionally reintegrated into their target activity, the practitioner must be certain that the individual has the appropriate physical qualities to underpin the demands of each progressive task. If achieved, the transition back to performance is optimized with maximum efficiency and minimum risk of further injury.

REVIEW AND REVISE QUESTIONS

1. Name the five qualitative responses to physical stress depending on the level of load applied.
2. What is Wolff's law?
3. What are the main differences between active and passive resistance to tissue elongation?
4. Motor learning is measured by assessing an individual's performance with the consideration of which three distinct factors?
5. What are the two key elements required to establish the starting point from which tissues can be reloaded?
6. What is the SAID principle?
7. What factors can be monitored to establish if the injured tissue is coping with the applied loads?

REFERENCES

Aagaard, P., Simonsen, E.B., Andersen, J.L., et al., 2002. Increased rate of force development and neural drive of human skeletal muscle following resistance training. J. Appl. Physiol. 93, 1318–1326.

ACSM, 2009. American College of Sports Medicine (ACSM) position stand. Progression models in resistance training for healthy adults. Med. Sci. Sports Exerc. 41, 687–708.

Agresta, C., Brown, A., 2015. Gait retraining for injured and healthy runners using augmented feedback a systematic literature review. J. Orthop. Sports Phys. Ther. 45, 576–584.

Behm, D.G., Chaouachi, A., 2011. A review of the acute effects of static and dynamic stretching on performance. Eur. J. Appl. Physiol. 111, 2633–2651.

Bell, D., Guskiewicz, K.M., Clark, M.A., et al., 2011. Systematic review of the balance error scoring system. Sports Health 3, 287–295.

Benjaminse, A., Welling, W., Otten, B., et al., 2015. Novel methods of instruction in ACL injury prevention programs, a systematic review. Phys. Ther. Sport 16, 176–186.

Blanch, P., Gabbett, T.J., 2016. Has the athlete trained enough to return to play safely? The acute:chronic workload ratio permits clinician to quantify a player's risk of subsequent injury. Br. J. Sports Med. 50, 471–475.

Cormie, P., McBride, J.M., McCaulley, G.O., 2009. Power-time, force-time, and velocity-time curve analysis of the countermovement jump: impact of training. J. Strength Cond. Res. 23, 177–186.

Dempsey, A.R., Elliott, B.C., Munro, B.J., et al., 2012. Whole body kinematics and knee moments that occur during an overhead catch and landing task in sport. Clin. Biomech. (Bristol, Avon) 27, 466–474.

Dye, S.F., 2005. The pathophysiology of patellofemoral pain: a tissue homeostasis perspective. Clin. Orthop. Relat. Res. 436, 100–110.

Finch, C., 2006. A new framework for research leading to sports injury prevention. J. Sci. Med. Sport 9, 3–9.

Gabbett, T.J., 2016. The training-injury prevention paradox: should athletes be training smarter and harder? Br. J. Sports Med. 50, 300–303.

Gajdosik, R.L., 2001. Passive extensibility of skeletal muscle: review of the literature with clinical implications. Clin. Biomech. (Bristol, Avon) 16, 87–101.

Gokeler, A., McKeon, P., Hoch, M., 2020. Shaping the functional task environment in sports injury rehabilitation: a framework to integrate perceptual-cognitive training in rehabilitation. Athle. Train. Sports Care 12 (6), 283–292.

Gribble, P., Hertel, J., Plisky, P., 2012. Using the star excursion balance test to assess dynamic postural-control deficits and outcomes in lower extremity injury: a literature and systematic review. J. Athl. Train. 47, 339–357.

Guissard, N., Duchateau, J., 2004. Effect of static stretch training on neural and mechanical properties of the human plantar-flexor muscles. Muscle Nerve 29, 248–255.

Herrington, L., Comfort, P., 2013. Training for prevention of ACL injury: incorporation of progressive landing skill challenges into a programme. Strength Cond. J 36, 59–65.

Herrington, L., Horsley, I., Rolf, C., 2009. Evaluation of shoulder joint position sense in both asymptomatic and rehabilitated professional rugby players and matched controls. Phys. Ther. Sport 11, 18–22.

Herrington, L., Myer, G., Horsley, I., 2013. Task based rehabilitation protocol for elite athletes following anterior cruciate ligament reconstruction: a clinical commentary. Phys. Ther. Sport 14, 188–198.

Hodges, P.W., Moseley, G.L., 2003. Pain and motor control of the lumbopelvic region: effect and possible mechanisms. J. Electromyogr. Kinesiol. 13, 361–370.

Iverson, G.L., Koehle, M.S., 2013. Normative data for the balance error scoring system in adults. Rehabil. Res. Pract. 1, 1–5.

Kal, E., Ellmers, T., Diekfuss, J., et al., 2021. Explicit motor learning interventions are still relevant for ACL injury rehabilitation: do not put all your eggs in the implicit basket! Brit. J. Sports Med. 56, 63–64. https://doi.org/10.1136/bjsports-2020-103643.

Khan, K.M., Scott, A., 2009. Mechanotherapy: how physical therapists' prescription of exercise promotes tissue repair. Br. J. Sports Med. 43, 247–252.

Krebs, E.E., Carey, T.S., Weinberger, M., 2007. Accuracy of the pain numeric rating scale as a screening test in primary care. J. Gen. Intern. Med. 22, 1453–1458.

Langevin, H.M., Sherman, K.J., 2007. Pathophysiological model for chronic low back pain integrating connective tissue and nervous system mechanisms. Med. Hypotheses 68, 74–80.

Linke, W.A., Leake, M.C., 2004. Multiple sources of passive stress relaxation in muscle fibres. Phys. Med. Biol. 49, 3613–3627.

Magnusson, S.P., Aagaard, P., Simonson, E.B., et al., 2000. Passive tensile stress and energy of the human hamstring muscles in vivo. Med. Sci. Sports Exerc. 10, 351–359.

Magnusson, S.P., Simonsen, E.B., Aagaard, P., et al., 1996. A mechanism for altered flexibility in human skeletal muscle. J. Physiol. 497, 291–298.

Magnusson, S.P., Simonsen, E.B., Aagaard, P., et al., 1997. Determinants of musculoskeletal flexibility: viscoelastic properties, cross-sectional area, EMG and stretch tolerance. Scand. J. Med. Sci. Sports 7, 195–202.

Mueller, M.J., Maluf, K.S., 2002. Tissue adaptation to physical stress: a proposed 'Physical Stress Theory' to guide physical therapist practice, education, and research. Phys. Ther. 82, 383–403.

Munro, A.G., Herrington, L.C., 2010. Between session reliability of the star excursion balance test. Phys. Ther. Sport 11, 128–132.

O'Sullivan, K., McAuliffe, S., Deburca, N., 2012. The effects of eccentric training on lower limb flexibility: a systematic review. Br. J. Sports Med. 46, 838–845.

Page, P., 2012. Current concepts in muscle stretching for exercise and rehabilitation. Int. J. Sports Phys. Ther. 7, 109–119.

Ralston, D.J., 2003. The RAMP system: a template for the progression of athletic-injury rehabilitation. J. Sports Rehabil. 12, 280–290.

Relph, N., Herrington, L., 2016. The effects of knee direction, physical activity and age on knee joint position sense. Knee 23, 1029–1034.

Riemann, B.L., Schmitz, R., 2012. The relationship between various modes of single leg postural control assessment. Int. J. Sports Phys. Ther. 7, 257–266.

Sahrmann, S., 2002. Diagnosis and Treatment of Movement Impairment Syndromes. Elsevier Health Sciences, St Louis, MO, pp. 12–13.

Salaffi, F., Stancati, A., Silvestri, C., et al., 2004. Minimal clinically important changes in chronic musculoskeletal pain intensity measured on a numerical rating scale. Eur. J. Pain 8, 283–291.

Sherman, D., Sherman, S., Norte, G., 2020. The power of language: using the OPTIMAL theory to coach your patients to recovery. Athl. Train. Sports Health Care 12 (6), 246–248.

Shrier, I., 2015. Strategic Assessment of Risk and Risk Tolerance (StARRT) framework for return-to-play decision-making. Br. J. Sports Med. 49, 1311–1315.

Siff, M.C., 2003. Supertraining. Supertraining Institute, Denver, CO, pp. 32–33.

Spencer, S., Wolf, A., Rushton, A., 2016. Spinal-exercise prescription in sport: classifying physical training and rehabilitation by intention and outcome. J. Athl. Train. 51, 613–628.

Stone, M.H., Sands, W.A., Carlock, J., et al., 2004. The importance of isometric maximum strength and peak rate-of-force development in sprint cycling. J. Strength Cond. Res. 18, 878–884.

Vleeming, A., Albert, H.B., Östgaard, H.C., et al., 2008. European guidelines for the diagnosis and treatment of pelvic girdle pain. Eur. Spine J. 17, 794–819.

Wainner, R.S., Whitman, J.M., Cleland, J.A., et al., 2007. Regional interdependence: a musculoskeletal examination model whose time has come. J. Orthop. Sports Phys. Ther. 37, 658–660.

Wall, B.T., Dirks, M.L., van Loon, L.J.C., 2013. Skeletal muscle atrophy during short-term disuse: implications for age-related sarcopenia. Ageing Res. Rev. 12, 898–906.

11 Considering Serious Pathology

Laura Finucane, Sue Greenhalgh, Chris Mercer, and James Selfe

LEARNING OUTCOMES

After studying this chapter, you should be able to:

- Understand the role of red flags in identifying serious pathology.
- Have a framework to manage your clinical decisions about red flags.
- Understand how to recognize the most common spinal red flags.

CHAPTER CONTENTS

INTRODUCTION

This chapter focuses on the importance of identifying potential serious pathology early within the clinical setting; it provides an approach and practical tools that aim to avoid causing unnecessary anxiety in both the patient and the clinician. Case studies are presented at the end of the chapter to illustrate key points and to aid the reader in adopting a pragmatic approach to working with complex patients in the presence of uncertainty.

The majority of individuals receiving care from clinicians have benign musculoskeletal conditions that respond well to evidence-based conservative management. However, a small number of patients, around 2%, may present with an underlying serious pathology (Budtz et al., 2020). Serious pathology is a term used to describe a variety of conditions that may present as benign musculoskeletal conditions but that are actually due to more serious underlying conditions. These include, but are not exclusive to, primary and secondary cancers, fractures, infections, aneurysms and inflammatory conditions. Therefore the ability to screen for a serious pathology that masquerades as a benign musculoskeletal condition is vital in ensuring safe practice and is crucial to ensuring that the patient receives the right treatment in a timely manner. Missed or delayed diagnosis of serious pathology can have devastating consequences for individuals and, in rare cases, can be fatal. However, an integral component of the clinicians' duty of care is not to subject patients to unnecessary and sometimes worrying investigations (Darlow et al., 2017), as these can affect the patient's perception of their problem and the outcome of treatment. Striking the right balance between 'clinical prudence' and 'alarmist over-investigation' can be a challenge and is one that occurs daily.

Clinical decisions on the presence (or not) of potential serious pathology are complex and go far beyond checking through standardized lists of red flags. They

TABLE 11.1 Four Most Common Serious Spinal Pathologies

Cauda equina syndrome (CES) 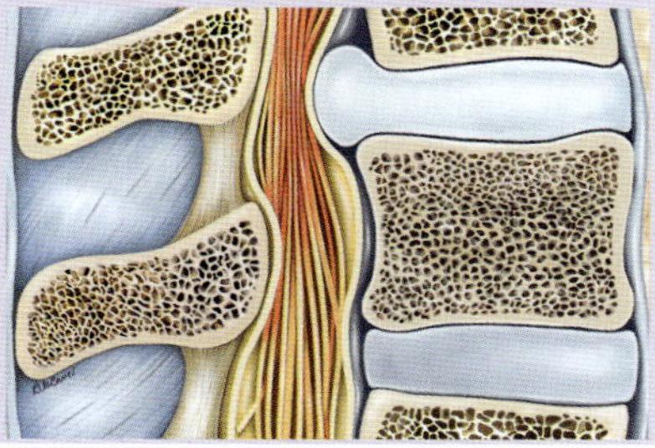	Anatomically, the cauda equina is made up of 20 nerve roots that originate from the conus medullaris at the base of the spinal cord. CES occurs as a result of compression of these neural structures. Compression of the cauda equina usually occurs as a result of an intervertebral disc prolapse (Dionne et al., 2019). Relevant symptoms which can be a precursor to CES are: • Unilateral or bilateral radicular pain • And/or dermatomal reduced sensation • And/or myotomal weakness
Spinal Fracture 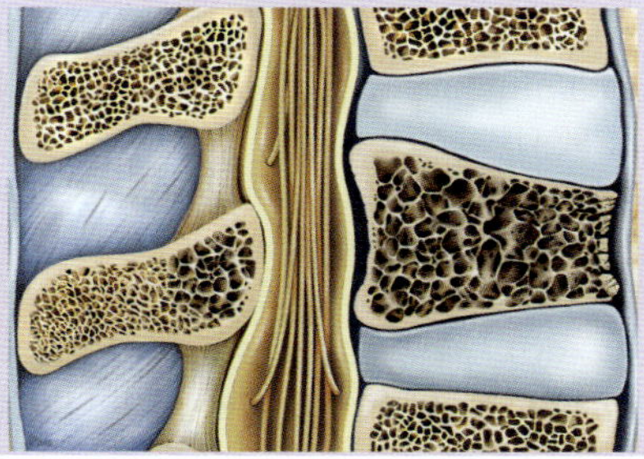	Spinal fractures make up the largest number of serious pathologies in the spine. These are predominantly a risk for older patients, especially females. Low-impact or nontraumatic fractures are the most common serious pathology in the spine, with vertebral fractures being the most common osteoporotic fracture. Approximately 12% of women between 50 and 79 years of age have vertebral fractures, and in the over 80-year-old age group, this rises to 20% (NOS, 2017).
Spinal Malignancy 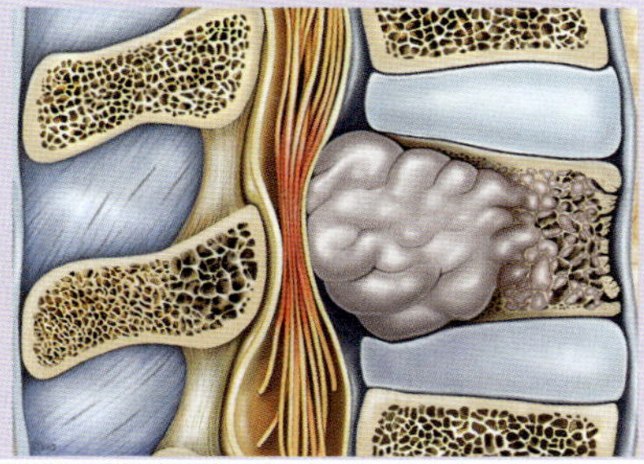	The most common malignancies seen in spines are metastatic. Metastases are cancer lesions that have spread from the primary cancer site to a new and different site in the body. Bone is a common site for metastases, known as metastatic bone disease (MBD). A number of primary cancers (breast, prostate lung, kidney and thyroid) are more likely to metastasize to the spine (Sutcliffe et al., 2013).
Spinal infection 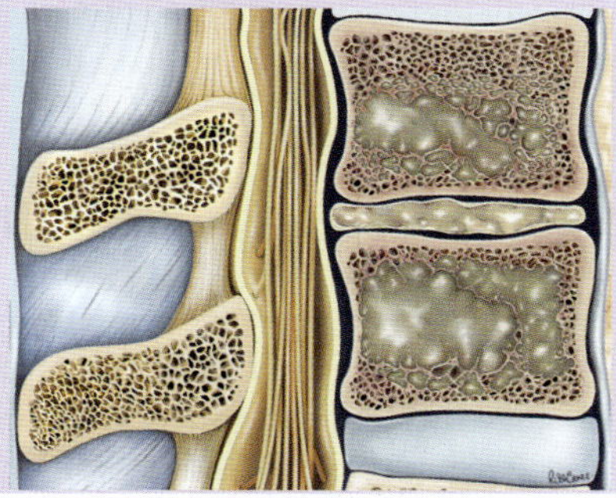	Spinal infection (SI) refers to an infectious disease that affects the spinal structures including the vertebrae, intervertebral discs and adjacent paraspinal tissues (Nickerson & Sinha, 2016). In high income and upper middle income countries SI has steadily increased over recent years. It is thought that this is related to an ageing population and an increase in intravenous drug abuse (Nagashima et al., 2018). In lower middle income and lower income countries, SI has increased due to the dual epidemic of HIV/AIDS and tuberculosis (TB).
Other spinal red flags	Whilst the four listed above are the most common red flags in the spine, other serious pathologies can cause back and leg symptoms. These include abdominal aortic aneurysm (Tohoku et al., 2013), pain referred from the viscera to the spine (Pacheco-Carroza, 2021), neurological conditions such as multiple sclerosis, syrinx or amyotrophic lateral sclerosis (Borsook, 2012).

Images Courtesy: Ruth Eaves.

require the use of a number of clinical reasoning skills, combined with emotion (gut feeling), understanding of the physiology of serious pathologies, and the cause of symptoms, to build a holistic clinical picture (Langridge et al., 2015, 2016). In the early stages, subclinical and prodromal phases (Gould, 2006), of a serious pathology of a disease process, the subjective examination provides clearer clues for causes for concern rather than the physical examination, where often there are fewer or no signs present (Finucane et al., 2020). The physical examination can provide helpful information, but this is often later in the disease process (Greenhalgh & Selfe, 2006). Therefore, good communication skills are central and key to the successful identification and management of potential serious pathology (Finucane et al., 2020).

Red flags have traditionally been used within musculoskeletal practice to help identify patients who may have serious pathology. They are findings in the patient history and examination that raise the suspicion of the potential presence of serious pathology (Goodman & Snyder, 2013). The main role of red flags is to raise the clinician's index of suspicion (Greenhalgh & Selfe, 2006) or level of concern (Finucane et al., 2020) and to potentially guide the management of the patient. However, the evidence supporting the usefulness of red flags has been challenged because of the lack of high-quality evidence for their diagnostic accuracy (Downie et al., 2013; Henschke et al., 2013). Where evidence does exist, it only supports a limited number of red flags to raise suspicion of serious pathology. With a few exceptions, the prognostic strength of individual red flags or combinations of red flags is not known (Verhagen et al., 2016). A good example of a red flag with moderate diagnostic accuracy is a past history of cancer. However, this only increases the chance of malignancy to around 10% (positive likelihood ratio ~15) (Downie et al., 2013). Knowing which cancers are more likely to develop metastatic bone disease (MBD) is helpful when assessing a patient within the context of a thorough subjective patient history and an appropriate physical examination (Finucane et al., 2017).

In recognition of this problem and to address some of these limitations, an International Federation of Orthopaedic Manipulative Physical Therapists (IFOMPT) endorsed framework focusing on spinal serious pathology which has been produced by Finucane et al. (2020). This has been translated into Portuguese and French. The four main spinal pathologies are summarized in Table 11.1.

This framework was informed by the available evidence and augmented by a formal international consensus process that included academics and clinicians involved in the management of musculoskeletal conditions. It provides a robust and clinically reasoned approach to the use of red flags in clinical practice. Whilst the framework focuses on four specific serious spinal pathologies, the underlying clinical principles are the same irrespective of the type of serious pathology or location. It focuses on the key components of clear and appropriate communication (Greenhalgh & Selfe, 2019; see Chapter 2 on communication in companion text, Ryder & Barnard, 2024).

Clinicians must be aware of potential red flags at all stages during every patient encounter, including face-to-face and telehealth appointments. In most situations, one new red flag on its own may not be enough to cause immediate concern, but it must be closely monitored throughout the patient's journey (Finucane et al., 2020).

KNOWLEDGE CHECK

1. How common is serious pathology in physiotherapy clinics?
2. Which of these examinations provides the most useful information about serious pathology in the early stages:
   a. Subjective examination
   b. Objective examination

The decision as to whether serious pathology may be present or not and the subsequent action is based on a two-step process.

STEP ONE: ESTABLISH LEVEL OF CONCERN (FIG. 11.1)

Consider whether the individual is at risk for the presence of serious pathology by combining the level of evidence supporting red flags with a person's determinants, e.g. age, sex, lifestyle. This will help to establish an index of suspicion and, in particular, the level of concern for any individual patient. Risk factors (determinants) are factors causally related to a health condition, e.g. a past history of cancer would increase the risk of malignancy but on its own would not trigger further investigation. It should be considered in conjunction with the presenting

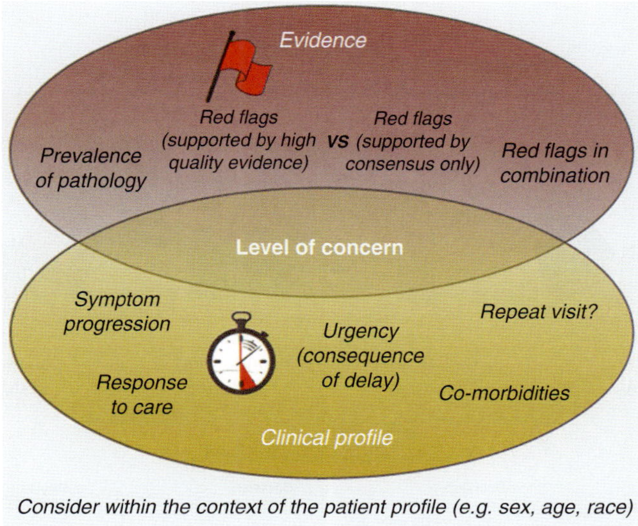

Fig. 11.1 Level of concern. Clinicians should consider both the evidence to support red flags and the individual profile of the person's health determinants, e.g. age, sex, to decide level of concern (index of suspicion) for presence of serious pathology. (*Finucane et al., 2020.*)

clinical features. In spinal infection risk factors such as intravenous drug use and diabetes, they are much more informative than clinical features and have a high sensitivity (98%) and negative predictive value (99%), making them better predictors of spinal infection than clinical features (Yusuf et al., 2019).

STEP TWO: MAKE CLINICAL DECISION (FIG. 11.2)

Based on the level of concern, the clinician needs to determine if physiotherapy intervention is indicated or not (keep or refer decision) and the speed at which appropriate action needs to be taken. Lackenbauer et al. (2017) highlighted that making accurate keep/refer clinical decisions related to serious medical conditions and benign musculoskeletal problems is a significant challenge that is shared internationally. It is important to understand whether a patient with suspected serious pathology can wait for onward referral/investigation or not, and whether any action needs to be taken immediately, or whether a short delay is acceptable and unlikely to affect the outcome for the patient. A good example of where it is acceptable to wait is presented in the case of Belinda, and where in the case of Brian, emergency action is required. The decision on whether the patient should be referred on or whether conservative treatment is appropriate (keep) is multifactorial and complex. It is dependent on the clinician's ability to clinically reason the relevance of specific red flags in the context of the individual patient's presentation. Using recognized strategies such as safety netting and watchful waiting will help to reduce missed or delayed diagnosis. These are important tools which should be used to help identify serious conditions early. These strategies are not only helpful in managing the uncertainty of whether a patient may or may not have a serious pathology, but also support the clinician in managing their own anxiety around the potential of missing or delaying a serious diagnosis.

SAFETY NETTING

Safety netting is a tool designed to help the clinician and patient manage risk and uncertainty. It requires working with patients to enable them to monitor their symptoms over time (Greenhalgh et al., 2020). The three principles of safety netting that the patient needs to know are illustrated in Fig. 11.3.

Effective implementation of safety netting requires the clinician to be aware of serious pathology as a differential diagnosis and understand the natural history of the serious pathology of concern. It also relies on the patient to monitor their symptoms which can be

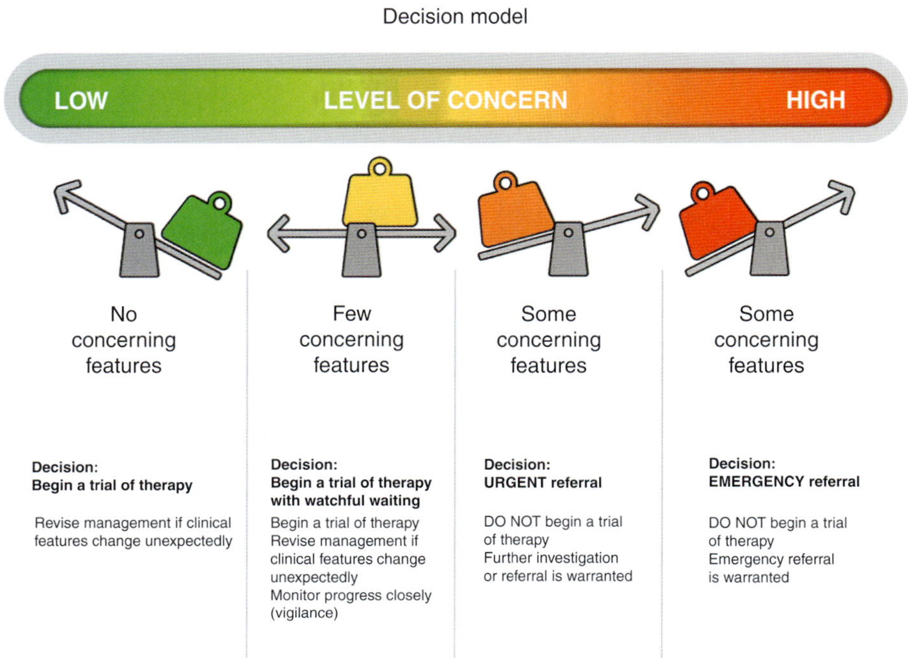

Fig. 11.2 Decision model. The choice of clinical action should be based on the level of concern. (*Finucane et al., 2020.*)

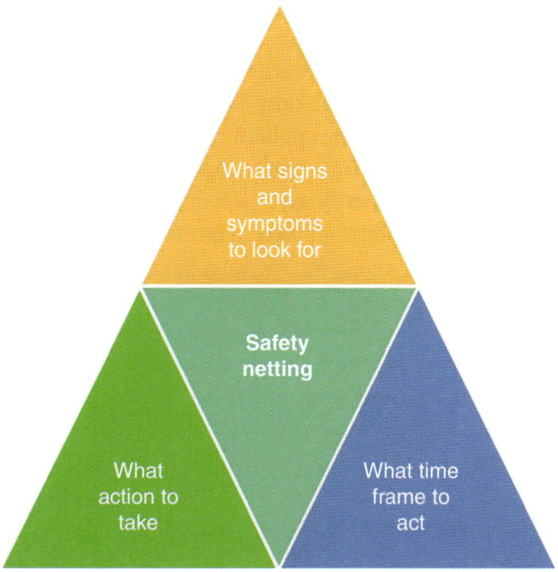

Fig. 11.3 The three key components of safety netting. (*Selfe et al., in press.*)

challenging as patients often underestimate the significance of symptoms and hesitate to seek advice for fear of 'wasting' clinical time (Evans et al., 2018). The clinician needs to clearly communicate the importance of red flags and encourage patients to consult with ongoing symptoms and provide easy access to follow-up consultations. Table 11.2 lists key advice and actions that contribute to successful safety netting.

EXAMPLE OF SAFETY NETTING

Becky is 36 years old and has developed an exacerbation of back pain and a recurrent episode of left leg pain 1 week ago. The leg pain is now severe, constant and extends to the top of her foot, with pins and needles in the middle three toes. Symptoms have been getting worse each day, with pain increasing peripherally. Reassuringly, however, on examination, Becky is neurologically intact. Importantly, the subjective history

TABLE 11.2 Safety Netting Advice for Patients and Actions for Clinicians

Advice for Patients
What Red Flag symptoms do they need to be aware of (e.g. Fig. 11.3)
What to do if these Red Flag symptoms develop (Verbal and written advice where possible) (e.g. Fig. 11.3)
Clear timescale for when they need to act (Urgent: within 5 days versus Emergency: on the same day) (e.g. Fig. 11.3)
When to come back if symptoms not resolved.
The reason for tests or referrals.
How test results will be obtained.
Likely time scale of current symptoms.
Action for Clinicians
Check to ensure that the patient understands safety netting advice.
Health care professionals retain the responsibility for reviewing and acting on results of investigations that they have requested.
Consider accuracy of diagnostic tests (N.B. False negatives). Review patients even when tests are negative.
Communicate test results to patient and General Practitioner (GP). Follow up as necessary (provide easy access to follow up consultations). Document test findings clearly.
Consider referral after repeat consultation for new symptoms (e.g. Three strikes and you are in)
Have systems in place that can highlight: (i) change in health seeking behaviour. (ii) multiple escalating health seeking behaviour. (iii) repeat consultations for unexplained recurrent signs and symptoms.
Offer patients with low risk, but not no risk, a review in an agreed timeframe.
Document safety netting advice carefully.
Debrief/reflect on all serious pathology cases.

Selfe et al. (in press).

revealed that she has no problems with her bladder, bowel, or sexual function and has no saddle numbness. Becky needs to be safety netted about Cauda Equina Syndrome (see Chapter 12 on Advanced Practice). The warning signs depicted on Fig. 11.4 are carefully discussed with Becky, and a card (or leaflet) containing this information is given to her to take away to help her to remember what symptoms to remain aware of (Fig. 11.4). Importantly, Becky needs to understand that if any of these symptoms develop in the context of progressing back and leg pain, then she needs to seek help that day. It is important to point out that the symptoms relate to a rare condition, Cauda Equina Syndrome, but that this condition is a potential surgical emergency, so health seeking must not be delayed. It is essential to establish that Becky clearly understands the advice and understands the speed at which an opinion needs to be sought. Documentation in the clinical notes should then take place, stating clearly that Becky has been safety netted about Cauda Equina Syndrome and a CES card should be given.

WATCHFUL WAIT

Watchful wait refers to the act of close monitoring of the patient's symptoms whilst undergoing treatment as required, but allowing time to pass before considering further intervention or investigation (Cook et al., 2018). A good example is a patient presenting with back pain and a history of prostate cancer. Despite being one of the five most common cancers to metastasize (Table 11.3) (Coleman & Holen, 2014), the history of prostate cancer alone would not trigger immediate further investigation, and the clinician would normally expect to start a course of treatment but ensure careful monitoring of symptoms at each episode of care.

Successful treatment and management of a patient requires more than careful clinical reasoning. It requires many aspects to come together to get things right. On rare occasions when things go wrong, the patient may consider litigation. Clinical negligence claims are an increasing burden on the NHS in the UK, with the annual cost of harm rising to £8.3 billion in 2019/2020. For example, between 2009 and 2021 there were 15 CES claims recorded against physiotherapists which is 0.7% of all CES claims recorded in the UK (Leech et al., 2021). Whilst at present the number of litigation cases involving physiotherapists in the UK is relatively small, it is predicted to rise and not just for those in NHS settings but in all settings. It is important to consider the emotional drivers and physical perspective of a patient who has chosen to pursue litigation.

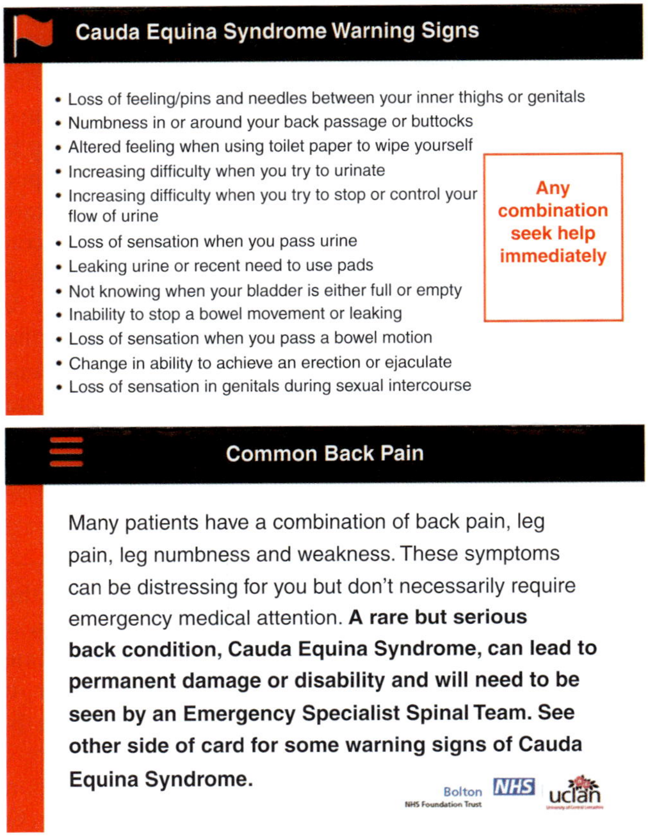

Fig. 11.4 Safety netting cauda equina syndrome (CES) credit card for patients. (*Link to online version of the CES cards. These are available in 31 languages for free download: https://www.eoemskservice.nhs.uk/advice-and-leaflets/lower-back/cauda-equina*)

TABLE 11.3 Five Commonest Cancers to Metastasize
Breast
Prostate
Kidney
Lung
Thyroid

Emotional turmoil is also clearly described by a CES sufferer.

> *My worst worry was that I was becoming incontinent… and in a wheelchair and my wife having to look after me…I have an arrangement with a friend where if either of us end up like this, we'll give 'the necklace treatment' and so save the family.*

In addition, not only is litigation costly from a purely financial perspective, but even the threat of litigation can be an emotionally difficult and challenging experience for the clinician too.

Here is how one physiotherapist described their experience of undergoing litigation related to a CES patient's management:

> *a whole lot of emotions, the fear, the worry, the doubt, the unknown I think, a big thing is the unknown, you don't know what I need to do next and what's going to happen, what's likely to happen but yes, it was very, very stressful, a lot of anxiety*

With this in mind, it is clearly and increasingly important to get the basics right.

KNOWLEDGE CHECK

1. What are the three key components of safety netting?
2. Which of these two statements best describes watchful waiting:
   a. Giving the patient an advice leaflet and a contact phone number
   b. Close monitoring of the patient's symptoms, whilst undergoing treatment

CASE STUDIES

The following cases present four different patient scenarios. Each one poses a series of questions to prompt your clinical reasoning to help you establish a level of concern and ends by asking you to make a clinical decision for each patient.

CASE STUDY 11.1

Brenda

Brenda is a 55-year-old woman who lives alone and is a cleaner. She has a sedentary lifestyle, is an ex-smoker of 15 cigarettes a day, and is a social drinker. Brenda suffers from Type 2 Diabetes, high blood pressure, anxiety and depression and has a BMI of 40. She has had chronic low back pain for 29 years and has previously been under the Pain Team on two separate occasions. Three months ago, she was discharged from the Pain Team. Brenda has attended her GP surgery today to see her First Contact Practitioner about her back pain which she describes as her usual pain that she has experienced for many years.

	Clinical Reasoning	Action Required
What risk factors does Brenda have for possible serious pathology? Which serious pathologies do each of these risk factors relate to?	Brenda's age puts her in the risk category for several serious pathologies such as metastases, myeloma and osteoporosis (spinal fracture). She is female and thus at higher risk of vertebral fracture. She has diabetes which may increase her risk of vertebral infection and vertebral fracture. Brenda is morbidly obese (BMI = 40), and has diabetes and hypertension which puts her at risk of vascular problems. Abdominal aortic aneurysm (AAA) is more common in men than women but is potentially a cause of LBP in people over 65	These are all theoretical risks and need to be considered in Brenda's case, but her symptoms are unchanged over many years so no specific action is required in relation to possible serious pathology. It is safe to proceed with treatment as planned.
What further questions do you want to ask Brenda?	Smoking is a risk factor for cancer and vertebral fracture, so it is important to ask Brenda how long she smoked for and how long ago she gave up. Similarly, alcohol intake of more than 3 units a day for a female is a risk factor for vertebral fracture, so it is important to ask Brenda how much she drinks.	These are all theoretical risks and need to be considered in Brenda's case, but her symptoms are unchanged over many years so no specific action is required in relation to possible serious pathology. It is safe to proceed with treatment as planned, but some general health and lifestyle advice may be appropriate.
What is your level of concern about Brenda?	Low level of concern about Brenda as nothing has changed or is new about this episode of back pain.	Monitor signs and symptoms and response to treatment and reassess level of concern at each appointment if they change.

Continued

CASE STUDY 11.1—cont'd

	Clinical Reasoning	Action Required
What is your clinical decision about Brenda?	Plan to treat as planned and no onward referral or further investigation required at this stage.	Monitor signs and symptoms and reassess clinical decision if they change.

Discussion

In Brenda's case, nothing has changed. There is nothing new about the back pain that Brenda is complaining of. She has chronic mechanical back pain.

Outcome

Therefore the level of concern is low (Fig. 11.5). The appropriate clinical action is to treat as planned and, in line with good practice, re-evaluate any change in symptoms at each consultation.

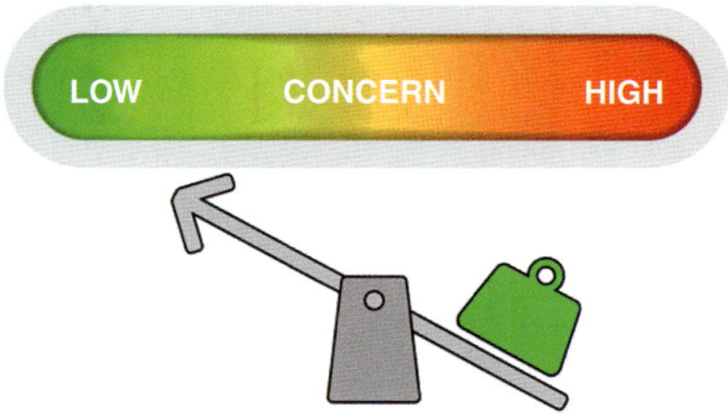

Fig. 11.5 Level of concern for Brenda.

CASE STUDY 11.2

Belinda

Belinda is a 68-year-old retired nurse. She has had low back pain episodically throughout her working life and has benefited from physiotherapy in the past. This episode of back pain began 6 weeks ago following gardening for 2 h the day before its onset. She is trying to stay active and has paid for several massages but is not improving as she had hoped. Belinda cares for her 2-year-old grandson 1 day a week and is struggling to manage. Belinda is a nonsmoker and drinks moderate amounts of alcohol (10 units a week). She is fit and well but has a history of breast cancer 10 years ago. She does not take any medication to relieve her pain as she does not like taking tablets.

	Clinical Reasoning	Action Required
What risk factors does Belinda have for possible serious pathology? Which serious pathologies do each of these risk factors relate to?	Belinda has the onset of back pain after a specific physical activity, and it is not improving with reasonable passage of time. Her age and sex put her at risk of vertebral fracture. She has a past history of breast cancer. Thus she is at a risk of metastatic bone disease in the spine, which could cause a vertebral fracture.	Whilst Belinda does have some risk factors, she has not had a lot of treatment, and a course of physiotherapy over 6 weeks or so would be appropriate. Signs and symptoms should be monitored and reassessed during this treatment period

CASE STUDY 11.2—cont'd

What further questions do you want to ask Belinda?	Belinda should be asked about her cancer in more detail, so that the type and stage of the cancer is clear, as this changes the risk of metastases.	Belinda had grade 1 cancer with a 1 cm tumour and no lymph node involvement, so she is at low risk for metastatic disease.
What is your level of concern about Belinda?	Some potential concerns as outlined above, so more information needed.	Low level of concern due to the further reassuring information about the size and type of tumour.
What is your clinical decision about Belinda?	Clinically low risk so safe to treat.	Treat as planned and reassess at each appointment. Safety net Belinda.

Discussion

In Belinda's case, she has a past history of cancer and is at risk of MBD.

Approximately 30% of patients with a past history of breast cancer go on to metastasize and can occur at any time, with 50% within the first 5 years after a primary diagnosis of cancer, with the other 50% developing 10 years and beyond (Lee et al., 2011). In Belinda's case, she was diagnosed 10 years ago, but she has no other symptoms suggestive of MBD. On its own, it would not cause concern at this point.

Outcome

Therefore the level of concern is one that requires a watchful wait approach (Fig. 11.6).

The appropriate clinical action is to treat as planned but to safety net. Belinda was advised to look out for any changes in her pain severity and pain behaviour, such as unremitting pain or constant night pain, forcing her to get out of bed and pace the floor, or band-like pain around her trunk. She was also advised to look out for any gait disturbance or loss of control of her legs (see Fig. 11.8). If she experienced any of these things, she was advised to contact the clinician immediately.

In line with good practice, re-evaluate any change in symptoms at each consultation.

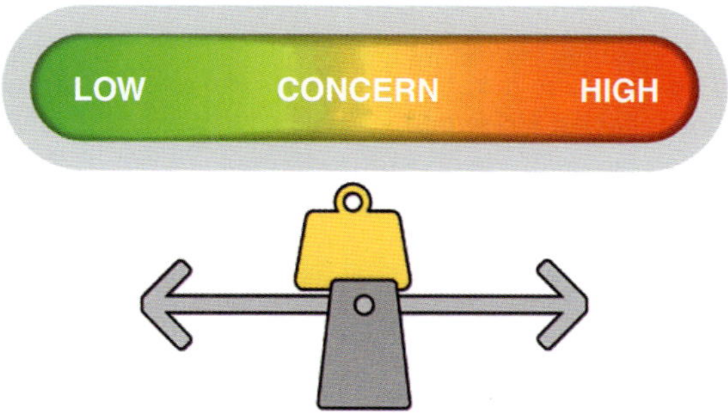

Fig. 11.6 Level of concern for Belinda.

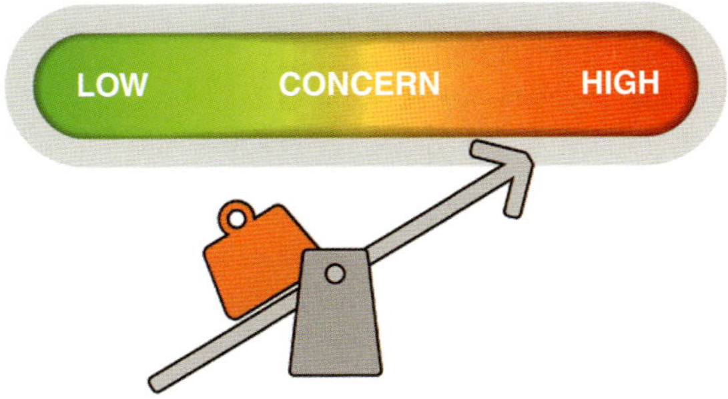

Fig. 11.7 Level of concern for Barry.

EARLY WARNING SIGNS OF MSCC
Greenhalgh S, Turnpenny J, Richards L, Selfe J (2010)

- **R** Referred pain is multi-segmental or band-like
- **E** Escalating pain which is poorly responsive to treatment (incl medication)
- **D** Different character or site to previous symptoms
- **F** Funny feelings, odd sensations or heavy legs (multi-segmental)
- **L** Lying flat increases pain
- **A** Agonising pain causing anguish and despair
- **G** Gait disturbance, unsteadiness, especially on stairs (not just a limp)
- **S** Sleep grossly disturbed due to pain being worse at night

NB – Established motor / sensory / bladder / bowel disturbances / late signs →

Fig. 11.8 Clinicians cue card for metastatic spinal cord compression (MSCC).

CASE STUDY 11.3

Barry

Barry is a 77-year-old gentleman referred with back pain. He has a history of prostate cancer with a Gleason score of 3+3 at the time of diagnosis. A Gleason score reflects the degree of abnormality of cells at two points within the prostate. A score of 8 at the time of diagnosis suggests a high risk of metastatic disease (Carter et al., 2012). In this case, he has some risk (Greenhalgh & Selfe, 2019). He currently describes himself as being in remission. On his attendance both Barry and his wife were very anxious. He described fluctuating back and neck pain, and at the time that he arrived at the clinic, his neck was acutely painful with his low back pain having settled. He gives a history of sunbathing in a deckchair on holiday for around 1½ hours 3 months earlier. He got up suddenly and collapsed, hitting his skull on the floor. His wife describes it as a very heavy fall, hitting his head. He apparently did not put out his hands to break the impact. Since the fall, he has been unable to move his neck fully, and the level of pain has escalated, with particular difficulties in turning to the left. Observation through the consultation revealed a gross limitation of movement in most directions. In addition, forward flexion reproduces paraesthesia in both hands. He feels no medication is helping his severe neck pain and describes it as a 9–10/10 on a Visual Analogue Scale (VAS). His sleep is disturbed due to the severe pain, and he has significant difficulty moving from lying to sitting and vice versa due to the weight of his head. He has had some occipital headaches and pain referral from the cervical spine into the mastoid process. He describes a 1-week history of being unable to drive. He has no arm pain but does have bilateral hand paraesthesia affecting all of the digits; no dizziness, no nausea, no tingling in the face. Although he usually sees an osteopath for his low back pain, he has not seen an osteopath for this present neck condition.

CASE STUDY 11.3—cont'd

On examination, cervical spine movements were almost negligible and hardly improved in supine lying. Flexion was limited to around a 1/5th of its range, provoking paraesthesia in both hands, but the lower limbs were not affected. Examination of the shoulders was unremarkable and myotomes, dermatomes and reflexes were intact in the upper and lower limbs. The clinician was concerned about the severe restriction of movement in the context of severe pain and a history of the fall with a clear correlation of neck flexion and bilateral paraesthesia.

Socially, Barry is a retired bus driver and a nonsmoker. He does like to drink socially (but is unsure of his units) and plays regular crown green bowls.

	Clinical Reasoning	Action Required
What risk factors does Barry have for possible serious pathology? Which serious pathologies do each of these risk factors relate to?	Barry's age puts him at a higher risk of serious pathology such as fracture, metastases and myeloma. He has a history of prostate cancer, which is the third most common cancer to metastasize to the spine. He has had a fall and has injured his neck. He has a significant loss of range of movement, which may indicate a fracture. He also gets paraesthesia into both hands with neck flexion, so there is a possibility of cervical cord injury or bilateral radiculopathy.	Further information is needed from Barry about the staging and classification of his prostate cancer and his Gleason score when he was diagnosed with prostate cancer (Greenhalgh & Selfe, 2020). Further questioning about his symptoms is needed in order to establish the relationship between his neck symptoms and upper limb symptoms, as well as exploring any lower limb symptoms.
What further questions do you want to ask Barry?	It would be helpful to know Barry's Gleason score when he was diagnosed with his prostate cancer. His was 3+3 which puts him with some risk of metastases. It would be good to know if Barry has had any x-rays or imaging done of his neck. X-ray would help to exclude fracture, and MRI would help to exclude cord/nerve root involvement. Also, it is important to know about any gait disturbance and any lower limb symptoms, which may indicate cord involvement.	Further imaging is required in the form of x-ray of the cervical spine and magnetic resonance imaging (MRI) of the whole spine.
What is your level of concern about Barry?	Barry has several concerning features so the level of concern is high.	Imaging of the cervical spine as an urgent case, but not requiring same day/emergency imaging.
What is your clinical decision about Barry?	Clinical decision is that Barry needs further investigation with a neck x-ray and whole spine MRI scan.	Barry needs urgent imaging, which was done. It revealed a tumour at C4/5 as a result of myeloma unrelated to his prostate cancer.

Discussion

Barry had a concerning presentation. The history of prostate cancer is significant as prostate, breast and lung cancer are the most common cancers that metastasize to the spine (Sutcliffe et al., 2013). However, don't forget that the new condition could be from an unrelated cause. Barry had developed a second type of malignancy. Barry had had an x-ray 3 months earlier that had been reported as normal. It is important to recognize that re-evaluation and clinical reasoning

Continued

CASE STUDY 11.3—cont'd

of the patient's presentation at each consultation is important. Tests such as x-rays and blood tests can be falsely reassuring, especially early in a serious disease process (Watson et al., 2019). Monitor Red Flags over time and do not be falsely reassured by a test being reported as normal.

MRI Whole Spinal

Metastatic spinal disease with abnormal marrow signal throughout the spine and a large lesion seen mainly at C4/5 with a posterior soft tissue extension causing moderate spinal canal stenosis. Multiple myeloma is the likely diagnosis.

Barry was admitted to the hospital. The large soft tissue swelling at C4/5 causing destruction of the C4 vertebral body was discussed with the spinal surgical team, and nonsurgical management with best supportive care was the treatment of choice.

Final Diagnosis

Myeloma

Myeloma, also known as multiple myeloma, is a blood cancer arising from plasma cells. At any one time there are around 24,000 people living with myeloma in the UK. It accounts for 15% of blood cancers and 2% of all cancers. Myeloma mainly affects those over the age of 65; however, it has been diagnosed in people much younger. https://www.myeloma.org.uk/understanding-myeloma/what-is-myeloma/

Outcome

Therefore the level of concern is high (Fig. 11.7).

The appropriate clinical action is to ensure the patient is investigated urgently (within 5 days) so no treatment would be offered.

CASE STUDY 11.4

Brian

Brian is a 67-year-old gentleman, still working as the managing director of his own company. He is normally fit and well, smokes 10 cigarettes a day and is a moderate drinker. He has a long history of intermittent episodes of mechanical back pain which usually respond to medication, staying active and private physiotherapy. This episode began 8 weeks ago and is different. It is not responding to his usual treatment approach, and so his GP referred him to the musculoskeletal triage service. An x-ray of the lumbar spine was reported as normal, and no abnormalities had been identified on any blood tests. Barry was contacted by telephone for a remote consultation. Barry was not anxious and was reassured that the recent investigations were normal. However, he was now struggling to stay at work. He was now waking at night with pain. In the last week, his legs had begun to feel weaker, which he attributed to lack of exercise, and he had developed a band of paraesthesia bilaterally around his ribs in the region of the tenth rib.

	Clinical Reasoning	Action Required
What risk factors does Brian have for possible serious pathology? Which serious pathologies do each of these risk factors relate to?	Brian's age puts him in the risk category for several serious pathologies such as metastases, myeloma and osteoporosis (spinal fracture). He has band-like paraesthesia around his abdomen in the lower thoracic region. The thoracic spine is where 70% of metastatic disease occurs, so this may be a concern.	These are all theoretical risks and need to be considered in Brian's case. His current pain is different from his usual back pain, and he is waking at night with the pain. Brian needs further investigation in the form of whole spine MRI scan.
What further questions do you want to ask Brian?	Smoking is a risk factor for cancer and vertebral fracture, so it is important to ask Brian how long he has smoked for and when he started.	These are all theoretical risks and need to be considered in Brian's case, but as his symptoms are worsening, further investigation is appropriate.

CASE STUDY 11.4—cont'd

	Similarly, alcohol intake of more than 3 units a day is a risk factor for vertebral fracture, so it is important to ask Brian how much he drinks.	
What is your level of concern about Brian?	High level of concern about Brian, as symptoms are different from his normal pain and are escalating. Although he has had blood tests and x-rays that are normal, these should not reassure you given the worsening clinical presentation.	MRI scan of the spine needed to exclude metastatic spinal cord compression (MSCC).
What is your clinical decision about Brian?	Need to investigate to exclude serious pathology	MRI scan requested. This showed multilevel metastatic bone disease throughout the spine, with metastatic cord compression at T10.

Discussion

Just like in Barry's case, Brian had negative tests relating to his condition. Brian had an undiagnosed lung cancer, one of the most common cancers to refer to the spine (Table 11.3). Twenty-five percent of patients presenting to primary care services with MSCC do not know they have cancer (NICE, 2008). Some useful clinical features to help you spot MSCC early are set against the mnemonic RED FLAGS in Fig. 11.8.

MSCC is an emergency oncological condition and must be acted on very quickly to avoid significant spinal cord damage, paralysis and an earlier than expected death (NICE, 2008).

Outcome

Therefore the level of concern is high (Fig. 11.9).

The appropriate clinical action is Brian requires emergency (same day) investigation.

Fig. 11.9 Level of concern for Brian.

CONCLUSION

This chapter has outlined the complexities of identifying serious pathology early when it masquerades as a musculoskeletal condition. It is particularly challenging in the early stages of a serious pathology. However, as clinicians, we are best placed to identify these pathologies and can make a huge difference to a patient's prognosis and outcome.

There are many more serious pathologies that have not been covered in this chapter, but the application of some basic principles outlined below will support the identification of most serious pathology.

Clinicians should:

- Understand how various serious pathologies may present.
- Consider serious pathology as a differential diagnosis.
- Appreciate that the patient is the expert and living with their own symptoms.
- Consider any red flags in the context of the specific patient (clinical profile).
- Consider serious pathology as the cause of symptoms where there is escalating pain and progressively worsening symptoms that do not respond to conservative management or medication as expected, i.e. the combination of red flags is increasing!
- Evaluate potential red flags at all stages during every patient encounter and be aware that symptoms may change as disease progresses.

Serious pathology represents a level of uncertainty and risk within clinical practice. It is important that you are able to minimize that risk and seek support when there is uncertainty. The following essential pointers will help support you to do this within the clinical setting:

- Make sure you understand the established clinical pathways in your area of work. Our experience has shown that these can vary considerably depending on your location.
- Speak to someone senior immediately if the situation is a potential emergency or if you are unsure.
- Communicate clearly to the patient the agreed management plan and safety net, wherever necessary, for those at risk of progressing to a more serious condition.
- Always document carefully and clearly. Remember, if it is not written down, 'it did not happen'!
- Always document who was spoken to and at what time if advice was sought. Clearly annotate the outcome of the conversation.

Identifying serious pathology is far from black and white, and the application of red flags in the context in which the patient presents will help to reduce their formulaic use. Grieve (1994) suggested that the identification of serious pathology depended largely on

> *awareness, vigilance and suspicion rather than a set of rules.*

REVIEW AND REVISE QUESTIONS

1. What are the two steps that will help to establish if a serious pathology is present?
2. Describe four cauda equina warning signs.
3. Name three of the five cancers that commonly metastasize to the spine.
4. Which of the following are not risk factors for an osteoporotic fracture.
   A. Smoking
   B. Long-term use of NSAIDs
   C. Alcohol consumption (female)
5. Name two factors that increase the risk of spinal infection?
6. All women with a history of breast cancer are at a risk of developing MBD within the first 5 years following diagnosis. True or false.

REFERENCES

Borsook, D., 2012. Neurological diseases and pain. Brain 135, 320−344.

Budtz, C.R., Hansen, R.P., Thomsen, J., et al., 2021. The prevalence of serious pathology in musculoskeletal physiotherapy patients - a nationwide register-based cohort study. Physiotherapy 112, 96−102. https://www.researchsquare.com/article/rs-11772/v1.

Carter, H.B., Partin, A.W., Walsh, P.C., et al., 2012. Gleason score 6 adenocarcinoma: should it be labeled as cancer? J. Clin. Oncol. 30 (35), 4294−4296.

Cook, C.E., George, S.Z., Reiman, M.P., 2018. Red flag screening for low back pain: nothing to see here, move along: a narrative review. Br. J. Sports Med. 52 (8), 493−496.

Coleman, R.E., Holen, I., 2014. Chapter 51 bone metastases. In: Abeloff's Clinical Oncology, fifth ed. Elsevier.

Darlow, B., Forster, B.B., O'Sullivan, K., et al., 2017. It is time to stop causing harm with inappropriate imaging for low back pain. Br. J. Sports Med. 51, 414−415.

Dionne, N., Adefolarin, A., Kunzelman, D., et al., 2019. What is the diagnostic accuracy of red flags related to cauda equina syndrome (CES), when compared to magnetic resonance imaging (MRI)? A systematic review. Musculoskelet. Sci. Pract. 42, 125−133.

Downie, A., Williams, C.M., Henschke, N., et al., 2013. Red flags to screen for malignancy and fracture in patients with low back pain: systematic review. BMJ. 11 (347), 7095.

Evans, J., Ziebland, S., MacArtney, J., et al., 2018. GPs' understanding and practice of safety netting for potential cancer presentations: a qualitative study in primary care. Br. J. Gen. Pract. 68 (672) e505−e511.

Finucane, L., Greenhalgh, S., Selfe. J., 2017. What are the red flags to aid the early detection of metastatic bone disease as a cause of back pain? Physiother. Pract. Res. 38, 73−77.

Finucane, L.M., Downie, A., Mercer, C., et al., 2020. International framework for red flags for potential serious spinal pathologies. J. Orthop. Sports Phys. Ther. 50 (7), 350−372.

Goodman, C., Snyder, T., 2013. Screening for immunologic disease. In: Differential Diagnosis for Physical Therapists. Screening for Referral, fifth ed. Elsevier, St. Louis, MO, pp. 464−467.

Gould, B.E., 2006. Pathophysiology for the Health Professions, third ed. Saunders, Philadelphia.

Greenhalgh, S., Finucane, L.M., Mercer, C., et al., 2020. Safety netting; best practice in the face of uncertainty. Musculoskelet. Sci. Pract. 48, 102179.

Greenhalgh, S., Selfe, J., 2006. Red Flags: A Guide to Identifying Serious Pathology of the Spine, first ed. Elsevier, Edinburgh, London, New York, Oxford, Philadelphia, Sydney.

Greenhalgh, S., Selfe, J., 2019. Red Flags and Blue Lights: Managing Serious Spinal Pathology, second ed. Elsevier, Edinburgh London, New York, Oxford, Philadelphia, Sydney.

Grieve, G.P., 1994. The masqueraders. In: Boyling, J.D., Palastanga, N. (Eds.), Grieve's Modern Manual Therapy: The Vertebral Column, second ed. Churchill Livingstone, Edinburgh, pp. 841−856.

Henschke N, Maher C, Ostelo R, et al. 2013 Red flags to screen for malignancy in patients with low-back pain (Review), (2). The Cochrane Collaboration. Wiley Publishers.

Lackenbauer, W., Janssen, J., Roddam, H., et al., 2017. Keep/refer decision making abilities of European final year undergraduate physiotherapy students: a cross-sectional survey using clinical vignettes. Eur. J. Physiother. 20 (3), 128−134.

Langridge, N., Roberts, L., Pope, C., 2015. The clinical reasoning processes of extended scope physiotherapists assessing patients with low back pain. Man. Ther. 20 (6), 745−750.

Langridge, N., Roberts, L., Pope, C., 2016. The role of clinician emotion in clinical reasoning: balancing the analytical process. Man. Ther. 21, 277−281.

Lee, S.J., Park, S., Ahn, H.K., et al., 2011. Implications of bone-only metastases in breast cancer: favorable preference with excellent outcomes of hormone receptor positive breast cancer. Cancer Res. Treat. 43 (2), 89−95.

Leech, R.L., Selfe, J., Ball, S., et al., 2021. A scoping review: investigating the extent and legal process of cauda equina syndrome claims for UK physiotherapists. Musculoskel. Sci. Pract. 56, 102458.

Nagashima, H., Tanishima, S., Tanida, A., 2018. Diagnosis and management of spinal infections. J. Orthop. Sci. 23 (1), 8−13.

National Institute for Health and Care Excellence Clinical Guideline 75, 2008. Metastatic spinal cord compression: diagnosis and management of adults at risk of and with metastatic spinal cord compression. https://www.nice.org.uk/Guidance/CG75.

National Osteoporosis Society (NOS), 2017. Clinical Guidance for the Effective Identification of Vertebral Fractures. https://theros.org.uk/media/3daohfrq/ros-vertebral-fracture-guidelines-november-2017.pdf.

Nickerson, E.K., Sinha, R., 2016. Vertebral osteomyelitis in adults: an update. Br. Med. Bull. 117 (1), 121−138.

Pacheco-Carroza, E.A., 2021. Visceral pain, mechanisms, and implications in musculoskeletal clinical practice. Med. Hypotheses 153, 110624.

Ryder, D., Barnard, K. 2024. Petty's Musculoskeletal Examination and Assessment: A Handbook for Therapists, sixth ed. Elsevier, Oxford.

Selfe, J., Greenhalgh, S., Mercer, C., Finucane, L. Red flags and masqueraders. In: Grieve's Modern Musculoskeletal Physiotherapy, fifth ed. Elsevier. in press.

Sutcliffe, P., Connock, M., Shyangdan, D., et al., 2013. A systematic review of evidence on malignant spinal metastases: natural history and technologies for identifying patients at high risk of vertebral fracture and spinal cord compression. Health Technol. Assess. 17 (42), 1–274.

Tohoku, J., Tsuchie, H., Miyakoshi, N., et al., 2013. High prevalence of abdominal aortic aneurysm in patients with chronic low back pain. J. Exp. Med. 230 (2), 83–86.

Verhagen, A.P., Downie, A., Popal, N., et al., 2016. Red flags presented in current low back pain guidelines: a review. Eur. Spine J. 25 (9), 2788–2802.

Watson, J., Jones, H.E., Banks, J.B., et al., 2019. Use of multiple inflammatory marker tests in primary care: using Clinical Practice Research Datalink to evaluate accuracy. Br. J. Gen. Pract. 69 (684), e462–469.

Yusuf, M., Finucane, L., Selfe, J., 2019. Red flags for the early detection of spinal infection in back pain patients. BMC Musculoskelet. Disord. 20 (1), 1–10.

12

Advancing Practice

Tim Noblet, Matthew Low, and Giles Hazan

LEARNING OUTCOMES

After studying this chapter, you should be able to:

- Define the term advanced practice (AP).
- Identify the four pillars of AP.
- Develop a broader understanding of clinical presentations that initially appear to be musculoskeletal conditions.
- Appreciate the diversity of scope of advancing practice across musculoskeletal physiotherapy conditions and settings.

CHAPTER CONTENTS

THE HISTORY OF MUSCULOSKELETAL ADVANCED PRACTICE

Musculoskeletal advanced practice (AP) physiotherapists are experts in the assessment, diagnosis, treatment and management of musculoskeletal conditions (Chartered Society of Physiotherapy (CSP), 2016b; Noblet et al., 2021). Advanced musculoskeletal physiotherapy job roles have existed in the United Kingdom for more than 30 years, playing an integral part within the delivery of musculoskeletal health services (James & Stuart, 1975; Byles & Ling, 1989; Noblet et al., 2021). Advanced practice was initially recognized in the 1980s when physiotherapists were adopted into orthopaedic and neurosurgical clinics where the availability of medical and surgical doctors did not meet the demands of the local community (Suckley, 2012; CSP, 2016b). These highly skilled clinicians were then termed 'Extended Scope Physiotherapists' or 'Extended Scope Practitioners' (ESPs) (CSP, 2016a).

Through local education, ESPs were able to develop knowledge and skills previously outside the traditional scope of physiotherapy, such as the ordering and interpretation of blood tests and diagnostic imaging (x-rays, ultrasound scans, MRI, CT, etc.), listing patients for surgery, provision of injection therapy and prescription of medicines (Noblet et al., 2021; Tawiah et al., 2021). In 2008, the term ESP was replaced by 'Advanced Physiotherapy Practitioner' or 'APP' as all the knowledge, skills and behaviours demonstrated by ESPs were at this point deemed within the normal scope of practice for physiotherapists in the UK (Noblet et al., 2021; Tawiah et al., 2021). The emergence of advanced practice roles within the fast-developing UK National Health Service (NHS) and the ongoing evolution of the physiotherapy scope of practice has led to the development and implementation of education and training programmes to better prepare the physiotherapy workforce at an advanced practice standard (Rushton et al., 2016; Noblet et al., 2021).

Since 2008, APPs have continued to expand the scope of physiotherapy practice for the benefit of their patients through further education and capability development. Individual APPs in specialist health services complete spinal diagnostic and therapeutic injections, diagnostic imaging, surgical procedures and complex psychological interventions as part of their multimodal physiotherapeutic management (CSP, 2016a; Noblet et al., 2020, 2021; Tawiah et al., 2021). By utilizing full and extended scopes of practice, APPs have been shown to be clinically and cost-effective across musculoskeletal patient pathways, working in a diversity of settings including emergency, rheumatology, persistent pain, paediatric and rehabilitation therapies departments, as well as in primary care as first contact practitioners and in musculoskeletal community secondary care interface services (Stanhope et al., 2012; Suckley, 2012; Saxon et al., 2014; Noblet et al., 2020). Musculoskeletal advanced physiotherapy practice is now being utilized in countries across the world, such as Australia, Canada, Ireland and New Zealand (Noblet et al., 2021; Tawiah et al., 2021).

What Is Advanced Level Practice?

It is important to recognize that advanced practice is a level of practice, not a specific job role. Clinicians working at an advanced practice level will have developed their abilities through their individual career journey. Following the introduction of the term 'advanced physiotherapy practitioner' in 2008, the CSP defined advanced practice as *'synthesising knowledge and skills to support comprehensive clinical reasoning to manage patients (often with complex, recurring, challenging and unusual presentations) in an unpredictable and often high-risk situation'* (CSP, 2016a). This definition has been further developed for use across all professions and specialties Fig. 12.1.

The Four Pillars of Advanced Practice

Musculoskeletal advanced physiotherapy practitioners demonstrate expertise across four pillars of advanced practice:

1. Clinical practice
2. Leadership and management
3. Education
4. Research (Table 12.1) (NHS-England, 2017)

All advanced practitioners are expected to demonstrate the knowledge, skills and behaviours of an advanced practitioner through post-registration master's level learning and years of clinical and professional experience. However, they will use their skills in different ways depending on their specific role or area of practice (Stanhope et al., 2012; Suckley, 2012; Saxon et al., 2014; NHS-England, 2017; Noblet et al., 2020).

KNOWLEDGE CHECK

1. Define advancing practice.
2. What are the four pillars of advanced practice?
3. Identify one of the knowledge skills and behaviours for each pilar of advanced practice.

Advanced clinical practice is delivered by experienced, registered health and care practitioners.
It is a level of practice characterised by a high degree of autonomy and complex decision making.
This is underpinned by a master's level award or equivalent that encompasses the *four pillars of clinical practice,* leadership and management, education and research, with demonstration of core capabilities and area specific clinical competence. Advanced clinical practice embodies the ability to manage clinical care in partnership with individuals, families and carers. It includes the analysis and synthesis of complex problems across a range of settings, enabling innovative solutions to enhance people's experience and improve outcomes.

Fig. 12.1 Definition of advanced practice across professions and specialties. (NHS-England, 2017.)

TABLE 12.1 The Four Pillars of Advanced Practice

Clinical Practice	Musculoskeletal advanced physiotherapy practitioners can assess, diagnose, treat and manage the spectrum of musculoskeletal presentation across all sectors of healthcare (primary, secondary, tertiary care and public and private sectors). They work with complex patient presentations, dealing with high risk, uncertainty and incomplete clinical and social information. Using advanced-level communication skills, the clinicians are able to support people to make complicated decisions while holistically planning care. Advanced practitioners use their expert decision-making skills, advanced physical examination skills and diagnostic tests such as imaging, blood tests, nerve conduction studies and electromyography (EMG) to inform clinical reasoning when dealing with undifferentiated complex individual presentations in complex multifaceted situations. They synthesize the information gained from many sources to make evidence-based judgements and diagnoses and therefore can initiate, evaluate and modify a range of interventions which may include manual and or exercise or psychological therapies, medicines, electrotherapies and complementary therapies, and social prescribing, all within a dynamic multimodal physiotherapeutic management plan.
Leadership & Management	Advanced practitioners are true leaders across health services and professions. They proactively initiate and develop effective relationships which leads to new practices and service design solutions. Advanced practitioners supervise and mentor other healthcare professionals, acting as role models to inspire future generations of clinicians. As part of their job role, they provide consultancy across professional and health service boundaries, leading teams to be receptive to challenges and proactive in challenging others in the name of best practice and patient care. Advanced practitioners will engage with communities to provide health services specific to the needs of their local community through co-design and co-production.
Education	Healthcare Consumers: Advanced practitioners work with healthcare consumers to promote joint decision-making about their health and empower them to optimize their health and well-being. Patient, relatives and carer education may take place on both an individual or group basis with the clinician appraising and responding to the individual's developmental stage, mental capacity and motivation. The Individual Advanced Practitioner: Advanced practitioners critically assess their own learning needs, engaging in self-directed learning and critical reflection across the four pillars of advanced practice. Other health professionals: Advanced practitioners identify the learning needs and progress of other healthcare providers and students, acting as an educator, role model, supervisor, coach and mentor to help develop confident, quality practitioners of the future.
Research	Advanced practitioners critically engage in research, audit and quality improvement activity. They critically appraise and synthesize the outcomes of relevant research and audit to underpin their practice and to inform the practice of colleagues and peers. Advanced practitioners actively disseminate best practice research findings and facilitate collaborative links between clinical practice and research groups and universities.

From NHS-England, 2017; Noblet et al., 2021; Tawiah et al.,2021.

CASE STUDIES

Advanced practitioners work in a range of settings, often needing to liaise and work closely with a range of allied health practitioners in managing complex patients dealing with diagnostic uncertainty. What follows are four cases taken from real life to illustrate the application of clinical reasoning in advanced practice: the first from an advanced practitioner working in a first contact practitioner (FCP) role in general practice; the second from an advanced practitioner working in a community pain clinic; the third from a community spinal service; and lastly, in a secondary care setting around a Physiotherapy department.

CASE STUDY

First Contact Practitioner in General Practice

Mr JK, a 65-year-old gentleman, presents with shoulder pain that has gradually worsened over the last few months, initially affecting the left shoulder to then involve both.

The pain was generally worse with activity and eased with rest; his sleep was unaffected. He had no small joint pain or swelling and no neck or lower back pain. He had normal gait and balance, no neurological symptoms in the upper or lower limbs and no disruption of bladder or bowel function.

He had a history of moderate hip osteoarthritis and previously saw a physiotherapist and found the exercises helped him although he describes some worsening in the aches in his hips and knees more recently.

He had a history of mild hypertension and took a regular dose of amlodipine (a medication for blood pressure) and simvastatin (to lower cholesterol). He had no history of cancer, drank only modest amounts of alcohol and was not a smoker.

Initial assessment showed a reduced range of movement in both shoulders in a capsular pattern. Neurological assessment of the upper limbs and cervical spine was normal. His general practitioner (GP) had ordered an x-ray a few weeks previously that showed mild osteoarthritis in his left shoulder.

KNOWLEDGE CHECK

1. What do you think the diagnosis is?
2. What might be your treatment plan and timing of follow-up?

Working on a presumption of possible glenohumeral joint osteoarthritis, he was given some advice on the diagnosis and exercises to improve range of movement and strength in the upper limbs.

At review 2 weeks later, his shoulder pain had worsened significantly, he described worsening pain in his hips, his mobility was reduced, and he felt like he was '100 years old' and admitted to feeling lower in mood and was unable to engage with activities he enjoyed.

KNOWLEDGE CHECK

1. What do you think is going on?
2. What would you do next?
3. Who else might you involve in his care?

His case was discussed with his GP as the FCP was concerned he was not responding to therapy and raised the possibility of serious pathologies. A screen of blood tests was ordered including FBC, erythrocyte sedimentation rate (ESR), bone profile, myeloma screen, liver function tests (LFTs) and urea and electrolytes (U&Es).

The results came back with normal FBC, LFT, U&E and myeloma screen but the ESR was raised at 50. (As ESR increases with age, most work on what the upper limit of normal is, which is: Male: age $\div$ 2; Female: (age + 10) $\div$ 2.) It was agreed a trial of steroids would be suitable with a working diagnosis of polymyalgia rheumatics, and he was commenced on 15 mg of prednisolone daily. He was followed up by the FCP 1 week later and found to have seen an almost complete resolution of symptoms (much to his delight), and the diagnosis of polymyalgia rheumatica was confirmed.

KNOWLEDGE CHECK

1. What would be the significance of him subsequently developing a headache and visual disturbances?
2. What would you do?

Both polymyalgia rheumatica (PMR) and giant cell arteritis (GCA) are forms of inflammatory disease. GCA involves inflammation of the vessels supplying the head and neck, i.e. it is a type of vasculitis. They have overlapping features

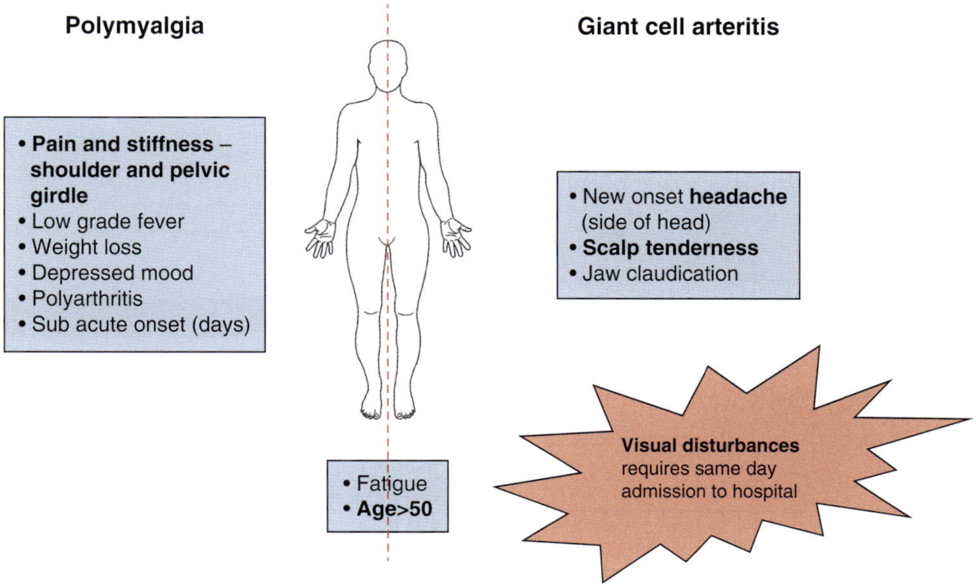

Fig. 12.2 Features of polymyalgia and giant cell arteritis.

that tend to affect the same population, so it is worth considering both pathologies as around 20% of patients with PMR have GCA symptoms and 50% of GCA patients show symptoms of PMR (Buttgereit et al., 2016) Fig. 12.2.

The symptoms can be widespread and vague, and as a clinician you need to consider the broader differential to screen for serious pathologies that can mimic the symptoms. They respond well to rapid use of steroids but can be significantly disabling if left undiagnosed and unmanaged.

CASE STUDY

Advanced Practitioner–Community Pain Clinic

Mr H was referred to the spinal clinic by their GP with concerns over bilateral upper limb paraesthesia querying whether the symptoms may be referred from the cervical spine.

He reported a year of progressively worsening pins and needles affecting both hands, principally the thumb and first two fingers. This was more noticeable at night, often waking him (and he described feeling increasingly tired/listless) as well as when driving long distances.

He described no significant neck pain nor any lower limb symptoms of note. He had occasional back pain related to heavy gardening that was eased with rest. There was no change in gait, balance, nor any disturbance of bladder or bowel function, nor any change in sensation in the saddle region.

He was an ex-smoker who drank 20–25 units of alcohol a week and used no illegal drugs. He was overweight and had seen his GP recently, who advised him on lifestyle factors and discussed some features of depression. He had no history of diabetes or any other significant medical history.

Examination showed a normal cervical spine with a negative Spurling's test; the upper limbs showed normal tone, power, sensation, reflexes and no upper motor neurone signs were elicited. Symptoms were reproducible with both wrists held in flexion with added compression over the carpal tunnel. Assessment of the rest of the spine and lower limbs was normal.

KNOWLEDGE CHECK

1. What do you think the diagnosis is?
2. Is there any more information that might help with the differential?

Further questioning revealed he had become so tired he often went to sleep when he got back from work (6–7 pm) and admitted to losing his libido. He felt his hands were not only tingling but swollen too. There was no obvious synovitis (squeeze test was negative), but his hands were objectively enlarged, and he mentioned he had had to have his wedding ring resized twice in the last 18 months.

On in-depth questioning, he says he had been slightly concerned that his vision has changed somewhat; he realized he was less aware of things off to either side. He had no history of cancer nor any personal or family history of spondyloarthropathy/inflammatory arthritis.

KNOWLEDGE CHECK

1. What might be going on here?
2. What differential diagnoses can you offer for bilateral carpal tunnel syndrome?
3. Who would you involve in the patients care now?

The AP discussed the case with the referring GP, who agreed to run further blood tests that showed very low testosterone and raised growth hormone. He was referred to endocrinology, who went on to run further blood tests, confirming a diagnosis of acromegaly (Fig. 12.3). An MRI of the patient's head identified a pituitary macroadenoma (a benign pituitary tumour) with involvement of the optic chiasm (where the left and right optic nerves intersect), and he was referred to neurosurgery for subsequent excision.

CASE STUDY

Advanced Practitioner—Community Spinal Service

In the early phase of the COVID-19 pandemic in 2020, a 38-year-old bar worker contacted their GP with worsening low back pain and left-sided leg pain in the gluteal and lateral calf region associated with paraesthesia in the left foot. She also reported similar right-sided gluteal pain but no radiation beneath the buttock. Prior to this, she had episodes of back pain over a five-year period with no clear onset or history of injury. The GP referred the patient to a spinal AP team who contacted her via telephone call and took a detailed history.

The patient had previous treatment with Chiropractic and Physiotherapy which appeared to help to a degree, but the symptoms persisted. Her pain was worse when sitting and certainly worse in the morning, with some

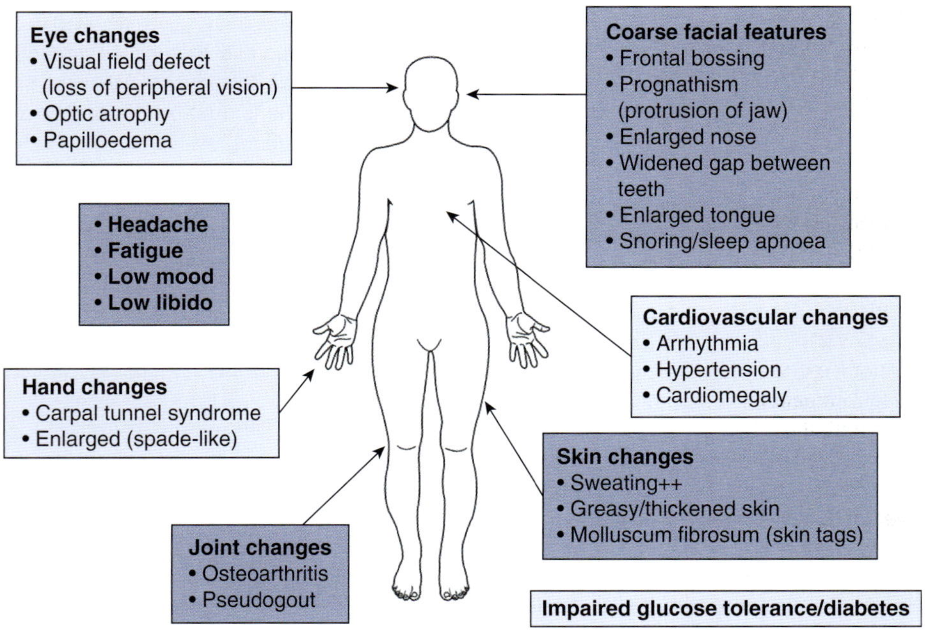

Fig. 12.3 Clinical features of acromegaly.

positive improvement when walking short distances. Longer periods of walking increased both her back pain and leg pain.

There were no red flags or features of cauda equina syndrome (please refer to Table 12.1).

PMH: Nil

Medications: Amitriptyline, diazapam, ibuprofen and paracetamol.

Social history: Lives with two children and a current smoker of 20 cigarettes a day.

There was no physical examination performed due to the nature of the encounter being a telephone contact. The patient was keen to have a medical opinion on possible interventions and due to the persistent nature of the pain and lack of progress made through usual conservative care.

KNOWLEDGE CHECK

1. What do you think is going on?
2. What would you do next?
3. Who else might you involve in her care?

In summary:

- Persistent back pain.
- Worsening back pain leg pain with signs of symptoms becoming bilateral.
- Requires safety netting.

The patient was advised about the rare nature of a condition called cauda equina syndrome (CES) and advised of its symptoms but also what to do if symptoms worsened (to attend the emergency department as per locally agreed pathway for the emergency assessment of patients with suspected cauda equina syndrome). The patient was provided with information to review the BASS (British Association of Spinal Surgery) website, and a routine lumbar spine MRI was requested.

What Happened Next?

Over the period of time waiting for the scan, the patient's symptoms fluctuated but did not progress. She had her MRI scan with the following findings (Fig. 12.4A and B).

Report:

"At L4/L5 level there is a degenerative disc bulge with a large central disc protrusion/extrusion causing severe central canal stenosis and severely compressing the cauda equina nerve roots. At this level there is minimal anterior spondylolisthesis. No significant foraminal narrowing. Degenerative disc bulges at L5/S1 and L3/L4 levels with posterior annular tears/fissures but no overt nerve impingement at these levels. Elsewhere disc hydration is well preserved. Normal vertebral height with no marrow infiltration. Normal lower cord and conus. Report to be communicated to the referrer."

The radiologist immediately informed the AP physiotherapist of the result. The AP contacted the patient and was again asked questions surrounding the risk of developing cauda equina syndrome (Table 12.2).

The patient reported some altered sensation in the peri-anal region in the last two days but was uncertain if they were symptoms. She could not recall if she had gone to the toilet recently. The AP asked the patient to perform a self-sensory examination over the phone, and the patient reported that the sensation around her anal and genital area was not intact.

KNOWLEDGE CHECK

1. What do you think is going on?
2. What would you do next?
3. Who else might you involve in his care?

In summary:

- Evidence of progressive incomplete cauda equina syndrome with concordant imaging.
- Requires immediate referral to emergency surgical pathway.

The patient was referred to the local emergency spinal surgical team and had an emergency lumbar spine decompression at L4/5 with resolution of her symptoms and an excellent final outcome. The reader is referred back to Chapter 11.

CASE STUDY

Physiotherapy Department–Secondary Care Setting

A 40-year-old gentleman self-referred to Physiotherapy due to disabling widespread back and a one-year onset of right-sided leg pain in the L5 dermatomal distribution. At the time, the patient was contacted by telephone

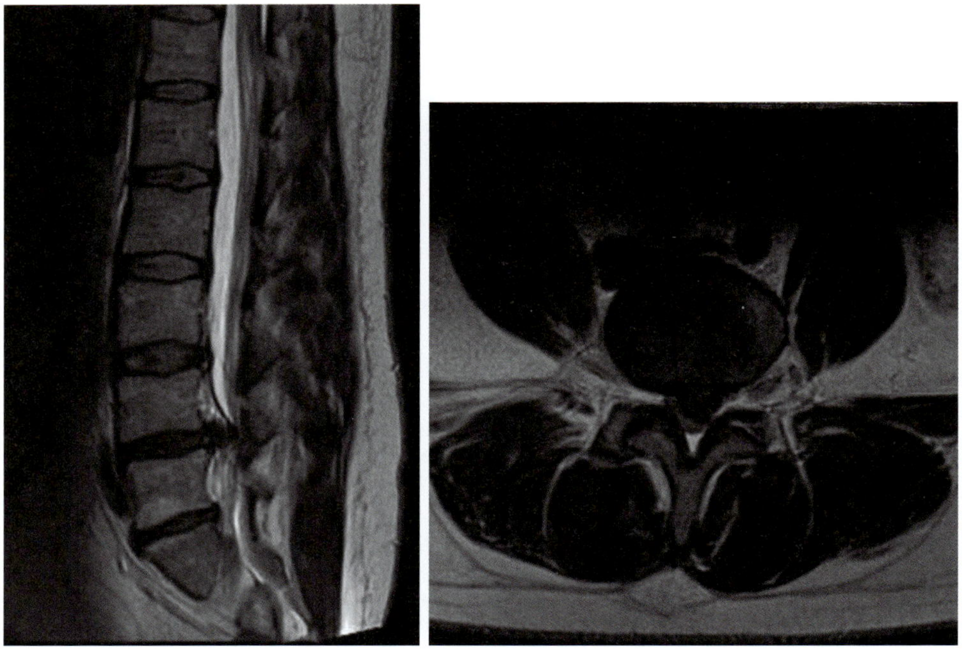

Fig. 12.4 Lumbar spine magnetic resonance imaging demonstrating a significant L4/5 disc protrusion causing severe central canal stenosis compressing the cauda equina nerve roots. The images on the left are T2 weighted sagittal images and on the right are T2 weighted axial images taken through the midline of L4/5.

call during the midst of the COVID-19 pandemic, and there was considerable uncertainty with regard to the relevance and inconsistent information around his symptoms which included changes in bladder control. The patient reported normal sensation around the saddle area and could feel his bladder/bowel and had no issue with bowel control.

The Physiotherapist discussed this with the spinal AP service, who then referred the patient for urgent spinal imaging. The spinal MR imaging demonstrated no cauda equina compression and no evidence of serious pathology. The imaging showed a broad-based disc at the L4/5 level which was touching the left L5 nerve root in the lateral recess and some mild foraminal narrowing with no impingement of the right L4 level. The L5/S1 level had a shallow disc bulge that contacted but was not impinging the left S1 nerve root with no foraminal nerve impingement.

Social history: The patient used to be a builder but had not worked for the last eighteen months. He lived in a caravan with his son.

In summary:

The MR imaging results were not concordant with the patient's symptoms, and further considerations needed to be made.

What Happened Next?

The spinal AP service reviewed and reassured the patient with regards to the MRI results. The patient expressed to the AP that he had had back ache and stiffness for several years and that although his right sciatica symptoms had been present for the last year, he also had paraesthesia in his right arm in a non-specific region. He also complained of his hand being stiff and 'sticking' when returning from flexion.

The AP identified, according to the medical notes, previous blood tests that identified *Borrelia* antibodies (a response to a tick bite that causes Lyme disease). The patient reported that there was no family history of arthritis on his mother's side. However, his father suffered from vasculitis with kidney involvement, and two of his brothers have been diagnosed as having ankylosing spondylitis.

TABLE 12.2 Risk Factors for Cauda Equina Syndrome

Risk Factor/ Level of Evidence	Context	Further Questions	Low Clinical Suspicion	High Clinical Suspicion
Herniated intervertebral disc Low Lumbar spine stenosis Low	The most common cause arises from a large central disc herniation at the L4/5 or L5/S1 level. Those under 50 years of age carry a higher risk, as do obese people. Relevant symptoms that may be precursors to CES: • Unilateral or bilateral radicular pain and/or • Dermatomal reduced sensation and/or • Myotomal weakness	How old are you? Do you have any leg pain? Where exactly is the pain in your legs (above or below knees)? Is the pain down both legs at the same time? Do you have any pins and needles or numbness in your legs, inner thighs, bottom, or genitals? Do you feel any weakness in your legs? Can you describe any worsening symptoms, including your level of pain or symptoms in your legs? If 0 is no pain and 10 is the worst pain you have ever had, how low does the pain go?	No leg pain, normal neurology, and no cauda equina syndrome (CES) symptoms. Stable or no neuropathic leg symptoms	Unilateral or bilateral radicular pain and/or dermatomal reduced sensation and/or myotomal weakness. • Reduced saddle sensation (subjective or objective pinprick) • Bladder disturbance • Bowel disturbance • Reduced anal tone/absent squeeze • Sexual disturbance Presentations that increase the probability of acute threatened CES: • Back pain with: Presence of new saddle anaesthesias, bladder or bowel disturbance Age, <50 years Unilateral onset progressing to bilateral leg pain Alternating leg pain Presence of new motor weakness
Spinal surgery	The degenerative changes in the lumbar spine that are responsible for lumbar spine stenosis (LSS) have the potential to lead to a gradual compromise of the cauda equina nerve roots. This can result in slow-onset CES being overlooked or dismissed in older people.	How high does the pain go? What makes it worse? What makes it better? N/A	N/A	Recurring and insidious but increasing back pain, with gradual onset of unilateral or bilateral lower-limb sensory disturbance and/or motor weakness Incomplete bladder emptying, urinary hesitancy, incontinence, nocturia or urinary tract infections. Bladder and/or bowel dysfunction may progress gradually over time Nerve injuries and paralysis can be caused by a number of problems, including

Continued

TABLE 12.2 Risk Factors for Cauda Equina Syndrome—cont'd

Risk Factor/ Level of Evidence	Context	Further Questions	Low Clinical Suspicion	High Clinical Suspicion
	11 CES symptoms associated with degenerative LSS are generally much less clear than with a herniated disc or claudication. A range of typical leg symptoms (e.g., aching, cramping, tingling, and heaviness) provoked by walking and eased by sitting should be considered as important in LSS CES is a risk with any lumbar spine surgical intervention			• Bleeding inside the spinal column (extradural spinal hematoma) • Leaking of spinal fluid (incidental durotomy) • Accidental damage to the blood vessels that supply the spinal cord with blood • Accidental damage to the nerves when they're moved during surgery

From Finucane et al. (2020).

Alongside the patient's history of prolonged pain and stiffness in the morning, the AP requested blood tests including a full blood count, inflammatory markers, rheumatoid factor and human leukocyte antigen B27 (HLA B27, an antigen located on the surface of white blood cells that could be indicative of the presence of a spectrum of inflammatory disorders).

KNOWLEDGE CHECK

1. What do you think is going on?
2. What would you do next?
3. Who else might you involve in his care?

The AP considered the diffuse neurological aspects of the symptoms might be related to Lyme disease, and in view of the patient's unusual symptoms, the spinal AP referred the patient to the Rheumatology department for an opinion and organized a face-to-face follow-up.

Subsequently, the Rheumatologist reviewed the patient and felt that several of the patient's symptoms could be indicative of fibromyalgia, namely, generalized pain including the elbows and shoulders, having non-refreshed sleep and general fatigue. He also reported a boom/bust activity cycle corresponding with his pain with generalized weakness, impaired concentration and memory, increased sensitivity to touch and movement and nocturnal urinary urgency (Bellato et al., 2012). The Rheumatologist found that none of his joints have been red, warm or swollen and that he did not have any skin psoriasis or other rashes. The blood results had returned with normal full blood count, no evidence of raised inflammatory markers and negative rheumatoid factor and HLA B27.

The Rheumatologist found that the patient had two prolonged courses of doxycycline after his Lyme serology came back as positive last year.

Following a physical examination, the Rheumatologist identified no focal abnormal neurology, no evidence of synovitis in any joints, limited spinal movement due to pain, negative pain provocative tests of the sacroiliac joints, normal straight leg raise/sciatic stretch test and tenderness over the lumbar spine but none around the sacroiliac joints.

The blood tests returned with normal inflammatory markers, a negative rheumatoid factor and connective tissue disease screen, as well as a negative HLA B27 test.

KNOWLEDGE CHECK

1. What do you think is going on?
2. What would you do next?
3. Who else might you involve in his care?

The Rheumatologist felt that the likely diagnosis was that of a persistent pain presentation, therefore a diagnosis by medical exclusion, fibromyalgia, was given. He provided an education leaflet and information on pacing, relaxation and sleep hygiene. For completeness, the Rheumatologist requested an MRI scan of the hands and sacroiliac joints, x-rays of the hands and chest, as well as vitamin D, thyroid function test and serum creatine kinase (CK). The reason was to exclude any potential medical diagnosis, including systemic autoimmune disorders, thyroid impairments, myopathy and malabsorption disorders. Finally, the Rheumatologist suggested the GP prescribe amitriptyline 10 mg at night-time with the potential benefit of gradually increasing up to 30 mg depending on the patient's response. Amitriptyline is used in cases such as this to improve sleep hygiene and can help moderate widespread pain.

What Happened Next?

- The MRI scans of the hands and sacroiliac joints, the x-rays of the hands and chest wall and all blood tests were normal.
- The spinal AP reviewed the patient considering all the medical investigations and referred the patient to the local pain service and to AP rehabilitation physiotherapy.

Advanced Practice Rehabilitation

With all the available information gleaned so far, the patient was referred to an AP in rehabilitation where the therapeutic encounter focused upon a greater relational emphasis. The relational emphasis of rehabilitation allowed a space for considering the unique biographical, biological, psychological and social contexts into account to bring a sense-making co-constructed process to occur (Low, 2017). This process takes time to allow trust and facilitation of a therapeutic alliance to explore a situational understanding of the patient's predicament and avenues toward the patient's goals, meaningful activities, and aspirations.

The patient disclosed that they had several persistent stressful situations occurring in the background and that they had experienced several adverse childhood experiences. These circumstances are associated with a greater likelihood of experiencing persistent pain (Ranjbar & Erb, 2019; Groenewald et al., 2020). However, the patient was very focused on the possible relationship between having a positive Lyme disease serology and his symptoms and that a course of antibiotics that he had in the past helped him. It was important to accept and understand the patient's perspective and to recognize that his experience is valid even if the instinct and reasoning of the therapist disagree. The process of sense-making in all its uncertainty is a fluid process and not one that resides within clear diagnostic criteria and distinct categorical treatment algorithms. A useful framework to consider this is based upon Levanthal's common sense model (Leventhal et al., 2012) (Fig. 12.5).

As can be seen in Fig. 12.5, the sense-making process is not a clear and linear one. A key part of rehabilitation is to facilitate cohesion between the interpretation, embodied sense-making, actions, response, and the appraisal of symptoms. In this way, both the patient and the therapist engage with this process, one that demands empathy.

Through careful and considerate communication, the patient elicited their perspectives on their current predicament. This appeared to reflect a person out of control of their circumstances, their bodily experiences of pain, their identity and relationships, which appeared to be becoming toxic within a fluctuant environment. The association between the patient's current situation was also mirrored by their challenging upbringing, which was distantly alluded to within and between the patient's narrative.

It was of no surprise that the patients' movements appeared stiff, guarded and restrained. This was partly due to the experience of pain but also the apprehension of causing further pain. A careful and attentive examination demonstrated a normal neurological examination, but all movements of all limbs and the trunk were associated with an underlying high tone and resistance to movement. The pain was mainly focused on the lower back, and the therapist palpated this area and appreciated the way in which the soft tissues felt co-contracted. The patient often held their breath during low load movements which did not demand such bracing. All the while, the therapist reflected back to the patient what they were seeing, feeling, and observing. A tentative relationship was described to the patient in the way of a vicious cycle between movement, overguarding, tension and experiencing pain. The therapist used gentle palpation to communicate with the patient and provide feedback to them about the way in which they were holding their trunk. Using a steady breathing pattern, the patient was asked to breathe toward the area being palpated in the lower back where the pain was being experienced. As the patient did this, he was

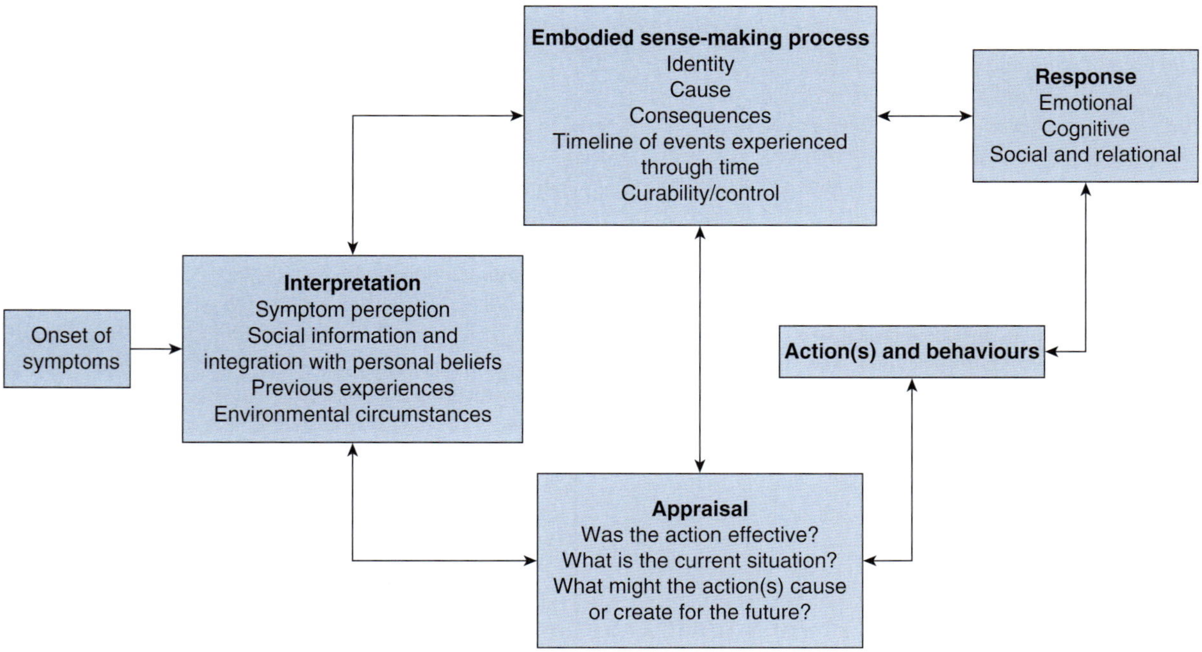

Fig. 12.5 Sense making process based upon common sense model. (From Levanthal et al., 1980).

asked to 'let go' after every outward breath. Within a few breaths, the patient could appreciate that they could relax, but almost immediately they started to panic and could not understand why. It was hypothesized that this could be important, and the patient was open to the idea of talking to a psychologist who had the specialist skills to support the patient. This reflected an important moment where the patient started to make sense of their own situation in an embodied way. The patient started to challenge and reflect on their experiences and understood how to move in relaxed and fluid ways while partaking in different and varied environments. Steadily, over time, the patient began to regain all their movements with less pain and started to participate in meaningful activities such as cycling with his son.

The reader is referred to Chapter 9 Understanding and managing persistent pain in the associated text Ryder & Barnard, 2024.

CONCLUSION

The above case studies have described the broad skill sets that Advanced Practice Physiotherapists can provide healthcare services from diagnostic, treatment to management in diverse settings. It is important to note that advanced practitioners, despite working within different areas and sectors, share common dispositions towards a person-centred approach using embodied, empathetic, and careful communication skills and a willingness to embrace a reflective multi-dimensional perspective to care.

REFERENCES

Bellato, E., Marini, E., Castoldi, F., et al., 2012. Fibromyalgia syndrome: etiology, pathogenesis, diagnosis, and treatment. Pain Res Treat 2012, 426130. https://doi.org/10.1155/2012/426130.

Buttgereit, F., Dejaco, C., Matteson, E., et al., 2016. Polymyalgia rheumatica and giant cell arteritis. JAMA 315 (22), 2442.

Byles, S., Ling, R., 1989. Orthopaedic out-patients—a fresh approach. Physiotherapy 75, 435–437.

Chartered Society of Physiotherapy (CSP), 2016a. Advanced practice in physiotherapy, understanding the contribution of advanced practice in physiotherapy to transforming lives, maximising independence and empowering populations.

Chartered Society of Physiotherapy (CSP), 2016b. Scope of Practice [Online]. Chartered Society of Physiotherapy, London. (Accessed 3 December 2017).

James, J.J., Stuart, R.B., 1975. Expanded role for the physical therapist: screening musculoskeletal disorders. Phys. Ther. 55, 121–132.

Leventhal, H., Bodnar-Deren, S., Breland, J.Y., et al., 2012. Modeling health and illness behavior: the approach of the commonsense model. In: Baum, A., Revenson, T.A., Singer, J. (Eds.), Handbook of Health Psychology. Psychology Press, New York, pp. 3–35.

Low, M., 2017. A novel clinical framework: the use of dispositions in clinical practice. A person centred approach. J Eval Clin Pract 23 (5), 1062–1070. https://doi.org/10.1111/jep.12713. Epub 2017 Feb 21. PMID: 28220638.

NHS-England, 2017. Multi-professional framework for ACP in England. NHS England.

Noblet, T., Heneghan, N.R., Hindle, J., et al., 2021. Accreditation of Advanced Clinical Practice of Musculoskeletal Physiotherapy in England: a qualitative two-phase study to inform implementation. Physiotherapy 113, 217–244.

Noblet, T., Marriott, J., Hensman-Crook, A., et al., 2020. Independent prescribing by advanced physiotherapists for patients with low back pain in primary care: a feasibility trial with an embedded qualitative component. PloS One 15, e0229792.

Rushton, A., Beeton, K., Jordaan, R., et al., 2016. IFOMPT educational standards. International Federation of Orthopaedic Manipulative Physical Therapists.

Ryder, D., Barnard, K. 2024. Petty's Musculoskeletal Examination and Assessment: A Handbook for Therapists, sixth ed. Elsevier, Oxford.

Saxon, R.L., Gray, M.A., Oprescu, F.I., 2014. Extended roles for allied health professionals: an updated systematic review of the evidence. J. Multidiscip. Healthc. 7, 479.

Stanhope, J., Grimmer-Somers, K., Milanese, S., et al., 2012. Extended scope physiotherapy roles for orthopedic outpatients: an update systematic review of the literature. J. Multidiscip. Healthc. 5, 37–45.

Suckley, J., 2012. Core Clinical Competencies for Extended-scope Physiotherapists Working in Musculoskeletal (MSK) Interface Clinics Based in Primary Care: a delphi consensus study Professional Doctorate. University of Salford.

Tawiah, A.K., Desmeules, F., Wieler, M., et al., 2021. Advanced practice in physiotherapy: a global survey. Physiotherapy 113, 168–176.

INDEX

Page numbers followed by " *f* " indicate figures, " *t* " indicate tables, and " *b* " indicate boxes.

D

E

N